Talc and glove powder p14

SECOND EDITION

WOUND REPAIR

ERLE E. PEACOCK, JR., M.D.

WALTON VAN WINKLE, JR., M.D.

1976
W. B. SAUNDERS COMPANY
Philadelphia, London, Toronto

W. B. Saunders Company: West Washington Square
Philadelphia, PA   19105

1 St. Anne's Road
Eastbourne, East Sussex BN21 3UN, England

833 Oxford Street
Toronto, Ontario, M8Z 5T9, Canada

Library of Congress Cataloging in Publication Data

Peacock, Erle E

Wound repair.

First ed. published in 1970 under title: Surgery and biology
of wound repair.

Includes bibliographies and index.

1. Wound healing.   2. Wounds – Treatment.   I. Van
  Winkle, Walton, joint author.   II. Title.

RD94.P4 1976   617'.14   76-8584

ISBN 0-7216-7124-1

Wound Repair   ISBN 0-7216-7124-1

Last digit is the print number: 9   8   7   6   5   4   3   2   1

To

JAMES LOWREY PEACOCK
SUSAN LOUISE PEACOCK
VIRGINIA GAYLE PEACOCK
and
TINA VAN WINKLE MACBETH

— a new generation of "healers"

PREFACE
to the
Second Edition

The first edition of *Surgery and Biology of Wound Repair* was intended to bridge, where possible, many of the basic biological disciplines contributing to knowledge of wound healing and regeneration and the clinical discipline of surgery. There are some reasons to suspect that the words Biology and Surgery in the title of the first edition may have retarded rather than accelerated progress toward that goal. The use of such words seems to stake out claims and define territorial rights rather than meld interest and information. Biology and Surgery have been dropped from the title of the second edition, therefore; it was the strongest action we could devise to signify our belief that in the decade ahead the healer must come to the fore in this field if the brilliant accomplishments by fundamental biologists are to be translated into health and happiness for human beings recovering from wounds. Stated more explicitly, our greatest expectations in 1971 have been fulfilled, in determination of the final sequencing of the collagen molecule; much has been accomplished in understanding relationships within different structures. In addition, most if not all of the important cross-links in biological systems have been identified and located. Interrelations between various collagens and other substances such as mucopolysaccharides, macrophages, and endothelial cells, always a difficult problem, still are not clearly understood but considerable progress has been made. Ability to type collagens by biochemical and immunological means has provided still another tool for study of the behavior of these extraordinary proteins. Identification of procollagen peptidases and discovery of dermatosparaxis and identification of the biochemical defects in various types of Ehlers-Danlos syndrome are other examples of the wealth which has been added to our understanding of synthesis and assembly of connective tissue. But where is it all taking us?

As stated in the preface to the first edition, it seems to the authors that ultimately the road must lead to the control of scar tissue in human beings. Animals do not have serious health problems because of a scar, but people are beleaguered by and sometimes even die because of the presence of unwanted scar tissue or the abnormal physical properties that scar tissue imparts. Control of scar tissue, therefore, is still the treasure at the end of the rainbow for those who are concerned primarily with the health of human beings. The goal is within our grasp but the physician must assume more responsibility in the years ahead if the terribly difficult step between Phase II (animal testing) and Phase III (human testing) is to be taken. Encouraging as basic contributions have been, the pall which currently hangs over human biology because of present attitudes concerning even legitimate research on human disease cannot be denied. Difficult as such attitudes may make research in human disease, the possibility of expanding connective tissue research to include control of scar formation in human beings need not be retarded or halted in the next few years. Progress, however, depends to a great extent upon interest as well as the continued support of productive basic scientists. Speculation as to the direction such "good things" may take is easy.

The area that seems most ready to send a penetrating phalanx into human biology is the control of physical properties of scar tissue. After all, scar tissue causes many of the problems injurious to human health by virtue of physical properties. Thus the applied scientist, for whom this book is directed now, can take advantage of a great deal of basic information related to the control of physical properties of collagen without interfering with or controlling synthesis and deposition of scar tissue. For example, now that a preparation of β-aminopropionitrile, apparently without toxicity for human beings other than upon newly synthesized connective tissue, is available, clinical testing in surgical patients is possible and indeed has already started in several centers. Other similar lathyrogenic agents are becoming and will continue to become available. Such agents will require individual as well as combination testing in human trials. Although Phase II studies on the use of three proline analogs to inhibit synthesis and deposition of collagen have not been encouraging from the standpoint of supporting clinical trial in human beings, other analogs and rate-limiting agents either are available or can be developed in the immediate future. Such investigations undoubtedly will include different approaches such as the development and utilization of anti-ascorbic acid agents as well as control of enzyme kinetics and use of trace metal inhibitors. Extremely toxic substances and strong teratogenic agents must be avoided at first; what is needed now is some modicum of success—even though it be relatively small—in improving the health of a human being through manipulation of even a small property of unwanted scar tissue. It appears now that the principle of controlled induced lathyrism (relatively selective for newly synthesized scar tissue because of the rapid kinetics of wound healing compared to normal tissue turnover) offers the best possibility for controlling physical properties of wound collagen without damaging mature connective tissue in the immediate future. Hence, the spotlight is on the surgeon and the change in title for the second edition of the book is the signal to accelerate the pace. It is in surgical patients that the healing wound can best be manipulated selectively without damage to the rest of the body. Biologists have shown at least one way that such a manipulation is possible in this decade; the final step must be taken by those for whom the title of the second edition was selected.

Finally, the greatest pleasure in writing a book, acknowledging gratitude to all whom gratitude is due, is not such a pleasure in the preface to the second edition as it was five years ago. There simply are too many now and the debt is too great to be paid in this way. Because of seemingly unprecedented conditions which have consumed so much of the authors' time and energy during the last three years, preparation of the second edition of *Wound Repair* has been dependent literally upon a host of individuals — more than can possibly be named. As an example, in addition to our renowned colleagues in the wound healing field, Dr. Milos Chvapil, Dr. John Madden, Dr. Edward Carlson, Dr. Ron Misiorowski, and Dr. Arnold Arem and their brilliant students and assistants, the loyalty and raw courage of the magnificent men and women comprising many of the faculty and literally all of the house staff in the Department of Surgery at the University of Arizona must, for reasons known only to them, be acknowledged with devotion as well as deep appreciation. The second edition of *Wound Repair* could not have been produced without them. Miss Elizabeth Taylor of the W. B. Saunders Company has continued to provide part-time authors with technical and professional support needed to bring out a second edition. As before, the final price for whatever contribution the second edition may make was paid mostly by Mary Peacock and Frankie Van Winkle. To all these individuals and to so many others too numerous to identify here, we are deeply grateful.

EEP
WVW
Tucson, Arizona

PREFACE
to the
First Edition

"A definitive book on wound healing is needed," said our advisers. "By all means write one as soon as possible." "You should be able to finish the job in two years," said our publishers.

These statements were made more than ten years ago, when silver nitrate was the topical agent of choice for preventing infection in burned tissue, lathyrism was primarily a disease of poultry, and zinc was of no more concern to wound healing biologists than as a material used in the battery-powered spectrophotometer. The naïveté with which such advice was given and received reflects the fact that a study of the biology of wound healing seemed a dull and nonproductive venture in those days, when so little of modern cellular and subcellular biology had found its way into surgical practice.

The concept that the goal of applied research in healing and regeneration is the "spot weld" of disrupted tissues is responsible for much of the apathy engendered in the past: most papers published in surgical journals have been directed at shortening the time required for surgically repaired tissue to regain tensile strength.

But the decade during which we have worked on this book has come to be dominated by a larger concept. It has not been only that major breakthroughs in basic research have achieved broader practical application (although this is occurring too). Rather, there has been the generation and acceptance of the idea that there are rewards in the field of applied wound healing research every bit as spectacular and possibly even more useful than "spot welding" of injured tissues. As our horizons have widened to encompass the numerous influences on health that healing exerts aside from the time it takes to occur, research in wound healing has become one of the most exciting and, in our judgment, promising fields in surgical biology.

And why should this not be so? To limit our interest in healing to the speed of its various reactions is almost as restrictive as it would be to continue embryological investigation in the hope that a baby can be produced in less than nine months. Wound healing can in fact be accelerated, but analysis of surgical problems at the moment strongly suggests that, with the exception of bone, the length of time required to reestablish the physical integrity of an injured tissue is not a major problem. The alteration of function in a vital organ that results when a simple scar replaces complex tissue is of paramount importance to the future health and welfare of the patient. Scar tissue is a real killer disguised by its appearance as a product of a valuable homeostatic mechanism.

The changes in our plans, objectives, and thoughts about this book can be summed up by the panic we have sometimes felt as the world of healing and regeneration spun by while we were trying to write about it. Publication has become almost an act of desperation, brought about in the end by the feeling that we had too much in the book to abandon it, and that a page was inadequate literally before we had lifted our pens. By our initial standards, the manuscript is woefully incomplete; we have had to realize that we cannot produce a definitive work on healing and regeneration in human begins at this time.

We did agree, however, to terminate our work in an orderly fashion by November 15, 1969, as suggested by an unbelievably patient, although practical, publisher. To do so has meant a painful but, we believe, wise change in basic objectives. We ask that the book be judged against the goal we have now accepted, which is to bring together some of the work, thoughts, investigations, and clinical experiences of an exciting decade of biological research. It is dedicated to the proposition that healing by synthesis of scar, although undoubtedly important as a pristine function (perhaps even pivotal in such vital processes as natural selection) is no more than a second best solution to the problem created by interrupting tissue integrity.

The importance of such a concept becomes readily apparent. In so many patients it is not the lye burn of the esophagus, the inflammation of the heart valve, or the injury to the liver that kills; unappreciated though it may be, it is the scar that forms during healing that impairs health and, in some patients, may even cause death. Paré's old concept "I dressed the wound; God healed it" is simply not one under which we are willing to live.

The process of healing is the result of cell movement, cell division, and cellular synthesis of various proteins—basic biological processes which are under intensive study in laboratories throughout the world. The end product is primarily a crystalline fibrous protein which behaves predictably and which can be manipulated according to presently understood basic principles of crystalline protein chemistry.

Control of synthesis and degradation of collagen and manipulation of the physical properties which it imparts to scar are not science fiction. Such manipulations are already possible under controlled conditions, both in laboratory animals and in human beings. The therapeutic implications are enormous. In addition, although it is pure speculation at this time, complete control of fibrous scar production might open an entirely new approach to tissue regeneration — particularly in the liver and bladder, where unusual kinds of regenerative potential appear to be expressed in various ways.

We would point out to all who are responsible for the care of human wounds that there are rewards in modern biological research that can put such work on a higher plane than it has ever been in the past. In 1970 wounds do not have to be treated solely on the empirical basis of dogmatic teaching by master surgeons. To understand *why* and *how* certain therapeutic regimens work is to make a great advance in the ability to utilize more fully some of the lessons that have been learned by trial and error.

Moreover, some of our past teaching has been erroneous, and many principles have been taught as fact even though they are simply based upon the attempt of surgeons to explain and understand clinical observations. Research has exposed some of these errors in a way that is refreshing to the inquisitive student with far better preparation than most of his teachers.

Finally, in certain areas, such as deformity caused by wound contraction, neoplasia initiated by wound healing, and complications caused by reopening a wound at an inopportune time, recent data have provided knowledge which is useful in caring for patients today. This book attempts to focus on these areas in particular, with the thought that the information presented may help practicing surgeons to treat wounds more intelligently and thus more successfully.

Just as important, we also have attempted to demonstrate to basic scientists that there is a real discipline known as human biology, and that wound healing is an area of investigation in which the best of scientific thought and practice can be truly utilized with gratifying results. As in most scientific disciplines, there is a sickening gap between brilliant research accomplishments and practical clinical applications. Perhaps it is in human biology, more than in any other discipline, that the gap between laboratory and bedside needs to be bridged. It is our fondest hope that this book will begin the work on that bridge.

Authors, particularly those who have full time occupations, need a great deal of help. One of the real privileges accorded us, therefore, is the right to acknowledge our debt to those who have made this book possible. Appreciation is due first to the faculty and house staff of the University of North Carolina School of Medicine and to Dr. Nathan Womack and Dr. Richard Peters in particular. Because the most time-consuming portion of the task was completed during the first year of development of a new Department of Surgery, a word of special thanks must be said to the surgical faculty and residents of the University of Arizona, not only to our brilliant colleagues in the wound healing field, Dr. John Madden, Dr. Milos Chvapil, and Miss M. F. Thompson, but also to Dr. William Trier, Dr. Charles Witte, Dr. Charles Zukoski, Dr. Scott Clark, and Dr. Leonard Weiner, who helped in so many ways to make our book a reality. Similar thanks are due to our colleagues at Ethicon, including Mr. Richard B. Sellars, who gave one of us the freedom to undertake this project, to Dr. Richard Kronenthal and Dr. Irving Oneson, who helped with scientific advice, and to Dr. Emil Borysko, who provided photographs and electron micrographs.

As novice authors we are especially indebted to Miss Gloria Fitz, Mrs. Evelyn Brady, and Mrs. Jean Szymborski who cheerfully and skillfully typed countless pages of manuscript. Additional thanks are due Dr. Eddy Martin and Dr. Sam Barnes for invaluable aid in library research and editorial advice. The patience and professional skill of Mr. Robert Rowan and Miss Elizabeth J. Taylor of the W. B. Saunders Company are appreciated, as is the generosity of many authors who have allowed us to reprint illustrations from their work. Finally, to Mary Peacock, Frankie Van Winkle, and our children, the people who really paid the price for whatever contribution our book may make, we express gratitude for patience and understanding.

EEP
WVW
Tucson, Arizona

CONTENTS

Chapter 1

INFLAMMATION AND THE CELLULAR RESPONSE TO INJURY

It is almost axiomatic that injury is followed by inflammation. Inflammation can be characterized as a vascular and cellular response designed to defend the body against alien substances and to dispose of dead and dying tissue preparatory to the repair process. The quantitative extent of inflammation depends upon the severity of the injury. Within limits, the inflammatory response shows a typical "dose-response" curve when related to the severity of the trauma. The qualitative nature of the inflammatory response may vary with the kind of injury produced. However, these qualitative differences are more readily discernible in chronic than in acute inflammatory reactions.

An understanding of the nature, mechanisms, and consequences of inflammation is important to the surgeon. Every surgical procedure results in an inflammatory reaction. The surgeon who understands the nature and mechanism of this reaction to injury has within his power the ability to minimize the adverse consequences and to utilize the reaction to the benefit of his patient.

THE ACUTE INFLAMMATORY REACTION

Inflammation resulting from trauma may initially appear to differ from that resulting from bacterial infection or from physical agents such as heat, cold, and radiant energy. This is only apparent; the basic response is the same regardless of the inciting cause. However, in the case of most trauma, there is physical interruption of blood vessels with immediate hemorrhage, more or less extensive cell destruction at the immediate site of injury, and in many instances a path to the external environment permitting body fluids, including blood, to drain off and allowing bacteria and other foreign substances to gain access to the wound. The response of the body to injury, regardless of its nature, is basically the same, and the most significant element of that response is seen in the local vasculature.

THE VASCULAR REACTION. The immediate response of small vessels in the area of injury is vasoconstriction. At the point of injury, actual vascular occlusion may occur, which combats the tendency to hemorrhage. This vasoconstriction usually lasts only five to ten minutes at the most, and is followed by an active vasodilatation. All elements of the local vasculature appear to be involved in this dilatation.

Almost immediately after injury, leukocytes in the local vessels appear to become "sticky" and begin to adhere to endothelium, particularly of venules. Within 30 minutes to one hour, the entire endothelium of the local venules may be covered with adherent leukocytes. At the same time there is a lesser, but definite adhesion of erythrocytes and platelets. The erythrocytes also tend to adhere to each other and form rouleaux. These tend to plug capillaries, but since platelet-fibrin thrombi do not form until later, this occlusion can be reversed.

Coincident with vasodilatation, leakage of fluid from venules occurs. This fluid has the same composition as plasma with its full complement of macromolecules. This occurs before any cells leave affected vessels and also occurs in the absence of obvious "gaps" in the vessel walls. Electron microscope observation of vessels, however, indicates that there is a separation of endothelial cells so that they are no longer in direct contact with each other. The basement membrane is now exposed to the luminal contents of these vessels.

MOVEMENT OF CELLS. Soon after the onset of leukocyte sticking, these cells are seen to move through the vessel wall by a process of diapedesis. This phenomenon involves active motion; by some not yet proved mechanism leukocytes force their way through the basement membrane to the extravascular space. There is a visible indication that at least a temporary defect is produced in the vascular wall since often a second cell will follow in the path of the first one and erythrocytes, which move only passively, appear to escape through the same channels.

After passing the blood vessel wall, leukocytes exhibit a positive, but somewhat random, motion. Eventually, by one means or another, they concentrate at the site of injury. The predominant cell form is the polymorphonuclear leukocyte, and at one time it was thought that these cells migrated first and were followed at a later time by the mononuclear cells. However, careful studies have shown that the migration of cells is in the same proportion that they occur in the bloodstream. However, the polymorphonuclear cells are very short-lived compared to the mononuclear cells so that in the older inflammatory reactions, the mononuclear cells predominate.

The escape of fluid from local vessels, combined with migrating leukocytes and dead tissue at the site of injury, constitutes the inflammatory exudate. As the polymorphonuclear cells die and are lysed, the exudate assumes the character of pus. It is important to realize that pus can occur in nonbacterial inflammations.

LOCALIZATION OF THE INFLAMMATORY REACTION. The major factors determining whether an area of inflammation will produce enough pus to constitute what is termed an abscess are (1) the extent of injury to normal tissue, (2) the extent of the cellular reaction, and (3) the extent to which polymorphonuclear cells accumulate and die. These last two factors are, in turn, determined by the state of the local circulation and, in particular, lymphatic drainage.

Lymphatics are more fragile than blood vessels. Thus, in any injury, damage to local lymphatics is usually greater than to the vasculature. Furthermore, leakage of fluid from venules provides fibrinogen and other elements of the blood clotting system. Fibrin plugs quickly form in damaged lymphatics, effectively stopping any drainage from the injured area. Thus, the inflammatory reaction is localized to an area immediately surrounding the injury. Eventually, of course, activation of fibrinolysin relieves the stoppage and drainage can again take place.

Local vasodilatation, leakage of fluid into the extravascular space, and stoppage of lymphatic drainage produces the classic signs of inflammation — redness, swelling, and heat. Pressure, and perhaps chemical stimulation, produces the fourth sign — pain.

The Mechanism of Acute Inflammation

A vast amount of literature in the last 20 or 30 years has dealt with the mechanism of inflammation. Discovery of the anti-inflammatory action of corticosteroids provided a useful tool in the analysis of the many factors alleged to be responsible for the various components of the inflammatory reaction. More recently, the development of antisera against each of the cell types involved in the inflammatory reaction has given insight into the specific functions of each cell and has provided a basis for study of interactions of these cells with one another. For instance, it was shown that certain cells important in defense against infectious agents are of no significance in healing of noninfected wounds. It is also suggested that one cell type may initiate or aid in migration, differentiation, and functional activity of another cell type. These in-

ing observations will be dealt with when we discuss the cellular
nse to inflammation.

It is convenient to concentrate on two major aspects of the acute
inflammatory reaction: alteration of vascular permeability and forces
responsible for movement of leukocytes into the injured area. In a
subsequent section, the consequences of inflammation and its role in
repair will be considered.

THE VASCULAR RESPONSE. Increased vascular permeability, which
is usually referred to as increased capillary permeability, but which is
actually confined to small venules, is the key to all subsequent events in
inflammation. In 1924 it was postulated that this was brought about by
locally released histamine, emanating from destroyed cells, or by a
closely related chemical termed H-substance. The proof that histamine
or H-substance was present or responsible for increased capillary permeability was far from satisfactory.

In 1936 isolation of a substance called leukotaxine was described; it
was claimed that this substance was the agent responsible for increasing
capillary permeability, and also acted as a chemotactic agent, attracting
leukocytes into the injured area. Leukotaxine appears to be a polypeptide and is formed in damaged tissue by enzymatic destruction of albumin. Cortisone was reported to prevent the permeability and chemotactic action of leukotaxine. However, the precise role of leukotaxine in the inflammatory process is still a matter of debate.

That there might be more than one factor involved in the induction of increased capillary permeability was suggested when some
careful observations of graded thermal injury showed that increased
capillary permeability occurred in two phases: the immediate reaction
and a delayed reaction which occurred one to two hours after injury.
These reactions appeared to be separate and independent phenomena
suggesting separate mediators. The biphasic reaction was also observed
in carefully controlled experimental bacterial inflammation.

It has been demonstrated that the permeability effect and the
chemotactic effect can be clearly separated and are probably not due to
the same substance. There is increasing evidence that the initial, short-
lived increase in vascular permeability may be a result of histamine action. A number of endogenous and exogenous compounds will release
histamine or cause histamine to be formed through the action of histidine decarboxylase on intracellular histidine. Local increases in capillary permeability are seen following injection of these substances. In
addition, wound tissue fluid shows appreciable histamine content and
blood histamine rises immediately after injury.

Since about 1955 a large number of substances have been isolated
which can cause increases in capillary permeability. The precise role of
these substances is as yet not clearly elucidated. The more important
ones are discussed individually.

Histamine. As has been mentioned, it appears probable that the earliest change in vascular permeability following injury is brought about by histamine. The major but not the sole source of histamine is the mast cell. These cells lose their characteristic granules at the time of injury; granules contain a wide variety of active materials including 5-hydroxytryptamine (serotonin), heparin, and histamine. Histamine is also found in platelets, but there is wide species variation in platelet histamine content. In the rat, the platelet may be a major source, but in the human the histamine content of platelets is low. Other sources are granulocytes and possibly other white cells.

Histamine action is very short-lived, probably lasting not longer than 30 minutes. Furthermore, injury will deplete local sources of histamine so that considerable time is required before sufficient endogenous histamine can be synthesized to bring about further reactions. However, since the vascular permeability increase lasts long beyond the time of histamine action, other permeability-increasing factors have been sought.

Serotonin. Serotonin, or 5-hydroxytryptamine, has an action almost indistinguishable from that of histamine. It also is discharged from mast cells. In some species, such as the rat, it is the dominant vascular amine, rather than histamine. Although it is found in inflammatory exudates, its role in species other than the rat is questionable. In humans and many other animals, serotonin has a negligible effect on vascular permeability.

It is important to emphasize that the effect of these amines, histamine and serotonin, is *not* on capillaries. This was amply demonstrated by electron microscopy. The effect is on vessels 20 to 30 μ in size on the venous side of capillary loops. Vessels 4 to 7 μ, true capillaries, are unaffected by these amines. The action appears to result in a separation of contacts between endothelial cells, possibly owing to a swelling and "rounding" of these cells. The basement membrane is not visibly affected, but acts as a filter at the points of exposure.

Serotonin also has been found to stimulate DNA synthesis in granuloma cells in the late phase of cell population growth. Evidence obtained in polyvinyl sponge-induced granulomas suggests that the principal effect is on the fibroblast population. Although synthesis of collagen appears to be suppressed, but not abolished, there is an increase in the ratio of insoluble to soluble collagen, suggesting that cross-linking of collagen is enhanced. More direct evidence that this may be the case has recently been obtained. Serotonin in concentrations of 10^{-6} M has been shown to induce a marked increase of lysyl oxidase activity in tissues and in fibroblast cultures. As will be discussed in Chapter 4, this enzyme is responsible for initiating reactions leading to collagen cross-linking.

The question arises whether serotonin is involved in later phases of wound healing *in vivo.* Certainly, in many fibrotic lesions such as cirrhosis of the liver and lung fibrosis, the association of large numbers of mast cells has been reported. Mast cells, along with platelets, are the major sources of serotonin. However, in ordinary healing wounds, although mast cells may be present, one is not impressed that they are there in significant numbers. Whether or not the macrophage can synthesize and liberate serotonin does not appear to have been studied. It is, of course, interesting to speculate about the possible role of serotonin in wound healing, particularly in the activation of lysyl oxidase. However, before such a hypothesis can be entertained one needs to show that serotonin is actually present in the wound after the inflammatory reaction has subsided, and that, if serotonin is inhibited or destroyed, cross-linking is also inhibited. Certainly, here is an area for further study.

Kinins.   Kinins are biologically active peptides that appear to be involved in the inflammatory process and are found in areas of tissue injury. The kinins (bradykinin or kallidin) are released from α_2-globulin of plasma, which has also been termed a kininogen, by a plasma enzyme, kallikrein. Kallikrein is activated by Hageman factor (Factor XII) which, in turn, is activated by contact with glass or by other negatively charged insoluble substances. Kallikrein was described over 30 years ago and was thought to be a blood pressure-controlling substance. A similar material was found in the pancreas and urine and subsequently in the salivary glands. It was generally overlooked until the mid-fifties when its enzymatic nature was recognized and its relation to bradykinin established. More recently, a kallikrein has been found in granulocytes, and it is suggested that release of this kallikrein initiates an inflammatory response.

A number of kinins have been described, but their separate identities are questionable. Certainly two, bradykinin and kallidin, have been shown to be nearly identical. The terminology in this field is confusing and, until the substances are better characterized, it would seem best to refer to them collectively as kinins. Bradykinin and two kallidins have been characterized as identical peptides except that the two kallidins have one and two extra terminal amino acids, respectively. Their structure has been elucidated, and bradykinin contains nine amino acid residues.

The kinins appear to act on the microvasculature in a manner quite similar to histamine and serotonin. The kinins are short-lived since they are rapidly destroyed by plasma and tissue proteases. Thus, it appears unlikely that they are involved in producing the late phase of vascular response.

Prostaglandins.   Although the first prostaglandin was discovered in 1930 it was not until nearly 40 years later that the ubiquitous nature of these substances was recognized and the role of certain members of this group of compounds in inflammation delineated. These substances act as mediators of inflammation. Prostaglandins E_1 and E_2 (PGE_1 and PGE_2) possess strong vasodilative, permeability-increasing and lymph-flow-promoting properties. These two prostaglandins, along with $PGF_1\alpha$ and $PGF_2\alpha$, induce wheal and flare response in human skin. PGE_2 has been isolated from rat inflammatory exudates and PGE_1 exerts a chemotactic effect on rabbit polymorphonuclear cells.

It is now suggested that prostaglandins, particularly PGE_1 and PGE_2, are terminal mediators of the acute inflammatory response. Release of these substances requires the presence of the complement system and follows the phase of kinin formation. Aspirin and indomethacin are potent inhibitors of prostaglandin biosynthesis, and it is suggested that this is the principal mechanism of the anti-inflammatory action of these drugs.

Although prostaglandins have been shown to play an important role in producing and prolonging the inflammatory reaction, paradoxically they also have been implicated as important mediators of wound healing. PGE_1 and PGA_1 have the ability to increase adenyl cyclase activity in T-lymphocytes, and since cAMP is believed to stimulate mitosis and post-injury cell proliferation, prostaglandins may play a part in wound healing.

The mechanism by which prostaglandins are formed is believed to be as follows: Injury activates the phospholipase of cell membranes in the affected area. This enzyme hydrolyzes phospholipids to release prostaglandin precursors such as arachidonic acid. These polyunsaturated fatty acids are coverted by prostaglandin synthetase, a group of intracellular enzymes, to various prostaglandins. Prostaglandins are eventually inactivated by prostaglandin dehydrogenase which converts them to less active or inactive metabolites.

The mode of action of prostaglandins has not been completely elucidated. However, the principal effect appears to be upon the enzyme responsible for synthesis of cyclic AMP from ATP, adenyl cyclase. Among the substances whose action may be mediated by cyclic AMP and modulated by prostaglandins are serotonin and histamine. In addition, prostaglandins are in some way involved in displacement of membrane-bound Ca^{++}, thus altering membrane reactions and cell permeability.

Not all of the actions of prostaglandins in inflammation can be explained by serotonin or histamine release. Since some prostaglandins have anti-inflammatory roles, the problem is complicated by the possible presence of prostaglandins having opposite actions in the area of injury. The net effect will thus depend upon the relative concentrations, relative activities, rates of synthesis and rates of destruction of each member of this group of mediators. Evidence now available indicates that the initial effect in the inflammatory reaction is due to stimulatory prostaglandins of the E series and that later, anti-inflammatory effects may be due to prostaglandins of the F and perhaps the A series.

Macromolecular Mediators.   Several ill defined large molecule "permeability factors" have been described which are alleged to be responsible for delayed permeability changes in the microvasculature at the site of an injury. It is difficult to assess the validity of these substances since the kinins are derived from macromolecules as is leukotaxine. Thus, some of these "factors" may merely be precursors of already known vasoactive materials. It is likely, however, that one or more of these may be responsible for late vascular reactions.

Chemotactic Agents. It has been shown that although many substances affecting vascular permeability also have mild leukotactic action, this is insignificant at concentrations present locally at the site of an injury. For example, leukotaxine, which was originally thought to be the principal substance causing leukocyte emigration, does not show any marked chemotactic activity at levels of concentration seen in lesions *in vivo.*

Three substances have been shown to have the greatest effect in promoting influx of leukocytes into the inflammatory zone. One of these is the so-called "lymph node permeability factor" (LNPF). This is derived by extraction from lymph nodes which have been disintegrated by ultrasonic means or by freeze-thawing. White cell emigration commences immediately after injection of this material and lasts for less than 24 hours. A substance with a similar action is derived from rat serum incubated with minced rat liver. Also, an extract of leukocytes is reported to produce a similar action. None of these substances have been isolated in pure form, and their identity and mode of action are unknown. Some believe that the LNPF may be important in chronic inflammation and in inflammation of the delayed hypersensitivity type.

The relation of prostaglandins, particularly PGE_2, to these various chemotactic agents is unclear. It is possible that the leukotactic substances mentioned before are actually prostaglandins. It is also possible that the lymph node permeability factor may be one of the prostaglandins, since certain of these do increase cell membrane permeability.

Summary of the Acute Inflammatory Process

At present, the best evidence indicates that the acute inflammatory reaction comprises the following sequence of events:

Injury, either mechanical, chemical, or bacterial, causes release of intracellular materials into the extracellular compartment of injured tissue. These cell-derived materials now react directly upon the local microcirculation. Some of these materials, such as histamine and serotonin, directly increase permeability of this microcirculation. Simultaneously, certain intracellular enzymes can destroy norepinephrine (normally found extracellularly) which is required to maintain tonus of the microcirculation. Vasodilatation is the result.

Proteolytic enzymes can attack directly the endothelial (or basement membrane) lining of the microcirculation, rendering it "leaky"

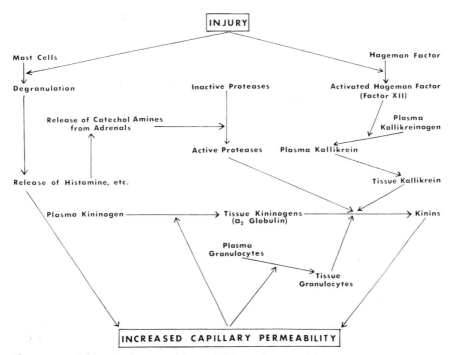

Figure 1–1. Schematic diagram of the probable mechanism of the acute inflammatory reaction. It is important to note that there are at least three pathways involved in release of tissue kinins, and that in the case of two of them there are postulated feedback mechanisms that act to prolong the effect. Thus, although the duration of histamine and kinin actions on capillary permeability is short, the feedback mechanism may play a role in producing the prolonged effect actually observed.

with respect to circulating macromolecules and cells. Some of these released proteases may also be capable of activating kallikrein which, in turn, releases bradykinin from α2-globulin substrate found normally in the circulation. These proteases may also act directly in a kallikrein-like manner to release kinins from appropriate extracellular substrate. These kinins increase markedly the permeability of the microcirculation, causing an increase in concentration of proteins and cells within the wound space. Following release of the kinins and in the presence of complement, prostaglandins, principally PGE_1 and PGE_2, are synthesized by injured cells. Prostaglandin levels increase in the course of inflammation, whereas those of the primary mediators decrease. Prostaglandin E_1 may antagonize vasoconstriction and thus increase vascular permeability. Prostaglandin E_2 attracts leukocytes by its chemotactic action. Prostaglandins also regulate the reparative process and may be involved in synthesis of mucopolysaccharides found in early phases of healing. Thus, prostaglandins appear to be responsible for late stages of the inflammatory reaction while simultaneously initiating early phases of injury repair.

Tissue Destruction by the Inflammatory Reaction

A very mild injury will produce only a transient inflammatory reaction and may not result in further damage. However, if trauma is extensive, resulting in destruction of a considerable amount of tissue, or if the wound is contaminated with either irritants or viable bacteria, the reaction may be extensive and this has certain unfavorable consequences.

Granulocytes have been shown to contain within their lysosomes a wide variety of proteolytic enzymes, including a collagenase. Normally, serum contains an inhibitor of tissue collagenase, but this inhibitor can be destroyed by released proteases. Furthermore, there is recent evidence that granulocytic collagenase is not inhibited by serum. Granulocytes are extremely sensitive to lowering of pH. With plugging of lymphatics, vascular stasis, and resulting anoxia at the site of injury, glycolysis produces excessive lactic acid and local pH drops. Granulocytes are lysed and release their enzymes, among which is a collagenase that becomes active. This collagenase acts upon local connective tissue and solubilizes it. Proteases digest it further. Since drainage from the area is impaired, necrotic debris, lysed granulocytes, and so forth, accumulate and become a necrotic abscess. This constitutes severe destructive inflammation.

Destructive inflammation is encouraged by the presence of dead tissue, bacteria, blood clots, and poor circulation. Thus, gentle handling of tissue, meticulous hemostasis, aseptic technique, and avoidance of tight sutures will prevent this type of inflammation in the ordinary surgical procedure.

CHRONIC INFLAMMATION

In most noncontaminated wounds, particularly those produced by the surgeon's knife, the acute inflammatory reaction subsides and recognizable repair commences in three to five days. Unfortunately, some wounds, even those produced by surgeons, become contaminated, or contain foreign material that cannot be removed during the acute inflammatory reaction. A condition of chronic inflammation then exists.

The predominant cell in the chronic inflammatory process is the mononuclear cell. As we pointed out, in early stages of acute inflammation, the mononuclear cell is only rarely seen. This is not because it fails to migrate at the time granulocytes are invading the zone of injury, but because the relative numbers in the circulation are far fewer than granulocytes. As granulocytes disappear through destruction or migration, however, mononuclear cells, which are much more resistant to lysis than granulocytes, persist at the site of injury. Thus, their relative number increases. For a time they are augmented by additions from the circulation.

These mononuclear cells modulate into cells we recognize as macrophages and become actively phagocytic. Some coalesce and become multinucleated giant cells, which are also phagocytic. The mononuclear cell is the scavenger of those materials in the injured area which are not readily solubilized by enzymes released by granulocytes or activated from the local circulation. This process is usually the terminal phase of the acute inflammatory reaction. However, continued presence of foreign materials, development of delayed hypersensitivity, or action of other unknown factors can cause a persistence and an evolution of this monocytic inflammatory reaction. This we recognize as chronic inflammation.

A similar type of reaction, except that from its inception granulocytes are not present in significant numbers, is that seen in delayed hypersensitivity due to infections, allergy, cutaneous reactivity to purified proteins, and the reaction of rejection of homologous or heterologous tissues and organs. A more complex type of delayed hypersensitivity is the tuberculin reaction. Characteristic of these reactions is the early appearance of perivascular accumulations of mononuclear cells. This is true of skin graft and organ graft rejections. In the rejection reaction, lymphocytes also play a major role. The relations of lymphocytes, macrophages, complement, and possibly other immune factors with each other are complex and will not be discussed here. Nevertheless, macrophages play an important role in this type of reaction. As we shall see later, the macrophage is also one of the key cells in early stages of wound healing.

It must be emphasized that persistence of mononuclear cells at a site of injury is indicative of the presence of some foreign material which the granulocytes have been unable to dispose of. Although mononuclear cells are derived from the circulation, with subsidence of the acute inflammatory reaction, local vascular permeability is restored toward normal and blood cells cease to pass into the extravascular space. It can be demonstrated that if an inciting agent is still present, then mononuclear cells undergo local proliferation. This mononuclear cell proliferation can be considered as characteristic of a chronic inflammatory reaction and is a response to the continued presence of foreign materials, including bacteria.

These mononuclear cells, besides becoming phagocytes, also evolve into histiocytes and, in certain types of lesions, into epithelioid cells. In chronic lesions, such as a tubercle, these cells may die without subsequent autolysis. A coagulative necrosis involves them and the surrounding tissue, producing caseation. This type of lesion appears to incite a fibroplasia and typically it is walled off by a collagenous capsule. A similar type of reaction is occasionally seen around nonbacterial foreign bodies.

There is evidence, which will be discussed later in this chapter, that there exists some sort of chemotactic mechanism between macrophages

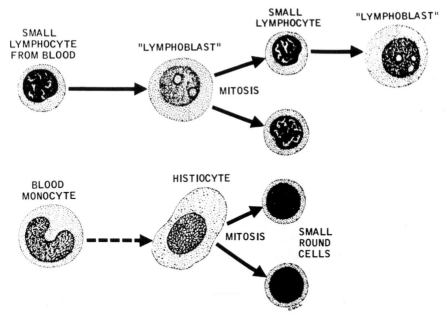

Figure 1–2. Two possible pathways for derivation of local small-round-cell or lymphoid collections in chronic inflammatory lesions or granulomas. Compare this diagram with Figure 1–4 to see the possible interrelationships of various cell types seen in chronic inflammatory lesions. (Reproduced by permission from W. G. Spector and A. W. J. Lykke, J. Path. Bact. 92:163, 1966).

and fibroblasts. In the absence of macrophages, fibroblasts migrate to the site of injury in markedly reduced numbers, and those that are found appear to be relatively immature.

Lymphocytes are also characteristically found in sites of inflammation. Both the thymus-derived or T-lymphocytes and the bone-derived or B-lymphocytes, sometimes referred to as gut-derived lymphocytes, are found in chronic inflammatory reactions. These are of importance in inflammation caused by microorganisms, but are probably relatively unimportant in traumatic inflammation. Traumatic inflammation in the absence of sepsis is not chronic and soon disappears to be replaced by the repair reaction.

The evidence that is accumulating suggests that most, if not all, chronic inflammation has an immunogenic component. This is readily apparent in reactions to bacteria such as tubercle bacilli and others that cannot be disposed of by the body's primary defenses, and to foreign proteins such as homograft material. However, it is more difficult to relate chronic foreign body reaction, nonbacterial granulomas, and so forth, to an immune response. It has been suggested that tissue destruction produced by such foreign bodies as silica and glass may result eventually in an autoimmune reaction.

Although most chronic inflammatory lesions, such as tubercles, are of only occasional interest to the surgeon, such problems as typical foreign body reaction and suture granulomas are problems of healing with which he must deal. The purpose of the foregoing discussion is to suggest that the mechanism and result of chronic inflammation may be the same regardless of the particular incitant. This should be borne in mind when we consider fibrous adhesions and peritoneal granuloma in Chapter 12.

GRANULOMAS. The type of chronic inflammatory process with which surgeons most frequently have to contend is granuloma. Most, but not all, granulomas are the end result of chronic inflammation, due to the presence of a foreign substance. The formation of a granuloma is a slow process and can be viewed as a sort of "last-ditch" defense by the body against an invader which cannot be dislodged.

The key to the persistence of the chronic inflammatory reaction which is the basis of granuloma formation is the observation that macrophages which have ingested foreign particulate matter will persist at the site of injury if they are unable to solubilize the material. This does not mean that these cells live forever. They can be seen to die and discharge their cytoplasmic contents, which are promptly engulfed by another macrophage. These cells have been shown to persist for years at the site of particulate insoluble foreign bodies.

There is now good evidence that some sort of chemotactic substance is released by macrophages which not only attracts mesenchymal cells to the area of inflammation or injury, but also influences their differentiation into fibroblasts. Studies on silica-induced fibrosis suggest

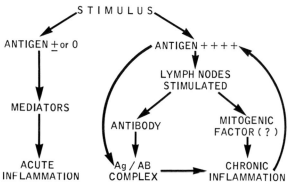

Figure 1–3. Tentative hypothesis to suggest how immunological factors may contribute to the chronicity of inflammation. Not all chronic inflammatory reactions necessarily have an immunological component; for example, persistent indigestible foreign bodies can produce chronic inflammation without the intervention of antigen-antibody complex. Nevertheless, many chronic inflammatory reactions may be primarily immunological in character, i.e., tuberculous granulomas. (Reproduced by permission from D. A. Willoughby and W. G. Spector, Biochem. Pharmacol., Suppl., 1968, p. 123.)

that activation of macrophages by foreign materials is a prerequisite for release of chemotactic material. In granulomatous reactions, the macrophage is usually found immediately adjacent to the inciting material or it may actually have phagocytosed it. Fibroblasts move into the area and surround the cluster of macrophages. Collagen is laid down, eventually enclosing the lesion in a dense fibrous capsule. These hard spheres of fibrous tissue constitute the granuloma.

The types of granuloma resulting from surgical procedures are chiefly those associated with deposition into the wound of starch or talc from glove powders, particularly in the peritoneal cavity. These are preventable if the surgeon takes the precaution of washing his gloves thoroughly. Formerly glove dusting powders were applied in the operating room. These fine dusts pervaded the atmosphere and inevitably found their way onto everything, including the surgeon, the patient, and the wound. When talc was used, the complications of granulomas were severe. Starch powder was substituted for talc in the hope that if some accidentally found its way into the wound, it would be hydrolyzed and absorbed. Unfortunately, hydrolysis is slow and the macrophage response is fast. Starch did not solve the problem. Powdering of gloves in the operating room was largely abandoned, and the manufacturers of surgeons' gloves powder them at the time of packaging. Since the powder is practically invisible, some surgeons forget that it is still there and fail to take the simple precaution of washing their gloved hands in sterile saline before commencing the operation. Thus, there are still far too many granulomatous reactions due to starch glove powders reported in the literature.

A second type of granulomatous reaction familiar to surgeons is that seen around sutures. Any suture material is a foreign body. It incites a typical foreign body reaction. Nonabsorbable sutures are the worst offenders, but catgut likewise can cause granulomatous reactions. Fortunately, most such reactions are minor, consisting of a layer of macrophages around the suture, surrounded by a few fibroblasts and a thin fibrous capsule. This usually is unimportant to the patient or surgeon. Only when the suture is located in the superficial layers of the skin and the reaction is more extensive does this present a problem. The use of fine, nonreactive sutures, or of skin-closure tapes, will usually obviate this problem.

Advantage has been taken of these foreign body granulomatous reactions to achieve correction of two troublesome defects. Aphonia due to damage to one of the recurrent laryngeal nerves, occasionally produced during lung resections or neck dissections, can be distressing. The affected vocal cord becomes immobilized in a retracted position. It has been found that relatively normal phonation can be produced if the paralyzed vocal cord can be brought to the midline. This has been accomplished by careful injection of a suspension of a Teflon powder (50 to 100 μ in diameter) directly into the edge of the paralyzed cord.

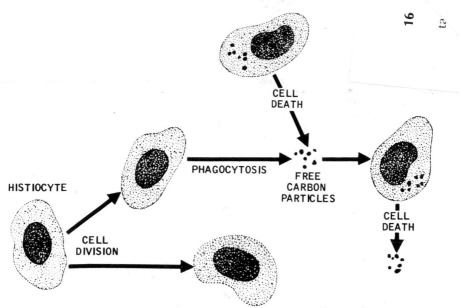

Figure 1–4. Schematic diagram of the suggested sequence of events whereby insoluble particulate matter is retained within a granuloma. (Reproduced by permission from W. G. Spector and A. W. J. Lykke, J. Path. Bact. 92:163, 1966.)

This produces a confluent granulomatous reaction which appears to be permanent, since the Teflon particles are not removed from the site. The therapeutic results are dramatic. A Teflon paste (Polytef paste) has been approved for treating vocal cord paralysis and has been widely used for selected cases.

A similar approach to the correction of velopalatine insufficiency has also been tried. Relatively large quantities of Teflon suspension have been injected into the posterior pharyneal wall, bringing it forward so that the soft palate will close off the nasal cavity during speech. This procedure is more hazardous than injection of the vocal cord because of the difficulty of confining the injected material to the desired site and because injection into a blood vessel can be fatal. This application of Teflon paste has not received FDA approval although in selected centers investigations are still continuing. Other possible applications of the principle of correcting anatomical deformities or functional disabilities by induction of granulomatous reactions are being studied. It is likely that any new applications will be limited because of difficulty in confining the granulomatous reaction to a specific location, and possible involvement of other important structures such as nerves or blood vessels in the granulomatous reaction.

These procedures are quoted to illustrate how a particular type of chronic inflammatory reaction and its sequelae may be used for the benefit of the patient instead of being an adverse reaction. It is impor-

motion is usually achieved even though the induced sheath is not anatomically identical to the structure it replaced.

THE CELLULAR PHASE OF REPAIR

It has long been argued that inflammation is a necessary concomitant to repair. In fact, in some very early work in which total inflammatory response to injury was inhibited, there appeared to be a delay in the healing process. However, with development of specific antibodies against specific cells involved in the inflammatory response, it has been possible to elucidate more precisely the role of each cell type in the process of repair.

Neutrophilic granulocytes are the first cells to appear in numbers in the area of a wound. These cells contain lysosomal enzymes which are released as these cells are damaged by lowered pH or other environmental factors. The question arises whether these cells are necessary for the repair process to proceed normally. This has been tested by administration of specific antineutrophil serum to animals during the first 10 to 14 days of wound healing. It was observed that although virtually no neutrophils were present in the wound, macrophages made their appearance on schedule, phagocytosed dead cells and debris, and appeared to be performing normally in all respects. Fibroblasts migrated into the wound area and deposited collagen on schedule. It appears that wound healing proceeds normally and on schedule in the complete absence of neutrophils. Obviously, if sepsis is present, neutrophils are important and wound healing will not progress until infection is under control. However, in the absence of infection, granulocytes are not necessary for wound healing to proceed normally.

Similar experiments have been performed with anti-macrophage serum. Unfortunately, anti-macrophage serum appears to be effective only against activated macrophages, and in order to prevent migration of blood-borne monocytes into the wound, anti-macrophage serum must be administered with cortisone. In experiments on wound healing, there was no observable effect on the healing wound in control animals in which only cortisone was used. Not all parameters of wound healing were studied quantitatively and thus the experiments are not truly definitive. Nevertheless, the combination of anti-macrophage serum and cortisone inhibited migration of monocytes into the wound so that virtually no macrophages were present during the first 10 to 14 days of healing. It was observed that the appearance of fibroblasts in the wound area was delayed; those that were eventually seen were mostly immature and the amount of collagen laid down seemed to be diminished. It was concluded from these experiments that the presence of active macrophages is essential to proper wound healing. Their major function appears to be that of disposing of dead and necrotic tissue, removal of foreign bodies, and by some mechanism that is not understood, attracting fibroblasts to the wound and perhaps influencing them to undergo maturation and maximal collagen synthesis.

Similar experiments with antilymphocyte serum indicate that lymphocytes, like neutrophils, are not necessary for wound healing. Wounds heal perfectly well in patients receiving large doses of antilymphocytic serum for suppression of immune rejection phenomena after organ transplantation.

Recently a specific antiserum to surface antigen of fibroblasts has been prepared. *In vitro* and *in vivo* studies have shown that administration of this antifibroblast serum has a cytotoxic action on fibroblasts, decreases collagen synthesis, and inhibits development of wound strength.

Repair commences almost immediately after injury, although to the casual observer this is not apparent. We shall discuss epithelial response to injury in another chapter. Shortly after injury and at some distance from the injured site, undifferentiated mesenchymal cells begin to modulate into migratory fibroblasts. As rapidly as necrotic tissue, blood clot, and so forth, are removed by granulocytes and macrophages, these fibroblasts move into the injured area. In the initial stage of inflammation, the inflammatory exudate contains a considerable amount of fibrinogen and, with release of enzymes from blood and tissue cells, fibrin is formed and laid down in the area of injury. This fibrin acts as a hemostatic barrier and as a framework for the elements of repair.

The migrating fibroblasts appear to use strands of fibrin as a scaffold. Whether or not fibrin strands are oriented in some particular direction and whether they provide contact guidance for migrating fibroblasts is still a matter of some argument. However, there is a close association between migrating and proliferating fibroblasts and the fibrin network. In fact, this close association has led some investigators in the past to conclude that fibrin was "converted" to collagen. This would be quite a feat considering the fundamental chemical differences between the two proteins. Actually, fibrin disappears coincidentally with collagen deposition. The mechanism for this has only recently been elucidated.

Although fibrin appears to provide a scaffold for fibroblast migration, the large quantity present in a wound actually inhibits cell migration, not only of fibroblasts but also of epithelial cells. Fibroblasts do not contain fibrinolytic enzymes. However, when fibroblasts migrate into a wound they are closely followed by new capillary formation. These capillaries are formed by endothelial budding and these new capillaries are a prominent feature of granulation tissue. It has been found that these endothelial cells contain a plasminogen activator. Thus, as capillaries grow into the wound area immediately behind migrating fibroblasts, fibrinolysis occurs and the fibrin network is broken down and removed.

The presence of extensive hematomas, necrotic tissue, and bacteria will block migration of fibroblasts and formation of new capillaries. If such areas are small and discrete, fibroblasts may surround and wall them off. In uncomplicated simple wounds, however, debris is usually removed by the third to fifth day and by that time fibroblasts and capillaries are invading the entire wound area.

New capillaries are extremely fragile at this stage of healing. They are also more numerous than in normal tissue and are easily traumatized. In handling wounds at this stage, great care must be taken not to damage delicate granulation tissue.

Fibroblasts not only have migrated but have also proliferated. Initially they manufacture and secrete elements of ground substance: protein-polysaccharides and various glycoproteins. About the fourth or fifth day post wounding, collagen synthesis commences and the stage of fibroplasia begins.

During the fibroplastic phase of repair, the cell population probably does not change appreciably. Collagen is laid down at a very rapid rate. Epithelium either has moved or is moving across the granulating wound. Proliferating epithelial cells liberate a collagenase which is important in controlling the collagen content of the wound. Fibroblasts coming in contact with new epithelium are also induced to secrete a collagenase. This lays the foundation for subsequent wound remodeling.

The fibroplastic phase of repair lasts approximately two to four weeks, depending on the site and size of the wound. At the end of this phase, a large number of new capillaries regress and disappear. The glycoprotein and mucopolysaccharide content of scar tissue decreases and the number of synthesizing fibroblasts diminishes markedly. Thus, the rate of total collagen synthesis decreases and eventually balances the rate of collagen destruction. The maturation phase of wound healing is then fully under way.

The length of time in which active collagen synthesis is proceeding in a wound varies with the tissue in which the wound occurs. In the bladder, for instance, the wound heals quickly and elevation in collagen synthetic rate lasts for only four to eight weeks. On the other hand, wounds of the stomach or intestines show exceedingly high rates for collagen synthesis for over 120 days.

The biochemical events in these various stages of wound healing will be discussed in greater detail in Chapter 5. The description of the healing process given in this chapter is that seen in most tissues of the body. Exact timing of the various steps in repair differs from one tissue to another—skin heals quickly, viscera heal very rapidly, and fascia and tendons heal more slowly—and the reasons for this will become apparent when repair of these tissues is discussed in detail.

Certain tissues show certain unique aspects of repair or regeneration, and these are discussed in separate chapters. However, the description of inflammation and of cells involved in repair given here is basic to all forms of repair regardless of site.

SUGGESTED READING

Bazin, S., Pelletier, M., and Delaunay, A. Influence of Chemical Mediators of Acute Inflammation on the Cells of Subacute Inflammation. Agents Actions 3:317, 1973.

Bhoola, K. D., Calle, J. D., and Schachter, M. The Effect of Bradykinin, Serum Kallikrein, and Other Endogenous Substances on Capillary Permeability in the Guinea Pig. J. Physiol. 152:75, 1960.

Boucek, R. J., and Alvarez, T. R. 5 Hydroxytryptamine: A Cystospecific Growth Stimulator of Cultured Fibroblasts. Science 167:898, 1970.

Burke, J. F., and Miles, A. A. The Sequence of Vascular Events in Early Infective Inflammation. J. Path. Bact. 76:1, 1958.

Harington, J. S. Fibrogenesis. Environ. Health Persp. 9:271, 1974.

Heppelston, A. G., and Styles, J. A. Activity of a Macrophage Factor in Collagen Formation by Silica. Nature 214:521, 1967.

Houck, J. C. A Personal Overview of Inflammation. Biochem. Pharmacol., Suppl., 1968, p. 1.

Hurley, J. V. Substances Promoting Leukocyte Emigration. Ann. N.Y. Acad. Sci. 116:918, 1964.

Lack, C. H. Some Biological and Biochemical Consequences of Inflammation in Connective Tissue, Biochem. Pharmacol., Suppl., 1968, p. 197.

Leibovich, S. J., and Ross, R. The Role of Macrophages in Wound Repair. Amer. J. Path. 78:71, 1975.

Majno, G., and Palade, G. E. Studies on Inflammation. I. The Effect of Histamine and Serotonin on Vascular Permeability: an Electron Microscope Study. J. Biophys. Biochem. Cytol. 11:571, 1961.

Majno, G., Palade, G. E., and Schoefl, G. L. Studies on Inflammation. II. The Site of Action of Histamine and Serotonin along the Vascular Tree: a Topographic Study. J. Biophys. Biochem. Cytol. 11:607, 1961.

McLean, A. E. M., Ahmed, K., and Judah, J. D. Cellular Permeability and the Reaction to Injury. Ann. N.Y. Acad. Sci. 116:986, 1964.

Menkin, V. Biology of Inflammation, Chemical Mediators and Cellular Injury. Science 123:527, 1956.

Miles, A. A. Large Molecular Substances as Mediators of the Inflammatory Reaction. Ann. N.Y. Acad. Sci. 116:855, 1964.

Page, A. R., and Good, R. A. A Clinical and Experimental Study of the Function of Neutrophils in the Inflammatory Response. Amer. J. Path. 34:645, 1958.

Paz, R. A., and Spector, W. G. The Mononuclear Cell Response to Injury. J. Path. Bact. 84:85, 1962.

Rocha e Silva, M. Chemical Mediators of the Acute Inflammatory Reaction. Ann. N.Y. Acad. Sci. 116:899, 1964.

Ross, R. Inflammation and Formation of Granulation Tissue. In: Inflammation. Mechanisms and Control. Edited by I. H. Lepow and P. A. Ward. New York, Academic Press, 1972.

Schild, H. O., and Willoughby, D. A. Possible Pharmacological Mediators of Delayed Hypersensitivity. Brit. Med. Bull. 23:46, 1967.

Spector, W. G. Substances Which Affect Capillary Permeability. Pharmacol. Rev. 10:475, 1958.

Spector, W. G., Heesom, N., and Stevens, J. E. Factors Influencing Chronicity in Inflammation of Rat Skin. J. Path. Bact. 96:203, 1968.

Spector, W. G., and Lykke, W. J. The Cellular Evolution of Inflammatory Granulomata. J. Path. Bact. 92:163, 1966.

Uvnas, B. Release Processes in Mast Cells and Their Activation by Injury. Ann. N.Y. Acad. Sci. 116:880, 1964.

Webster, M. E., and Pierce, J. V. The Nature of the Kallidins Released from Human Plasma by Kallikreins and Other Enzymes. Ann. N.Y. Acad. Sci. 104:91, 1963.

Weeks, J. R. Prostaglandins. Ann. Rev. Pharmacol. 12:317, 1972.

Willoughby, D. A., and Spector, W. G. Inflammation at the Cellular Level. Biochem. Pharmacol., Suppl., 1968, p. 123.

Chapter 2

EPITHELIZATION AND EPITHELIAL-MESENCHYMAL INTERACTIONS

Epithelium covers all surfaces of the body, including such internal surfaces as the gastrointestinal tract, respiratory tract, and genitourinary tract. Because of its location, epithelium is constantly exposed to the physical and chemical trauma of living. The surface layer of cells must constantly be renewed; this is accomplished by cell regeneration. Thus, the response of epithelium to severe injury or wounding is merely a quantitative extension of a process which occurs normally from the time we are born until we die.

We can learn a great deal about the response of epithelium to severe injury by study of the normal process of cell replacement, and in this chapter we shall discuss many aspects of this phenomenon including the important and interesting question of how the repair process is initiated. In any consideration of the repair process, regardless of what tissue or cell groups are involved, we must be aware of the ultimate function of that tissue or cell population; otherwise, no assessment can be made of the efficiency of repair or its long-term effect on the organism.

The major function of epithelium is to act as a selective barrier between the body and its environment. This barrier prevents bacteria, toxic materials, and long wave (ultraviolet) radiations from gaining access to the body. Conversely, it prevents or lessens loss of fluid, electrolytes, and other essential materials from underlying tissues. This barrier function is not absolute since, for example, toxic materials can penetrate the barrier when in appropriate solvents, and ionizing radiations such as x-rays or gamma rays can penetrate epithelium easily. Nevertheless, epithelium is our primary defense against a hostile environment and it is a major factor in maintaining an internal homeostasis.

Only slightly less important are functions of epithelium that reside in specialized cells and organs of epithelial origin. Examples of such specialized cells and functions are mucus-secreting cells of the gastrointestinal and respiratory tracts which provide lubrication, sebaceous and sweat glands of the skin, chief and parietal cells of the stomach which provide acid and enzymes for digestion, and cells of the intestinal villi through which absorption of nutrients occurs.

In assessing efficacy of repair and regeneration, the restoration of each function must be judged. It is insufficient to restore the barrier function of gastric mucosa if regenerated cells cannot differentiate into chief and parietal cells and perform their important functional chores. Furthermore, the rate of regeneration is likewise important since this process is in competition with a repair process involving connective tissue and, as we shall discuss later, this form of repair, while restoring structure, may seriously interfere with function. This is well illustrated in the end result of repair of third degree burns of the skin when skin grafts are not used, or the end result of chronic ulcerative lesions of the gastrointestinal tract.

A somewhat less obvious but extremely important epithelial structure that must be restored following injury is the cilium of the respiratory tract epithelial cell. If such cells were to be replaced by nonciliated cells, the patient would literally drown in his own secretions. Cilia perform the very important function of moving tenacious mucous secretions upward to the pharynx where they may be cleared.

EPIDERMAL REPAIR

The skin is the largest organ of the body. It is likewise the most exposed, and hence the organ most subject to trauma, both major and minor. Skin is composed of layers. The deepest layer, binding skin to superficial skeletal muscle, is a bed of loose areolar tissue called the *tela subcutanea*. In animals other than man, a layer of skeletal muscle, the *panniculus carnosus*, overlies this areolar tissue. In man, however, this is vestigial and the *platysma* is the only remaining reminder of this useful adjunct to skin mobility. Underlying the dermis is a layer of fatty tissue, the *panniculus adiposus*, whose thickness varies with site and sex, being much thicker in the female than in the male. Dermis is composed primarily of connective tissue through which blood vessels and lymphatics nourish this tissue and overlying epidermis. Within dermis are bundles of smooth muscle fibers, the *arrectores pilorum*, attached to hair follicles. Specialized epidermal structures, hair follicles, and cutaneous glands project into dermis.

Epidermis and specialized epidermal structures are composed of epithelium. This epithelium consists of stratified layers of epithelial cells resting on each other, and the lowermost, or basal cells, rest on the connective tissue of dermis. Epidermis consists of two principal layers of cells, the *stratum malpighii,* consisting of living cells, and the *stratum corneum,* consisting of dead horny cells. The stratum malpighii can be further subdivided into the basal cell layer, sometimes called the *stratum germinativum;* a layer of variable thickness, called the prickle cell layer or *stratum spinosum;* and the granular layer, or *stratum granulosum.* This latter layer is not always included as part of the stratum malpighii since it represents cells that are in late stages of differentiation and are about to die and pass into the stratum corneum.

Regeneration After Minimal Trauma

As we have mentioned previously, epidermis is subject to constant wear, and dead, horny cells of the outermost stratum corneum are constantly being shed. These are replaced by keratinizing cells which migrate upward to the surface. In any given location on skin this process of replacement is slow, and it is difficult to study the entire process of regeneration in detail. However, a number of years ago a simple procedure was devised which accelerates normal regenerative process in epidermis, and it has provided us with a clear picture of the sequence of events that takes place.

If one takes a piece of clear adhesive cellophane tape and applies it to a surface of skin and then quickly removes it, it will be found that approximately one layer of cells of the stratum corneum will adhere to the tape and be removed. This has been termed "stripping." If stripping is repeated in the same area, successive layers of cells will be removed; it is thus possible to remove completely the stratum corneum by this technique. The events that follow this trauma can be observed by means of small punch biopsies taken at the site of stripping at various time intervals.

Stripping experiments have shown that resting dermis responds quickly and vigorously to denudation of the stratum corneum. The mechanism of regeneration is mitosis of preexisting cells. This occurs mainly in cells of the basal layer, but also, to a varying extent, in prickle cells immediately above the basal layer. Many of the daughter cells, formed by cell division, migrate into the upper layers of the stratum malpighii, and without further division differentiate into keratinizing cells. Some daughter cells remain in the basal and lower prickle cell layers; they do not undergo differentiation. Cells in the basal layer show enlargement after the trauma of stripping; this apparently squeezes other cells upward into the prickle cell layer. The maximal increase in mitosis is noted 48 to 72 hours after injury.

It is apparent from these studies that the main regenerative activity occurs in the basal cell layer. For this and other reasons that will become apparent, the dermis-epidermis junction is of considerable importance in healing of epithelial wounds. This junction is not a flat surface, but is characterized by projections of epidermis down into dermis in well defined ridges which are called "rete pegs." The portion of dermis immediately under the basal cell layer consists of delicate collagenous elastic and reticular fibers, enmeshed with superficial capillaries and surrounded by a viscous ground substance. This portion of dermis is called the "papillary layer" or "body"; it is a negative imprint of the ridges, folds and projections of epidermis into dermis. Basal cells are normally firmly attached to the papillary layer, but following injury this adhesion to dermis is lessened and the cells can migrate upward or, as we shall see later, outward.

Not only does enlargement of basal cells force some cells into the stratum spinosum but, following trauma, epidermal ridges or rete pegs tend to flatten, thus forcing cells from the basal layer upward. We shall have occasion to refer again to this flattening of rete pegs when we discuss some of the consequences of epithelial repair in more extensive wounds.

This brief description of epidermal response to minimal trauma contains all of the essential elements of epithelial regeneration in both mild and severe wounds regardless of the location of epithelium. These are: mobilization, or loosening of basal cells from their dermal attachment; migration, or movement of cells to a position of cell deficit; proliferation, or replacement of cells by mitosis of preexisting cells; and differentiation, or restoration of cellular function. In the case of epidermis, the function is production of keratin. We shall now examine these steps of regeneration in more detail, and discuss factors which influence them, and the relative importance of each in the healing of wounds.

Epithelial Repair of Incised Wounds

During the period 1955 to 1965 meticulous studies of healing of cutaneous wounds were made and, by careful observations and refinements in techniques, many of the existing incomplete descriptions of both early and late events in repair of skin were extended and corrected. Even though the surgeon exerts extraordinary care to evert the skin edges while suturing a wound, the epidermal edges will always be found to turn downward into the dermal portion of the incision. If hemostasis is perfect around the incision, then the dermal and subcutaneous parts of the incision will be held together by an acellular fibrin clot.

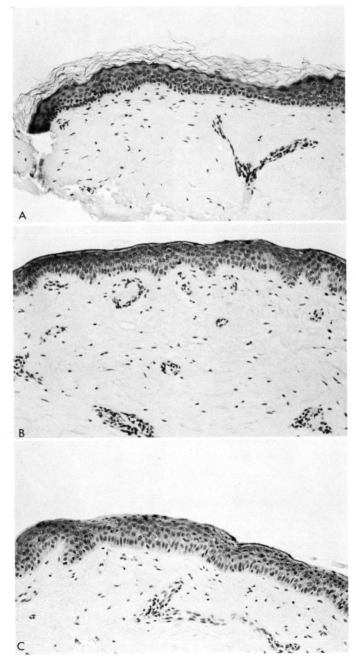

Figure 2–1. Epidermal response to minimal trauma produced by tape stripping. *A,* Control. *B,* Response 12 hours after stripping. *C,* 24 hours after stripping.

Illustration continued on opposite page.

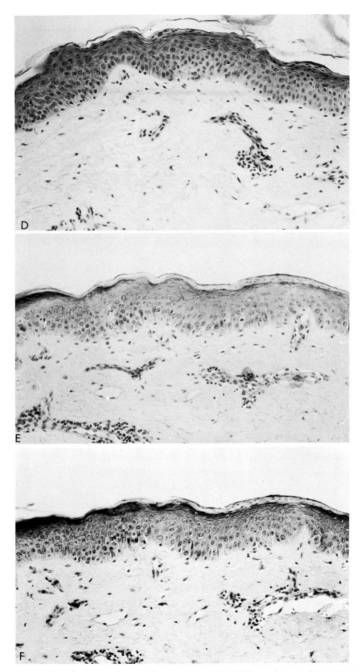

Figure 2–1. *Continued* *D,* 36 hours after stripping. *E* and *F,* 48 hours after stripping. At 12 hours and thereafter, many dividing cells can be seen in the basal cell layer and in the layer immediately above it. The picture is one of intense proliferative activity. Hematoxylin and Eosin, × 225. (Reproduced by permission from H. Pinkus and A. H. Mehregan, *A Guide to Dematohistopathology,* New York, Appleton-Century-Crofts, 1969.)

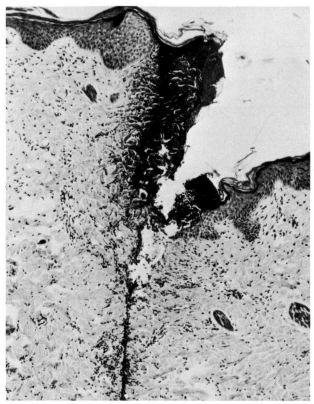

Figure 2–2.   Skin incision in young pig at day 1 showing step face at wound surface. A band of polymorphonuclear leukocytes with round cells marks the boundary between normal and darker-staining dead dermis at the right. Downgrowth of epithelium has not yet started. × 96. (Reproduced by permission from L. J. Ordman and T. Gillman, Arch. Surg. 93:857, 1966.)

Within 24 to 48 hours after wounding, the inverted portion of epidermis shows thickening. Marginal basal cells show mobilization; they no longer are firmly attached to underlying dermis. These cells enlarge and flatten, and, because of the increased area occupied, they extend out and downward over the incised dermis. As these cells enlarge, rete ridges adjacent to the wound tend to flatten, thus diminishing the area to be covered by basal cells. The excess cells commence to migrate over the defect. In the case of a clean, incised and sutured wound, migrating epithelial cells move down over the exposed portion of dermis and across the base of the wound. By 48 hours epithelial cells have bridged the gap. It is important to remember that during this 48 hour period no new connective tissue has been formed in the wound, and that epithelial migration occurs on the incised parts of the original dermis.

Sometime between 24 and 48 hours after wounding, increased mitosis of basal cells in a zone very near the cut edge of inverted epidermis is seen. In the case of epidermis, this increase in mitosis is initially confined to fixed, basal cells and to some prickle cells in the layer immediately above the basal cells. After migrating epithelium has bridged the gap, migrated cells become more columnar in character and commence mitosis, and daughter cells migrate upward within the V-shaped inverted surface of the wound. Simultaneously, the wound edges show hyperplasia of epithelium. Some spurs of the hyperplastic epithelium invade subepithelial tissues around the surface portions of the incision. At the same time, surface cells that have covered the incision begin to keratinize.

Of importance to the surgeon is the observation that downward growth and epithelial invasion occur not only at the incision, but also in

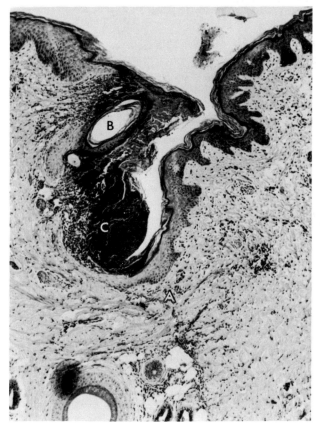

Figure 2–3. Skin incision in young pig at day 2. Epithelium from the lower step *(A)* has already grown across the incision as a thin sheet and has even begun to ascend the step face. There is some epithelial downgrowth from the surviving part of the injured hair follicle *(B)* lying within the upper step face. Upper surface epithelium has just started to grow down toward the injured hair follicle *(B)*. Dark-staining altered sloughed collagen in the scab is well shown at *(C)*. × 77. (Reproduced by permission from L. J. Ordman and T. Gillman, Arch. Surg. 93:857, 1966.)

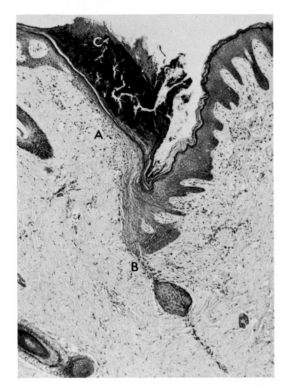

Figure 2–4. Skin incision in young pig at day 3. Epithelial union has now occurred at the middle of the upper step face *(A)*. Step-face epithelium itself is thin compared with that of transincisional epithelium *(B)* which shows some thickening and a small invasive spur. The scab of sloughed collagen *(C)* is still attached to step-face epithelium. × 49. (Reproduced by permission from L. J. Ordman and T. Gillman, Arch. Surg. *93*:857, 1966.)

Figure 2–5. Skin incision in young pig at day 5. Healing epithelium is similar to that shown in Figure 2–4. However, step-face epithelium *(A)* is now beginning to thicken and differentiate into layers. Keratinization and scab separation are consequently imminent above this zone. × 38. (Reproduced by permission from L. J. Ordman and T. Gillman, Arch. Surg. *93*:857, 1966.)

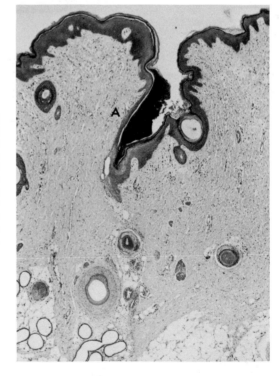

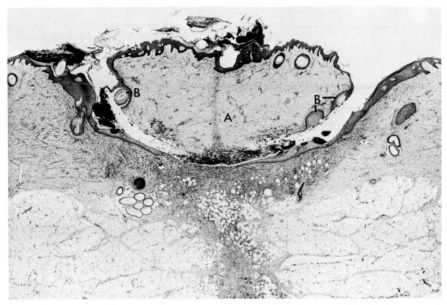

Figure 2–6. A sagittal section of a suture tract at seven days showing its length, the extent of epithelial downgrowth, and the perisutural cellular and fibrotic reactions on the outer aspect of the tract compared with those on the inner side. On the inner side, the depth of epithelial downgrowth is attributable mainly to surviving epithelium *(B)* from hair follicles injured by the suture needle and hence lying along its tract in dermis. That the cellular reaction is far less above than below the suture also is noteworthy. Intradermal part of scalpel incision at *(A)*. Hematoxylin and Eosin, × 19. (Reproduced by permission from L. J. Ordman and T. Gillman, Arch. Surg. *93*:883, 1966.)

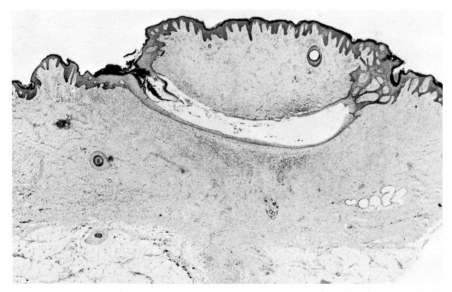

Figure 2–7. A sagittal section showing that the suture tract at day 17 is here completely lined with epithelium on its outer and deep surfaces only and that the incision is not visible here. The suture tract, in this case, lies entirely within dermis. The suture itself was removed after biopsy. Hematoxylin and Eosin, × 20. (Reproduced by permission from L. J. Ordman and T. Gillman, Arch. Surg. *93*:883, 1966.)

uture tracts, which can be considered small individual incised wounds. Even if subcuticular stitches are used, wherever these traverse an epithelial appendage extending downward into dermis, migration of epithelial cells along the suture tract will occur. Keratinization of epithelial cells which are in direct contact with components of connective tissue induces an intense localized inflammatory reaction. These reactions frequently have been mistaken for infections of the suture tract and are referred to as stitch abscesses. Culture of the tract usually reveals no viable organism; reaction is due to the presence of active keratinization in immediate contact with connective tissue. By the tenth to fifteenth day after wounding, the invasive spurs of epithelium regress; they are replaced by internally keratinizing epithelial pearls which represent detached epithelial cells derived from the regressing invasive spurs.

Recently, suture tracts other than in dermis have been studied in order to compare epithelial responses in various sites. Investigations of sutured wounds of stomach, colon, and bladder have been made. No evidence of epithelial migration along the path of the suture was found in any stomach or colon wounds. However, in several bladder wounds, sutured with nonabsorbable sutures, epithelium was found to have migrated and proliferated along the suture tract. The appearance was

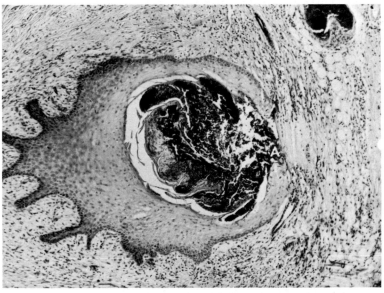

Figure 2–8. A perisutural reaction at day 10. Note that collagen related to that part of the circumference of the lining of the suture tract deficient in epithelium has lost its fibrillar character and is acellular (A). Opposite (A), epithelial spurs are prominent on the outer aspect of the suture tract lining and there is an extensive connective tissue reaction related to these invasive spurs. Hematoxylin and Eosin, × 62. (Reproduced by permission from L. J. Ordman and T. Gillman, Arch. Surg. 93:883, 1966.)

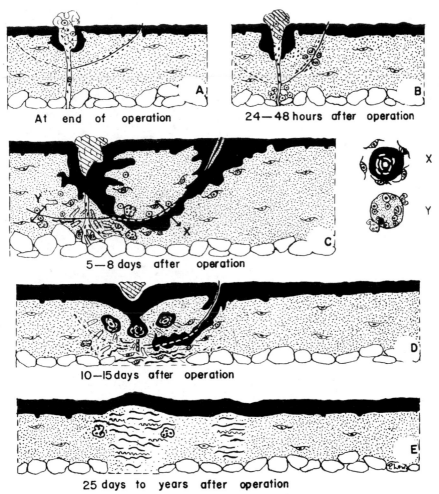

Figure 2–9.   The healing of an incised, sutured, skin wound.

A, Note inverted epithelial edges immediately after operation. Fibrinous exudate can be seen between cut edges of the incision, above which is a small surface clot.

B, Epithelial edges are thickened and are beginning to grow down in contact with the cut surface of dermis. Note round cell infiltration around the suture tract (reactions to the suture are shown only on the right, for simplicity).

C, Epithelial hyperplasia and invasive "spur" formation are marked. This growth also extends down the suture line. Fibroblasts are invading the wound from subcutaneous fat, but dermis and dermal fibroblasts are inert. Fibroblasts *(X)* also surround the epithelized suture tract. In other areas, giant cells *(Y)* are noticeable.

D, Capillary growth is proceeding upward from subcutaneous tissue and fibrosis is far advanced. Invasive epithelial spurs have regressed, leaving small round keratinizing epithelial "pearls" behind. Epithelium is beginning to straighten at the line of incision and the scab is being pushed off the wound. Epithelization of the suture tract is being narrowed by vigorous round cell and fibrotic reactions.

E, Epithelial and connective tissue reactions have abated and epithelium thins and assumes the late scar-like appearance. Deeper, collagen deposition is marked although elastic fibers are absent until very late in the course of healing. (Reproduced by permission from T. Gillman and J. Penn, Med. Proc. 2:121, 1956.)

very similar to that seen in skin wounds. Bladder epithelium is of the transitional type, but in some areas of the suture tract epithelium appeared to be squamous in character. It was also noted that epithelial lining in older wounds appeared thicker along the suture tract than in normal surface lining of the bladder lumen.

The major points of importance in the events comprising epithelization of incised wounds are: mobilization and migration of epithelial cells occurring before connective tissue regeneration, and closure of the gap by migrated epithelium before the other events of wound healing occur; mitosis of epithelial cells occurring in the basal layer adjacent to the wound, and, subsequently, in migrated cells covering the wound bed; migrating epithelium invading the subepithelial tissues at wound margins and along suture tracts; and keratinization of epithelial cells in direct contact with connective tissue, invoking an intense inflammatory reaction which can be mistaken for infection.

Epithelial Repair of Excised Wounds

Although epithelization of excised wounds follows the general pattern just described for incised wounds, certain differences due to connective tissue regeneration, presence of blood clots and scab, and so forth, are observed. These differences are more apparent than real, and the repair process is, perhaps, more under control of the surgeon, provided he has a grasp of underlying mechanisms.

In an excised wound, epithelial regeneration commences by cell mobilization and migration at the wound edges, exactly as it does in the incised wound. In addition, if the full thickness of dermis has not been removed, epithelial cells of the skin appendages, notably hair follicles which extend deep into dermis, will also commence to migrate. In such an excised wound, one is apt to see numerous "islands" of new epithelium on the surface.

Almost invariably, an excised wound initially is covered by a blood clot. Migrating epithelium does not move through the clot but under it, in direct contact with the original wound bed. Epithelial cells appear to secrete a proteolytic enzyme which dissolves the base of the clot and permits unhindered cell migration. The manifestation of this undermining of the clot and, later, the scab by migrating epithelium is seen in the peripheral separation of the scab from the healing wound as epithelization progresses.

In large excised wounds, all stages of epithelial repair may be seen simultaneously. At the margin of migrating epithelium, a single layer of flattened cells is moving across the wound. Farther back, some cells will be undergoing mitosis and just beyond them, upward cell migration is occurring, producing stratification. Where several layers of cells cover the wound, differentiation and keratinization occur; at the origi-

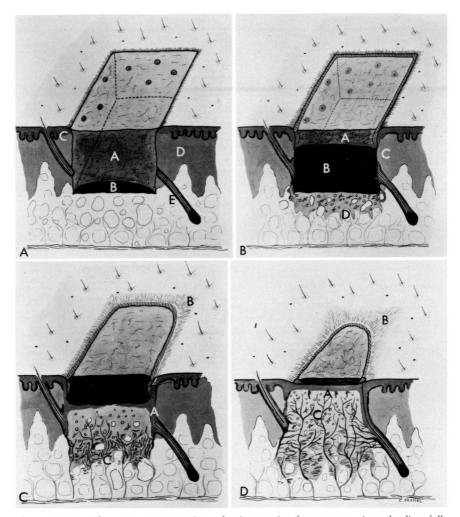

Figure 2–10. Schematic representation of microscopic changes seen in a healing full-thickness excised wound.

A, Immediately after operation. The wound cavity is filled with a blood clot (A). At the base is a cell-rich exudate (B). Epithelium at the edge shows thickening (C). Dermis is the shaded area (D) and a transected hair follicle is present (E). Similar transected appendages can be seen in the wall of the excision.

B, Two to three days after injury. The surface clot (A) has retracted, and subclot cellular exudate (B) has increased. Epithelium is advancing mainly from edges of the wound (C), but also from transected appendages. New connective tissue (D) is beginning to form at the base of the wound and the fatty layer shows increased cellularity.

C, By about the sixth day after injury, new epithelium from all sources has extended almost across the wound (A, B). New connective tissue at the base of the wound is proliferating and new capillaries (C) are invading granulation tissue from underlying fatty tissue.

D, Wound between eight and ten days after injury. Epithelium (A) has covered the excision and has thickened considerably. The wound is being further closed by active contraction of surrounding tissue (B). New connective tissue, in the form of highly vascular granulations, has filled the wound cavity. Later, vascularity will diminish and a dense collagenous scar will underlie new epithelium. (Modified from T. Gillman, in *Treatise on Collagen,* vol. 2B, edited by B. N. Gould, New York, Academic Press, 1968.)

nal wound margin a hyperplastic thickening of the original epithelium is seen.

Of equal importance to covering of the wound by new epithelium are the events occurring at the epithelium-wound base junction. Within four to five days after wounding, invasion of the wound bed by fibroblasts is well underway, new capillaries are being formed, and the typical picture of a granulating surface appears. New connective tissue, principally collagen, mucopolysaccharides, and glycoproteins, is formed in this bed. It is over this bed that subsequent migrating epithelial cells pass.

About 10 to 12 days after wounding, hyperplastic epithelium, covering the wound bed and newly formed connective tissue, appears invasive. Numerous projections of epithelial cells move downward into this new connective tissue, giving rise to "pseudo rete pegs." These projecting ridges do not persist, however, and by the fifteenth to twenty-fifth day they become separated from surface epithelium and form internally keratinizing epithelial pearls. These usually degenerate and disappear at a later date.

With the regression of pseudo rete pegs, the dermal epithelial border becomes straighter. True rete ridges never develop at the injured site; thus, for a given area of scar epithelium there are far fewer basal cells attached to underlying dermis than in normal epidermis. By 30 to 40 days the surface of the reepithelized wound is covered by "scar epithelium" characterized by thinness, fragility, or lack of strong attachment to underlying dermis. Microscopically, epidermis covering a healed wound can always be distinguished from normal epidermis by its lack of papillary layer in dermis and the straight epidermal-dermal junction.

Regeneration of Epithelial Appendages

For many years it was thought that specialized epithelial structures of the skin, such as hair follicles and sebaceous glands, did not regenerate if they were totally destroyed. However, it has been demonstrated conclusively that in the rabbit, at least, these appendages can be regenerated by differentiation of migrated epidermal epithelium.

Regeneration of skin appendages occurs late in healing, usually after surface epithelization is complete. About 30 days after wounding, in the rabbit, downward projections of new epithelium into underlying dermis may be seen. These are indistinguishable from pseudo rete ridges previously mentioned. Some of these, however, instead of receding, become radially arranged bars of thickened epithelium. Cell condensations develop under these epidermal bars and form dermal papillae. These appear to have been regenerated from the connective tissue. As the downward-thrusting buds of epithelial cells develop and mature into hair follicles, the epithelial ridges disappear as do other pseudo rete ridges.

Sebaceous glands, which are specialized structures attached to hair follicles, appear about the time newly formed follicles start to produce hair. They first appear as bulbous swellings in the neck of hair follicles near their attachment to surface epithelium. They then proceed to differentiate rapidly into fully functional sebaceous glands.

The question of whether eccrine sweat glands can regenerate has not been fully explored. It has been stated that sweat glands are not formed after birth. However, if the duct of a sweat gland is injured or severed, basal cells of ductal epithelium migrate and divide, and a new duct is formed. The fate of injured sweat glands cannot be studied in the usual laboratory animals since they do not have sweat glands. Definitive studies in man do not appear to have been made.

REGENERATION OF NONEPIDERMAL EPITHELIUM

Having shown that epidermal epithelium is capable of regeneration, and that, in all respects but one, repair of epidermal wounds is complete and efficient, we shall now look at the situation with respect to major epithelial surfaces elsewhere in the body. At the outset it can be stated that epithelium, no matter where it is located, undergoes essentially the same steps in regeneration as does epidermis. Differences in rate, and occasionally in order, do occur and appear to be related to the original epithelial structure and to its normal state of regenerative activity.

Trachea

Tracheal epithelium differs from most other epithelia in that cells of the surface layer are columnar and ciliated. Among these are goblet cells whose function is to secrete mucus. Immediately beneath the basal layer of tracheal epithelium lies an elastic lamina of connective tissue. We have already commented on the important function performed by cilia in removing accumulated secretions and foreign particles.

If tracheal mucosa is removed by curettage, intact epithelial cells at the margins of the wound flatten out, lose their cilia, and commence to migrate. This occurs sooner than the corresponding phenomenon in epidermis; the first phase can be noted as early as two hours after wounding and is usually well under way by eight hours. Migration of the flattened cells appears to be guided by the elastic lamina since, if this is destroyed, cell migration is abruptly halted and then proceeds at a much slower rate than when the elastic lamina is intact.

In contrast to the case with epidermis, basal cells of tracheal epithelium do not migrate; cell mobilization and migration appear to involve only marginal ciliated columnar cells and those immediately beneath them. Another difference is that two cell layers may migrate together in the trachea. As in epidermis, these migrating cells appear to secrete a fibrinolytic or proteolytic enzyme capable of dissolving the fibrin clot that covers the denuded area.

Cell migration precedes cell mitosis, and mitosis commences in both basal and ciliated columnar epithelium close to, but not at, the wound margin. Mitosis in migrated epithelium commences at about 48 hours, and in the next 24 hours the thickness of the epithelial layer over the wound doubles. At this time epithelium looks like transitional epithelium and the normal architecture of the mucosa is not restored.

At 96 hours, organization and differentiation of tracheal epithelium begins. Transitional epithelium arranges itself into a layer of low cuboidal cells overlying one or more layers of flattened basal cells. The upper layer of cuboidal cells lengthens at right angles to the surface and the nucleus assumes its characteristic position at the base of the cell. Cilia develop in these columnar cells while others differentiate into goblet cells and commence mucus secretion. Thus, in the trachea, epithelial regeneration is complete, provided underlying structures are relatively intact.

If there is extensive loss, not only of tracheal epithelium but also of underlying supportive tissues, scarring and poorly differentiated epithelium may close the wound. Attempts to prevent scarring or to bridge a gap in the trachea with artificial prostheses may be successful in maintaining an airway, but the patient will likely succumb to pulmonary infection, atelectasis, or other complications because of the absence of ciliated epithelium necessary for removal of dust and secretions. There is considerable evidence, as will be discussed later in this chapter, that functional differentiation of epithelial cells is controlled, to some extent, by the nature of underlying mesenchymal structures. If normal structures are replaced by indifferent scar tissue, or by synthetic substitutes, cells may cover the surface, but they do not differentiate into epithelium characteristic for that organ.

Regeneration of bronchial epithelium is essentially similar to that of trachea. The importance of epithelium to lung function and patient survival can be well illustrated by the problems encountered in lung transplantation. Even if a lung is removed and immediately reimplanted in the same individual, two major problems are encountered. Denervation, incident to the operation, causes cessation of activity of mucus-forming cells in bronchial epithelium, although ciliary activity is not interfered with. At the sites of bronchial or tracheal anastomosis, a short area of denuded connective tissue is present which acts as a bar to upward movement of bacteria and particulate matter. Mucus is needed to protect epithelium and provide lubrication for upward movement of foreign particles. Thus, in the transplanted lung, bacterial invasion and infection are the usual end results.

Esophagus

Esophageal epithelium, like that of skin, is of the stratified squamous type, except that it is not keratinized. The process of regeneration is essentially the same as that seen in epidermis except that flattening of migrating cells is less pronounced, and usually migrating cells consist of two or more layers. Further stratification and differentiation of esophageal epithelium is slower than in epidermis, possibly owing to the invariable presence of inflammatory cells and irregular spaces in migrated layers.

Stomach

Grossly, epithelium of the resting stomach appears to be arranged in deep folds. This is due to underlying musculature, however, and on distention the surface appears relatively smooth. Microscopically epithelium is characterized by the presence of pits, at the base of which are highly differentiated functional cells. In the fundus these are chiefly mucus-secreting cells, but in the body and pylorus, the pits also contain parietal cells which produce hydrochloric acid, and chief cells, which produce pepsin. Surface cells are of the simple columnar type. Thus, epithelium of the stomach contains four distinct functional cell types.

Normally, the entire epithelium of the stomach is being replaced continuously. This appears to start by mitosis of cells at the neck of gastric glands at the base of pits. These new cells migrate upward and differentiate into surface epithelium, or mucus-producing cells. In the fundus, the cell turnover cycle is about five days, but in the body of the stomach, the whole cycle occurs in only one day.

When a wound is made in gastric mucosa, considerable disorganization occurs at the margin of the wound. Glands in the vicinity of the wound margin contain no cells identifiable as chief or parietal cells. All marginal cells are the mucus-secreting variety. These are cells that migrate over the wound defect. In the case of a wound, mitosis is not confined to the necks of glands, as in normal cell replacement, but occurs at all levels, in glands and in surface epithelium. New glands form in the resurfaced wound by downgrowth of tubularly arranged epithelial cells of the mucus-secreting variety. As glands form and increase in size, certain cells differentiate into new chief and parietal cells.

In normal stomach, discharge of mucus occurs sequentially in various cells so that some are discharging while others are in various stages of mucus formation and storage. This staggered discharge of mucus provides a continuous cover and protects the epithelial lining from attack by hydrochloric acid and proteolytic enzymes. However, in injury or shock, this orderly sequential secretion of mucus is disturbed and many or all of the cells discharge it simultaneously. As this mucus is swept away, the cells cannot replace it and areas of epithelium are

.eft exposed to gastric juices. The result is the formation of ulcers. When due to repeated or prolonged injury, they are referred to as "stress ulcers."

The observed pattern of events suggests that under the stimulus of a wound, highly differentiated chief and parietal cells undergo a partial dedifferentiation to mucus-secreting cells and, after repair is effected, undergo differentiation back to their original functional state.

Small Intestine

Epithelium of the intestine is formed into villi, finger-like folds which project into the lumen, and which are subject to mechanical and chemical trauma during the course of digestion. These cells are highly specialized to perform the functions of absorption and secretion. Regeneration of intestinal epithelium is a constant process; it is the result of continuous mitotic activity of cells in crypts of Lieberkühn. The mitotic cycle has been found to be one hour and 15 minutes, and the time required for complete renewal of intestinal epithelium is 2.25 days for the duodenum and 2.75 days for the ileum.

Repair of mucosal lesions in the intestinal tract differs from that of epidermis in one important respect. Preexisting cells do not migrate; migrating cells are ones formed by mitosis of crypt cells. About the fourth day after injury, flattened cells covering the defect begin to divide, and crypts are formed by epithelial downgrowth into underlying connective tissue. The organizing tissue remaining between developing crypts becomes the stroma of new villi. If the muscularis mucosae is damaged, it does not regenerate, and the submucosa in the area of injury is thicker than normal because of an increased content of collagen fibers. Mitotic activity in response to wounding is not greater than that seen in normal crypts; this suggests that, normally, mitotic activity of intestinal epithelium is occurring at a maximal rate.

An interesting question that can be considered here is the effect of

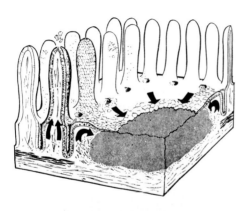

Figure 2–11. Diagrammatic representation of early stages of repair in an epithelial wound in the small intestine. Flattened epithelium, derived in part from mitotic activity in the crypts of Lieberkühn, can be seen migrating over the floor of the wound. In surrounding undisturbed epithelium mitotic activity in the crypts gives rise to cells which migrate along the sides of villi to be lost eventually at the extrusion zone. (Reproduced by permission from F. R. Johnson, Sci. Basis Med. Ann. Rev., p. 276, 1964.)

intestinal resection and end-to-end anastomosis on remaining functional epithelium. It is well known that if certain organs, such as liver, are diminished in size by removal of 60 to 80 per cent of their mass, a compensatory hyperplasia occurs, and almost the entire lost mass is replaced. In the case of resected intestine, it is obvious that no such restoration of tissue occurs. However, there is evidence that when more than 75 to 80 per cent of the intestine is removed, the average number of epithelial cells per unit length of the remaining intestine increases by 20 to 22 per cent. This certainly appears to be an attempt by the body to replace lost absorptive and secretory cells, and thus compensate for part of the functional, if not anatomical, loss.

Colon

Colon epithelium heals much like the remainder of the intestine, but the process is considerably slower, for some reason not well understood. At first, a flat layer of epithelium migrates over the wound bed, and later this transforms into the normal columnar type. As with the small intestine, downward invaginations develop and crypts are formed. Epithelization and restoration of normal morphology may take as long as three months.

Rectum

Although healing of rectal lesions follows the same general pattern as elsewhere in the intestine, two other processes modify this. Extensive granulation tissue tends to form in denuded rectal lesions and this appears to inhibit epithelization to some extent. Usually, wound contraction occurs in extensive lesions before epithelization is complete, and the wound is closed by contraction. If cicatrization and contraction are extensive, rectal stricture will result.

Urinary Bladder

Regeneration of bladder mucosa, while following the general sequence of events seen in regeneration of other types of epithelium, shows one notable difference. Epithelization of mucosal defects is rapid; it is accomplished by migration of a single or double layer of marginal epithelial cells. However, after one day, mitosis is seen in both surrounding epithelium and migrating epithelium. Mitosis in migrating cells is not usually seen in other types of epithelial regeneration.

The question of whether bladder can regenerate as a functional organ has been hotly debated in the literature. There are numerous papers reporting that, following extirpation of the entire bladder, except for a small portion of the trigone, more or less complete regeneration of bladder with restoration of partial function has occurred. Other investigators have reported, however, that only a fibrous sac, lined by regenerated epithelium, is formed and so-called "function" is merely an overflow phenomenon when hydrostatic pressure exceeds resistance of the bladder-neck sphincteric mechanism.

It will be pointed out in subsequent chapters that in granulating open wounds and in granulomatous tissue, a particular form of contractile fibroblast is present. Structurally, this cell has attributes of both a fibroblast and a smooth muscle cell. It is likely, therefore, that this cell has been mistaken for a smooth muscle cell, and the fact that it can contract has led observers to conclude that the entire organ has regenerated.

Certainly, it is well known that denervation of the bladder leads to marked impairment of function. There is no evidence that these so-called "regenerated" bladders ever become reinnervated. Other observations of synthesis of proteins in bladder wounds have shown that only collagen is being synthesized and that the rate of synthesis of non-collagenous protein is no different in the wound than in nonwounded bladder wall. It seems unlikely, therefore, that the bladder can regenerate as an organ.

Bladder epithelium, on the other hand, does regenerate rapidly. This is readily seen after removal of epithelium in treatment of extensive transitional cell cancers of the bladder. The fact that both undamaged and migrating epithelium undergo mitosis aids in the rapidity of epithelial regeneration.

Gallbladder

Epithelium of gallbladder behaves much like that of urinary bladder following wounding. Mitosis is seen in migrating cells. However, regeneration is not complete since the new epithelium remains flat and the normal convolutions do not appear to be restored.

Bile Duct

Bile duct epithelium regenerates in a manner similar to that of small intestine. Experiments in which all but a small remnant of the common bile duct has been removed and replaced with a stent have shown that a tube-like structure is formed rapidly. On removal of the stent, the duct appears to perform in a satisfactory manner. This is probably not a true regeneration of all elements of the duct. A fibrous tube lined with epithelium, while functionally satisfactory in this site, cannot be equated with a "regenerated" bile duct.

CELLULAR RESPONSES TO TRAUMA

Responses of epithelial cells to a wound will now be discussed in detail, since these responses appear not to be confined to this class of cells, but represent a general response of all cells in the body that are capable of such response. At the outset it should be noted that, in general, the greater the functional differentiation of a cell, the less likely it is that it will respond in a meaningful and purposeful way to a wound. This is most strikingly observed by contrasting epithelial regeneration with response of nerve cells to trauma. In almost every instance, epithelium responds to trauma by complete regeneration of cells and replacement of lost tissue, although in some instances the precise anatomical or histological relationships of the new tissue to adjacent tissues may be altered. Nerve cells, however, do not undergo regeneration if the cell body is lost. The cellular deficit is never corrected. The only regeneration that can occur in nervous tissue is regeneration of a cell process, the axon, if it has been severed. As we shall see in subsequent chapters, other elements of the repair process can seriously interfere with restoration of function even though this small amount of regenerative activity exists.

Mobilization and Migration

The first response of cells immediately adjacent to a wound is mobilization. This involves detachment from their substrate and preparation for migration. Normally a cell, such as an epidermal basal cell, adheres strongly to the underlying papillary layer of connective tissue of dermis. Likewise, cells adhere to each other. The nature of these adhesive forces is unknown, but in the case of prickle cells in epithelium it was once believed that direct mechanical connections existed between cells. This belief arose from the observation of intercellular bridges and desmosomes among cells in the stratum spinosum. Electron microscopic studies, however, have shown that these bridges are, in fact, small regions of contact between adjacent cells, characterized by a thickening of each adjacent cell membrane. No cytoplasmic continuity exists between adjacent cells.

The attachment of basal cells to underlying connective tissue can be severed cleanly by treatment of living tissue with trypsin. This enzyme will also separate adherent cells. This suggests that some readily hydrolyzable protein is involved in cell adhesion. It is also possible that such proteolytic action is involved in cell mobilization at the site of a wound, the enzyme being supplied by damaged cells or by leukocytes which quickly invade the area of trauma.

Cell migration appears to be initiated by a negative feedback mechanism. Isolated epithelial cells and fibroblasts, for example, will move if they are not in contact with other cells. Such motion is entirely random, if the substrate on which they are placed is not oriented. Motion is accomplished by formation of a cytoplasmic extension termed a ruffled membrane. This extends outward from the cell and adheres to the solid substrate. The body of the cell loosens from the substrate and the cell streams in the direction of the extended ruffled membrane. If a mobile cell comes in contact with another similar cell, motion ceases abruptly. This is termed contact inhibition. If a free edge is still present, a new ruffled membrane will form, cell adhesion is broken and the mobile cell will move off in another direction.

Orientation of the substrate, such as that provided by the presence of collagen fibers, will direct the movement of migrating cells. This is termed contact guidance and is an important factor in epithelial migration. Thus, it can be seen that orientation of the substrate on which cells move, and the presence of other cells of the same type, determines the extent and direction of cell movement. If two relatively clean and even surfaces are present, cell migration will be enhanced. However, if the surfaces are not oriented, as in the case of some plastic films, cells tend to pile up rather than move across the surface. In some instances, neoplastic changes occur. The mechanism by which such changes are induced is still unknown.

Of considerable interest and importance is the observation that cells of two different types do not exhibit mutual contact inhibition. Thus, epithelial cells can move across and between fibroblasts and vice versa. It has been shown that neoplastic cells, for instance fibrosarcoma cells, do not show contact inhibition when in contact with fibroblasts, but will freely invade masses of fibroblasts in tissue culture as well as in the animal body. This is only one aspect of the invasiveness of malignant cells, however.

Epithelial cells, in migrating over a wound surface, appear to move as a sheet. Individual cells maintain contact with each other. But it is not just cells at the edge that are responsible for the movement, dragging the others with them; all of the cells in the sheet contribute to the motion. The rate of movement may amount to several millimeters in a 24 hour period.

Mitosis and Its Control

In normal epidermis, very few basal cells are in mitosis at any given time. This is in contrast to cells in the crypts of Lieberkühn in which mitosis is nearly always seen. A number of years ago it was discovered that the incidence of mitosis in epidermal epithelium has a diurnal rhythm, being greatest during rest and inactivity (sleep), and least during wakefulness and activity. Such a diurnal rhythm is not seen in intestinal epithelium, probably because the mitotic activity is at a maximum at all times.

Epidermal wounds result in abolition of the diurnal mitotic rhythm in cells immediately adjacent to the wound, with an absolute increase in mitotic activity. This increase in mitotic activity of cells adjacent to the wound was observed nearly a century ago and led some investigators to postulate the release from the wound of some substance which diffused into adjacent tissues and directly stimulated cells to divide. Such a hypothetical substance was termed a wound hormone, and much effort has been expended to isolate and characterize it.

Most of the evidence on which the concept of a wound hormone is built involves the response of cells to crude extracts of mashed tissue. For instance, it has been shown that extracts of orbital glands of rats, if injected parenterally in other rats, will lead to a burst of mitotic activity in the recipients' orbital glands. Injection of extracts of other tissues had no effect. It has also been shown that similar effects in skin can be produced by injection of skin homogenates. It has been reported that extracts from young animals are more active than those from older animals, and that tissues of young animals are more responsive to these extracts than those of older animals. However, no clear dose-response curve has been obtained with any of these extracts; in fact, in most instances the effect is abolished or reversed with large doses of extracts. This is a strong argument against the existence of a specific wound hormone.

If such a wound hormone exists, it should be capable of exerting its effects at a distance from its site of production. This, of course, is suggested by the ability of orbital glands to respond to an intraperitoneal injection of an orbital gland extract. However, it has been shown that the rate of healing and tensile strength of each of two wounds in the same animal, made 5 to 15 days apart, are unaffected by the presence of the other wound.

None of the various tissue extracts used have ever been purified; nor has any specific chemical entity been identified as the local tissue stimulant. The equivocal evidence—the heterogeneous nature of the extracts, the lack of a dose-response relationship, and the wide variability of responses—argues against the concept of a wound hormone. Certainly, more convincing and critical evidence will have to be assembled before the concept can be entertained. This does not mean, however, that the response of injured tissue is not under humoral control. Just one example will illustrate that humoral control can be extremely important in specific situations. If a large amount of the thyroid gland is extirpated, there is a fall in circulating thyroid hormone. The pituitary responds to this deficit by secretion of thyrotropic hormone. The remaining thyroid tissue responds to the increased circulating thyrotropic hormone by regeneration of thyroid tissue. This is what Abercrombie calls a compensatory stimulus.

There is no doubt that some substances can stimulate cell growth and proliferation. These may be specific nutriments, or they can be substances which combine with or inactivate an inhibitor. It is with the question of a mitosis inhibitor that a great deal of interesting and potentially important work has recently been concerned.

Before a cell can undergo mitosis, several prerequisites must be met. A store of energy must be built up, since, during mitosis, neither glycolysis nor aerobic respiration appears to be involved. Cell growth is not a trigger for mitosis, but a certain minimal amount of growth appears to be necessary before cell division can take place.

Prior to mitosis, nuclear deoxyribonucleic acid (DNA) must double. Likewise, a store of nuclear ribonucleic acid (RNA) is synthesized. This takes place during interphase. Since materials needed for cell division occupy more than half of the cell, a cell that is performing numerous functional syntheses, i.e., fibroblasts producing collagen or epithelium producing keratin, does not have the resources to undergo mitosis. Conversely, a cell preparing for or undergoing mitosis has insufficient resources to undertake a functional chore. This may explain why it is usually the least differentiated cells that undergo proliferation in a tissue and why extremely differentiated cells do not divide often.

Shock inhibits epidermal mitosis. This observation led to the investigation of the effect of adrenal hormones on mitotic rate. It was found that both cortisone and epinephrine are powerful mitotic inhibitors. The blockage produced by epinephrine is not due to an action on glycolysis, the Krebs cycle, or the cytochrome system, all of which are active in the early phases of the mitotic cycle. The block appears to occur in late interphase.

If shock and outpouring of adrenal hormones produce mitotic inhibition, one would expect that wounds would produce the same response. However, the converse is observed. In seeking an explanation for this, radial cuts were made in the ears of mice and it was observed that increased epidermal mitotic activity was confined to a 1 mm. width of epidermis immediately adjacent to the wound. No diurnal rhythm was seen, and muscular exercise did not inhibit this activity, as it did in adjacent normal epithelium.

If a small wound was made on one side of the ear, down to cartilage, it was observed that on the opposite side of the ear, a zone of increased mitosis was found directly opposite the wound, with the greatest activity immediately opposite the wound center. The width of this mitotic zone was less than the sum of the two mitotic zones (one on each side of the wound) on the wounded side of the ear. This suggested that the stimulus to mitosis was due not to a diffusible material originating in damaged tissue, but to absence, or removal, of some inhibiting substance. This inhibiting substance could not be epinephrine or cortisone since the act of wounding would either not change their concentration in the circulation or, more likely, increase it.

On the assumption that whatever is responsible for stimulation of mitosis in wounding, be it an inhibitor or stimulator, is present in the normal animal and might be involved in normal diurnal mitotic rhythm of epidermis, various factors influencing mitotic activity were studied. Starvation, a stress situation, was found to inhibit mitotic activity in both wounded and normal epithelium.

If epidermis adjacent to a wound, in a starved animal, was cultivated *in vitro*, inhibition of mitosis disappeared and the mitotic rate became as high as in normal wounded skin. Since added glucose was not needed, and since the response was prompt, it seemed likely that inhibited cells had proceeded through interphase before inhibition and that washing out of some substance in culture might have permitted them to go on and finish the mitotic cycle. It was next shown that if normal animals were "primed" with epinephrine, no mitoses were observed, but on removal and culture of epidermis, mitotic activity appeared promptly. This burst of mitotic activity could be completely prevented by addition of as little as 0.5 μg. of epinephrine per 4 cc. of culture media.

Further evidence of the role of epinephrine was adduced by the observation that adrenalectomy abolished diurnal mitotic rhythm, and also abolished the inhibiting effects of activity. However, if epinephrine was injected adjacent to an epidermal wound, no mitotic inhibition was observed, even though one-tenth the amount, injected into normal skin, completely inhibited mitosis in a large area around the injection. Thus epinephrine effects could account for diurnal rhythm and the effects of starvation and other stress situations, but its action on cells adjacent to a wound was paradoxical. It was obvious that something else was involved in initiation of mitosis around a wound.

In considering all the facts, it was concluded that the absence of some factor other than epinephrine is responsible for the effects on wounds. Extracts obtained from epidermis and hypodermis were shown to have an inhibitory effect on mitoses in their respective tissues. Partially purified extracts showed a clear dose-response curve. The material, which has been termed a "chalone," is water-soluble and heat-labile.

Chalone, to be effective, appears to require epinephrine and possibly exists as an epinephrine-chalone complex. In a wound, chalone concentration and production would fall; a decreasing concentration gradient would exist from normal tissue to the tissue defect, where presumably it would be zero. This would account nicely for the zone of mitotic activity around the wound margin and would explain the narrowness of this zone. It has also been shown that chalone is tissue-specific but not species-specific. Mouse epidermal chalone will inhibit mitosis in epidermis of the mouse, rat, and numerous other species, but has no action on other tissues.

The chalone-epinephrine complex appears to act at a point just previous to prophase, i.e., in late antephase, after DNA synthesis is complete. If the cell has entered prophase, chalone-epinephrine complex has no effect; if the cell is in antephase, blockage is complete. In this action, chalone-epinephrine complex does not appear to be a classic DNA repressor. Its exact mechanism of action is still unknown.

If further experimental work substantiates the chalone concept, and if this is shown to be a general mechanism of mitotic control, a number of interesting and exciting possibilities are obviously open. One can, for instance, speculate on the role of chalones in neoplastic growth. In any event, the hypothesis, even if it is later shown to be erroneous, is useful as a framework for future investigative effort.

The observations on neoplastic tendencies of epithelial pearls, or rests, in scar tissue fit well with the chalone concept. It will be recalled that these epithelial cell groups are separated from migrated epithelium by regression of invasive epithelial spurs. They are surrounded, not by normal dermis, but by imperfect connective tissue. Since, in the absence of the required concentration of chalone, cells undergo uninhibited mitosis, and since they are in a hostile environment, it is conceivable that, by some unknown mechanism, a malignant change is induced. Certainly, it is well known that actively multiplying cells, such as are found in wounds, are more susceptible to agents that induce malignant change. An example of this can be seen in the propensity of radiation-induced wounds to develop cancer.

The important facts to be remembered are: cells, if not inhibited by contact with like cells, or with their normal underlying or overlying connective tissue, tend to migrate and proliferate. Under these conditions they are susceptible to the effects of inducers (virus, chemicals, radiation) and may undergo malignant degeneration. They then lose their normal contact inhibition, become invasive, and also lose their normal adhesiveness. A malignant neoplasm is the result. Because of their exposure to hostile environmental factors, epithelial cells are most prone to such changes.

Differentiation

Cell differentiation is the process whereby an embryonic, nonfunctional cell matures and changes into a tissue-specific cell performing one or more functions characteristic of that particular cell. Thus, from the time of fertilization of the ovum to birth of the newborn, cell differentiation is taking place. In the adult, many tissues and organs contain cells which are undifferentiated to the extent that although they cannot change into a cell of another tissue, they have not differentiated to a fully functional state. Examples of such cells are stem cells of the bone marrow, mesenchymal cells around small blood vessels in connective tissue which may become fibroblasts, and basal cells of epidermis.

It is also possible for cells that are differentiated to the extent of having become functional to dedifferentiate and revert to a more primitive type. This is seen in hair follicles following injury, in liver cells following ablation of more than half of that organ, and in specialized epithelial cells of the stomach following mucosal injury. It has been suggested that this reversion of differentiated cells to a more primitive type is a necessary prerequisite to their undergoing cell division. A cell undergoing mitosis requires all its energy sources and synthetic apparatus for the process of cell division, and none of these are available for functional chores. This also explains the undifferentiated state of most malignant neoplasms.

It has been suggested that there are in any tissue four main categories of cells:

1.   Progenitor cells that are involved in mitotic cycles.

2.   Immature cells that have ceased or are ceasing to divide and are preparing for tissue function.

3.   Mature cells that may or may not be functional and that, if circumstances dictate, are capable of reversion to mitosis.

4.   Mature cells that are perhaps always functional but cannot revert to mitosis and are approaching death.

The important point is that at some stage during cell differentiation a point is reached at which the cell has no option but to continue performing a specialized function and ultimately die. Before that point, the cell can either move forward or revert to a stage at which it may undergo mitosis to produce daughter cells characteristic of that tissue.

Given the proposition that some cells can dedifferentiate and undergo mitosis, it is interesting to find out how far backward this dedifferentiation can be carried. Obviously, in the adult one does not expect an epidermal cell to become a primitive blood cell; but of some practical importance is the question of whether one type of epithelium can be made to change to another type. It has been demonstrated that within a. given organ this is possible, i.e., interconversion of chief and parietal cells with gastric mucus cells; but of more interest is the question of whether epidermis could convert to tracheal mucosa, or some other type.

Studies have been made of interconversion of various types of epithelia by transplanting them to denuded recipient sites in epidermis. The grafts were made smaller than the recipient site so that cell migration in both host and graft tissue could be observed. When two types of epithelium met, one of two kinds of reaction was observed. The first was termed "fusion," and was characterized by coalescence and intermingling of host epidermis and graft cells until no sharp distinction between the two types of cell was visible. Migration ceased, and a continuous sheet of epithelium with a smooth outer contour was established over the wound area.

The second kind of reaction, "nonfusion," differed in that there was a cell-sharp line of demarcation between graft and host epidermal cells with no intermixing of cells. Epithelial migration continued, and resulted in a piling up of epidermal cells along the area of contact with the graft. This was accompanied by signs of disorganization and disintegration of cells. After the piling up occurred, host epithelium continued its migration and forced itself between graft epithelial cells and the subepithelial connective tissue until graft epithelium was completely undermined and the graft lost.

In the case of epidermal grafts, fusion always took place, regardless of the skin region from which the graft was taken. The same was true for grafts of cornea in host epidermis. Oral epithelium, from the roof of the mouth, fused well with host epidermal epithelium, although both types of cells retained their characteristic morphology and could be distinguished from one another.

Esophageal epithelium, on the other hand, showed nonfusion. The same nonfusion reaction was seen between intestinal epithelium and epidermal cells, and between gallbladder epithelium and epidermal cells.

These experiments are significant in that they demonstrate the importance of tissue specificity in wound healing. Fusion between two epithelia occurs only if, normally, there is a continuity, or coaptive relationship, between these epithelia in the intact organism.

In the experiments just described, one important variable was held constant, namely, the type of mesenchymal base upon which the grafts were placed. However, there is some evidence that, in certain instances, epithelial differentiation may be influenced by inductive contact with various types of mesenchyme. This type of inductive differentiation has been demonstrated only in embryonic tissues. Chick embryo epidermal epithelium will not live if cultured alone and not in contact with mesenchyme. If placed on limb mesenchyme, it grows and keratinizes normally, but if placed on cartilage, it fails to become established and degenerates or undergoes total keratinization. Epidermal epithelium, if transplanted to gizzard mesenchyme, differentiates into a ciliated mucus-secreting epithelium. Epithelium from the stomach is unaffected by the type of mesenchyme upon which it is grown. It would appear then that, in the embryo, certain types of mesenchyme can induce tissue-specific epithelial differentiation, but this ability is apparently lost in the adult.

EPITHELIAL-CONNECTIVE TISSUE INTERACTIONS

Notwithstanding the lack of inductive effect of mesenchymal tissue on adult epithelium, there are important interactions between epithelium and its underlying connective tissue. We have mentioned the failure of wound epithelium to develop rete ridges, resulting in a less firm adherence of scar epithelium to the underlying connective tissue. We have also mentioned the incompatibility of actively keratinizing epithelial cells and connective tissue. We now want to allude to another functional aspect of epithelium which may have an important bearing on scar formation and scar remodeling.

Two observations were made many years ago, and well substantiated, but until recently have not been explained. One is that in the healing wound there is normally an overproduction of collagen fibers, leading to a temporarily hypertrophied scar which later regresses to a thin, dense, white tissue. The other, not now seen in this day of overadequate vitamin intake, is weakening and disruption of old scars after prolonged scurvy. A possible explanation for these observations is to be found in the discovery that epithelium of the metamorphosing tadpole secretes a collagenase that aids in the remodeling of connective tissue of that animal, and in the demonstration that human epidermis frequently shows collagenolytic activity, and epithelium covering scars always shows such activity. This then suggests that there may exist in scar tissue a homeostatic mechanism. On the one hand, we may have continuous collagen production in connective tissue of scar, and on the other, we may have a continuous collagenolysis brought about by secretion of a collagenase in overlying epithelium. In the early stages of scar formation, collagen production will exceed collagen breakdown, leading to hypertrophy. Later, as overlying epithelium thickens and matures, collagenase production may increase and collagen breakdown may exceed collagen formation. Finally, a balance is achieved between two opposing reactions and a steady state is reached. If, however, collagen production is inhibited, as in scurvy, and collagenase production remains constant, then eventually the scar will erode away; the time required for this depends on the turnover rate of collagen in the scar. On the other hand, one could imagine a condition in which collagen production was normal and collagenase production was deficient. This would obviously result eventually in a great overabundance of collagen in the scar—a condition we recognize as a keloid. Much more experimental work remains to be done before we can achieve a complete understanding of the important relationships existing between epithelium and its underlying connective tissue.

We shall now consider briefly other inductive effects produced by epithelial-mesenchymal interactions. We have just illustrated one kind of inductive effect, namely, enzyme induction. We also alluded to another kind, the control of cell differentiation. We now wish to discuss similar interactions which may be important in the repair process.

Inductive effects between epithelium and mesenchyme have long been recognized as important in organogenesis in the developing embryo. This subject is too vast to be discussed here, and we shall say only that during organogenesis the type of epithelium that ultimately develops and the organ structure are determined by the type of mesenchyme with which epithelium interacts.

Of more interest to the surgeon are the implications of some experiments on inductive effects operating across interface materials. It has been observed that if living epithelial cells are cultured on one side of a millipore membrane, and mesenchymal cells are cultured on the other side of the same membrane, fibers which can be identified as collagen appear on the epithelial side but not on the mesenchymal side. The question arose whether collagen was being produced not by mesenchymal cells but by epithelial cells. With ^{3}H-proline as a label, epithelial cells were tagged in one experiment and mesenchymal cells in another. It was found that when mesenchyme was labeled there was a higher number of grains at the filter interace with epithelium than in the filter or on the mesenchymal side. However, when epithelium was labeled there was no such concentration of label at that point, but rather a smooth gradient across the filter. Further experiments indicated that mesenchyme produced tropocollagen and this diffused across the membrane and was polymerized in close association with epithelium. Further evidence, acquired with the use of labeled hexosamines, indicates that a halo of hexosamine-containing material, perhaps a protein polysaccharide, exists around epithelial cells and it is in this environment that collagen fiber formation occurs.

These observations suggest that the kind of epithelium that is present and the kind of protein-polysaccharide produced may play an important role in the size, distribution, and organization of the underlying fibrous network. We shall return to this subject in more detail in Chapter 4.

SUGGESTED READING

Abercrombie, M. Localized Formation of New Tissue in an Adult Mammal. Sympos. Soc. Exp. Biol. *11*:235, 1957.

Abercrombie, M. Behavior of Cells Toward One Another. Advances Biol. Skin 5:95–112, 1964.

Baker, R., Tehan, T., and Kelly, T. Regeneration of Urinary Bladder after Subtotal Resection for Carcinoma. Amer. Surg. *25*:348, 1959.

Billingham, R. E., and Reynolds, J. Transplantation Studies on Sheets of Pure Epidermal Epithelium and on Epidermal Cell Suspensions. Brit. J. Plast. Surg. 5:25, 1952.

Bohne, A. W., Osborn, R. W., and Hettle, P. J. Regeneration of the Urinary Bladder in the Dog Following Total Cystectomy. Surg. Gynec. Obstet. *100*:259, 1955.

Breedis, C. Regeneration of Hair Follicles and Sebaceous Glands from the Epithelium of Scars in the Rabbit. Cancer Res. *14*:575, 1954.

Bullough, W. S. Mitotic and Functional Homeostasis. A Speculative Review. Cancer Res. *25*:1683, 1965.

Chiakulas, J. J. The Role of Tissue Specificity in the Healing of Epithelial Wounds. J. Exp. Zool. *121*:383, 1952.

Cohen, P. J. The Renewal Areas of the Common Bile Duct Epithelium in the Rat. Anat. Rec. *150*:237, 1964.

Grobstein, C. Epithelio-Mesenchymal Interactions in Relation to Reparative Processes. In: *Repair and Regeneration.* Edited by J. E. Dunphy and W. Van Winkle. New York, McGraw-Hill Book Co., 1969, p. 57.

Johnson, F. R. The Reaction of Epithelium to Injury. Sci. Basic Med. Ann. Rev., 1964, pp. 276–90.

Johnson, F. R., and McMinn, R. M. The cytology of Wound Healing of Body Surfaces in Mammals. Biol. Rev. *35*:364, 1962.

Joseph, J., and Townsend, F. J. The Contribution of Migratory Epithelium and the Relation of Wound Enlargement to Healing. J. Anat. *95*:403, 1961.

McLoughlin, C. B. Mesenchymal Influences on Epithelial Differentiation. Sympos. Soc. Exp. Biol. *17*:359, 1963.

Ordman, L. J., and Gillman, T. Studies in the Healing of Cutaneous Wounds. I. The Healing of Incisions through the Skin of Pigs. Arch. Surg. *93*:857, 1966. II. The Healing of Epidermal, Appendageal, and Dermal Injuries Inflicted by Suture Needles and by the Suture Material in the Skin of Pigs. Arch. Surg. *93*:883, 1966. III. A Critical Comparison in the Pig of the Healing of Surgical Incisions Closed with Sutures or Adhesive Tape Based on Tensile Strength and Clinical and Histologic Criteria. Arch. Surg. *93*:911, 1966.

Pinkus, H. Examination of the Epidermis by the Strip Method of Removing Horny Layers. I. Observations on Thickness of Horny Layer and on Mitotic Activity after Stripping. J. Invest. Dem. *16*:383, 1951.

Teir, H., and Nystrom, B. Organ Homogenates to Stimulate Wound Healing in Rats. Arch. Path. *74*:499, 1962.

Weiss, P. The Biologic Foundations of Wound Repair. Harvey Lect. Series *55*:13, 1959–60.

Chapter 3

CONTRACTION

The terms "contraction" and "contracture" are frequently confused. Contraction is the designation for an active process which tends to close a wound in which an actual loss of tissue has occurred. Such wounds are frequently referred to as "excised" wounds. Contracture refers to an end result which may, in some instances, be caused by the process of contraction or may be the outcome of fibrosis of muscle or other tissue damage.

Contraction may be defined as the process by which the size of a full-thickness open wound is diminished, and is characterized by the centripetal movement of the whole thickness of surrounding skin. In lower mammals, contraction is the major process by which surface wounds are healed; it seldom results in deformity or loss of function unless it occurs over a joint and scar tissue is fixed to underlying structures. On the other hand, in humans, contraction seldom goes to completion except in very small wounds, and it may result in deformity and loss of function, the extent of which depends upon size and location of the original wound.

Upon reflection, it is fairly apparent that unless skin is mobile and can be stretched over the wound, simple contraction will not accomplish closure. Thus, a test which may be applied to find out if a wound can close by contraction is to grasp opposite edges of the wound with forceps and see if gentle traction will bring the edges together.

The apparent difference between contraction as seen in lower animals and that seen in humans is not due to a fundamental difference in the process or its mechanism, but lies in an anatomical difference in subdermal tissues. Anyone who has seen a horse get rid of a fly on its flank will immediately recognize that skin is capable of considerable movement and has a well developed superficial musculature. Unfortunately, humans have lost that local dermal mobility in many areas. In man, skin is more or less firmly attached to relatively inelastic and immobilie fascia which in turn is attached to major musculature, bone, or other underlying structures, particularly on the extremities and anterior chest wall.

Lower animals possess a well developed layer of cutaneous striped muscle, the *panniculus carnosus,* of which only vestigial remnants remain in humans. This muscle and the lack of substantial attachment of integument to underlying structures permit contraction to occur to its fullest extent without interfering with mechanical function of underlying structures. The same process occurs in humans, but in contrast to other mammals, leads to constriction, distortion, or immobilization in some locations owing to tensions developed through attachment of the integument to underlying structures. Thus, unless controlled by the surgeon, wound contraction can be a detriment rather than a benefit to the patient.

Avoidance of contraction is particularly important when the defect involves skin over the flexor aspect of a joint. Tensions developed during contraction and formation of subcutaneous fibrous tissue may lead to permanent flexion of the joint, termed a "flexion contracture."

THE PROCESS OF CONTRACTION

With modern surgical treatment of wounds characterized by loss of tissue, the full effects of wound contraction are not frequently seen. Because of this, surgeons are apt to forget that the phenomenon is very real and contributes materially to the end result of the healing process. Nearly 200 years ago, John Hunter described contraction over the base of an amputation stump of the mid-thigh with a resulting cicatrix "no broader than a crown piece." Since that coin was about 1½ inches in diameter, the area covered by centripetally moving skin margins was about 20 times that of the residual scar. Surely such a remarkable spontaneous wound closure deserves attention by surgeons.

Unfortunately, the happy result observed by John Hunter does not always occur, or if it does, distortion and functional disability can occur. Since the basic elements of contraction and its mechanism are the same regardless of whether we consider lower animals or humans, it is convenient to study the process in animals where it may be observed without complicating factors introduced by the peculiarities of human anatomy. A thorough understanding of the process is essential to its control.

When a full-thickness segment of skin, including the panniculus carnosus, is excised in an animal, the wound edges retract, so that the wound enlarges up to 10 or 15 per cent. There is an immediate exudation of blood and tissue fluid which forms a fibrin clot, providing a temporary closure. Evaporation of fluid from this clot leads to formation of a scab. After a lag period of five to nine days, depending on the site, species, and age of the animal, centripetal movement of wound margins begins. At the same time, epithelial cells around the margin of the wound become detached from their substratum. These cells gradually move down the free edge of the wound, onto the granulating surface, and underneath the scab, as described in the preceding chapter. Their place is taken by new cells formed by cell proliferation about 1 mm. back from the wound margin. This process continues until the entire wound surface is covered with a thin layer of migrated epithelial cells.

Wound contraction involves movement of the entire dermis, not just epithelial cells. The processes of epithelization and wound contraction are independent; one can occur without the other. In a contracting wound, epithelization may be regarded as a temporary repair aimed at providing a barrier to infection from without and loss of fluid from within. In a fully contracted wound, much of this migrated epithelium is lost.

The wound bed is at first covered with extravasated blood and cell debris. Within 12 to 24 hours it is invaded by leukocytes, chiefly the polymorphonuclear variety. These are followed by small and large lymphocytes and macrophages, whose principal role is to clean up debris preparatory to new tissue formation. Within a few days, capillaries at the base and edges of the wound enlarge and form endothelial buds which rapidly elongate, forming a network of new capillaries in the wound bed. It is these that give healthy granulation tissue its pink color.

Concomitantly with capillary proliferation, fibroblasts invade the wound area, the greatest number usually being seen first at wound margins. Toward the end of the proliferative phase of fibroblastic activity, collagen fibers can be seen throughout the wound bed. These elements, with associated ground substance composed of mycopolysaccharides and glycoproteins, comprise what is termed granulation tissue. It is over this base that movement of skin occurs.

In the incompletely contracted wound, fibrous tissue formation may occur to an excessive degree. Collagen fiber deposition may outpace new capillary formation and the resultant mound of new tissue presents a dusky unhealthy appearance. Patients will refer to this mass of unorganized, unsightly tissue as "proud flesh." The development of this useless connective tissue can inhibit further contraction and must be dealt with as described in Chapter 6.

In a rectangular wound, not all edges move at the same rate. If such a wound is made on the torso of an animal, it will be observed that the dorsal and caudal edges contract at a faster rate than the lateral edges. Because of mutual interference at the corners, the final scar resembles two V's pointing toward each other, the points connected by a thin line along the body axis of the animal. Circular wounds are observed to contract at a slower rate than rectangular wounds, and the resultant scar is not circular, but linear.

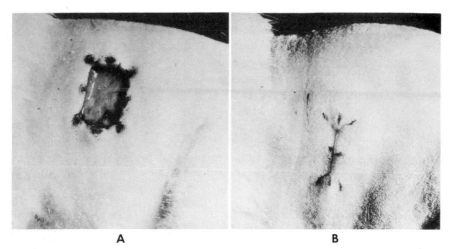

Figure 3-1. Wound contraction in the guinea pig. *A,* The fresh defect showing the eight tattoo marks at the margin. The base is the deep fascia. *B,* The fully contracted wound. The scar and tattoo points have assumed their characteristic alignment. Note the two V's pointing toward the central linear scar. (Reproduced by permission from H. C. Grillo, G. T. Watts, and J. Gross, Ann. Surg. *148*:145, 1958.)

It must be emphasized that contraction involves movement of existing tissue at the wound edge, not the formation of new tissue. It can be appreciated, therefore, that as contraction proceeds, tissue surrounding the wound is thinned, stretched, and under tension. These facts have been firmly established by relatively simple experiments. For instance, a square may be outlined on the skin of an animal with eight tattoo points, four at the corners and four at the midpoints of the lines

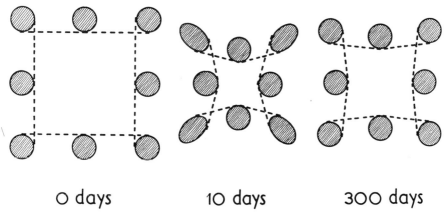

Figure 3-2. Schematic drawing of tattoo points around a square excised wound. At ten days, contraction of wound margins has displaced the center tattoo points inward and altered the shape of the corner tattoo marks. At 300 days, the resulting scar has expanded owing to collagen remodeling and intussusceptive growth. (Illustration by courtesy of D. W. James.)

joining the corners. By incision just within the borders outlined by these tattoo points, the full thickness of skin may be excised, down to the panniculus carnosus; the tattoo marks will then outline precisely the wound margins. This permits accurate measurement of changes in size of the wound due to movement of the wound margin, and eliminates errors of measurement which might be caused by epithelial growth over the wound bed. When this experiment was performed in rats it was found that the so-called "lag phase" during the first five days after wounding was more apparent than real. A small but significant diminution in wound size occurred. However, between day 5 and day 10 contraction was quite rapid, and thereafter further diminution in wound size was not seen.

Obviously, as wound margins move toward the center of the defect, the distance between adjacent tattoo marks should decrease. This happens, but the decrease is not in proportion to the decrease in area of the wound itself. This curious paradox results from the fact that tattoo marks at center points of wound margins move toward the wound center at faster rate and to a greater extent than do tattoo marks at the corners. The end result is not a square or punctate scar, but one in the shape of a four-pointed star. However, measurement of the final wound perimeter as determined by tattoo marks shows that the perimeter has decreased, and therefore some skin compression has occurred immediately around the wound.

The tissue deficit caused by stretching and thinning of skin surrounding a contracted wound is eventually compensated by what has been termed "intussusceptive growth." This involves production of new epithelial cells in areas of skin under tension and formation of new connective tissue in underlying dermis. This proceeds until the full thickness of stretched skin is restored. This statement, as it stands, can be misleading unless we examine the evidence upon which it is based and the nature of "intussusceptive growth." If a series of lines is tattooed parallel to the edge of a square skin wound prior to excision of the full thickness of skin, then the distance between adjacent parallel lines will furnish a semiquantitative measure of movement of skin surrounding the wound edge. Such observations have been made, and the results show clearly that as wound edges move toward the center of the defect, the lines on the skin also move toward the wound center. However, the increase in distance between adjacent parallel lines becomes less the further the measurement is made from the wound edge. This suggests a "stretching" of skin around the wound which is greatest in the region immediately adjacent to the wound margin.

If, instead of tattooing lines parallel to wound margins, adjacent skin is marked off in a series of small squares of equal area, it is possible to gain a more accurate measure of the distortion and stretching of skin during contraction of a wound. Such an experiment has been performed in the guinea pig, and one of the most striking observations

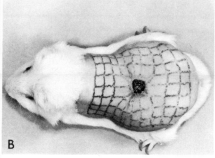

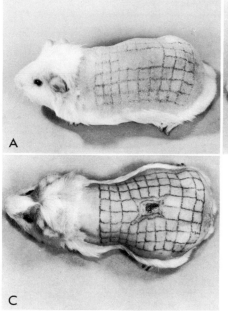

Figure 3–3. *A,* Photograph of a guinea pig taken 42 days after tattooing and prior to wounding. The squares provide a co-ordinate system from which movement of unwounded skin can be measured during the process of contraction.

B, Photograph of the same animal as in *A,* taken 104 days after wounding. Note that the squares in the anterior and posterior position have increased in area and that some of the squares in the lateral aspect have decreased in size. Wound contraction is maximal in this animal. This illustrates the relative distortions of skin surface that occur in a maximally contracted wound.

C, Photograph taken 103 days after wounding in another animal in which contraction was minimal. Diminution in size of the lateral squares is not seen, but expansion of the anterior and posterior squares is evident. Considerable epithelization has occurred. (Reproduced by permission from W. E. Straile, J. Exp. Zool. *141*:119, 1959.)

was that movement of wound edges occurred primarily in an anterior-posterior direction. A marked shortening of the lateral borders of the wound was the result, and this led to a relaxation in normal tension of lateral skin. There was an actual reduction in the surface area of skin lateral to the wound as shown by diminution in the areas of squares adjacent to the wound edge. Conversely, marked expansion of squares anterior and posterior to the wound during contraction was seen even at a considerable distance from the wound margin. The squares became rectangles with the long axis parallel to the anterior-posterior axis of the animal.

As mentioned previously, circular wounds contract incompletely or not at all. This is because all edges of the wound become compressed by the force of contraction. A practical application of this observation is the designing of skin wounds to accommodate a stoma, such as a colostomy opening. If the stoma is formed by making a square or elliptical incision in the skin, the process of contraction will constrict the stoma, and may cause an obstruction. A carefully designed circular skin wound will not contract and the stoma will not be constricted.

These experiments serve to demonstrate that wound contraction involves expansion and stretching of skin surrounding the defect; this involves skin at some distance from the wound. This expansion and stretching is not uniformly distributed around the wound; in the animals studied it was greater in the anterior-posterior direction than lateral to the defect.

In Chapter 2 regeneration of epithelium was discussed and from the evidence presented there it is evident that, although epithelial cells multiply in stretched skin around a contracting wound, they can only contribute an insignificant amount to replacement of tissue which has become stretched and thinned. Since the evidence available suggests that the tissue deficit is eventually supplied, the question arises: With what is dermis replaced?

A simple but ingenious technique for study of the growth of new tissue in stretched and expanded skin around a contracting wound has been devised. To use skin around the wound margin for biochemical studies introduces uncontrollable sampling variations; but if, when the original defect is made, an island of skin is left in the center of the wound, this provides a well defined sample of expanding skin for study. As outer margins of the wound move toward the geometrical center, the skin island expands by movement of its margins across the wound bed toward the advancing outer margins. Tissue in the island becomes thinned and stretched. Noteworthy is the observation that hair follicles spread apart as the island expands, but no new ones are formed. It is important to realize that as an "organ," the skin does *not*

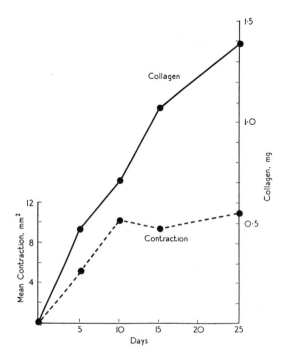

Figure 3–4. Relationship between contraction and collagen content of an excised wound. Note that collagen content increases long after the wound has ceased to contract. This is due to intussusceptive growth. (Reproduced by permission from M. Abercrombie, M. H. Flint, and D. W. James, J. Embryol. Exp. Morph. 2:264, 1954.)

regenerate. None of the specialized structures of skin increase to make their density in stretched skin equal to what it was before this expansion occurred. However, 50 to 100 days after wounding, the skin island can be shown, by histological examination, to be of the same thickness as normal skin; chemical examination shows that the new tissue is primarily collagen. Thus, at 100 days, the collagen content of the whole island is increased nearly fourfold over what it was estimated to be at the time of wounding. It must be remembered, however, that the area of the skin island also has increased, so that, although collagen per unit area of skin is slightly increased, the unit composition of skin, from a limited biochemical point of view, is not markedly different from that of normal skin.

The data just presented were obtained long after wound contraction had gone to completion and a stable histological and biochemical equilibrium had been established. Biochemical events occurring in skin surrounding a wound are of practical interest to the surgeon. During closure of a wound by a contraction, it has been found that the weight of surrounding skin actually increases, and this is due to an increase in water content. In contrast, however, actively expanding skin shows a large and significant deficit of collagen. This can be accounted for by dilution of already existing skin collagen, and failure of collagen synthesis to keep pace with skin expansion. With the "tattooed square" technique described earlier in this chapter, it was found that when one of the squares had expanded 30 per cent in area, 18 days after wounding, collagen content increased less than 4 per cent. This collagen deficit is not made up until late in the healing process. Thus, after all visible changes in the wound have ceased, there is still an active synthetic and reparative process going on beneath normal-appearing skin.

Although mobile skin involved in closing a defect by contraction may appear normal to the casual observer, observations on changes that occur in it, during and after wound contraction, should make it obvious that its quality has been impaired. Many elements of dermis are incapable of regeneration. Thus, only epithelium and collagen can fill in voids created by stretching out and expanding this skin. It is questionable whether collagen can be said to perform any useful function other than occupying space in this situation. Nevertheless, as will be discussed in Chapter 6, this covering of a wound is vastly superior to that involving only connective tissue covered with migrated epithelium.

The size of the wound does not affect the rate at which it will contract. The amount of available mobile skin will determine whether the wound will be completely closed or not. Contraction proceeds at a fairly uniform rate of about 0.6 to 0.75 mm. per day. If the wound is not completely closed by the twelfth to fifteenth day, contraction usually ceases.

Although the rate of movement is usually stated to be constant, close observation will show that during the first five to seven days, little change in size or shape of the wound occurs. This is often referred to as the "lag" phase and corresponds to a similar phase seen in the wound closed primarily with sutures during which little or no gain in tensile strength can be observed. Dunphy prefers to call this the preparatory phase, since significant cellular and biochemical changes are in progress.

After this preparatory phase, movement of skin edges commences and proceeds rapidly. Later, as elastic tension in the surrounding skin increases and opposes the force of contraction, movement of skin margin slows and stops. Two events may stop wound contraction. If the edges of the wound meet, contact inhibition of moving cells sets in and halts further advance. If before the edges meet the tension in the surrounding skin equals or exceeds the force of contraction, further centripetal motion will cease and, indeed, some backward movement may occur.

If, shortly after the wound has completely contracted, the residual scar with a small margin of the wound edge is excised, the wound will immediately gape because of tension of surrounding skin. Unlike the primary wound, however, centripetal movement of the wound margin commences without a preparatory period and the secondary wound will close in a shorter time than a primary wound of the same size. This acceleration of contraction in a secondary wound is not due to more rapid movement of the skin margins, but to the fact that all elements needed for this movement are already present, and the "lag" or preparatory phase is eliminated.

THE END RESULT OF CONTRACTION

If wound contraction results in apposition of skin margins, a relatively thin, stellate scar will remain as visual evidence of the former wound. Depending upon the extent of the surrounding mobile skin and structures in it, a variable amount of visible distortion may be apparent. This will be particularly apparent if the degree of mobility is less in one direction than another. In this instance the relative positions of various parts of the integument are altered and some parts of the skin are under greater tension than others.

It must be emphasized that the external appearance of a wound that has closed completely by contraction is misleading. Underneath the migrated dermis lies a connective tissue scar equal in extent to that of the original wound. Also, as we have discussed, the quality of the expanded skin has been altered by intussusceptive growth of collagen, restoring the thickness of the thinned out dermis.

If equilibrium is reached before wound edges meet, a defect remains. Collagen continues to be laid down in the uncovered area and this area begins to increase in size again. This expansion of the scar in unclosed wounds is a late phenomenon. The extent of scar expansion appears to be related in part to body growth; that is, it is greatest in growing animals and least in adult animals whose growth rate is minimal. This, as will be seen, has implications in the treatment of human wounds.

At least part of this late expansion of scar tissue can be related to the well known loss of elasticity of skin with increasing age. In young animals, elastic skin exerts continual tension on the scar. This tension exerts a stimulating effect on production of connective tissue fibers and also reorients and remodels them. Hypertrophic scars and keloids are more prevalent in young people than in old. This is not to say that skin tension is responsible for abnormalities in scar formation, only that it is one of many factors that play a role.

In the final phase of healing, the collagen becomes covered with a thin layer of epithelium. Some absorption and remodeling of the scar occurs, capillaries become greatly diminished, and water content of the wound diminishes. This results in the typical white scar which is firmly fixed to underlying tissue and which, because of this fixation, limits motion and, in critical areas, interferes with function.

Because fibrous connective tissue covered by a thin layer of epithelial cells is a very poor substitute for normal skin, every effort should be made to minimize the extent of scars. The procedures that are most likely to achieve satisfactory results are discussed in Chapter 6.

THE MECHANISM OF CONTRACTION

Having described the phenomenon of wound contraction and discussed its consequences, we must now turn our attention to the underlying mechanism responsible for movement of skin in covering a tissue deficit. It is only through an understanding of this mechanism that the surgeon can hope to exert rational control of the healing process.

When fibers were first identified in wounds it was thought that contraction was caused by shortening of collagen fibers which are laid down in granulation tissue in the wound bed. However, it has now been demonstrated that collagen fibers are not contractile and do not shorten except under extreme conditions. They may be stretched, particularly in dermis and subcutaneous tissue, but this is due to the fact that, in this location, they may be woven into a random mesh, kinked or coiled. Stretching is merely a straightening or reorientation of fibers, without a change in their dimensions. In contrast, a tendon, in which collagen fibers lie in a straight parallel array, is quite resistant to stretch.

The structure of collagen fibers will be discussed in detail in a later chapter, and it will suffice to say here that their structure makes them ideally suited for transmission of a force. In normal skin these fibers are interwoven in a more or less random fashion. When skin is stretched, these fibers tend to orient along the line of tension much in the way that cotton fibers in a ball of cotton will orient when the ball is pulled. The inelasticity of collagen fibers thus sets a limit on the amount of stretch to which skin can be subjected. The elasticity of skin is due not to its collagen content but to elastic fibers which are present. A scar is relatively inelastic because it has few, if any, elastic fibers and collagen fibers are denser than in normal skin and tend to be oriented in lines of original tension. It is apparent, therefore, that the role of collagen fibers in wound contraction is at best only a passive one and we must look elsewhere for the active mechanism.

Many theories regarding the mechanism of contraction have been advanced. Most of these attribute the force to activity of the fibroblast. They differ as to the location of the fibroblasts exerting this force. One school of thought finds evidence that fibroblasts immediately beneath the wound margin pull the wound edge toward the center as they migrate centripetally. This has been termed the "picture frame" theory. The other school of thought finds evidence that cells within the wound contents exert their force by cellular contraction, pulling the margin to the center of the wound.

If a wound is made in a scorbutic animal, fibroblastic proliferation proceeds at a normal or even an accelerated rate. It has been shown, however, that in the healing wound, and in such artificial situations as subcutaneous implantation of polyvinyl sponges or injected carrageenin, collagen formation is inhibited almost completely. This occurs, of course, only in animals that are unable to synthesize their own ascorbic acid and hence can develop scurvy. Among common laboratory animals, only the guinea pig can be utilized for such studies.

In the scorbutic guinea pig, it has been demonstrated that wound contraction proceeds at the same rate and to the same extent as it does in the normal guinea pig. Analysis of the collagen content of scorbutic wounds reveals that they contain only 15 per cent of the collagen of normal wounds. This evidence also implicates cells and eliminates collagen fibers as being involved in contraction. It is also compatible with either theory.

One curious finding, noted by investigators who examined scabs on normal and scorbutic wounds, was that the scab on the scorbutic wound was thicker and persisted longer than that on the normal wound. In fact, the scab appeared to delay the inward movement of the skin margins as evidenced by prompt and normal contraction after removal of the scab. Analysis of hydroxyproline content of the scab revealed a much higher amount in the scorbutic scab than in the normal scab. The source of this hydroxyproline is thought to be collagen from the base of the wound that was there at the time of wounding and not collagen formed after wounding; however, direct evidence as to the source is lacking. The presence of hydroxyproline does not aid wound contraction since movement of skin margins was normal after complete removal of the scab.

That the fibroblast is capable of both movement and contraction has been well demonstrated. Fibroblasts, like epithelial cells, tend to grow in syncytia. It has been observed that fibroblasts growing in tissue culture, when not in contact with another cell, show completely random movement. It has also been noted that cultures of adult fibroblasts show only slow and sluggish movement; explants of such cells expand quite slowly. However, if the cells are derived from wound tissue, they show greatly increased movement and cultured explants expand rapidly. This expansion of cell population is due to active movement of cells, since it is far greater in extent than can be accounted for by any observed change in mitotic rate.

As will be discussed later in this chapter, there is a specific reason for the differences between ordinary fibroblast cultures and those of wound fibroblasts. The differences are not observable with ordinary light microscopy. The experiments described here were all performed with light microscopy, and the true explanation of the motion of wound fibroblasts had to await study by electron microscopy and other experiments.

The increased rate of cell emigration from an explant is termed "mobilization." It is seen with cells other than fibroblasts, such as epithelium, and is believed to be an important response to production of a wound. What initiates this change in cellular activity is still unknown, but changes in cell surface which reduce cell adhesion are thought to be responsible. It is known that proteolytic enzymes will reduce cell adhesion, as will alterations in the charge on the cell surface. It has been suggested that wounding causes liberation of intracellular proteases and alters ionic balance in adjacent tissues, thus leading to cell mobilization.

Cell movement appears to be accomplished by formation of a "ruffled membrane" at one edge of the cell which extends and fixes itself to the substrate and, by contraction, pulls the cell over the underlying material. Nearly all cells that show migration appear to do so by this mechanism. Some cells, such as those of epithelium, have an undulating membrane that extends nearly around the cell body, while others, like the fibroblast, have one predominant membrane which extends only in the direction of movement.

If the ruffled membrane of one cell comes in contact with another cell, movement ceases, a phenomenon called "contact inhibition." When one cell comes in contact with another of the same kind, mutual adhesion occurs between their cell surfaces. Careful electron microscopic studies appear to indicate that cell membranes may not come into physical contact but may actually be separated by some 20 Å (so-called "close-adhesion") or 100 to 200 Å, a commonly observed separation. Cell adhesion, then, may be due not to some physical contact between cells, but to some other force. The nature of this force is not known, but increasing ionic concentration, increasing cation valency, and decreasing pH all favor adhesion. An element of mechanical stability is also involved in fibroblast adhesion since the cell wall may show many indentations and protuberances, especially at the surface of the ruffled membrane, and the wall of the adhering cell will conform closely to these irregularities, apparently "locking" cells together.

Recently, more detailed electron microscope observations of adhering fibroblasts have suggested that under certain conditions all extracellular space between adjacent fibroblasts may become obliterated and the outer lamellae of unit membranes may appear fused. Such observations are in keeping with a theory that movement of sheets of fibroblasts and contraction of a whole population of cells is initiated and propagated by transmission of information of an electrical nature. How important such a phenomenon may be in wound contraction will be discussed later in this chapter.

If an edge of a cell is free in another direction, a new ruffled membrane will develop and the cell will move in the direction of free space. In a whole population of cells, the population tends to expand in the direction of free space. When all cells are in contact with one another, movement ceases. This phenomenon is seen only when cells have a solid substrate on which to move. If the substrate is structureless, movement can occur in any direction in which there is free space. However, if the substrate has an oriented structure, such as might be provided by a fibrin network, the movement appears to be in the direction of substrate orientation. This is called "contact guidance." Syncytia of fibroblasts appear to be held together by mutual adherence of cell surfaces. Thus, when cells on a free edge move, the entire syncytium moves in that direction also.

Contact guidance may be a very important mechanism in repair of wounds. It is readily observable that fibers, such as fibrin and collagen, orient in lines of superimposed tension. In a skin defect, such as that brought about by tissue loss, a fibrin clot quickly develops on the surface of exposed tissue. The natural elasticity of surrounding skin places tension on the clot adhering to the margin; thus the fibrous components tend to orient toward wound margins. Direct observation of fibroblasts on fibrin clots has shown that they move along fibers, not across them. Thus, as fibroblasts move out into the wound they are guided by fibrous elements whose position and orientation make them ideally suited to bring cells toward the center of the defect.

Not only do cells adhere to each other, but the process of locomotion appears to involve first extension of the ruffled membrane along the oriented substrate and its adherence to the substrate. The cell can be seen to "round up" and advance toward the out-thrust pseudopod or membrane. The adhering mass of cells, in the wake of the lead cell, also appears to contract and advance in the same direction.

The question of the origin of fibroblasts will be dealt with in more detail in Chapter 4, and it will suffice to say that although some may be derived from large mononuclear cells coming from the general blood circulation, in a healing wound the majority are probably derived from resting mesenchymal cells and fibrocytes located in adventitia of small local blood vessels in subcutaneous tissue and subcutaneous fat. It would seem, therefore, that fibroblasts could originate in the wound base as well as in tissue immediately under the wound margin. Histological observations suggest that fibroblasts do come from both sources, but a greater number appear to move into the wound from the margins.

Since significant fibroblastic invasion of the wound bed does not occur until three to four days after wounding, the "lag" or preparatory phase of wound contraction could be accounted for by the time it takes for this fibroblastic proliferation. Thus, the observation that wound contraction is preceded by a lag phase is consonant with a cell-mediated phenomenon.

Experimental evidence demonstrates that any interference with the wound margin, by undermining in the horizontal plane, results in an immediate retraction of the wound to a size equal to, or larger than, that existing before contraction commenced. Using wounds in rats, tattooed so as to mark the margins of the wounds, and excising the newly formed tissue in the wound bed at 10, 15, and 25 days after wounding, results in an immediate reexpansion of skin margins; wound edges retreat about three-fourths of the distance over which they had moved. These experiments suggest that the motivating force for contraction lies within wound granulation tissue rather than in the wound margin.

Completely different results were obtained when these experiments were repeated on guinea pigs. When the central granulation tissue was excised on the seventh day after wounding, no change in wound size was found and no effect on the rate or extent of contraction was observed. Furthermore, repeated excision of central granulations every three days did not alter the size of the wound or affect the inward movement of wound margins. In these experiments, the line of incision for removing granulations was placed about 0.5 to 1.0 mm. inside the wound margin. If the incision was made right at the wound margin, however, equivocal results were obtained. In some animals contraction was delayed and in others no change occurred. No instance of wound enlargement was seen. If, however, excision of the granulation tissue was done so that 0.5 mm. of skin margin was included, immediate reverse movement of the wound edges was seen and the wound regained its original size. The same result was obtained when just the wound margin, the "picture frame" area, was excised, with central granulations left intact.

At this stage of the argument the weight of evidence appeared to be in favor of the "picture frame" theory. The case was strengthened by an ingenious experiment. Moderate doses (750 r) of x-ray delivered to wound contents and wound margin between 24 and 48 hours after wounding were found to retard contraction. Although closure by contraction ultimately occurred, there was a considerable delay in initiation of contraction. It had been shown that fibroblasts, as well as other cells, were most sensitive to effects of irradiation at the time of cell division. These observations suggest that the effect of these moderate doses of x-ray on wound contraction was to halt, temporarily, proliferation of fibroblasts.

This experiment had one difficulty; it was not possible, for technical reasons, to irradiate only central granulations or only the "picture frame" area. Thus, the observations did not settle the dispute between picture frame protagonists and central granulation defenders. The results did, however, support the concept of a cell-mediated phenomenon and suggested a local origin for fibroblasts concerned in repair.

Many observations have been made on biochemical constituents of the wound bed. Some of the observations are conflicting, but most of the difficulty can be traced to problems in sampling of tissue. It has been observed by several investigators that, in wound areas not covered by epithelium, formation of collagen fibers proceeds uninterrupted. However, as soon as the granulating area is covered by either migrating epithelium or contracting skin margin, further production of fibrous tissue slows or ceases; in fact, some resorption of collagen appears to occur. Thus, the original wound bed, when partially covered by advancing skin and viewed in cross-section, has the appearance of a truncated cone, with the major thickness of granulation tissue in the uncovered central portion.

Estimations of total collagen content of wound granulation tissue during the course of contraction indicate that it increases up to about the eighth to tenth day and then remains constant or falls. This does not necessarily mean that all collagen production has ceased, but there is evidence that, beneath the advancing skin edge, collagen fibers are being resorbed and remodeled and this may be proceeding at the same rate as, or faster than, new collagen formation in the exposed central portion of the wound.

The whole problem of collagen synthesis, absorption, and remodeling in wound healing is discussed thoroughly in Chapters 4 and 5 and will not be repeated here. However, it has been found that regardless of how much absorption and remodeling of collagen occurs in a wound, the extent of the original wound in skin can be estimated years later by careful microscopic examination. Collagen formed in response to the original injury does not assume the random pattern normally found in skin, but is denser and more oriented and can be found over the entire original base of the wound even though the movement of the wound margins has brought a covering of skin over much of the original defect.

If cell movement and cell contraction is responsible for centripetal movement of wound margins, the force of contraction should be within a range reasonable for a cell-mediated phenomenon. The force of contraction has been measured directly and was found to be of the order of 3.2×10^4 dynes per square centimeter. To make the measurement a square full-thickness wound was made in the skin of a rabbit. A "splint" was fashioned from clear rigid plastic strips, which were fixed to the skin with a glue immediately around the wound and joined each other at the corners. Thus, a frame was constructed around the wound which prevented, to a great extent, the centripetal movement of skin margins. The plastic strips forming the cranial and caudal sides of the frame were so prepared that on one a vertical plastic strip with a strain gauge could be fastened, and on the opposite member of the frame a vertical piece of steel tubing could be mounted. The two vertical limbs were connected by a steel tube. When the two lateral wound splints were removed, movement of the skin bent the flexible vertical strip and the force required to do this bending was measured by the strain gauge. No tension was detectable in four day old wounds, and tension in ten day old wounds was found to be about three times that in seven day wounds. If an incision was made across the wound through the center of the granulations and at right angles to the direction of tension measurement, the tension across the wound dropped to zero. The tension developed was found to correlate well with granulation tissue thickness but not with wound size or area.

Similar measurements have been made on cultured explants of chick frontal bone. When outgrowths of two adjacent explants meet and are mechanically detached from each other, they are immediately drawn toward each other. By direct measurement, the force exerted in this movement was found to be 3.4×10^4 dynes per square centimeter, a figure in good agreement with that found for the contracting wound.

It must be emphasized that there was a considerable spread in measurements, and technical problems in performing these experiments were considerable. However, sufficient repetitions were made and the data were treated statistically. The statistical parameters indicated that the differences observed were significant. Although the absolute force values may be in error, the striking agreement between the force of movement of an explanted cell mass and the force of wound contraction would appear to be more than fortuitous.

Although these measurements of the force of contraction appear to be consonant with a cell-mediated phenomenon, they do not tell us in what direction the force is acting. Information on this point can be gained from other experiments in which rectangular excised wounds are produced in rabbits and guinea pigs. Rectangular rigid plastic splints can be applied to skin around the wound margin, effectively preventing most of the contraction of wound edges. Removal of the splints after ten days results in an immediate rapid contraction of wound margins; half of the total contraction occurs within the first half hour and the amount of contraction at two hours is approximately equal to that of the unsplinted control wound. The central granulations show a marked bulging, indicating that contraction has also occurred within the wound contents.

If the granulations are incised just within the wound margins before removal of the splints, the central granulations immediately contract and bulge; on removal of the splints, the wound margins expand. This indicates that the force of contraction is derived from the wound bed. The rapid contraction observed on desplinting the wound margins could not be caused by migration of cells at the wound margins since the rate of movement is many times that ever observed for fibroblasts. The rapid movements are apparently due to preexisting tensions built up during the period of splinting.

These observations with splinted wounds appear to be most convincing as to the important role of central granulation tissue in causing and controlling the movement of skin margins during contraction. The observations of Grillo and his co-workers cannot be disregarded, however, and it is necessary to seek additional evidence to reconcile the "picture frame" hypothesis with effects exerted by the central granulations.

It has been observed that if the wound margin is undermined by incision of the horizontal plane between dermal and subdermal tissues, contraction ceases and, in fact, if this is done in a partially or fully contracted wound, rapid expansion of the wound to its original size occurs. These observations suggest that for contraction to occur there has to be an attachment between the movable skin margin and the underlying cell mass. These observations raised the question of whether contraction could occur if integrity of this cell population in the "picture frame" area were interrupted in the lateral direction. In other words, did this cell mass act as a "sphincter" through mutual cellular adhesion, and would contraction cease if this sphincter were cut? If multiple radially oriented incisions are made in the wound margin and repeated daily from day 5 onward, a significant reduction in the rate of contraction, as compared to control wounds, occurs. If portions of each lateral wound margin are excised, so as to leave a central peninsula of tissue with its original wound margin, contraction is even further reduced. On the other hand, if scar tissue in the fully contracted, and otherwise normal, wound is excised, the wound promptly retracts to its original dimensions and the wound again undergoes contraction. The rate of movement of skin edges in this secondary wound is not significantly different from that of the original primary wound.

These observations appeared to indicate that for wound contraction to proceed normally, the integrity of the cell mass immediately underlying the wound margin must be preserved. This provides powerful support for the "picture frame" hypothesis.

It now remains to consider another type of experiment designed to elucidate the mechanism of contraction. Several investigators have made experimental wounds in which an "island" of skin is left in the center of the wound. Initially, such an island decreases in size and its margins move away from the wound cavity. This would suggest that the initial force of contraction is directed toward the geographical center of the wound, the center of the island. This observed movement of edges of the skin island away from rapidly advancing outer wound margins is difficult to explain on the basis of the "picture frame" theory. Active cells beneath the margins of the skin island would be expected to behave in the same manner as those beneath outer wound margins if these cells were, in fact, the sole source of the moving force.

Later, the island was observed to expand and thin, and its edges eventually met advancing wound margins. The sequence of events is well illustrated in Figure 3–5. These observations are difficult to reconcile with any theories of wound contraction. However, careful histological studies of cellular events underneath the wound islands show that the wound cavity and its contents move toward the geographical center of the wound (center of the skin island) and undermine the edges of the island. Apparently this movement inhibits any tendency of the island to expand, and it is only late in the course of events that active movement of the margins of the island complete closure of the wound.

With all these data from various kinds of experiments before us, it would seem possible to reconcile various hypotheses regarding the mechanism of wound contraction and put the phenomenon on a sound biological basis. It would appear that movement of wound margins cannot be due to contraction of fibrous components of granulation tissue for at least two reasons: first, the principal fibrous component, collagen, is not a contractile protein and exhibits shortening only upon denaturation which disrupts its crystalline structure. This can be brought about only by unphysiological conditions not compatible with normal wound healing. Second, wound contraction proceeds normally in the scorbutic animal, in which collagen production is markedly inhibited. Thus, we are left with cells in and around the wound as the probable responsible agents for skin movement.

Aside from various blood cells which perform a scavenger function in any wound, the main moving and multiplying cells are those of epithelium and fibroblasts. Since epithelization and wound contraction have been demonstrated to be independent of each other, it follows that movement of epithelial cells is not responsible for movement of the full thickness of skin over the wound cavity. This leaves the fibroblast as the cell involved.

Electron microscopic studies of fibroblasts in contracting wounds have revealed that these cells differ in appearance from fibroblasts found in most other locations. They have the appearance of both fibroblasts and smooth muscle cells. Furthermore, immunofluorescence

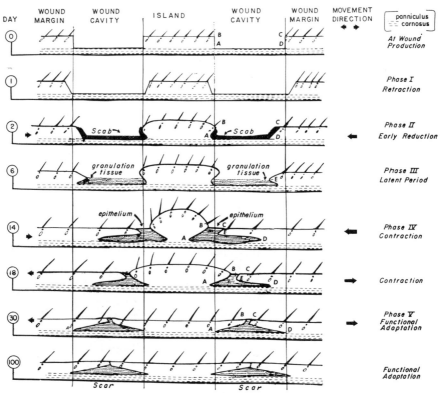

Figure 3–5. Schematic representation of closure of a full-thickness excisional wound with an island. Phase I: Retraction affects mainly the superficial portion. Phase II: Wound cavity with wound margins moves centripetally, undermining the island. Phase III: No gross movements occur; histologically, marked regeneration occurs. Phase IV: Composite centripetal movement occurs, consisting of a sliding of wound margins over the regenerate and a shift of wound cavity and its contents, further undermining the island. This causes the island to bulge above the surface of surrounding skin and move away from cavity. Day 18. During the latter part there is a rapid expansion of the island. Phase V: Day 30. Composite centrifugal movement occurs, consisting of a sliding of the approximated corium over the regenerate and a shift of the base of the wound cavity back to its original position. Day 100. Superficial location of the original wound is difficult to detect. There is an appreciable amount of deep scar, equal in width to the originally produced wound cavity. Hair follicles are spread apart. (Reproduced by permission from G. M. Luccioli, D. S. Kahn, and H. R. Robertson, Ann. Surg. *160*:1030, 1964.)

studies have shown that these cells, termed myofibroblasts, contain actin, a contractile protein. The syncytium of cells that develops in an open granulating wound are bound together by tight cell junctions or desmosomes in the same manner as in smooth muscle cells.

Careful examination of cells in the bed of a contracting wound reveals that not all are "myofibroblasts." There appears to be a spectrum of cell types ranging from those which could be classed as typical fibroblasts to those that are indistinguishable from smooth muscle cells.

However, a large population of the total cells present appear to have some evidence of contractile elements.

Of more importance is the pharmacological response of the tissue to smooth muscle stimulators and inhibitors. Serotonin (1×10^{-8} to 1×10^{-4} gram per milliliter) caused marked contraction of strips of granulation tissue. Prostaglandin $F_1\alpha$, promethazine hydrochloride, diphenhydramine hydrochloride, and morphine sulfate were also effective in causing contraction. Papaverine and prostaglandin E_1 caused relaxation of granulation tissue strips.

Experiments in rabbits with excised wounds showed that topically applied thiphenamid, a locally effective inhibitor of smooth muscle contraction, completely prevented wound contraction for as long as it was applied. After cessation of applications, the wound proceeded to contract normally. Thus, in effect, a chemical "splint" had been provided.

These contractile elements also appear to be concerned with cell locomotion. They are found in the "ruffled membrane" which forms on the leading edge of a motile fibroblast. The ruffled membrane attaches to the underlying substrate and, by contraction, the cell is pulled along. Cell migration can be inhibited by smooth muscle antagonists.

Discordant results have been obtained by different investigators who have excised central granulations in an actively contracting wound. Some report that wound margins retreat immediately to the position occupied at the start of wound closure. Others find no effect on wound margin movement. Resolution of these conflicting observations appears to lie in the extent of tissue removed. All agree that if the wound margin is detached or removed, the remaining wound margins will quickly retract, leaving a wound of the original size. Therefore, the cell population at, and under, the wound margin plays an important role in contraction. However, in order to move the skin margin, the cells must be attached to overlying dermis, just as they must have an attachment and exert tension on underlying fascia or panniculus carnosus of the wound bed. Destruction of either attachment would leave the normal tension existing in mobile skin, surrounding the wound, free to pull the skin margins back to their original position.

It has been demonstrated further that the syncytia of cells beneath the wound margin, as well as in central granulations, must be kept intact for maximal·movement of the wound margin. This seems reasonable when one considers that it must require mutual cooperation of a certain minimal number of cells before their combined force can overcome the elastic tension of skin. This is analogous to a team of horses being required to move a load that one horse cannot budge.

It seems possible to combine all these observations on wound contraction into a coherent theory on this subject. We can discard the notion that collagen fibers have anything to do with the phenomenon. They do not contract, and wound contraction proceeds without alteration in the presence of scurvy.

All the evidence points to contraction as a cell-mediated phenomenon. In the contracting wound the discovery of fibroblasts with characteristics of contractile cells provides us with the basic tool for understanding the event. The demonstration that contraction can be inhibited completely by local application of smooth muscle antagonists is very persuasive in the argument that the cause of contraction lies in cells of the wound bed.

However, no matter how cells contract or what the stimulus to contraction is, there must be some sort of attachment of the contracting mechanism to the wound edge, and there must be some mechanism for transmitting the contracting force between individual cells and between cells and wound margins.

Observations on contractile cells in the wound bed reveal that they have interconnections or desmosomes similar to those in smooth muscle. Furthermore, they have adherent processes tethering them to the underlying substratum and probably to structures overlying them at wound edges. Thus there exists the mechanical apparatus for exertion and transmission of the contractile force.

The question that remains is: Why do these cells contract? What is the stimulus that causes contraction? This is an area where knowledge is lacking. The easiest explanation is that the stimulus comes from exposure to a hostile environment, such as air. However, this cannot be the complete answer because in certain granulomatous or fibrous diseases characterized by contraction (i.e., Dupuytren's contracture and ischemic contracture of the intrinsic muscles of the hand), contractile fibroblasts are present but are not exposed to the same type of environment as cells in an open wound. Furthermore, myofibroblasts are ubiquitous and are found in many sites other than in open granulating wounds. Thus, although we have a much better understanding of the mechanism of wound contraction than we had in 1970, we still have much to learn. Fortunately, observations on the nature of the contractile fibroblast and its pharmacological behavior suggest that we may be able to exert some control over the process.

In experiments involving incision of granulation tissue at the wound margin, the reason why wound edges retracted is that the attachment of centrally located myofibroblasts to those adhering to the wound edge was disrupted. Thus, contraction of the central mass of myofibroblasts could exert no force on the wound edge. Unless skin tension was exceedingly low, the remaining myofibroblasts attached to the skin edge would not have sufficient contractile force to overcome the opposing skin tension.

FACTORS AFFECTING WOUND CONTRACTION

Having now developed a rational explanation of the mechanism of wound contraction, we can consider certain practical problems associated with this event. It becomes axiomatic that any substance, or procedure, that will interfere with fibroblast mobilization, migration, contraction, adhesion, or multiplication will inhibit wound contraction. On the other hand, diseases and noxious agents that do not interfere with fibroblast function in the healing wound will have little or no effect on the movement of skin margins in closing of a skin defect. As an example, scurvy, while affecting many aspects of wound healing, does not inhibit wound contraction, even though the fibroblast cannot perform its synthetic functions in the absence of vitamin C. Its mobilization, migration, multiplication, and contraction are not interfered with by vitamin C deficiency.

Cortisone has been shown to delay development of granulation tissue, depress proliferation of capillaries, and retard wound contraction. For instance, 10 mg. of cortisone administered daily to rabbits weighing 2 to 4 kg. retarded the rate of wound contraction by 50 per cent. Although this is admittedly a large dose, the possible adverse effects of smaller doses on wound healing should be kept in mind. Cortisone and related steroids, when given in large doses, suppress fibroblast proliferation. In animal experiments which demonstrated an inhibitory effect of cortisone on wound contraction, the dose was excessive. Smaller doses have been reported to be without effect on the fibroblast, and with these doses the expected wound contraction proceeded normally.

Cellular poisons, such as cyanide and dinitrophenol, have also been shown to inhibit movement of wound edges. In the case of dinitrophenol, the inhibiting dose was nonlethal. Likewise, drugs which are not lethal to cells, but which inhibit smooth muscle contraction, also inhibit wound contraction.

The influence of dressings on wound contraction seems to be largely mechanical. An adherent dressing, such as untreated gauze, will delay, but not prevent, contraction since it will act as a relatively inefficient splint. It has been reported that Vaseline gauze, or newer "nonadherent" dressings, if not taped close to the wound margins, do not appear to influence the rate or extent of contraction.

Notwithstanding the observation that some dressings do not affect contraction, it should be noted that their action appears to be related to the time, after wounding, when applied. If a synthetic film such as nylon or cellophane is applied to a wound surface during the lag phase, before active contraction has started, inhibition of contraction will be observed. Likewise, epithelization and fibroblast invasion are prevented.

The effect of skin grafts on contracting wounds has received considerable attention. It has been observed that if a full-thickness skin graft is applied to an excised wound before wound contraction commences, contraction is inhibited. However, if the graft is applied to a wound after contraction has started, contraction will proceed for several days before it is inhibited. The inhibition appears to be a mechanical blocking rather than an effect on the contraction mechanism. Split-thickness skin grafts have been reported to be ineffective in preventing wound contraction.

In an ingenious set of experiments, the effect of epithelization, splinting, and skin grafting on wound contraction in rabbits was studied. Two full-thickness wounds were made on the backs of animals. Both wounds were splinted so that contraction could not occur. One wound was allowed to epithelize while newly migrated epithelium was removed daily from the other wound. When the first wound was completely epithelized, splints were removed from both wounds and rate and extent of contraction measured. There was no difference in contraction of the two wounds. Thus, epithelization has no effect on wound contraction. This experiment also demonstrated that splinting of wounds for two weeks had no effect on the subsequent rate or extent of contraction.

In a second experiment, one wound was covered with a split-thickness skin graft and the other wound was left open. The presence of the graft minimally inhibited contraction, but by 31 days the grafted wound had lost up to 80 per cent of its original area.

In a third experiment, one set of wounds was grafted immediately and splinted. The control wounds were grafted but not splinted. Splints were removed after 14 days. At 31 days the splinted and grafted wounds had lost less than 20 per cent of their original area while the control wounds lost about 80 per cent of theirs. Thus grafting and splinting do have a marked effect on the contraction mechanism. It was also found that grafting and splinting for only seven days produced as much inhibition of contraction as did splinting for 14 days.

In the final experiment, splints were applied at the time of wounding, but grafting was delayed until the seventh day. The splints remained in place for 14 days and then were removed. At 31 days, the wounds had contracted to less than 30 per cent of their original area. Thus splinting and delayed grafting are ineffective in preventing contraction.

The question left unanswered is: What happens during the first seven days after wounding that cannot be inhibited by the combination of splinting and delayed grafting but only by splinting and immediate grafting? Whatever it is, it would appear that some interaction between graft and wound bed is possible during the first seven days, but after that time, even though contraction is prevented by splinting, events in the wound bed have proceeded to a point where such interactions do not occur or are ineffective. This is a subject for further investigation.

The practical lesson to be learned from these experiments is that wound contraction can be largely prevented if open wounds are grafted immediately and splinted for a week or more. Delayed grafting, even with splinting, will not prevent contraction.

WOUND CONTRACTION IN THE HUMAN

It has been pointed out that wound contraction can be both beneficial and detrimental, depending upon anatomical circumstances. Where the skin is highly mobile, wound contraction leads to closure with minimal scarring and no deformity. Where skin is attached to underlying structures, contraction cannot occur, but tension exists, cicatrization occurs, and eventual contractures with distortion and possible functional impairment are the end result. The skill of the surgeon in treating excised wounds lies in making use of contraction in appropriate locations and preventing it in others.

It must be emphasized that in man all the elements of the mechanism for wound contraction are present. The decision as to whether to allow a wound to close by contraction must be based on a sound knowledge of its mechanism and the anatomical factors that exist at the site

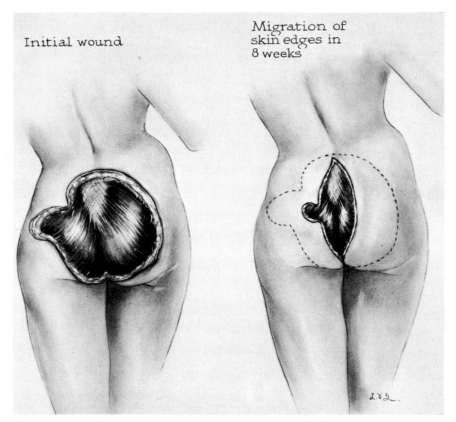

Figure 3–6.   Healing by contraction and intussusceptive growth. The patient was run over by a bus with traumatic loss of all of the skin of both buttocks. At eight weeks the wound has been reduced to 50 per cent of its original size by contraction. (Reproduced by permission from J. E. Dunphy, in *Repair and Regeneration,* edited by J. E. Dunphy and W. Van Winkle, Jr., New York, McGraw-Hill Book Co., 1969.)

of the wound. It must be remembered that stretched skin which has moved over an integumental defect is not of the quality of the original skin, owing to the "filling-in" by collagen and the lack of multiplication of normal skin structures. Nevertheless, this covering is vastly superior to a wide fibrous scar covered with a few layers of migrated epithelial cells. In man, contraction is most marked over the back, the back of the neck, buttocks, and abdomen. It is extremely limited over extremities and over the anterior chest wall and does not occur at all in circumferential wounds of the extremities. Thus, small full-thickness wounds of the back, back of the neck, buttocks, and abdomen can be allowed to close by contraction with assurance that scarring and deformity will be minimal.

Some distortion as a result of contraction is inevitable. As was pointed out earlier, skin elasticity and mobility are not the same in all directions. Thus, all edges of a wound will not move to the same extent or at the same rate. Similarly, the tensions developed in surrounding skin will not be the same in every direction. This becomes particularly apparent if a defect is produced in skin overlying the flexor aspect of a joint. Skin is more mobile and elastic in the direction of flexion and extension than at right angles to it. Thus, the major skin movement in closing a defect over a joint will be in the direction of flexion. This results in greater tension in this direction and the end result is a "flexion contracture."

In burn wounds contraction is delayed, and it is frequently poor and incomplete. The reason for delay is probably thermal damage to local fibroblasts near the visible burn. This would prevent their mobilization and migration. Nevertheless, burn wounds are characterized by extensive fibrous tissue production, and undoubtedly the first fibroblasts come from deeper, undamaged layers of tissue rather than from underneath wound margins. Until moving cells adhere to the wound margin in sufficient numbers, inward movement of the margin will not occur.

Excessive fibrous tissue production in a burn wound can also act as a mechanical barrier to closure by wound contraction. As this fibrous scar undergoes remodeling, as will be described in detail in Chapter 4, contracture with all its undesirable consequences will ensue. The handling of such problems is discussed in detail in Chapter 7.

The tendency to contraction which exists in mobile skin can be put to use in designing surgical incisions in these areas. It has been shown that contraction occurs mostly in the plane perpendicular to Langer's lines. Thus, an incision made at right angles to Langer's lines tends to shorten the resultant scar, but the edges, if not properly sutured, may gape. On the other hand, incisions made along Langer's lines tend to close quickly and place little or no tension on skin sutures.

Langer's lines are lines of tension in skin. On the back and flanks of the guinea pig, these run nearly circumferentially. As was discussed earlier, a square full-thickness wound on the back or flank of a guinea pig will show the greatest contraction in an anterior-posterior direction. This principle is illustrated in vivid fashion by the following experiment. In one set of guinea pigs a rectangular piece of skin with the long axis in the anterior-posterior direction is excised. In another set of guinea pigs a rectangle of similar size, but with the long axis running circumferentially, is made by removal of skin. In the first set of animals wound contraction converts the defect into a linear scar, but the direction of the scar is at right angles to the direction of the original wound. Although the scar is short, it is wide, and contraction is not complete. On the other hand, the defect that was oriented circumferentially closes rapidly and completely and a long linear scar, oriented in the same direction as the original defect, is the end result.

These experiments illustrate that the scar resulting from unimpeded wound contraction is markedly influenced by the differences in surrounding skin tension. It follows, then, that the pull on a sutured incision will be subject to the same tensions; the best closure can be made with incisions oriented so that tension on the edges is minimal.

Three important observations can be made by the surgeon relating to the probable outcome of a wound closure, whether it be made by the natural process of contraction or by mechanical closure with sutures. All that is needed is a pair of tissue forceps and a sensitive and gentle hand. By grasping opposite wound edges and gently pulling them together, the observant surgeon can judge:

1. Whether it is possible for the wound to close by contraction.
2. What distortion may be introduced by such closure.
3. How to revise a wound that is to be closed by sutures so that the best functional and cosmetic result is obtained.

Finally, the surgeon called on to treat large excised wounds should always be conscious of the consequences of allowing natural processes of repair to heal a wound. Scar tissue covered by a thin layer of poorly attached epithelium is a poor substitute for normal skin. Contraction will cover some wounds with a more functional, albeit somewhat defective, skin. However, mechanical tensions develop in the surrounding tissues and the consequences of such mechanical forces must be tested and evaluated before wound contraction is allowed to occur. If contraction is to be prevented, immediate skin grafting and splinting must be performed. If infection or some other contraindication to grafting is present, it may be necessary to remove the central granulations which contain the contracting mechanism when the time comes to graft the defect. However, optimal functional and cosmetic results will not always be obtained.

SUGGESTED READING

Abercrombie, M., Flint, M. H., and James, D. W. Collagen Formation and Wound Contraction during Repair of Small Excised Wounds in the Skin of Rats. J. Embryol. Exp. Morph. 2:264, 1954.

Billingham, R. E., and Medawar, P. B. Contracture and Intussusceptive Growth in Healing of Extensive Wounds in Mammalian Skin. J. Anat. *89*:114, 1955.

Grillo, H. C., and Gross, J. Studies in Wound Healing. III. Contraction in Vitamin C Deficiency. Proc. Soc. Exp. Biol. Med. *101*:268, 1959.

Higton, D. I. R., and James, D. W. The Force of Contraction of Full-Thickness Wounds of Rabbit Skin. Brit. J. Surg. *51*:462, 1964.

Higton, D. I. R., and James, D. W. The Effect of Potassium Cyanide on Wound Contraction. Studied in Vitro. Brit. J. Surg. *51*:689, 1964.

James, D. W., and Newcombe, J. F. Granulation Tissue Resorption during Free and Limited Contraction of Skin Wounds. J. Anat. *95*:247, 1961.

Madden, J. W., Carlson, E. E., and Hines, J. Presence of Modified Fibroblasts in Ischemic Contracture of the Intrinsic Musculature of the Hand. Surg. Gynec. Obstet. *140*:509, 1975.

Madden, J. W., Morton, D., Jr., and Peacock, E. E. Contraction of Experimental Wounds. I. Inhibiting Wound Contraction by Using a Topical Smooth Muscle Antagonist. Surgery *76*:1,8, 1974.

Montandon, D., Gabbiani, G., Ryan, G. B., and Majno, G. The Contractile Fibroblast. Its Relevance in Plastic Surgery. Plast. Reconstr. Surg. *52*:286, 1973.

Phillips, J. L., and Peacock, E. E. Importance of Horizontal Plane Cell Mass Integrity in Wound Contraction. Proc. Soc. Exp. Biol. Med. *117*:534, 1964.

Reynolds, B. L., Leveque, T. F., Codington, J. B., Mansberger, A. R., and Buxton, R. W. Wound Healing. II. Chemical Influence of Contraction and Migration of Regenerate. Amer. Surg. *25*:540, 1959.

Ryan, G. B., Cliff, W. J., Gabbiani, G., Iolé, C., Montandon, D., Statkov, P. R., and Majno, G. Myofibroblasts in Human Granulation Tissue. Hum. Path. *5*:55, 1974.

Ryan, G. B., Cliff, W. J., Gabbiani, G., Iolé, C., Statkov, P. R., and Majno, G. Myofibroblasts in an Avascular Fibrous Tissue. Lab. Invest. *29*:197, 1973.

Stone, P., and Madden, J. W. Effect of Primary and Delayed Split Skin Grafting on Wound Contraction. Surg. Forum *25*:41, 1974.

Straile, W. E. The Composition of Mammalian Skin Expanding Near Contracting Wounds. J. Exp. Zool. *142*:405, 1960.

Zahir, M. Contraction of Wounds. Brit. J. Surg. *51*:456, 1964.

Chapter 4

STRUCTURE, SYNTHESIS, AND INTERACTION OF FIBROUS PROTEIN AND MATRIX

In the mammal, repair occurs primarily by fibrous tissue proliferation rather than by regeneration of the original anatomical structures. Epithelial regeneration is an exception to this rule and has been discussed in an earlier chapter. Many tissues composed of a single cell type can regenerate. Some, such as nerve cells, are incapable of multiplication in the adult and do not regenerate. Others, such as endothelium and some glandular tissues, can regenerate after injury. However, most compound tissues or organs do not regenerate and are repaired by fibrous connective tissue deposition. Fibrous connective tissue is the single most prevalent tissue in the body and, in a variety of forms such as bone, tendon, cartilage, and fascia, it gives form and structural rigidity to the body. It is not surprising, therefore, that nature in seeking to repair damaged tissue, does so by replacing it with the strong and versatile connective tissue.

The principal components of connective tissue are three fibrous proteins—collagen, reticulin, and elastin—and ground substance composed of mucopolysaccharides, mucoproteins, and glycoproteins. The mechanical properties of connective tissue and of repair tissue, in par-

81

ticular, are due primarily to fibrous proteins; of these, collagen is the principal component. It is estimated that as much as 25 per cent of total body protein is accounted for by collagen. In repair tissue this proportion may be in excess of 50 per cent.

Healing by fibrous tissue replacement can be both beneficial and harmful, depending on the location of the injury and the tissue being replaced. In bone repair, for instance, deposition of a collagen matrix and its subsequent calcification restore the original structure and return the original function. Repair of damaged peripheral nerves by fibrous tissue growth, on the other hand, can interfere with regeneration of axons and thus prevent restoration of function. Frequently, an overproduction of fibrous tissue may lead to functional impairment even though damaged tissue is adequately repaired. Such is often the case in tendon repair or in intra-abdominal healing where fibrous adhesions may be formed.

Control and guidance of the repair process so that optimal functional and cosmetic results may be obtained is the objective of most surgical procedures. Therefore an understanding of underlying biochemical synthetic processes leading to formation of fibrous proteins is essential for a rational approach to wound repair. In addition, knowledge of how the synthetic process may be interrupted and the consequences of such interference can provide surgeons with a powerful tool to use in the control of scar formation.

THE STRUCTURE OF COLLAGEN

Up until 1968, collagen was considered to be a single protein, although it had been recognized that some heterogeneity existed among collagens derived from various species and from various tissues within the same species. Such heterogeneities usually consisted of minor substitutions of one amino acid for another in a few places along the peptide chains of the molecule.

With improved methods of separation and extensive sequencing of the peptide chains of collagen it became apparent that collagens of different tissues exhibited more marked differences, and today at least four distinct types of collagen are recognized.

There are, however, certain fundamental characteristics of collagen that enable us to identify a protein as being a collagen, and that distinguish all types of collagens into a well defined class. These characteristics are:

1. The presence of three linear peptide chains of equal length in a right-handed helical configuration, the three chains being arranged parallel to each other, and the assembly being twisted into a left-handed "super helix."

2. The presence of glycine in every third position along the pep-

tide chain, so that the chains (referred to as α chains) consist of repeating triplets Gly-X-Y, where X and Y may be any amino acid.

3. The presence of the unique amino acids, hydroxyproline and hydroxylysine. Hydroxyproline and hydroxylysine occur only in the Y position of the tripeptide Gly-X-Y.

Originally most of the biochemical studies on collagen were per formed on skin or tendon. It was early recognized that collagen derived from these tissues contained two identical α chains and one which was different. This was demonstrated by chromatographic separation of α chains in denatured collagen. Denaturation destroys the helical conformation of the chains and allows them to separate in solution. Subsequent studies of the amino acid sequences in these chains revealed that although the chains were homolgous, there were sufficient differences in the distribution of acidic and basic residues to account for the chromatographic separation. The two identical chains were termed $\alpha1$, and the dissimilar chain was designated $\alpha2$.

In 1969, a second type of collagen was discovered. In examining collagen derived from chick cartilage, it was found that the ratio of $\alpha1$ chains to $\alpha2$ chains approached 10:1 rather than 2:1 as found in other tissues. Further examination of $\alpha1$ chains revealed that there were two types that differed from each other by alterations in amino acid sequence. It was deduced that the new type of collagen was composed of three identical α chains differing from $\alpha1$ chains from collagen of other tissues by substitutions of amino acids in various parts of the peptide chains. Thus, two types of $\alpha1$ chains were recognized: $\alpha1(I)$ which was present in skin, tendon, and cartilage; and $\alpha1(II)$, which was apparently associated only with cartilage. The two types of collagen were identified as type I with the formula $\alpha1(I)_2\alpha2$ and type II, with the formula $\alpha1(II)_3$. The major differences in amino acid composition between these two types of collagen are larger numbers of threonine, glutamic acid, methionine, leucine, and hydroxylysine residues and fewer numbers of lysine and alanine residues in type II than in type I collagen. The most important difference, of course, is the absence of an $\alpha2$ chain in type II collagen.

In 1971, studies on infant dermis revealed a collagen with an $\alpha1$ chain distinctly different from the two just described. This was termed $\alpha1(III)$. This α chain contains large amounts of hydroxyproline, alanine, valine, phenylalanine, and histidine and, in addition, has two residues of cysteine, an amino acid not found in the helical portions of $\alpha1(I)$, $\alpha1(II)$, or $\alpha2$. Type III collagen does not have an $\alpha2$ chain.

Type III collagen was subsequently found in the aorta, in some parts of the lung, and in skin. In the last organ, type III collagen is present in high concentrations in embryonic dermis and the amount diminishes after birth. Adult skin is predominantly type I, although type III can be found in small quantities. Type III collagen has also been found in uterine leiomyoma.

It has been known for some time that the principal component of basement membranes, Descemet's membrane, and the anterior lens capsule is a collagen-like protein. Purification of this protein revealed that it too was composed of three identical α chains. The presence of eight residues of cysteine, with its high hydroxylysine content and low alanine content, and of large amounts of covalently linked carbohydrate clearly distinguished it from other types of collagen. This has been termed type IV collagen.

In summary, four types of collagen have been identified that appear to be tissue specific. Type III collagen, though observed in some adult tissues, appears to be found in greatest amounts in embryonic tissue. Synthesis of these collagens is probably directed by different structural genes, and it is possible that with aging there is suppression of one or more genes and activation of others. It is also possible that additional types of collagen with tissue-specific properties may be found.

Primary Structure

We have already characterized some essential features of the primary structure of collagen, for example, the presence of glycine as every third residue and of the unique amino acids, hydroxyproline and hydroxylysine. Proline and hydroxyproline together account for approximately one-third of the amino acids present. Until the discovery of types III and IV collagens, it was thought that the absence of cysteine or cystine was also a distinguishing characteristic of collagen.

The three α chains making up the collagen molecule are of approximately equal length, about 1000 amino acids to a single peptide chain. The molecular weight of collagen is approximately 270,000 daltons, which puts it in the class of larger proteins.

Collagen is not a simple protein. It belongs to the category of glycoproteins since it contains varying amounts of galactose or galactosylglucose, covalently linked by O-galactosidic bonds to certain hydroxylysine residues. The precise function of these carbohydrate residues is not known, but some investigators have speculated that they are required for transport of monomeric collagen across the cell membrane after synthesis.

It has been shown that the carbohydrate linked to soft tissue collagens is primarily the disaccharide, galactosylglucose. In bone collagen, however, the monosaccharide, galactose, is the major component. Because in the metabolic degradation of collagen small hydroxylysine-containing peptides with glycosidic mono- or disaccharides are excreted in the urine, it is possible to tell whether soft tissue or bone collagen is being preferentially degraded by determining the ratio of monosaccharide to disaccharide in excreted peptides. A high excretion of monosaccharide as compared to disaccharide indicates catabolism of bone collagen.

As we indicated previously, one of the important differences between type I collagen and types III and IV collagens is the content of hydroxylysine. In types III and IV collagens there is considerably more hydroxylysine than in types I and II collagens. It is also found that types III and IV collagens have a much larger carbohydrate content.

One important difference between type III and type I collagens is the presence of cysteine in type III. In order to separate the individual chains of type III collagen, reduction is necessary prior to denaturation. This is evidence that the molecule is stabilized by one or more disulfide cross-links in addition to hydrogen bonding.

It was mentioned previously that individual peptide chains of the collagen molecule were twisted into a right-handed helix. This helical twist is a result of the presence of a large number of imino-acid residues, proline and hydroxyproline. Because one side of the five-sided ring structure of these imino acids constitutes part of the peptide backbone of the molecule, free rotation of the chain cannot occur at these sites and the backbone of the chain is bent at these points. The net result of the presence of these residues is that the chain of amino acids is forced into the helical configuration. However, there is a short sequence of amino acids (15 in the case of type I collagen) at the N-terminal portion of the molecule that does not contain any imino acids and does not have glycine as every third residue. This is known as the "telopeptide" region. This region is not helical, can be attacked by ordinary proteolytic enzymes, and is important in cross-linking, as we shall discuss later.

Secondary Structure

The three peptide chains of collagen must be held together in some fashion to make a molecule. We will discuss the means by which this is accomplished in the next section. However, we shall note here that when first assembled, the three chains are held together by relatively weak forces. The molecule thus formed, and before it has become polymerized into fibrils and fibers, is referred to as "tropocollagen." The term collagen usually refers to the polymeric aggregation of a number of tropocollagen units to form a long polymer chain.

As will be discussed in more detail later, covalent cross-links can form among the three chains. When two of the three chains are linked, the resulting combination is called a beta (β) form and the appropriate numbers are used to designate between which chains the bond occurs, i.e., $\beta11$ or $\beta12$. All three chains may become cross-linked, resulting in the gamma form or $\gamma112$.

It has been mentioned that certain of the different types of α

chains are homologous with each other or that parts of the chain are homologous with similar parts in another type of α chain. Homology means that usually one or a few amino acids differ between the chains, but that long sequences are identical. Such substitutions usually do not affect materially the distribution of polar and nonpolar residues in the overall α chain.

If the sequence of amino acids in one peptide is totally different from that in another, they are not homologous even though, in collagen, all peptides have glycine as every third residue. In comparing sequences in various regions of the peptide chains, use is made of the fact that cyanogen bromide (CB) will break the bond between the carboxyl group of methionine and the amino group of the amino acid to which it is linked. Since there are nine methionine residues in $\alpha1(I)$, for instance, treatment produces ten peptides of varying lengths depending upon the positions of methionine residues along the chain. The peptides may be separated and isolated by column chromatography. By convention, the peptides are numbered (CB1, CB2, and so forth) in the order in which they are eluted from the column. All but one peptide will have a carboxyl terminal homoserine group (methionine is converted to homoserine in the reaction with cyanogen bromide). This peptide, lacking homoserine, is located at the C-terminal position in the α chain. The order of the other peptides may be determined in various ways but one ingenious method involves renaturation of isolated peptides to form the triple-helix structure. Electron micrographs of these reconstituted peptide segments can be matched with regions in an electron micrograph of the normal total α chain. This is possible because an electron micrograph of collagen reveals an asymmetrical banding owing to grouping of polar and nonpolar amino acids along the chain. Matching the band pattern of a cyanogen bromide-derived segment with that of the whole molecule will enable one to show precisely from what region of the α chain the segment was derived.

Analysis of the sequence of amino acids in comparable segments from two α chains from different collagens will reveal whether or not these are homologous. Such matching has been done for some segments from different collagens. This reveals that type II collagen is homologous to the $\alpha1$ chain of type I collagen throughout the major portion of the chain. In the case of type III collagen, which has 12 methionine residues, thus yielding 13 fragments on treatment with cyanogen bromide, many of the peptides are homologous with the peptides derived from the $\alpha1$ chain of type I collagen, but several are distinctly different.

These major variations are reflected by differences in solubility, carbohydrate content, fiber size, organization, and so on. Thus it seems possible that during evolution, the type of collagen produced was adapted to the particular functional needs of the tissue or organ in which it was located.

It is very curious that there is a greater interspecies homology of collagens from the same tissue than among different tissues of the same species. In all but a few instances, the substitution of one amino acid for another in a particular position of homologous collagens involves only a single base pair in the DNA molecule. Rarely, two base pairs may be involved. In general, interspecies homology is of the order of 85 to 95 per cent, contrasting with other proteins, such as the hemoglobins, in which the homology is only 72 to 78 per cent.

Tertiary Structure

The spatial arrangement of three chains in the molecule also is unique to collagen. Other linear proteins exist as single helical coils or as flat pleated sheets. Some nonprotein molecules such as deoxyribonucleic acid (DNA), which has two chains, exist as two intertwined helical coils. Each of the collagen chains exists as a helical coil, and they are arranged parallel to each other. The α chains are right-handed helices, and the three helices are then twisted into a left-handed "super helix." This entire structure is held together by hydrogen bonds.

Hydrogen bonds are formed between a hydrogen atom and a strongly electronegative atom such as F, O, or N. In proteins, a hydrogen attached to an amino group or a hydroxyl group may form a bond with an adjacent oxygen derived from a carboxyl group. Hydrogen bonds are quite weak and can be broken by mild heat or by concentrated urea or guanidine solutions. When this happens, the helical structure of the molecule is destroyed and individual chains separate as randomly coiled structures. In the case of collagen, mild heating, which leads to hydrogen bond rupture, produces what is termed "denaturation"; parent gelatin is the resulting product.

Because of the triple helix structure and total number of amino acids, tropocollagen exists as a rigid rod-like molecule 3000 Å in length, 15 Å wide, and with a molecular weight of approximately 270,000. It is quite large as protein molecules go.

Quaternary Structure

Knowledge of the quaternary structure, the way tropocollagen is aggregated into a stable biological unit of great mechanical strength, is important to an understanding of the mechanical properties of connective tissue, particularly scars. When collagen fibrils stained with phosphotungstic acid are examined under the electron microscope, the fibrils appear striated; that is, alternate light and dark stripes of varying widths are present at right angles to the long axis of the fiber. These bands have a definite pattern which repeats at approximately 640 Å in-

HYDROGEN BONDING
AND
DENATURATION OF COLLAGEN

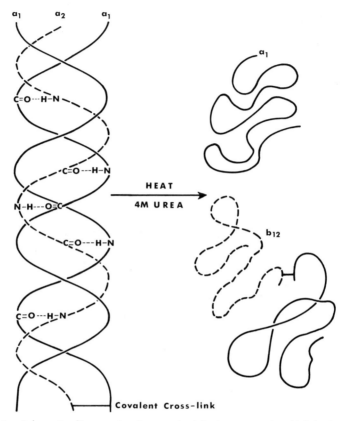

Figure 4–1. Schematic diagram showing, on the left, the manner in which hydrogen bonds form between α chains in the tropocollagen molecule, thus providing stability to the triple helical structure. Heat ($>60°$ C.), 4M urea, 2M potassium thiocyanate, or 5M guanidine hydrochloride will denature collagen. Denaturation involves collapse of the helical configuration and separation of individual α chains into random coil configuration. Note that the covalent intramolecular cross-link is unaffected and the two chains remain linked in the denatured state, as illustrated.

tervals. The band pattern is caused by selective binding of electron-dense dye to polar groups in the collagen molecule and appears as light bands. The dark bands are nonpolar regions. The band pattern is not symmetrical, and hence specific regions in the molecule can be identified.

For some time it was puzzling how to reconcile the 640 Å repeating sequence in the electron micrograph with the 3000 Å length of the tropocollagen molecule. However, by precipitation of collagen from solutions with highly charged substances, two other forms of collagen aggregates were identified by their electron microscope appearance; one form was called FLS (fibrous long spacing), and the other, SLS (segment long spacing). Although these curious forms of collagen are of only academic interest, they have elucidated the organization of the tropocollagen molecule in the mature fiber and, as we shall see later, have helped explain some aspects of maturation of scar tissue. On this basis, they deserve a brief description.

The FLS form of collagen appears as long fibrils under the electron microscope, but, instead of the 640 Å periodic banding seen in native collagen, it shows a repeating band pattern approximately 2800 Å in length. The SLS form, on the other hand, appears as short segments about 2800 to 3000 Å long with a characteristic asymmetrical band structure which permits one to distinguish each end of the segment. It

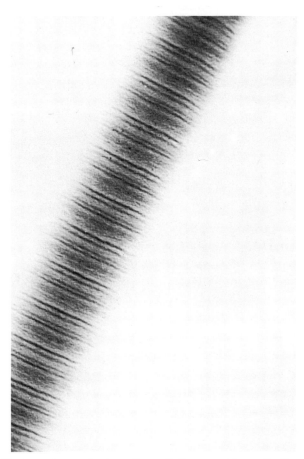

Figure 4–2.   Electron micrograph of a collagen fibril prepared by purification of steer tendon collagen. The repeating band pattern of 680 Å can be seen, and the finer band structure, corresponding to areas containing polar and nonpolar amino acid residues, is evident. Positive staining with uranyl acetate. × 154,000. (Electron micrograph by courtesy of Dr. Emil Borysko.)

has been shown that by simple manipulation of the solution environment, the SLS, FLS, and native forms of collagen can be interconverted.

A series of elegant experiments showed that the SLS form of collagen represents a later aggregation of tropocollagen molecules, all arranged so that similar ends are adjacent. The FLS form is brought about by end-to-end polymerization of tropocollagen molecules, but the molecules are arranged randomly. Finally, it was shown that the band pattern of native collagen could be reproduced if tropocollagen molecules were polymerized into chains in a head-to-tail arrangement with each adjacent chain overlapping the other by one-fourth its length.

Later, it was discovered that actually within a chain, the tail of one molecule overlaps the other by 10 per cent. Looking closely at this structure, one can see "holes" in the fibril between the head of one molecule and the tail of another in an adjacent chain. These "holes" appear

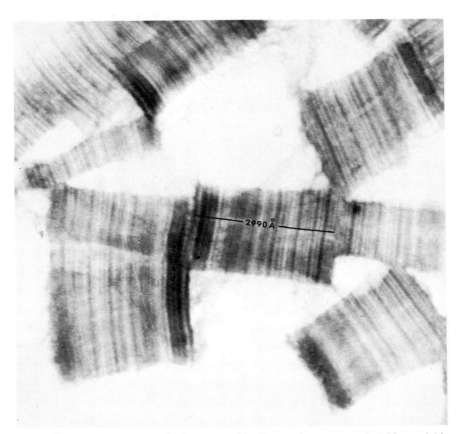

Figure 4–3.　Electron micrograph of SLS forms of collagen. These were produced from soluble collagen by precipitation with adenosine triphosphate. Each segment is approximately 2990 Å in length and the band pattern can be seen to be asymmetrical. (Electron micrograph by courtesy of Dr. Emil Borysko.)

TROPOCOLLAGEN AGGREGATION PATTERNS

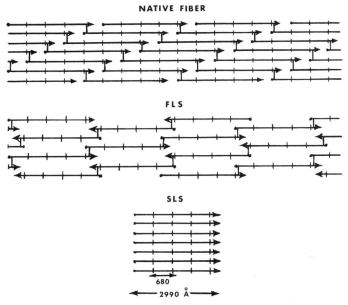

Figure 4–4. Schematic representation of principal forms of tropocollagen aggregation. The upper figure shows the quarter-stagger arrangement of tropocollagen molecules in the native fiber. Each molecule overlaps an adjacent one by 10 per cent of its length, and in the fiber there is a repetition of these overlaps every 680 Å. This gives rise to the characteristic 680 Å banding seen in electron micrographs of native collagen fibrils. Note also that because of the quarter-stagger arrangement and the 10 per cent overlap, "holes" appear between the ends of molecules. The intermolecular bond illustrated in Figure 4–19 is shown holding polymer chains together. If these bonds are in the Schiff-base form, they will be broken by acid and collagen will be solubilized (acid-soluble collagen). In the reduced form, the bonds resist acid attack and collagen remains insoluble.

The center figure represents the fibrous-long-spacing (FLS) form of collagen. The repeating band period in the electron micrograph is approximately 2700 Å. Note that the same intermolecular cross-links are present as in the native fiber. This form of collagen is produced by treatment of soluble collagen with a highly charged glycoprotein and subsequent dialysis. This changes the charge profile of the molecule so that the usual, native-type, aggregation is prevented.

The lower figure represents the segment-long-spacing (SLS) variety of collagen. Here tropocollagen molecules are aggregated side to side in parallel array. No fibers are formed, and no intermolecular cross-links are present. This form of collagen is produced by precipitation of soluble collagen with adenosine triphosphate.

real and are of importance, as we shall see when we discuss bone repair and calcification.

In the course of aggregation and, as we shall discuss later, during cross-linking, the solubility of collagen undergoes change. Tropocollagen is soluble in water. However, *in vivo*, tropocollagen probably exists only momentarily and most of it is rapidly aggregated into fibrils. Initially, the forces holding chains of tropocollagen molecules together are electrostatic; that is, the force of attraction of oppositely charged groups in adjacent tropocollagen molecules binds the monomers together. When so aggregated, collagen is no longer soluble in water but can be solubilized in neutral salt solutions such as 0.45M NaCl. Salt serves to neutralize the electrostatic forces holding molecules together and thus solubilizes them. As intermolecular cross-links form, collagen loses its salt solubility, but can be solubilized in dilute acid, such as 0.5M acetic acid. As will be discussed in a later section, the major intermolecular covalent cross-links that form are aldimines which hydrolyze in acid solution. As these aldimine bonds become reduced or substitutions occur across the double bond, collagen fibrils become completely insoluble, even in acid.

Models of Collagen Fibril

Anyone who looks at a flat, two-dimensional picture of the quarter-stagger array of tropocollagen polymers forming a collagen fibril does

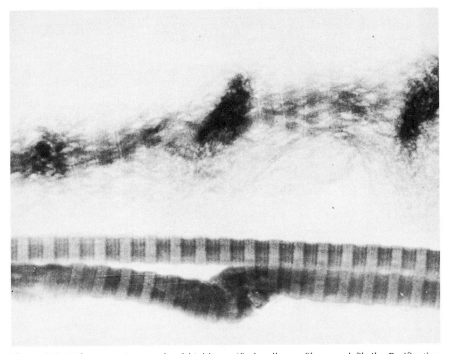

Figure 4–5. Electron micrograph of highly purified collagen fibers and fibrils. Purification was accomplished by treatment with crude alpha amylase. Fibers in the lower portion of the illustration show one fiber in the intact state and another being attacked by normal hydrochloric acid. In the upper portion of the illustration, a similar fiber has been unraveled by hydrochloric acid into its component protofibrils which may be identical to the "limiting" microfibril proposed in various models discussed in the text. Note that banding can be seen only where fibrils have maintained their spatial relationships and are close together. Negative staining with 1 per cent phosphotungstic acid in normal hydrochloric acid. × 260,000. (Reproduced by permission from F. S. Steven and D. S. Jackson, Biochem. J. *104*:534, 1967.)

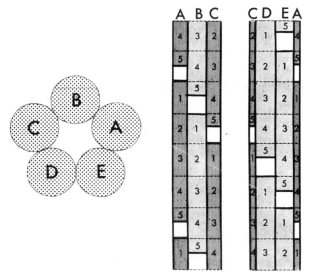

Figure 4–6. A proposed model for a collagen fibril. On the left is shown a cross-section of five tropocollagen molecules arranged in pentagonal fashion. On the right are shown two views in longitudinal array: the first as viewed from above, where molecules D and E are hidden; the other from below, where only partial visualization of molecules C and A is possible. For convenience, each tropocollagen molecule is subdivided into five sections, Nos. 1 to 4 showing the "quarters" and No. 5 indicating the "overlap" zone. Intermolecular bonds form between segments 1 and 5 where they are adjacent to each other. "Hole" zones are clearly indicated as white spaces. (Reproduced by permission from J. W. Smith, Nature *219*: 157, 1968.)

not immediately see one of the basic difficulties with this model. However, if one takes three match sticks and makes a mark on each, one-quarter of the length from the end, and lays them on a flat plane, it can be seen that this permits all three to be in the staggered array. However, if the match sticks are now arranged in a bundle so that each mutually touches the other two, one will find that two contacts out of three are quarter-stagger, but the third cannot be so arranged. When worked out mathematically for any number of chains, it develops that at a maximum only two-thirds of the chain contacts will be in the quarter-stagger array. Calculations based on electron microscope resolution and band density information predict that the band pattern will become apparent when a fibril reaches 70 Å in diameter if *all* contacts are in register, whereas the fibril will have to be 100Å in diameter before the pattern is visible if only two-thirds are in register. It has been shown that this is precisely the diameter at which the band pattern actually becomes visible under the best conditions in the electron microscope.

However, another model of the collagen fibril, based on physical chemical studies, suggests that the "limiting" microfibril may be composed of four or five polymer chains arranged (in cross-section) in a square or pentagonal arrangement where the contacts between individ-

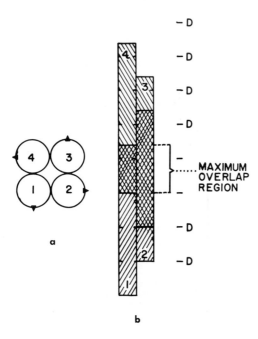

Figure 4–7. A unit fibril assembly according to the model of Veis et al. a, An end view of the tetrad unit indicating the proposed cubic packing of tropocollagen monomers and the relative rotational phasing of monomer units. b, A side-view projection along the long axis of a tetrad showing the quarter stagger (D) from the B-end region. (Reproduced by permission from A. Veis, A. R. Spector, and D. J. Carmichael, Clin. Orthop. 66:188, 1969.)

ual chains are more limited. It is envisioned that the microfibril is held together by covalent cross-links and the bundles of microfibrils are "cemented" together to form fibrils by protein polysaccharides or glycoproteins. It is possible that with high-resolution electron microscopy the true arrangement may be visualized in the future.

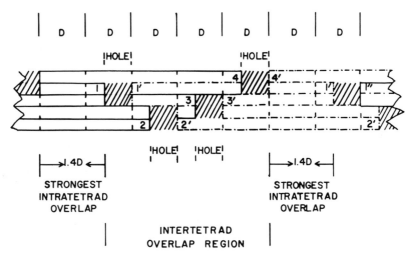

Figure 4–8. Assembly of unit fibrils into limiting microfibrils according to the model of Veis et al. A schematic view of the junction between tetrad units within a single limiting microfibril. "Hole" zones are clearly marked, as are regions of maximal overlap. (Reproduced by permission from A. Veis, A. R. Spector, and D. J. Carmichael, Clin. Orthop. 66:188, 1969.)

RANDOMIZED   COMPOSITE

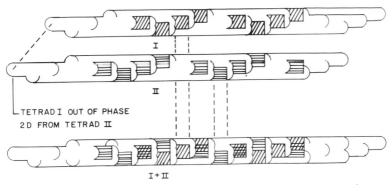

Figure 4–9. Assembly of two unit microfibrils, out of phase by 2D (D = 680Å, yielding a composite 1D repeat of "holes" over the entire structure. (Reproduced by permission from A. Veis, A. R. Spector, and D. J. Carmichael, Clin. Orthop. 66:188, 1969.)

As we shall discuss later in this chapter, fibrils increase in diameter by slow (sometimes rapid) accretion of polymer chains of tropocollagen, and probably by simultaneous addition and polymerization of tropocollagen monomer. If these polymer chains are arranged in a straight parallel array, each one is equivalent to every other one, with the exception of the outermost ones. Under such conditions there would be no limit to the diameter of a fibril—it could go on growing forever and attain enormous size provided building blocks were available.

This uninhibited growth of fibrils is not seen, however; each tissue and each species seems to have one or more characteristic fibril diameters. How does this happen? No one really knows the answer, but a

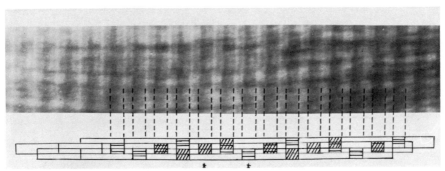

Figure 4–10. Relationship between a collagen fiber and a composite fiber assembled from two limiting microfibrils as in Figure 4–9. The two hole regions marked with an asterisk in the schematic drawing have one "filled" hole region in one of the limiting fibrils. A hole region appears in the fiber in each place in spite of this defect. The electron micrograph is of a collagen fiber from rat-tail tendon, stained negatively with uranyl acetate and phosphotungstic acid. (Reproduced by permission from A. Veis, A. R. Spector, and D. J. Carmichael, Clin. Orthop. 66:188, 1969.)

scheme has been suggested that appears to provide a simple and logical explanation.

Careful microscopic studies of collagen fibrils indicate that collagen chains may not lie in straight parallel array, but may be twisted into a helix. This arrangement can best be seen using the scanning electron microscope. It has been found that the location of bonding zones along the polymer chain requires a slight helical distortion of the chains to bring them adjacent to each other. As a fibril grows, each succeeding chain is distorted or twisted a bit more because of increasing surface of the fibril. This introduces a stress into the polymer and it requires force to maintain this stressed position. This force is provided by ionic or charge attraction between bonding sites in the tropocollagen chain. However, when the fibril reaches a certain size, the force necessary to distort the chain becomes greater than the bonding force and chains are no longer added. As one can readily appreciate, this model by itself would imply that all fibrils will eventually reach the same diameter. We know that this is not the case. It is likely that the interposition of mucopolysaccharide chains or protein-polysaccharide complexes, which we shall discuss a little later, can alter both binding sites and extent of strain necessary to conform to binding sites. Thus, ultimate fibril size may really be determined by components of ground substances.

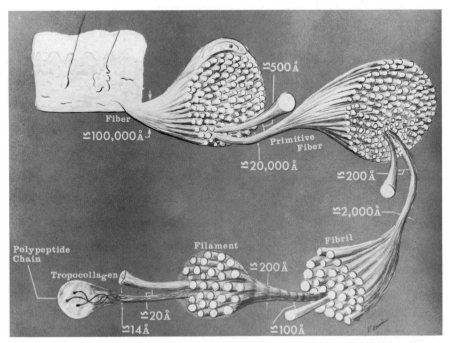

Figure 4–11. Schematic diagram of the assembly of components of a collagen fiber. (Reproduced by permission from W. M. Bryant, J. E. Greenwell, and P. M. Weeks, Surg. Gynec. Obstet. 126:27, 1968.)

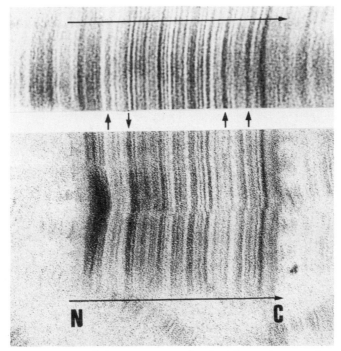

Figure 4–12. Comparison of electron micrographs of SLS forms of type I collagen (*top*) and type III collagen (*bottom*). Type III collagen was prepared from the 1.8M salt fraction of pepsin-solubilized aortic collagen. Major differences in band pattern are marked by arrows which point to the more heavily stained band. N and C indicate the amino-terminal and carboxy-terminal portions of the tropocollagen molecule. (Reproduced by permission from J. Rauterberg and D. B. Von Bassewitz, Z. Physiol. Chem. *356*:95, 1975.)

The hypothesis that ground substance may influence fiber size is well illustrated by the observation that in the cornea collagen fibrils are of small diameter and are arranged in a regular pattern. The principal mucopolysaccharide in cornea is keratosulfate. In skin, where dermatan sulfate exists in high concentration, the collagen fibrils are large and are arranged as a randomly oriented mesh. While such evidence is only circumstantial, it is, nevertheless, suggestive.

Almost all the studies on the tertiary and quaternary structure of collagen were done on type I collagen. The question arises as to whether other types of collagen differ in their higher organization. Type II collagen appears to differ least from type I collagen, even though it lacks an $\alpha2$ chain. It has been shown, however, that there is a high degree of homology between $\alpha1(I)$ and $\alpha2$ and between $\alpha1(I)$ and $\alpha1(II)$. Thus, for instance, one would not expect to find notable differences in electron micrographs of these collagens, but in fact it is extremely difficult to visualize a typical band pattern in electron micrographs of cartilage collagen, which is type II. The fibers are small and appear amorphous. Only occasionally can small areas with a distinctive band pattern be observed. This suggests that fibril organization of type

II collagen may be different from that of other types of collagen. However, only portions of the $\alpha1(III)$ and $\alpha1(IV)$ chains are homologous to the $\alpha1(I)$ chain. Thus one might expect differences in the electron micrograph appearances of these collagens, particularly if the distribution of charged groups in nonhomologous regions was different. This also has been found to be true. Comparison of electron micrographs of type I collagen with type III collagen shows significant differences in band pattern which permit ready recognition of the two types of collagen. The basic 690 Å spacing is not altered, however, suggesting that the polymeric organization of tropocollagen units is not altered.

We still do not know what alterations in fibril and fiber bundle aggregation result from differences among collagens. It is reasonable to presume that changes in numbers or positions of charged groups might influence fiber aggregation and fiber size. Future studies will probably throw more light on this subject.

Although we have now described the various levels of collagen structure, from the primary amino acid chain to molecular assembly of the fiber, there are certain other small but very important features of the structure to be discussed. These will be reserved until after we have seen how the body assembles this complex protein fiber from small building blocks, the amino acids, since it is by control of the synthetic process and manipulation of small additional structural features that the surgeon may be able to influence the ultimate results of the repair process.

SYNTHESIS OF TROPOCOLLAGEN

Fibroblast Origin and Function

It has been well established that the cell primarily responsible for the synthesis of collagen is the fibroblast. In cartilage and bone, the closely related cells (the chondroblast and the osteoblast, respectively) serve this function. Although it has been shown in tissue cultures that certain nonfibroblastic cells can produce collagen, there is no evidence that this happens in the body either as part of the normal growth process or as part of the repair process.

Although the fibroblast, osteoblast, and chondroblast are the principal cells involved in collagen synthesis, under certain circumstances non-mesothelial cells are capable of synthesizing collagen. During embryogenesis, the stroma of the cornea is produced by epithelial cells. Endothelial cells of the major arteries respond to injury by formation of collagen and this may be an important factor in the pathogenesis of atherosclerosis.

The fibroblast is a pleomorphic cell. In the resting, nonfunctional state, at which time it is usually called a fibrocyte, it has scanty cytoplasm and a deeply staining nucleus and may be of a varied shape. At times the cell wall seems to extend into and among various fibrillar elements of the connective tissue, like a reticulum. In the resting state it is frequently difficult to identify the fibroblast, but when it is called upon to perform its major function, collagen synthesis, it takes on a more characteristic appearance.

The active fibroblast is usually described as stellate or spindle-shaped. However, observations of living preparations have shown that it can assume almost any shape depending on circumstances. The electron microscope appearance is more characteristic. The nucleus is usually oval and slightly indented. The Golgi apparatus is located diffusely throughout the cytoplasm and mitochondria are large with irregular cristae. The most characteristic feature, however, is extensively developed dilated rough endoplasmic reticulum. This takes the form of long intercommunicating cisternae, which appear to be bounded by curved double rows of polysomes attached to ergastoplasmic membranes. These structures are important because they are the site of protein synthesis within the cell.

When a wound is made anywhere in the body, the first cells to be found in the area, other than locally damaged tissue cells, are those derived directly from the bloodstream. Usually the predominant cell in the early phases is the polymorphonuclear leukocyte. This is gradually replaced by small and large lymphocytes. Fibroblasts do not usually appear until about the third day, but thereafter their number increases rapidly.

In the chapter on wound contraction we have discussed the locomotor ability of the fibroblast. The problem we wish to consider here is where the fibroblast originates in wounded tissue, a matter of controversy for years that has only recently been definitively settled. The evidence indicates that the more primordial mesenchymal cells, some of which circulate in blood as large mononuclear cells and some of which are located in extravascular tissues, such as in fat, adventitia of blood vessels, and tendon sheaths, and are frequently described as undifferentiated mesenchymal cells, have the capacity to transform into fibroblasts. However, there is good evidence that the majority of fibroblasts seen in a healing wound are derived from local tissue mesenchymal cells, particularly those associated with blood vessel adventitia. These cells differentiate, move into the wound area, multiply, and start their synthetic activity. The sequence of events for any given cell is in just that order.

Recently very convincing evidence as to the origin of the fibroblast in wounds has been presented. Parabiotic rats were prepared. Both rats were given sufficient radiation to destroy the blood-forming organs, except that a leg of one rat was shielded. This rat provided all of the blood cells for both animals. The anastomosing flap between the two animals was clamped and tritiated thymidine was injected into the "pro-

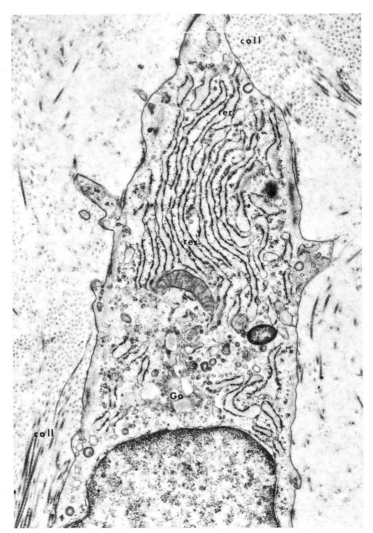

Figure 4–13.   Electron micrograph of a portion of a fibroblast. At the bottom is seen a portion of the nucleus. Immediately above is the Golgi complex *(Go)*. A crescent-shaped mitochondrion and numerous vesicles and vacuoles are also seen. The characteristic extensive and well developed rough endoplasmic reticulum *(rer)* with its dilated cisternae fills the upper part of the cell. Lying close to the cell wall, collagen fibrils *(coll)* can be seen in both longitudinal and cross-section. (Illustration by courtesy of Prof. Russell Ross, University of Washington.)

tected" rat. Simultaneously, wounds were made in both rats. Following disappearance of free labeled thymidine from the circulation in the injected rat, the clamp on the anastomosis was removed. Labeled blood cells appeared in the circulation of both rats. However, no labeled fibroblasts were detected in any of the wounds of the rat that did not receive the label directly, although fibroblast production, after the third day of wounding, was abundant.

The primary function of the fibroblast is to synthesize and lay down major components of connective tissue. There is good evidence for production of collagen and mucopolysaccharides by the fibroblast; in the case of elastin production, its role is less clear. However, the fibroblast is the only cell found in tissues predominantly elastic, such as ligamentum nuchae. Recently, electron microscopy of fibroblasts in wounds older than 28 days has shown the production of elastic tissue. Apparently in the older, negative reports the periods of observation were insufficient. Little is known, however, regarding the quality or organization of this elastic tissue in wound scars, and certainly scars are characteristically inelastic. Whether the fibroblast produces the protein component of the protein-polysaccharides, and also whether it synthesizes glycoprotein is, as yet, unanswered.

Less is known about the origin and biochemistry of the contractile fibroblast, the myofibroblast. This cell, when viewed with the electron microscope, has attributes of both smooth muscle cell and fibroblast. It has a wrinkled nuclear membrane similar to that seen in smooth muscle cells. The cytoplasm contains numerous microfilaments, mostly arranged in bundles and sprinkled with dense bodies, again similar to those seen in smooth muscle cells. On the other hand, large amounts of rough endoplasmic reticulum are seen and, in this respect, the cell has characteristics of a fibroblast. It has been demonstrated that the myofibroblast will produce collagen, but as we discussed in Chapter 2, it reacts pharmacologically as a smooth muscle cell. Myofibroblasts are also connected by various junctions and attach themselves firmly to the substrate on which they lie.

It is presumed that the myofibroblast arises from the same stem cell as the fibroblast. The intriguing question is: What determines whether a stem cell becomes a fibroblast or a myofibroblast? The fact that myofibroblasts are characteristically found in open granulating wounds whereas fibroblasts are found in closed incised wounds suggests that environmental factors, such as exposure to air, might be the determining factor. The observation that myofibroblasts are found in Dupuytren's contracture and in a number of induced granulomas argues against such a simple explanation, however. This is not an academic question since, if one knew what determined which path in differentiation the cell takes, one might be in a position to influence wound contraction and development of granulomatous lesions.

It has also been shown that smooth muscle cells may in some circumstances produce collagen. Thus fibroblasts and smooth muscle cells appear to be closely related insofar as their potential for biochemical activities are concerned. Whether smooth muscle cells can produce mucopolysaccharides and other components of ground substance is not known.

The functions of collagen production and mucopolysaccharide production are independent. Strains of fibroblasts have been grown in tissue culture that produce mucopolysaccharide but not collagen. Strangely enough, the reverse has not been observed. It should also be noted that, during the phase of proliferation, fibroblasts do not produce collagen or mucopolysaccharide. Probably the cell is too busy synthesizing its own structural components and enzyme systems to run also a building materials factory. The relation of energy requirements for mitosis and for function has been discussed in Chapter 2 in connection with epithelial cells. These requirements also must be met by fibroblasts. Cells other than the fibroblast have been shown to be capable of synthesizing collagen. Schwann cells of the nervous system, epithelial cells of the notochord, and epithelial cells in the developing cornea all have been shown to produce collagen.

Synthetic Pathway for Collagen

As with any protein, synthesis of collagen commences with the making of a "pattern" or "blueprint" within the nucleus of the cell. What triggers this mechanism is unknown, but there is some evidence that a metabolite, perhaps a diffusible, extracellular material, blocks a normally present repressor substance. This permits synthesis, within the cell nucleus, of certain ribonucleic acid (RNA) molecules, termed messenger RNA (m-RNA), from a template of DNA; these RNA molecules contain nucleotide sequences which are complementary to those in a portion of one strand of DNA. The m-RNA molecules are mobile, passing from the nucleus to the cytoplasm. They bear a "blueprint" for the synthesis of a particular protein, in this case collagen, consisting of a particular sequence of purine and pyrimidine nucleotides which specifies the amino acid sequence of protein. The m-RNA attaches itself to one or more ribosomes located around the border of the endoplasmic reticulum. The ribosome, which also contains an RNA and a protein, in some not yet understood manner translates the nucleotide sequence of the m-RNA into an amino acid sequence by selecting a specific transfer RNA (t-RNA, or sometimes called soluble RNA, s-RNA) with its attached amino acid corresponding to a sequence of nucleotides in the m-RNA. The t-RNA is believed to contain a critical nucleotide sequence, specifying just one particular amino acid, which it picks up from a cytoplasmic amino acid pool. The synthesis of the polypeptide chain on the ribosome begins at the amino terminal end and proceeds sequentially toward the carboxyl terminal end. On completion of the polypeptide chain, an event which is probably signaled by some special nucleotide sequence in the m-RNA, the protein is detached from the ribosome and enters the cisternae of the endoplasmic reticulum. It is now thought that the procollagen molecule passes from the cisternae of the endoplasmic reticulum to the Golgi apparatus. Here may be the site of glycosylation of hydroxylysine residues. From here it is reported to

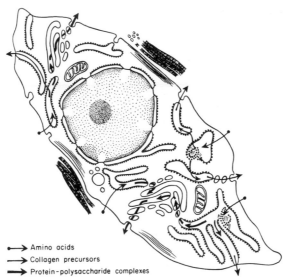

Figure 4–14. The cell in this figure represents an idealized diagram of a fibroblast. Two postulated pathways of amino acid incorporation into protein in this cell are shown by three types of arrows. The arrow attached to the black dot represents the entrance of amino acids, presumably through the cell membrane, to aggregates of ribosomes attached to the rough endoplasmic reticulum. These amino acids are picked up by specific transfer RNAs and are incorporated into growing peptide chains, attached to ribosomes, according to the coding sequence of messenger RNA which is also attached to ribosomes. Depending upon whether the finished proteins are collagen precursors or proteins to be complexed with polysaccharides, they may follow at least two different routes through the cell. It is suggested that collagen precursors are secreted directly from cisternae of the rough endoplasmic reticulum (*small black arrow*) either via direct, intermittent cisternal communications with the plasma membrane and release their material. It is proposed that proteins to be complexed as protein-polysaccharide are also sequestered in cisternae of the rough endoplasmic reticulum, but that these proteins separate by vesicle formation from the rough endoplasmic reticulum in regions adjacent to saccules and vesicles of the Golgi complex. These vesicles are presumed to merge with Golgi cisternae where their contents may be complexed with substances such as polysaccharide and are subsequently secreted from the cell, again by the process of vesicle formation, migration, and fusion with the plasma membrane. (Reproduced by permission from R. Ross, Biol. Rev. *43*:51, 1968.)

pass to the extracellular space at points where the external cell membrane is in close apposition to Golgi vesicles.

The preceding is a general and abbreviated statement of the intracellular course of protein synthesis. There are some special features of collagen synthesis that require closer examination, for an understanding of these is essential to an understanding of defective repair either due to disease or induced by chemicals. Furthermore, an understanding of those parts of the synthesis that are peculiar to collagen may suggest ways in which the repair process can be controlled and regulated by the surgeon.

The intracytoplasmic amino acid pool, from which various t-RNAs pick up specifically needed amino acids, is formed from two sources. The body can synthesize, from carbohydrate metabolites and ammonia, all but ten amino acids known to occur in proteins. These ten, known as the "essential" amino acids, must be derived from dietary intake. They are brought to synthesizing cell by the circulation, and diffuse into the cytoplasm.

We have mentioned previously that collagen contains two amino acids not found to any extent in other mammalian proteins: hydroxyproline and hydroxylysine. The question may naturally be asked: Where do these come from? Are these also "essential" amino acids required in the diet? Are they synthesized from proline and lysine and then incorporated into collagen? Or is the hydroxylation a process which occurs after formation of a polypeptide precursor?

Early in the 1940's it was determined, by the use of isotope tracer techniques, that hydroxyproline, when administered as such, is not incorporated into newly synthesized collagen. On the other hand, labeled proline appears in collagen as both proline and hydroxyproline. Later the same relationship was found for lysine and hydroxylysine. The question now was: Where does the hydroxylation occur: in the free amino acid pool, on the t-RNA, or after formation of the polypeptide chain?

To answer these questions, a number of investigators began examining certain aspects of ascorbic acid deficiency. It has long been known that the major manifestations of scurvy involve the connective tissue. It had been shown that lack of ascorbic acid in some way interferes with collagen synthesis, and because of marked decrease in strength of old wounds observed in severe scurvy, it was thought that ascorbic acid might be required to maintain collagen once it had been deposited in tissues in fiber form.

Early investigations on the effect of ascorbic acid depletion in embryonic tissue cultures led to the surprising finding that, in the absence of this vitamin, collagen production proceeded normally. In fact, addition of ascorbic acid to the growth medium did not change the rate until excessive amounts were added; then collagen production was inhibited. In stark contrast to this finding was the observation that injection of carrageenin into guinea pig subcutaneous tissue, or implantation of polyvinyl sponges subcutaneously in that species, produced in the normal animal copious deposition of new collagen, but in the scorbutic animal little or no identifiable collagen was produced. Similarly, guinea pig granuloma tissue slices or adult human dermal fibroblasts in tissue culture showed a marked inhibition of collagen production which could be corrected immediately by addition of ascorbic acid to the media.

The best explanation for the difference in behavior of embryonic and adult tissues with regard to the need for ascorbic acid rests on the observation that, in scorbutic animals, there is evidence of collagen formation, particularly replacement of tissue as a result of normal metabolic degradation. Inhibition of collagen synthesis seems to occur when there is a demand for rapid synthesis of connective tissue as in a healing wound. A dual mechanism has been postulated: one for normal growth and maintenance, not requiring ascorbic acid; and one for repair processes which are ascorbic acid-dependent.

Since collagen appears to be the main protein requiring ascorbic acid for its synthesis, it was only natural to hypothesize that ascorbic acid was in some way concerned with hydroxyproline and hydroxylysine synthesis, since it is in these two amino acids that collagen differs from all other proteins. Studies with radioactive proline suggested that this amino acid was incorporated into protein in scorbutic animals, but no tagged hydroxyproline was found. Other workers, however, found evidence that proline was not incorporated into a collagen precursor in ascorbic acid deficiency. Recent evidence suggests that in uncomplicated vitamin C deficiency, proline incorporation will occur, but the protein so formed will not be released from the cell unless the cell is destroyed.

The need for ascorbic acid in the hydroxylation of proline appears now to be well established. Various investigators have noticed large amounts of amorphous material accumulating around fibroblasts, in tissue culture or in artificially induced granulomas. It has been suggested that this material is a non-hydroxyproline-containing precursor of collagen. Analysis of the amorphous material did not, however, show an exceptionally high proline content, nor was the glycine content as large as would be expected for a collagen-type protein. We shall return to this question after considering some other facts with regard to proline and lysine hydroxylation.

If proline is hydroxylated before incorporation into the growing peptide chain, then one might expect to find a particular t-RNA-hydroxyproline in the fibroblast. Two possibilities appear to exist in this case. First, proline in the amino acid pool could be separated into two compartments. One compartment would contain proline destined for direct incorporation; the second would contain "activated" proline, possibly as prolyladenylate, which would then be hydroxylated and coupled to a specific t-RNA for incorporation into the collagen. The second possibility was that prolyl t-RNA was formed and subsequently part of this would be converted to hydroxyproline-t-RNA and incorporated into the protein. Both theories present some difficulties.

In the first theory, it is hard to visualize a process which would select part of the proline pool for hydroxylation. How would a specific t-RNA select hydroxyproline formed intracellularly rather than dietary or metabolic hydroxyproline from the circulation, since there is evidence that extracellular hydroxyproline can diffuse into the cell? The difficulty with the second theory is that t-RNA for proline and hydroxyproline would have the same base sequence, or code, and hence errors

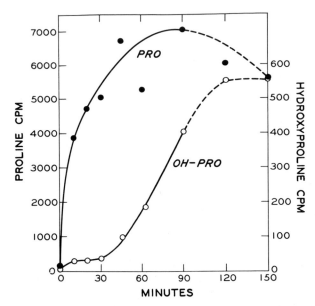

Figure 4–15. Time course of incorporation of ^{14}C-proline into protein-bound imino acids in the hot trichloroacetic acid-extractable, nondialyzable fraction of microsomes. The results are the average of two overlapping experiments. The dotted-line curves represent portions of the second experiment which have been extrapolated to coincide with values obtained for the first experiment since, although the two curves were parallel, absolute values differed by about one-half. The time lag in formation of hydroxyproline is clearly shown. (Reproduced by permission from B. Peterkofsky and S. Udenfriend, Biochem. Biophys. Res. Commun. *12*:257, 1963.)

could arise in incorporating the two amino acids. The finding that hydroxyproline occurs only in the third position in any sequence of Gly-X-Y, argues strongly against use of the same t-RNA for both proline and hydroxyproline.

Several laboratories tried to develop a cell-free synthetic system for collagen. The advantage of such a system is that known substances can be added or subtracted from such a mixture and their effect on synthesis can be measured. This was finally accomplished by using a purified microsomal fraction from chick embryo as an enzyme source and magnesium ion as a co-factor plus a number of other components. It was shown that this system could incorporate ^{14}C-proline into a peptide which proved to contain ^{14}C-hydroxyproline. There was a lag phase of 30 minutes from the time ^{14}C-proline began to be incorporated into the peptide before ^{14}C-hydroxyproline appeared. This observation was not consonant with hydroxylation of proline prior to incorporation into the peptide.

Puromycin will block the transfer of amino acids from t-RNA to ribosomal-bound peptide, by combining with the peptide and terminating synthesis. Puromycin added at the beginning of incubation completely inhibits both proline incorporation and hydroxyproline formation. However, if puromycin is added after incubation has proceeded for 30 minutes, there is no significant inhibition of hydroxyproline formation. Similarly, if ribonuclease, an enzyme which depolymerizes both t-RNA and m-RNA, is used at the start of incubation, no proline incorporation occurs, but when it is added after 30 minutes' incubation, little effect is seen and hydroxyproline is formed. All of this is strong evidence that hydroxylation occurs after formation of a proline-rich peptide.

It has been shown that molecular oxygen and not water is the source of the oxygen atom in the hydroxyl group. To a cell-free system for collagen synthesis ^{14}C-proline was added in the absence of oxygen. A second system was then obtained which contained polysomes, a hydroxylating enzyme, some dialyzable co-factors, and a peptide containing bound labeled proline. The co-factors were contained in an embryonic extract which could be heated without altering its activity; thus no additional enzymes were involved. The co-factors were removed and the system was studied with the addition of various known substances. It was found that Fe^{++} was necessary for hydroxylation. Neither puromycin nor ribonuclease inhibited hydroxylation, and it could be concluded that this was occurring on a ribosomal-bound peptide and that a specific hydroxyproline-t-RNA was not involved.

Subsequently, the hydroxylating enzyme, prolyl hydroxylase, was isolated and characterized. It appears to be localized in the endoplasmic reticulum. A similar but probably distinct enzyme, also found in the same location, is responsible for hydroxylation of certain lysine residues. This enzyme is known as lysyl hydroxylase and requires the same co-factors and conditions as prolyl hydroxylase.

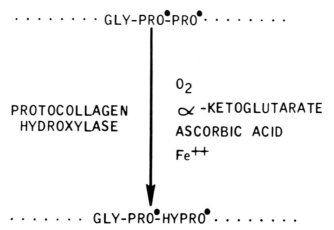

Figure 4–16. Schematic representation of mechanism of hydroxylation of proline in collagen. Only the proline in position 3 (glycine being in position 1) will be hydroxylated. The sequence Gly-X-Pro-Gly is apparently necessary for the enzyme. Also shown are the necessary co-factors and co-substrate.

Once a system for hydroxylation of proline was developed, it was necessary to define it more precisely. Not only was Fe^{++} needed, but an electron donor was required. Ascorbic acid could fulfill this function. Interestingly enough, ascorbic acid could be replaced by 2-amino-4-hydroxytetrahydrodimethylpteridine but the rate of collagen synthesis was diminished. This may be why, in the embryo and in normal tissue maintenance, ascorbic acid is not required, but in the demand for rapid collagen synthesis in wound healing, ascorbic acid is required. Another requirement for the hydroxylating system was α-ketoglutarate. Curiously, others had suggested that α-ketoglutarate was the precursor of proline in the cell.

Recent investigations have shown that ascorbic acid is probably not directly involved in the hydroxylating sequence. It has been demonstrated that prolyl hydroxylase exists in an inactive form. When activated, the inactive precursor aggregates into a trimer or tetramer and it is in this form that the enzyme becomes active. Apparently ascorbic acid is concerned with activation of prolyl hydroxylase and is more specifically concerned with catalyzing the aggregation process and perhaps maintaining the enzyme in the aggregated state.

α-Ketoglutarate is utilized in a 1:1 molar ratio when hydroxyproline is formed. By labeling experiments it has been shown that the ketoglutarate is converted to succinate and carbon dioxide. This conversion can be used as an assay technique for assay of the enzyme proline hydroxylase. Thus it would appear that α-ketoglutarate is a co-substrate in proline hydroxylation and not a co-factor for the enzyme.

The demonstration that molecular oxygen was used to oxidize both proline and α-ketoglutarate placed the enzyme prolyl hydroxylase in the class of dioxygenases. Several other enzymes belong to this newly discovered group. All require co-factors of molecular oxygen, ferrous iron, an α-keto acid, and a reducing agent, the most effective being ascorbic acid, and all are stimulated by catalase. Besides prolyl and lysyl hydroxylase, the enzyme γ-butyrobetain hydroxylase, oxygenases that catalyze oxygenation of thymine to 5-carboxyuracil and conversion of thymine riboside and deoxyuridine to uridine, and the enzyme p-hydroxyphenylpyruvic acid oxidase all belong to this class of dioxygenases.

α,α-Dipyridyl has been found to act similarly to anaerobiosis and prevent the hydroxylation reaction by forming a chelate with iron, thus removing a necessary co-factor. This fact has been made use of in attempts to isolate a non-hydroxyproline-containing collagen precursor. Impure material containing twice the normal ^{14}C-proline specific activity has been isolated from chick embryo slices after treatment with α,α-dipyridyl.

During the lag phase of 30 minutes before the start of hydroxylation, a peptide has been isolated from a cell-free synthesizing system which did not contain hydroxyproline. Because bacterial collagenase is specific for the linkage X-Gly-Pro-Y, this purified peptide has been treated with collagenase. Tripeptides containing glycine and proline have been isolated; this can be taken as evidence that, during the lag phase of synthesis, a proline-rich, hydroxyproline-deficient polypeptide is synthesized. Other evidence indicates that if such material is produced intracellularly by inhibition of hydroxylation with α,α-dipyridyl, the collagen precursor accumulates in the cell and is not found in the extracellular space. There is also evidence that the peptide must reach a certain minimal size before hydroxylation will take place.

It has been possible to separate the $\alpha1$ chains of collagen in pure form. In the N-terminal portion of the chain, there are six positions in which hydroxyproline is found. Two of these are sequences containing Gly-Pro-Hypro, two contain Gly-Glu-Hypro, and one each contains Gly-Leu-Hypro and Gly-Ala-Hypro. It has been found that the specific proline molecules in the third position in these peptides are not hydroxylated 100 per cent; that is, in the sequence Gly-Pro-Hypro, the

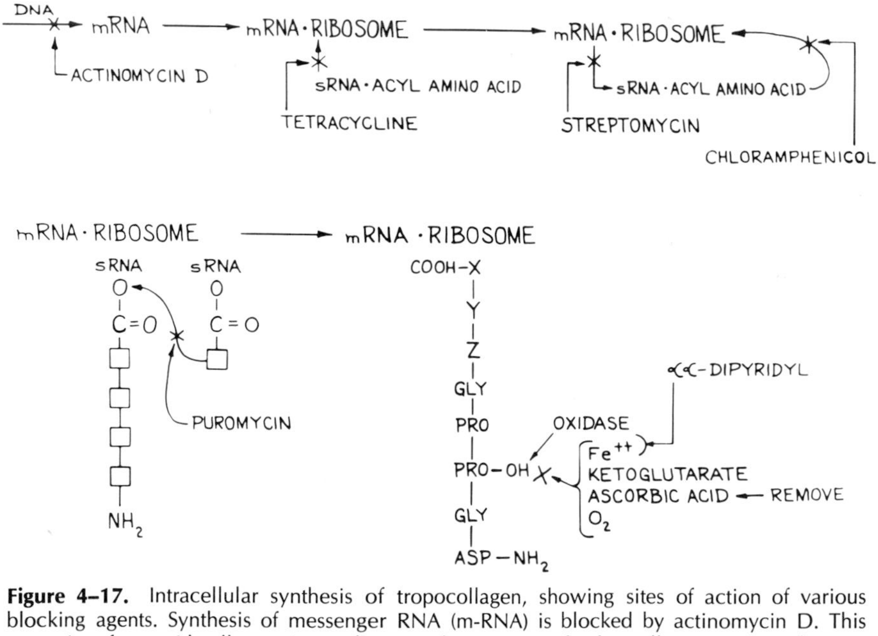

Figure 4–17. Intracellular synthesis of tropocollagen, showing sites of action of various blocking agents. Synthesis of messenger RNA (m-RNA) is blocked by actinomycin D. This agent interferes with all protein synthesis and is not specific for collagen. Tetracycline (in large concentrations) blocks the coupling of transfer RNA (s-RNA) with its attached acyl amino acid to the ribosome-m-RNA complex. Tetracycline is also a general inhibitor of protein synthesis and not specific for collagen. Streptomycin and chloramphenicol act somewhat similarly. Puromycin stops further formation of peptide chains on the ribosome by blocking the attachment of amino acids to the growing peptide chain. Again, this is nonspecific for collagen. α,α-Dipyridyl blocks the hydroxylation of proline by removing ferrous iron, a necessary cofactor for proline hydroxylase. Note that hydroxylation of proline occurs while the peptide is attached to the ribosome and that it requires the specific sequence Gly-X-Pro-Gly. The most common sequence that is hydroxylated is Gly-Pro-Pro-Gly, as shown in the diagram.

third amino acid will be Hypro 80 per cent of the time and Pro 20 per cent of the time. Furthermore, if one examines skin and tendon collagen, it is found that a given proline residue will be hydroxylated 80 per cent of the time in skin, but only 60 per cent of the time in tendon. The greatest difference between skin and tendon collagen has been noted in residues 43 and 46, where in skin these are 90 per cent Hypro and in tendon they are 80 per cent Pro. Until the entire primary structure of collagen is unraveled and the differences in occurrence of proline and hydroxyproline at particular sites are determined, the exact significance of these observations is not clear. However, it has been suggested that some proline molecules, because of the adjacent residues, are more readily hydroxylated than others. It is further suggested that when demand for collagen synthesis is high, many of these residues escape hydroxylation. This conceivably could explain some of the mechanical properties of scar tissue, particularly its lability and weakness.

It was mentioned earlier that type III and type IV collagens contain more hydroxyproline and hydroxylysine than types I and II collagen. This could be the result of either or both of two mechanisms. First, types III and IV collagen may have more sequences involving proline and lysine that are recognition sites for hydroxylating enzymes. At present the precise sequence for activation of these enzymes is not known. Second, the time for completion of the peptide chain on the ribosome may be prolonged, providing a greater opportunity for enzymatic conversion of proline and lysine to their respective hydroxylated derivatives. That time may be a factor is suggested by the observation that not all susceptible proline residues in type I collagen are always hydroxylated.

Another question of some interest is whether the three α chains of tropocollagen are synthesized simultaneously, or, if not, where they are assembled into the characteristic coiled coils. It has been shown, by sedimentation analysis, that a very large aggregate of ribosomes, termed a polysome, is involved in synthesis. If a single m-RNA was involved in the synthesis of one α chain, about 30 to 40 ribosomes would be required. However, the polysomes isolated were apparently composed of about 100 or more ribosomes. This would be consistent with simultaneous synthesis of the three α chains.

The observation that synthesis of tropocollagen is very rapid but that assembly of α chains into a triple helix configuration *in vitro* is very slow and usually incomplete led to the suggestion that α chains synthesized on ribosomes actually have an extension of their peptide chains which is not helical in character and which serves as "registration" peptides, thus facilitating assembly of the three α chains into the triple helix conformation. It was suggested that after assembly, "registration" peptides were hydrolyzed enzymatically, leaving a tropocollagen molecule. These predictions, made by P. T. Speakman, were shown to be true within a year after they were made. Collagens with nonhelical peptide extensions were isolated from fibroblast cultures. Subsequently such "elongated" collagens, termed "procollagen," were isolated from tissue culture. Almost simultaneously, examination of dermal collagen from skin of calves with dermatosparaxis revealed the presence of similar procollagen molecules. Dermatosparaxis is a recessive genetic disorder found in certain herds of Belgian cattle. The defect lies in failure to produce a specific proteolytic enzyme which cleaves the N-terminal nonhelical portion of the procollagen molecule, leaving native collagen. The disorder is characterized by extreme fragility of skin and, to a lesser extent, of other organs that depend on collagen for their structural stability. Microscopically, the collagen bundles are disorganized and the parallel packing of individual filaments within fibers is impaired. This disorganization of collagen filaments results in failure of intermolecular cross-links to form. As will be discussed later, intermolecular covalent cross-linking of collagen is necessary for strength of collagen fibers and makes collagen insoluble in neutral salt solutions.

Nonhelical extensions of the α chain are found at both N-terminal and C-terminal ends of the tropocollagen molecule. These nonhelical extensions contain less proline and less glycine than the helical portion of the peptide, and almost no hydroxyproline. They contain several residues of cysteine which apparently react with each other to form disulfide linkages in the C-terminal portion, thus binding and stabilizing adjacent pro-α chains. The pro-α peptides are acidic, having a higher content of serine and glutamic and aspartic acids than is found in tropocollagen.

The evidence suggests that these peptide extensions are, indeed, "registration" peptides and facilitate triple helix formation. They do, however, interfere with subsequent fibril aggregation to form collagen fibers.

A form of Ehlers-Danlos syndrome has been found to be associated with the continued presence of pro-α chains of collagen. Thus, failure to remove these peptides after assembly of the tropocollagen molecule can have serious consequences, not only in cattle, but also in man.

At least one and possibly more specific enzymes are required to cleave these terminal peptides. At the moment, it is unclear whether the identified procollagen peptidase removes terminal peptides in one stage or whether digestion of this portion of procollagen is accomplished in several sequential steps. Evidence now available suggests that the latter mechanism is correct.

COLLAGEN FIBRIL FORMATION

Site of Aggregation

Almost all microscopists who have described the fibroblast have mentioned the numerous intracytoplasmic filaments seen in the functioning cell. These appear to be heavily concentrated along cell margins. Frequently it is difficult to see a cell wall, and the filaments appear to be "extruded" into intercellular space. These filaments do not show the characteristic banding of collagen, but as has been pointed out, their diameters are always less than 80 to 100 Å, and the banding would not be visible until this width is exceeded. These intracytoplasmic fibrils have been found in cells not actively producing collagen. They do not stain as does collagen. The conclusion reached by most histochemists is that these are not collagen filaments, but perhaps represent polymerized mucopolysaccharides.

The careful work of several investigators has emphasized the possible importance of the cell surface in aggregation of tropocollagen. It has been suggested that the surface of the fibroblast may have a layer of mucopolysaccharide and that its charge and orientation direct the aggregation and orientation of the collagen polymer.

The very fine fibrils that are seen outside the cell, close to the cell surface, stain selectively with silver stains. Because they appeared different from the developing and larger collagen fibrils, they were thought to be of a different composition, although of fibroblastic origin. These argyrophilic fibers have been termed reticulin. This has led to considerable confusion, since fibers of basement membrane and certain other silver-staining structures have also been designated reticulin.

By chemical analysis, two groups of reticulins can now be distinguished: collagenous reticulins found in association with actively synthesizing fibroblasts and in basement membranes; and noncollagenous reticulins found in ovarian stroma and in the ciliary region of vitreous humor. The major distinction between the two forms is that the first group is digestible by collagenase, but not by trypsin, and the reverse is true for the second group. The staining reaction of reticulins appears to be due to associated carbohydrate or lipid components.

There is some evidence that a protein-polysaccharide complex stabilizes mature collagen fibers. Several workers have suggested that reticulin seen in newly forming connective tissue is in reality a combination of protein-polysaccharide around which tropocollagen molecules are aggregating in end-to-end and lateral array. Because of the proportionately higher ratio of polysaccharide to collagen, these fibers are argyrophilic, but as more collagen is bound to the growing fibril, it loses its ability to stain characteristically and takes up typically collagen stains. This is an attractive hypothesis which could explain many of the histological observations, but it awaits more definitive chemical proof.

Role of Ground Substance in Fiber Formation

Besides mucopolysaccharides, protein-polysaccharides, and glycoproteins, ground substance contains ions and considerable bound water. All of these may play a role in collagen aggregation, and there has been considerable speculation regarding this. Unfortunately, there is little solid evidence to support any of the theories.

There are seven substances which occur in various connective tissues of the body and that are classified as mucopolysaccharides. Heparin can also be included on the basis of composition, but it is not involved in the structural components of the body. Table 4–1 lists these substances, gives their composition, and also indicates their usual location in the body.

It is doubtful that polysaccharide moieties exist in appreciable concentrations by themselves. All of them, with the possible exception of hyaluronic acid, are covalently linked to a protein. Because of the close chemical similarity of various mucopolysaccharides, separation and analysis have been difficult problems. After the problem of separation had been solved, it was discovered that instead of being well defined chemical entities, each mucopolysaccharide was a heterogeneous mixture. The heterogeneity is manifest in three ways: individual chains of polysaccharide may have more than one type of disaccharide unit; the protein core may be heterogeneous; and there may be more than one kind of polysaccharide attached to protein. As examples of these types of heterogeneity, chondroitin sulfate protein regularly shows at least one keratosulfate chain also attached to protein. Similarly, dermatan sulfate, which characteristically contains iduronic acid, also contains small amounts of glucuronic acid. It has been shown that the polysaccharide chain is a hybrid molecule. Finally, skin dermatan sulfate and umbilical cord dermatan sulfate differ in the amount and nature of the protein core.

Many investigators have drawn conclusions regarding the role of mucopolysaccharides in healing wounds on the basis of changes in hexosamine content of healing tissues. However, serum glycoproteins, which will be present in a wound (coming into it from the circulation), also contain hexosamine. Thus, in order to understand the biochemical events, tissue mucopolysaccharides must be separated from other hexosamine-containing materials and identified specifically.

Recent studies utilizing specific chemical procedures to isolate and identify mucopolysaccharides in healing wounds have shown that in guinea pig skin wounds, hyaluronic acid was present in fairly high concentration initially, but decreased from the fifth to tenth day and leveled out at a low concentration thereafter. At about the fifth day chondroitin-4-sulfate and dermatan sulfate appeared and both increased up to about day 15 to 18. Chondroitin-4-sulfate, which was present in greatest concentration, declined after the eighteenth day, as did dermatan sulfate, but to a lesser extent. No chondroitin-6-sulfate could be found in skin.

In rabbit tendon, a similar picture with hyaluronic acid was obtained, and dermatan sulfate increased to become the major mucopoly-

Table 4–1. Mucopolysaccharides: Composition and Location in the Body

	Synonym	Disaccharide Repeating Unit	Significant Amounts In
Chondroitin		Glucuronic acid + galactosamine	Cornea
Chondroitin-4-sulfate	Chondroitin sulfate A	Glucuronic acid + 4-sulfo-galactosamine	Aorta Costal cartilage (newborn) Bovine nasal septum Cornea Bone
Chondroitin-6-sulfate	Chondroitin sulfate C	Glucuronic acid + 6-sulfo-galactosamine	Tendon Costal cartilage (aged) Umbilical cord Nucleus pulposus
Dermatan sulfate	Chondroitin sulfate B	Iduronic acid + 4-sulfo-galactosamine	Skin Heart valves Aorta
Heparin sulfate	Heparitin sulfate	Glucuronic acid + glucosamine	Aorta
Keratan sulfate	Keratosulfate	Galactose + 6-sulfo-glucosamine	Cornea Skeleton (fetal)
Hyaluronic acid		Glucuronic acid + glucosamine	Cartilage

saccharide. Very little chondroitin-4-sulfate was found, and chondroitin-6-sulfate was similar in concentration to that found in normal tendon and remained constant.

In wounded cornea, all mucopolysaccharides disappeared, and later chondroitin sulfate and dermatan sulfate appeared in the wound, but keratan sulfate, which is normally present in cornea, was not replenished even after three months. These results provide another example of the observation which will be made constantly in this book: repair tissue differs structurally and biochemically from the tissue it replaces.

In vitro studies of precipitation of collagen fibers in the presence of various mucopolysaccharides have shown that when dermatan sulfate is present, collagen fibers that are formed have a greater average diameter than those formed when chondroitin-4-sulfate is present. Likewise, it is notable that in the cornea, where keratan sulfate is the major mucopolysaccharide present, collagen fibers are extremely fine. The heavier fibers of skin appear to be associated with high content of dermatan sulfate. All of this evidence certainly suggests a definite relationship between the type of mucopolysaccharide present and the size, and possibly the orientation, of collagen fibers in different tissues.

There are, however, a number of persons who feel that ground substance has nothing to do with fibril formation. They point out that tropocollagen aggregation and fibril formation can be made to proceed in neutral salt solutions by merely warming such solutions to body temperature. Typical 640 Å-banded collagen fibrils are formed. Others, impressed with the orientation of collagen fibrils in tissue, assign a role to charged components of ground substance in bringing about orientation of the collagen fibril during aggregation and growth.

The discovery of several types of collagen and the location of certain of these in highly specialized tissues such as cartilage suggest that there may be a special relationship between collagen and the other substances composing the tissue. For instance, it has been found that type I collagen is found in perichondrium and type II in matrix of cartilage. Type II collagen contains about nine times as much hydroxylysine-linked carbohydrate as does type I collagen from bone. Some investigators have speculated that extensive glycosylation of hydroxylysine residues may promote collagen-proteoglycan interactions through carbohydrate side chains of both types of macromolecule. Such interactions could be of significance in maintaining the structural integrity of cartilaginous tissue. Since wounded cartilage shows little if any tendency to repair, it is interesting to speculate whether this is due to inability of repair cells to produce type II collagen. Much work remains to be done in this important area.

Corneal collagen is type I. However, corneal collagen has slightly more glycosylated hydroxylysine residues than type I collagen from skin. It is of interest that collagen in corneal scars is less glycosylated than normal corneal stromal collagen. It has been suggested that the presence of a high degree of glycosylation in collagen leads to formation of small fibers with a relatively constant fibril size. Scar collagen exhibits large fibers and size. However, it is not possible at present to say that glycosylation is the sole determinant of fibril size since, as we have indicated, there is equally strong evidence that the kind of mucopolysaccharide in the environment may influence fibril diameter. Perhaps both mechanisms are operative.

CORNEAL HEALING

Since we have previously alluded to events in corneal healing as an example of the effects of specific collagen-protein polysaccharide interaction, it would seem desirable to consider in more detail the problem of corneal healing in order to illustrate and emphasize this point.

Anatomy of the Cornea

In order to appreciate healing problems in the cornea, the anatomy must be well understood. The outer surface of the cornea is composed of stratified squamous epithelial cells, five or six layers thick. The outer surface consists of two layers of thin, flat cells, which in many ways correspond to the stratum corneum of skin, except that they are more active metabolically. The outermost layer of cells has minute microvilli which project into the tear film which continually bathes the surface.

The three layers immediately under the outer surface cells consist of semiflattened cells called "wing cells." Immediately under these is a layer of columnar basal cells which rest on a thin membrane (Bowman's membrane) which is believed to be composed of a collagen-glycoprotein substance.

Underneath the epithelial layer and Bowman's membrane is the corneal stroma, or substantia propria, which composes about 90 per cent of corneal tissue. The cellular portion of this part of the cornea is composed of a flattened cell, termed the keratocyte. This cell is functionally a fibroblast, but like the osteoblast, chondroblast, and other such cells, it receives a special name and since, when it is seen by light microscopy, its morphology is somewhat different from that of the fibroblast, it is often accused of "transforming" into a fibroblast following the stimulus of an injury.

The greatest bulk of stroma consists of collagen fibrils of uniform diameter gathered into bundles, or corneal lamellae. Each successive lamellar layer has collagen fibrils oriented at right angles to the ones above and below it. Each fibril is imbedded in a characteristic matrix, or ground substance, the composition of which will be discussed later.

On the inner surface of the cornea a single layer of mesenchymal epithelial (endothelium) cells lies on an important membrane, Descemet's membrane. This membrane, like Bowman's on the outer surface, is composed of collagen and glycoprotein. However, although it has no elastic fibers, it has a degree of elasticity that causes it to retract or roll away from penetrating wounds of the cornea.

Corneal stroma differs from other connective tissues in two major respects: collagen fibers are extremely uniform in diameter and exhibit remarkable orientation; and surrounding ground substance is distinguished by being composed of keratan sulfate and chondroitin, in addition to chondroitin-4-sulfate. As will be discussed, this may be an important factor in healing in the cornea as keratocytes, or corneal fibroblasts, appear to be the only cells programmed for production of this combination of mucopolysaccharides, and new cells formed by mitotic division of older cells do not commence to produce this combination of substances for many months after they mature.

Epithelial Abrasion

As in epithelial repair elsewhere in the body, corneal epithelium covers the surface of a defect by migration and proliferation. Migratory activity begins about an hour after injury to the cornea. Basal cells extend long pseudopods into the wound area and these pseudopods eventually make contact with each other and form a continuous one cell thick covering over the wound. If the wound is extensive, basal cells actually move out to cover the wound.

Basal cell proliferation begins some time after migration has been completed. Epithelial covering of the wound is gradually thickened, and true regeneration of the original epithelial structure occurs. If the whole cornea is denuded of epithelium, conjunctival epithelial cells migrate over the exposed stroma. However, the rate of migration is markedly slower than when repair can be effected by corneal epithelium.

Nonpenetrating Stromal Wounds

Some nonpenetrating corneal wounds heal by complete regeneration of corneal stroma with normal cellular and fiber architecture. A perfect functional eye is the end result. Unfortunately, other corneal wounds heal by means of a disorganized connective tissue scar which, while restoring the substance of the cornea, is opaque and causes varying degrees of disability.

Within 24 hours of wounding, keratocytes at the margin of the wound, and for a very short distance away, modulate into forms called keratoblasts. In many ways these are indistinguishable from fibroblasts found in wounds in other portions of the body.

Within four hours after injury, polymorphonuclear cells and macrophages will be found within the wound. These reach a maximal concentration on the second and third days. They are apparently derived from conjunctival vessels at the limbus, which show engorgement following injury. These cells, however, do not migrate quickly through the dense corneal stroma. They have been shown to be carried to the wound site by the tear film on the surface of the cornea.

There has been some dispute about whether monocytes or macrophages actually reach a corneal wound. The differences of opinion seem to be related to the distance of the observed wound from the limbus. Wounds in rat eyes, which are small, give a different picture from those of rabbit or dog eyes when the wound is centrally located. Wounds on the periphery of the cornea usually will be found to have mononuclear cells.

The importance of this question revolves around the source of many of the fibroblasts in the repairing corneal wound. It is difficult to account for the large number of fibroblasts in the wound on the basis of the observed rate of mitotic division of local keratocytes. Studies with tritiated thymidine indicate that migrated epithelial cells do not transform into fibroblasts. Likewise, polymorphonuclear cells do not become fibroblasts. As we have already mentioned, there is some evidence that under particular conditions macrophages or mononuclear cells may modulate into fibroblasts. Whether this occurs in a corneal wound is not definitely proved or disproved. The only other source for fibroblasts would be the adventitia of limbal blood vessels. However, there is as yet no definitive proof of their migration.

The reason for ascribing two sources of fibroblasts in a corneal wound is the two different courses which the healing process may take. A small wound, in which the local cell population can repair the damage within a few days, probably is exposed to only one kind of fibroblasts: that derived from adjacent keratocytes. Such wounds heal with full restoration of structure and function; no scar is formed. Biochemically, these wounds are abnormal initially in that only chondroitin-4-sulfate is synthesized and laid down by fibroblasts. However, between 15 and 30 days after wounding, keratan sulfate begins to appear and gradually increases until the content in the wound area is normal at about the third month.

In large wounds of the cornea, particularly if they are penetrating wounds, or if the wounds, for one reason or another, become vascularized, the mucopolysaccharides are the same as those laid down in scar tissue elsewhere in the body and collagen fibers are of random size and arranged in a disorderly fashion. A true scar forms.

Penetrating Wounds of the Cornea

If a penetrating wound of the cornea is large enough, the aqueous humor will be lost. This is replaced by a fluid which contains as much protein as blood plasma (a transudate). This fluid contains fibrinogen and a fibrin "plug" is quickly formed in the wound. This clot forms a fairly effective seal of the wound.

Contact with aqueous humor, as well as with blood or saline solutions, causes corneal stroma to swell several hundred per cent. Within an hour of wounding, basal cells of corneal epithelium have commenced to migrate and within a relatively short time (24 hours for small incisional wounds) an epithelial plug has covered the wound. This provides protection as the fibrin plug undergoes lysis within four to five days after formation.

Keratocytes begin to differentiate into active keratoblasts at about six hours and proliferation begins at about 30 hours. Mucopolysaccharide synthesis begins at about the third day and is maximal in about two weeks. Collagen fibers, randomly oriented, begin to appear in the anterior cornea and the healing proceeds posteriorly. Remodeling and maturation also commences in the anterior portion and spreads posteriorly and is not complete, even at 90 days.

If the wound in the cornea is large, the defect in Descemet's membrane, which is exaggerated by its tendency to roll back away from the wound edge, may show no signs of repair. However, endothelial cells will cover the defect fairly quickly. In smaller wounds, endothelial cells migrate across the wound and secrete a new Descemet's membrane. However, the full thickness of this membrane is never restored.

One important fact deserves mention in connection with corneal wound healing. If for some reason epithelial cells are prevented from migrating over the wound surface, keratocytes do not modulate and stromal healing is inhibited. Apparently, epithelium exerts an inductive effect on the underlying mesenchymal cells, as was discussed in Chapter 2.

A collagenase has been isolated from corneal ulcers. This collagenase is active at pH 7.0 to 8.0 and splits the collagen molecule into two fragments, similar to those produced by other tissue collagenases. Collagenase is not found in normal corneal epithelium or stroma; however, after injury, both migrating epithelial cells and underlying stroma produce the enzyme.

Corneal collagenase is irreversibly inhibited by cysteine which appears ideally suited to control the destructive action of the enzyme. $CaNa_2EDTA$ is also an inhibitor of corneal collagenase, but its action is reversible. Recently progesterone has been shown to inhibit collagenase and may now be the drug of choice in treatment of corneal ulcers.

Complications of Healing

Ingrowth of either epithelium or corneal stroma into the anterior chamber is a serious complication of corneal wounds. Ingrowth of corneal stroma is the more common and is particularly prone to occur after large penetrating corneal wounds. Such stromal tissue may come to line the anterior chamber, and in addition to blindness it can lead to intractable glaucoma.

Epithelial ingrowth is most prone to occur in penetrating wounds that fail to form a fibrin plug or in suture tracts where penetrating sutures have been used and where they have been left in too long. It is now rare for sutures to be used this way and epithelization of the anterior chamber has become quite rare. It may occur, however, in traumatic wounds of the eye in which epithelial tissue has been driven into the anterior chamber. The visual consequences of epithelization of the anterior chamber are usually less serious than those of stromal ingrowth; but immobilization of the iris can occur.

Thus, in the cornea, we have evidence of both epithelial-mesenchymal interaction and collagen-protein polysaccharide interaction. These have important consequences in determining the outcome of wound healing.

In other healing wounds, there is very little direct evidence concerning the role of the components of ground substance in the formation of the collagen fibril. All that can be said is that this is the environment in which fibrillogenesis takes place and this environment appears to differ from that of normal tissue. However, as we shall see, elements of ground substance may play an important role in the maturation of collagen; this will be discussed later in this chapter.

COLLAGEN MATURATION

We now come to the most significant discussion regarding collagen from the standpoint of the surgeon and his handling of a wound. The brief discussion we have given on structure and synthesis of collagen is important only insofar as it provides a sound basis for more practical concepts to be presented.

Maturation can be defined as the process by which the fragile, soluble fibrils of collagen change into strong, insoluble fibers and how they proceed from a disorganized, random, and not very useful arrangement to an oriented, organized structure providing mechanical strength to a tissue. We shall examine the nature and mechanism, as far as they are known, of this process and suggest ways in which they may be controlled and ways in which they may go awry.

Cross-Linking and the Properties of Collagen

Tropocollagen that has not yet polymerized into fibrils is quite soluble in cold water. Even after it has formed fibrils, these are readily soluble in neutral salt solutions. However, as time passes, the solubility decreases until only acid solutions will dissolve the fiber. Finally, a state of insolubility is reached in which only materials which break covalent bonds or totally destroy the fiber will bring collagen into solution.

These changes in the solubility of collagen fibers occur in newly formed collagen as it is deposited to form connective tissue structures in the body and scars in healing wounds. Simultaneously, tensile strength of the fibers increases dramatically and continues to increase even after the fibers have become insoluble. These changes in collagen fibers are of major importance to the surgeon. They determine the ultimate strength of a healed wound. The rate at which these changes occur determines how long sutures must retain their strength to prevent wound dehiscence. They also account for the toughness and intractability of unwanted fibrous adhesions. An understanding by the surgeon of the molecular events that are responsible for these changes during maturation of collagen fibers is essential in order that he may devise rational methods for controlling and directing the repair process. That such control is now becoming a reality will be discussed repeatedly in this book; this control became possible only when the mechanism of maturation could be explained on a biochemical basis.

In this section the structural aspects of maturation will be discussed, and mechanisms by which these structural changes are brought about will also be dealt with. It must be emphasized that our knowledge regarding the structural features of mature collagen fibrils is far from complete. Much of what we have to discuss is still speculative in the sense that the available evidence is suggestive—absolute proof of the structural concepts has not yet been presented.

When tropocollagen first aggregates, the force that holds the chains of tropocollagen molecules in the precise quarter-stagger arrangement appears to be due to electrostatic bonds between charged polar groups along the chain. As we mentioned in our discussion of the primary structure of collagen, these polar amino acids are located in "bunches" along polypeptide chains. The band pattern of collagen fibrils seen in the electron microscope suggests that these highly charged regions along adjacent molecules are in lateral "register." At the stage of fibril formation at which only the attraction of oppositely charged groups holds the structure together, altering the charge by introducing salts or other charged molecules can disrupt the fiber. The fiber can literally go into solution.

It should be noted that assembly of the three polypeptide chains that compose tropocollagen is directed by the N-terminal and C-terminal nonhelical peptides that make up procollagen. These are termed "registration" peptides but should not be confused with the term "registration" as used in the previous discussion. In fact, if these registration peptides are not removed from procollagen, assembly into fibers cannot take place since extra peptides in procollagen block the formation of the quarter-stagger arrangement of tropocollagen molecules and thus block the first stage of maturation.

When tropocollagen is first formed from procollagen, the individual α chains are held together only by hydrogen bonds. Similar bonds may also play a part in holding several molecules of tropocollagen together in the form of a fiber. Compared to electrostatic bonds, however, these are weak and relatively unimportant. However, early after the tropocollagen molecule is synthesized, certain of the lysine residues, notably near the amino terminal end of the $\alpha 1$ chain, undergo an oxidative deamination; that is, the amino group on the last carbon atom is lost and an aldehyde is formed in its place. Aldehydes are very reactive groups and they like to react with each other and with amino groups. A

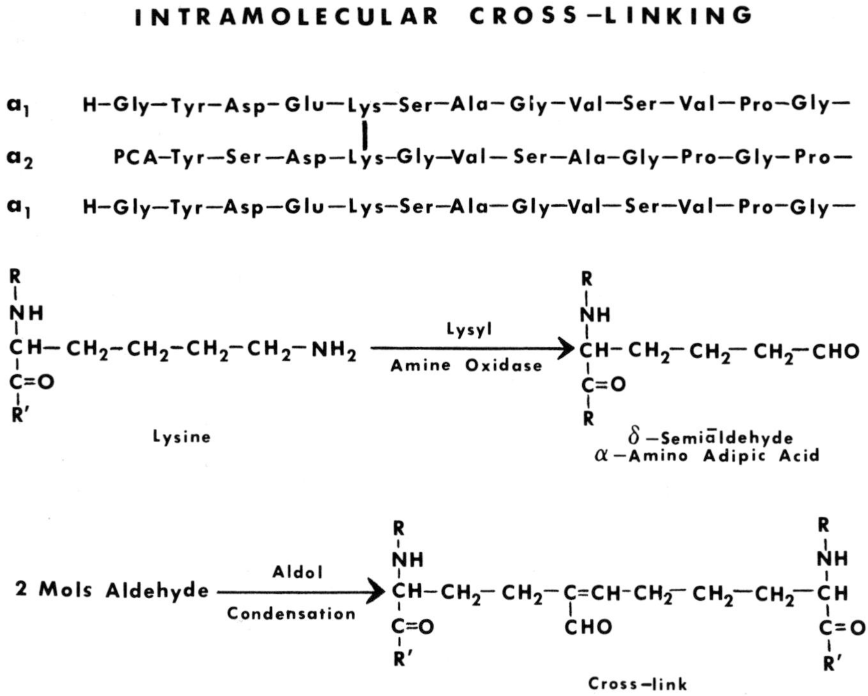
INTRAMOLECULAR CROSS-LINKING
a1 H-Gly-Tyr-Asp-Glu-Lys-Ser-Ala-Gly-Val-Ser-Val-Pro-Gly-
a2 PCA-Tyr-Ser-Asp-Lys-Gly-Val-Ser-Ala-Gly-Pro-Gly-Pro-
a1 H-Gly-Tyr-Asp-Glu-Lys-Ser-Ala-Gly-Val-Ser-Val-Pro-Gly-
Lysyl
Amine Oxidase
Lysine
δ-Semialdehyde
α-Amino Adipic Acid
2 Mols Aldehyde
Aldol
Condensation
Cross-link

Figure 4–18. Postulated formation of intramolecular cross-links. At the top is shown amino acid sequences of the amino terminal ends of the three peptide chains of the tropocollagen molecule. A cross-link between lysines in an $\alpha 1$ and the $\alpha 2$ chain is shown. Postulated steps in the formation of this cross-link are shown in the lower portion of the figure. Note that after formation of the cross-link, an aldehyde group is available for further interactions, including the possible formation of an intermolecular bond.

INTERMOLECULAR CROSS–LINKING

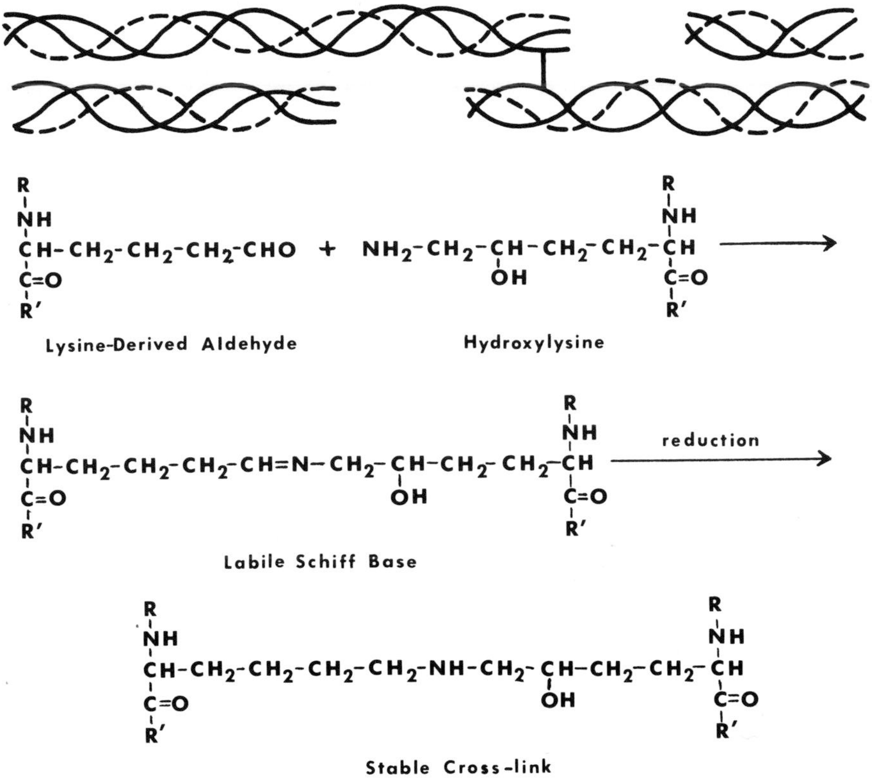

R
|
NH
|
$CH-CH_2-CH_2-CH_2-CHO$ + $NH_2-CH_2-CH-CH_2-CH_2-CH$ ⟶
| | |
C=O   OH   C=O
| |
R'   R'

Lysine-Derived Aldehyde   **Hydroxylysine**

R   R
| |
NH   NH
| | reduction
$CH-CH_2-CH_2-CH_2-CH=N-CH_2-CH-CH_2-CH_2-CH$ ⟶
| | |
C=O   OH   C=O
| |
R'   R'

Labile Schiff Base

R   R
| |
NH   NH
| |
$CH-CH_2-CH_2-CH_2-CH_2-NH-CH_2-CH-CH_2-CH_2-CH$
| | |
C=O   OH   C=O
| |
R'   R'

Stable Cross-link

Figure 4–19. Postulated formation of intermolecular cross-links. At the top, the cross-link is shown as bonding a lysine in the amino terminal of a tropocollagen molecule with an hydroxylysine near the carboxyl terminal of another tropocollagen molecule. Also illustrated is the quarter-stagger arrangement of molecules in a fibril and the "holes" between ends of linearly arranged tropocollagen molecules. In the lower part of the figure are proposed reactions leading to labile and stable intermolecular cross-links.

similar event occurs on the α2 chain and another aldehyde is formed from lysine. The two aldehydes react, possibly by a reaction well known to organic chemists, the aldol condensation, and form a covalent bond between the α1 and α2 chains or between two α1 chains. This is termed an intramolecular bond, since it occurs within a single tropocollagen molecule. From earlier discussions, it can be recognized that the two bonded chains constitute the β form or chain.

From the standpoint of number, the most common type of cross-link is that formed by reaction of an aldehyde produced from lysine or hydroxylysine with an amino group of another lysine or hydroxylysine. The resultant compound is termed a Schiff base. Schiff bases are readily disrupted by acid and, since solubilization or purification of collagen frequently involves the use of acid, these cross-links were not discovered by early workers. However, if these Schiff bases are reduced with such substances as sodium borohydride, they become stable and can be isolated.

It is believed that many of these Schiff bases become reduced gradually in the body. This can account for the resistance of old collagen to acids and other forms of solubilization. Cross-links involving two hydroxylysine residues appear to be particularly resistant to cleavage. Such cross-links are found in bone, and perhaps this is why bone collagen is the most insoluble of all collagens. They are also found in type III collagen, and embryonic collagen is also notably resistant to acid solubilization.

As far as is known, Schiff base formation occurs between lysine and hydroxylysine residues in α chains of different tropocollagen molecules. They are thus intermolecular bonds and are the major force holding fibrils and fiber bundles together. Their presence is the chief contributing factor in the tensile strength of collagen. It has been shown that lysine and hydroxylysine residues near the C-terminal portion of tropocollagen react with allysine or hydroxyallysine residues at the N-terminal region of another tropocollagen molecule, thus "locking" the end-to-end quarter-stagger polymeric chain of tropocollagen molecules.

It must be remembered that for these intermolecular bonds to form, the participating groups must be within 14 to 15 Å of each other. This requires tight packing of the polymer chains. There is some evidence that mechanical tension may play a role in packing the chains so that these cross-linking reactions are facilitated.

The formation of an intramolecular bond does not alter the solubility of collagen, but it does make the molecule much more stable and possibly increases its resistance to attack by enzymes. When a similar bond forms between α chains in adjacent tropocollagen molecules, there is a change in solubility. If only a few intermolecular bonds are formed, the fibril will dissolve in increasing concentrations of salt. However, as more such bonds are formed among adjacent tropocollagen molecules, acid solutions are necessary to dissolve the fibers. Finally, a highly cross-linked collagen becomes insoluble.

The formation of intramolecular and intermolecular cross-links involving aldehyde groups occurs early in the formation of collagen fibrils. The evidence for this statement rests on the observation that these cross-links are found in soluble collagens and on observations made on the connective tissue defect induced by lathyrogenic agents. The discovery of the mechanism of lathyrism has opened up possibilities for the surgeon to control, by chemical means, the formation of scar tissue. The usefulness and limitations of this control mechanism can best be understood by examining the biochemical events occurring in this disorder.

Lathyrism and the Blocking of Maturation

Animals that have the misfortune to eat the seeds of the sweet pea, *Lathyrus odoratus*, rather than their ordinary fodder, develop a most unpleasant condition known as lathyrism. The connective tissue of the body, particularly that which has a relatively high metabolic turnover, loses its structural properties, most notably its tensile strength. This results in skeletal deformities and aneurysms of major blood vessels. The effects are most noticeable and develop most rapidly in young, growing animals.

The active principle of sweet pea seeds has been shown to be one of a family of amino nitriles, of which β-aminopropionitrile is the most commonly used and active member. Administration of these agents, called lathyrogens, does not alter the quantity of collagen produced or found in affected connective tissue. Furthermore, electron microscope observations do not show any obvious abnormalities in collagen fibrils.

Chemical examination of collagen derived from lathyritic animals reveals no changes other than the solubility of fibrils. In fully developed lathyrism, the amount of salt-soluble and acid-soluble collagen increases markedly and the proportion of insoluble collagen decreases. Careful isotope tracer studies have shown that already existing insoluble collagen is not solubilized, but practically none of the newly formed collagen is converted to insoluble collagen. Lathyrism is, therefore, a defect in maturation.

Examination of the proportion of α, β, and γ components of lathyritic collagen, as compared to normal collagen, has shown an abnormally high percentage of the α form present, and a virtual absence of the γ form. This points to a defect in the formation of cross-links, both intramolecular and intermolecular. Separation of the various α components of lathyritic collagen and examination of the number of

Figure 4–20. Effect of β-aminopropionitrile on burst strength of rat abdominal-wall wounds. Wounds were made on day 1 and 100 mg. β-aminopropionitrile was administered intraperitoneally daily from day 14 through day 19. Burst-strength measurements were made on days 14, 19, and 22. Note that the strength of wounds of treated animals was significantly less than that of controls but that the strength did not decrease during the period of β-aminopropionitrile administration. (Reproduced by permission from E. E. Peacock, Jr., and J. W. Madden, Surgery 60: 7, 1966.)

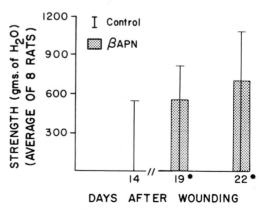

DAYS AFTER WOUNDING

* βAPN treated animals less than controls p < .001

Table 4–2. *Effect of β-Aminopropionitrile on Nonextractable (Insoluble)*
Collagen of Rat Abnormal-Wounds*

The drug was administered to group C from day 14 through day 19. No significant
increase in insoluble collagen between day 14 and day 19 is seen in either the control
or treated rats.

Group	Hydroxyproline†
A – 14 d. Control	108.0
B – 19 d. Control	116.8
C – 19 d. βAPN	106.4
No significant difference p > .6	

*From E. E., Peacock, Jr., and J. W. Madden, Surgery *60*:7, 1966, used by permission.
† Average of 8 rats.

available aldehyde groups has revealed a reduction of at least 50 per
cent in the α chain. This appears to be the major chemical difference
between lathyritic and normal collagen.

Investigations to elucidate the mechanism of the lathyrogenic effect led to discovery of a specific enzyme, lysyl oxidase, which catalyzes
the oxidative deamination of lysine and hydroxylysine, forming their respective aldehydes. It will be recognized that this enzyme belongs to the
class of monoamine oxidases. However, the relationship of this enzyme
to circulating monoamine oxidase in blood is not clear. There are
conflicting reports in the literature on the effect of amino nitriles on
amine oxidases other than lysyl oxidase. On the other hand, isoniazid,
a potent monoamine oxidase inhibitor, is only minimally effective
against lysyl oxidase, whereas amino nitriles are effective in millimole
concentrations. Nevertheless, lathyrogens of the amino nitrile class
exert their effect through selective inhibition of lysyl oxidase. In the
presence of lathyrogens, formation of lysyl and hydroxylysyl aldehydes
is blocked and cross-linking of collagen, as well as elastin, cannot occur,

The metabolic product of penicillin degradation, pencillamine (β,

Table 4–3. *Effect of β-Aminopropionitrile on 0.45M NaCl-Extractable*
Collagen in Rat Abdominal Wounds*

The drug was administered to group C from day 14 through day 19. The increase in
neutral-salt-soluble collagen at day 19 is nearly ten times that of the control animal.

Group	Hydroxyproline† μg./cc.
A – 14 d. Control	1.066
B – 19 d. Control	0.278
C – 19 d. βAPN	2.304‡

*From E. E. Peacock Jr., and J. W. Madden, Surgery *60*:7, 1966, used by permission.
† Average of 8 rats.
‡ Greater than A or B p < .01.

Table 4–4. *Specific Enzymes Involved in Collagen Synthesis and Destruction*

Enzyme	Substrate	Co-Factors	Action	Inhibitors	Failure Evidenced By
Prolyl hydroxylase	α-Chain peptides attached to ribosomes	F^{++} O_2 Ascorbic acid α-Ketoglutarate	Hydroxylates proline in Y position in sequence Gly-X-Y	Anoxia Vitamin C deficiency Iron chelators	Scurvy
Lysyl hydroxylase	α Chain peptides attached to ribosomes	F^{++} O_2 Ascorbic acid α-Ketoglutarate	Hydroxylates lysine in Y position in sequence Gly-X-Y	Anoxia Vitamin C deficiency Iron chelators	Scurvy
O-Lysyl galactosyl transferase	Hydroxylysine Hydroxylysine peptides α Chains	Mn^{++}	Glycosylates certain hydroxylysines		
Glucosyl transferase	Hydroxylysyl-O-Galactose in α chains	Mn^{++}	Attaches glucose to O-lysylgalactose		
Procollagen peptidase	Procollagen		Cleaves N-terminal non-helical registration peptides	SO_4^{++} Tris buffer (in vitro)	Dermatosparaxis Type V Ehlers-Danlos syndrome
Lysyl oxidase	Tropocollagen	O_2 CU^{++}	Deaminates and oxidizes lysine and hydroxylysine, forming respective aldehydes	Amino nitriles Hydrazines	Lathyrism
					Activity Evidenced By
Granulocyte collagenase	Collagen	Ca^{++}	Cleaves collagen into $1/4$ and $3/4$ segments	(Not serum) Peptidases Cystine, $CaNa_2EDTA$	Necrotic abscess
Tissue collagenase Synovial collagenase (type B)	Collagen	Ca^{++}	Cleaves collagen into $1/3$ and $2/3$ segments	Cystine, $CaNa_2EDTA$ Serum Low pH	Collagen remodeling
Synovial rheumatoid collagenase (type A)	Collagen	Ca^{++}	Cleaves collagen into several fragments	EDTA	Destruction of tendon and cartilage
Uterine collagenase	Collagen	Ca^{++} Plus M (unknown)	Cleaves collagen into $1/4$, $1/3$, $3/4$ and $2/3$ segments	Low pH NaEDTA (not cysteine) Serum	Failure of postpartum uterus to involute

β-dimethylcysteine), has also been shown to act very similarly to lath-yrogenic agents. Its effect was first noticed in patients being treated with penicillamine for Wilson's disease. Some of these patients developed mild symptoms of lathyrism while under therapy. Penicillamine is a copper-chelating agent, and it is for this reason that it finds some usefulness in Wilson's disease. The known monamine oxidases contain copper as an integral part of the enzyme. It was suggested that penicillamine causes lathyrism by chelating with copper in the enzyme, thus preventing it from performing its function. Later work has shown that penicillamine reacts with aldehyde groups and blocks cross-linking.

On the basis of recent studies with lysyl oxidase, β-aminopropionitrile, and penicillamine, the following pathway is postulated for the formation of the aldol-type cross-link in collagen:

$$2 \text{ Lys} \xrightarrow[(1)]{} 2 \text{ } \alpha\text{-aminoadipic acid semialdehyde} \xrightarrow[(2)]{} \text{aldol}$$

Step 1 is catalyzed by lysyl oxidase and blocked by β-aminopropionitrile. Step 2 may occur spontaneously, but is blocked by penicillamine.

The studies on lathyrism are significant because they illustrate the importance of covalent cross-linking in the development of mechanical properties of connective tissue. The cross-links that appear to be primarily involved in providing these mechanical properties, early in fibril formation, are those involving aldehyde functions in the collagen molecule.

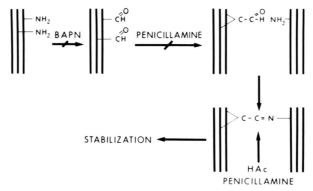

Figure 4–21. A schematic representation of the formation of intramolecular and intermolecular cross-links in collagen. It will be seen that β-aminopropionitrile (BAPN) blocks the formation of aldehydes. Penicillamine blocks the interaction of aldehydes to form the aldol condensation product. Also shown is a postulated reaction whereby free aldehyde formed in aldol condensation (see Fig. 4–18) may react with a lysine in another collagen molecule to form a Schiff base, thus making an *inter*molecular cross-link.

Other Cross-Links in Collagen

If covalent cross-linking is important in the maturation of collagen and in the tensile strength of wounds, the introduction of cross-links by local treatment of a healing wound with cross-linking agents might be expected to hasten the increase in tensile strength. This experiment has been performed, with formaldehyde in one instance and 1-ethyl-1-3(3-dimethylaminopropyl) carbodiimide hydrochloride in another. It was suggested that formaldehyde would introduce methylene bridges between adjacent tropocollagen chains. The carbodiimides had been shown to be useful in forming amide bonds during protein synthesis. With both agents there was a sizable increase in tensile strength of the wounds between the third and fourth days postoperatively in treated wounds as compared with controls. The thermal shrinkage temperature of the individual collagen fibers from the wounds was increased in treated wounds as compared to fibers from comparable control wounds. These facts, taken in conjunction with what is known of the

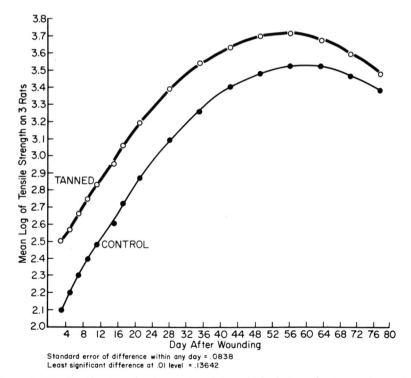

Standard error of difference within any day = .0838
Least significant difference at .01 level = .13642

Figure 4–22. Tensile strength of normal and formaldehyde-tanned rat wound scar tissue within 80 days after wounding. Semilog graph. Tanning was performed by immersing excised wound strips into the tanning solution. Note that the effect is greatest in early stages of healing, when natural cross-linking is least. At later stages, the effect of tanning is less, since natural cross-linking has already commenced. (Reproduced by permission from E. E. Peacock, Jr., Ann. Surg. *163*:1, 1966.)

mechanism of lathyrism, all suggest that cross-linking, after fibril formation, is an extremely important aspect responsible for the mechanical properties of collagen, particularly its tensile strength.

Three major types of intermolecular cross-links have been identified: (1) a Schiff base involving two lysine residues, termed lysinonorleucine; (2) one involving a hydroxylysine and lysine, called hydroxylysinonorleucine; and (3) one formed from two hydroxylysine residues termed dihydroxylysinonorleucine. This last cross-link is found primarily in bone collagen as well as in type III collagen.

There is some evidence that another cross-link, involving the cross-link formed during aldol condensation between two lysine groups that constitute the intramolecular cross-link and histidine, exists. This cross-link has been found only in cow skin collagen, and there is some question of its general importance.

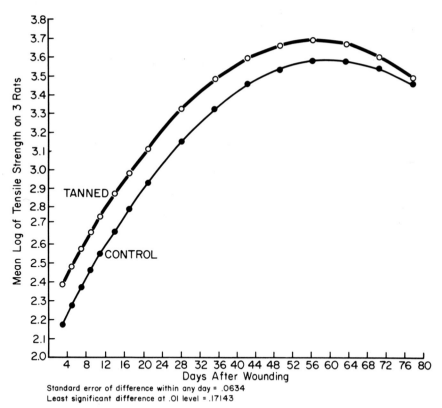

Standard error of difference within any day = .0634
Least significant difference at .01 level = .17143

Figure 4–23. Tensile strength of normal and carbodiimide-tanned rat wound scar tissue within 80 days after wounding. Semilog graph. Tanning was performed by immersing excised wound strips into 1 per cent 1-ethyl-3-(3-dimethylaminopropyl) carbodiimide hydrochloride for 22 hours. A significant increase in tensile strength of treated wound strips was seen through the twenty-first day. It is assumed that thereafter the sites favorable for amide bond formation were already blocked by conversion of lysine ε-amino groups to aldehydes or their involvement in natural cross-links. (Reproduced by permission from E. E. Peacock, Jr., Ann. Surg. *163*:1, 1966.)

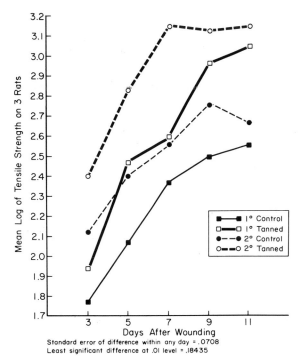

Figure 4–24. Semilog graph showing tensile strength of primary and secondary wound scar tissue following formaldehyde tanning during early phases of healing. Secondary wounds were produced by mechanically dehiscing seven day old wounds and resuturing immediately. Tanning was performed by immersing 1 cm. strips of excised wound scar into the tanning bath. Note that control secondary wounds show the expected increase in tensile strength over primary wounds at the same time periods. Tanning produces a comparable increase in tensile strength in both primary and secondary wounds. (Reproduced by permission from E. E. Peacock, Jr., Ann. Surg. *163*:1, 1966.)

Another type of cross-link, termed hydroxymerodesmosine, has been reported in collagen. This is analogous to the desmosine type cross-links found in elastin. This cross-link involves Schiff base formation between a hydroxylysine residue and the free aldehyde in the aldol intramolecular cross-link. The abundance of this cross-link is not known and, in fact, it may be present only temporarily. It is of interest, however, since it can involve three different α chains.

A more abundant type of cross-link has tentatively been identified. This is a combination of the histidine-aldol and hydroxymerodesmosine cross-links. This involves four separate α chains and is, in fact, a true network.

Lysine and hydroxylysine can also form Schiff bases with reducing sugars such as glucose and mannose. Such "cross-links" have been reported to occur in "older" connective tissues and in connective tissues that contain polysaccharides. Whether these are true cross-links or merely another means by which collagen is glycosylated remains to be elucidated.

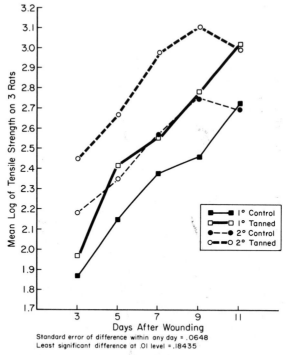

Figure 4–25. Semilog graph showing tensile strength of primary and secondary wound scar tissue following carbodiimide tanning during early phases of healing. The procedures were as described for Figures 4–23 and 4–24. Note that the carbodiimide effect is not observed at day 11. This is probably due to formation of natural cross-links at the sites of carbodiimide action. (Reproduced by permission from E. E. Peacock, Jr., Ann. Surg. *163*:1, 1966.)

Thus, seven distinct cross-links have been reported in collagen, all of them dependent for their formation on oxidative deamination of lysine and hydroxylysine residues. The aldol cross-link is strictly an intramolecular cross-link and occurs near the amino terminal of the tropocollagen molecule. Lysinonorleucine, involving one lysine aldehyde and one lysine residue, is common in all collagens and also is found in elastin. Hydroxylysinonorleucine, involving hydroxylysine and lysine, one or the other being in aldehyde form, is also abundant in most collagens. Dihydroxylysinonorleucine, involving two hydroxylysines, is found chiefly in bone collagen and is a more stable cross-link than the others we have discussed. Of the three other cross-links, aldohistidine has been reported only in cows, and hydroxymerodesmosine may be an intermediate in collagen during the formation of histidino-hydroxymerodesmosine. This last cross-link is reported to be abundant in most collagens, but it is said to form only after other cross-links have been made.

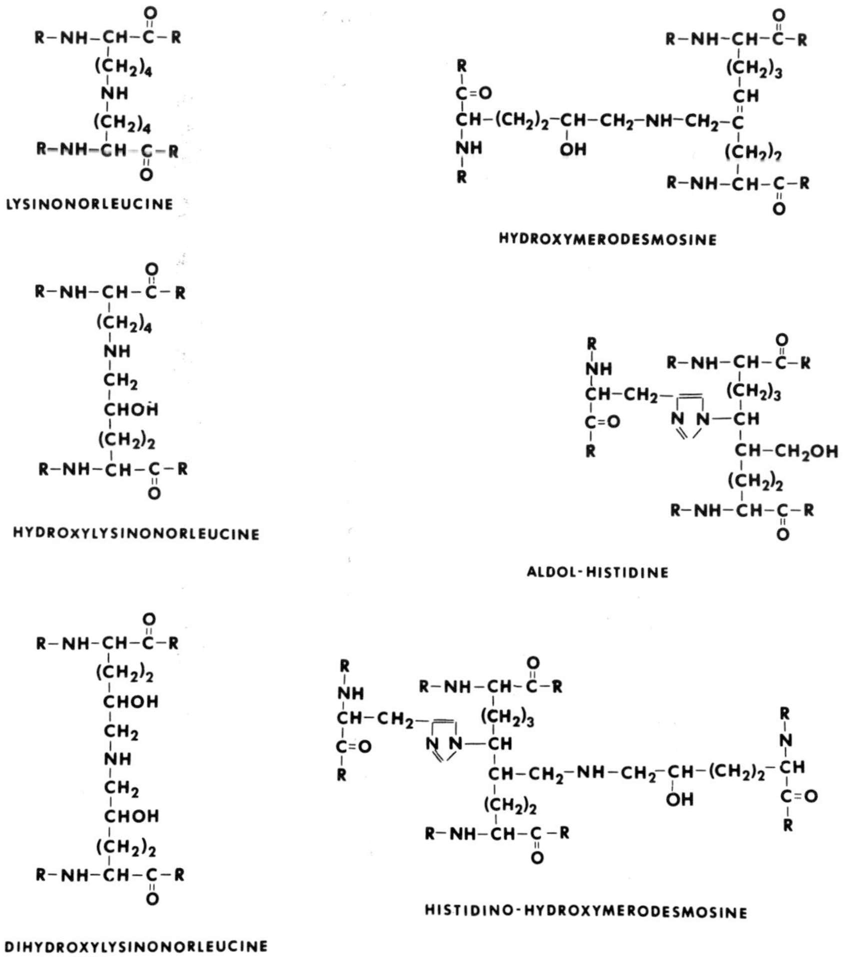

Figure 4–26. Intermolecular cross-links identified in collagen. *Lysinonorleucine* is present in both collagen and elastin and is common in both proteins. *Hydroxylysinonorleucine* is also common in most types of collagen, but particularly in type I collagen of soft tissues. *Dihydroxylysinonorleucine* is most abundant in type III collagen and type I collagen of mineralized tissues. *Hydroxymerodesmosine* is formed from an intramolecular aldol cross-link and is probably an intermediate stage or precursor of other cross-links. It is actually an inner- and intramolecular cross-link and is not abundant. *Aldol-histidine* has been found only in cow skin collagen. It also is derived from an aldol intramolecular cross-link and probably is an intermediate or precursor form of an intermolecular cross-link. *Histidino-hydroxymerodesmosine* links one intramolecular cross-link with two other α chains to form an intermolecular cross-link involving three collagen molecules. It exists in two isomeric forms and is abundant in most collagens, particularly adult types.

Collagen–Ground Substance Interactions

Earlier we mentioned the possible stabilization of the collagen fibril through electrostatic bonding with a protein-polysaccharide. While undoubtedly this plays a role in the physical properties of the collagen fibril and may regulate the size attained by the fibril, there are other interactions that collagen may undergo with materials in ground substance.

It is known that in special tissues, such as bone, cartilage, dentin, and cornea, collagen fibrils not only have certain structural features, but the fibrils may be covalently linked to glycoproteins, the precise nature of which may determine the exact properties of the particular tissue. The evidence for a chemical combination between collagen and glycoproteins in other tissues, such as tendon and skin, is at present quite tenuous. It has been shown, however, as we mentioned previously, that the most likely linkage of glycoprotein to collagen is through O-glucosyl-galactosidyl bond to hydroxylysine.

Some interesting experiments suggest that the tensile strength of skin may not be due solely to the tensile strength of mature collagen fibers. The tensile strength of rat tail dermis has been measured at various pH's and in the presence of a variety of ions. It was found that pH had a marked effect on the breaking strength, the maximal strength being observed around pH 7 to 8, with a sharp decrease below pH 7, reaching a minimal value at pH 5 or lower. This marked effect of pH, particularly the steep drop in breaking strength between pH 7 and 6, is hard to explain in terms of an effect on collagen, but it may be an effect on asssociated material in the dermis. It was also found that nitriles, penicillamine, and cysteamine, as well as a number of sulfhydryl compounds, shifted the pH curve to the right so that at pH 7 there was a marked decrease in tensile strength. Under similar conditions, but using relatively pure reconstituted collagen the effects of these substances were minor. It was also found that $10^{-3}M$ cyanide ion shifted the pH curve of breaking strength of rat dermis to the left, and at pH 6 the strength was markedly greater than in the control. Again, with purified collagen, cyanide ion had no effect.

Two explanations for the experimental results just described may be offered. The effects produced by penicillamine, nitriles, and sulfhydryl compounds might be due to breaking of unstable covalent intermolecular cross-links in collagen. The lack of effect on purified reconstituted collagen might be due to prior stabilization of the cross-links. Beef tendon collagen is normally more insoluble than rat collagen. A second, less likely, explanation is that nitriles and sulfhydryl compounds destroy or interfere with stabilizing forces between collagen and ground substance components.

It seems possible that nitriles and cyanide ion might react with aldimine cross-links. In the case of nitriles, the bond might be broken and in the case of cyanide, an addition product might be produced. The latter reaction would tend to stabilize the cross-link to the action of acid.

Although there is good evidence for covalent linkage of a glycoprotein to collagen, another possibility exists to explain the alteration in solubility and physical properties of collagen in maturing connective tissue. We have suggested that fibrils are formed outside the cell in a matrix that includes a variety of mucopolysaccharides, glycoproteins, and protein-polysaccharides. Most of the sulfated mucopolysaccharides are present in tissue in combination with protein. Hyaluronic acid, on the other hand, appears to exist primarily free. The chondroitin sulfates appear to exist as polymers of approximately 15,000 to 50,000 molecular weight, attached to an acidic protein of about 1.2×10^6 molecular weight. Of particular interest, because of its interaction with collagen, is a protein-polysaccharide in which about 60 chondroitin sulfate chains of about 45,000 to 50,000 molecular weight are covalently linked to an acidic protein whose length is about 4000 Å. This complex of protein and polysaccharide may be visualized as a "bottle-brush" with the protein being the central core and the polysaccharide being the bristles. Since chondroitin sulfate chains have a high negative charge they repel each other and this serves to stiffen the entire structure. Evidence exists that these "bottle-brush" molecules lie among collagen fibrils, and the highly charged chondroitin sulfate molecules form ionic bonds or complexes with polar groups in the collagen molecule. They do not appear to form covalent bonds; some recent evidence suggests that the sites of complex formation are at specific bands in the tropocollagen macromolecule as seen in the electron microscope. Most of the evidence for complexes of this type has been obtained from studies on cartilage where there is a 1:1 ratio between protein-polysaccharide and collagen. However, there is evidence that even in tendon, where the mucopolysaccharides compose only about 0.5 per cent of the tissue, they are important in stabilizing fibers. There is also evidence that the same may be true of skin. It is possible that this association with protein-polysaccharides occurs early in maturation, and covalent cross-linking with similar molecules occurs later.

Notwithstanding the paucity of facts regarding the precise mechanism of maturation of collagen, there appear to be enough to permit one to suggest a possible sequence of events. Tropocollagen, secreted by fibroblasts, is assembled into long polymer chains by staggered end-to-end interaction. Simultaneously, lateral aggregation of these polymer chains begins, and this appears to be controlled by the charge distribution along tropocollagen chains. These first events take place near or on the surface of the fibroblast, and it has been suggested, largely on the evidence of histological observation, that fiber orientation is controlled by the cell and possibly through a "template" of protein-polysaccharide.

Collagen fibrils grow in diameter by accretion of new polymer chains and possibly by surface aggregation of tropocollagen molecules. Simultaneously, collagen in the center of the fibril is compressed and the density of the center portion of the fibril increases. Intramolecular and intermolecular cross-linking commences in this region through interaction of aldehyde groups, formed previously by the oxidative deamination of ϵ-amino groups in lysine, mediated by lysyl amine oxidase. These aldehydes react with each other or with other free amino groups. Thus, a growing fibril is characterized by a center portion made up of intermolecularly cross-linked insoluble collagen, surrounded by less completely cross-linked material which shows progressively greater susceptibility to solution by acids and neutral salt solutions until, at the surface, low concentrations of salt at pH 7 can solubilize the outer layers.

The limits of fibril size may be established by the force required to distort the chains to match adjacent binding sites coming into equilibrium with the electrostatic binding forces. This equilibrium may be modified by the interposition of highly charged protein-polysaccharides. The presence of particular types of mucopolysaccharide may determine ultimate fiber size and, possibly, their arrangement in the tissue.

When fibrils have reached their normal size, cross-linking continues and the fibrils become increasingly insoluble. There is considerable evidence, however, that a second type of cross-linking begins to occur during the latter phases of maturation. It has been observed that as collagen matures, the content of aldol intramolecular cross-link decreases and the histidino-merodesmosine cross-link appears and increases. This suggests that late maturation involves formation of a network of cross-linked collagen molecules. It is also observed that the content of reduceable cross-links decreases with maturation. It is postulated that aldimine cross-links are slowly reduced and stabilized during maturation. This late type of maturation appears to be important both in stabilizing the connective tissue and in increasing its tensile strength. There is also evidence that this late maturation does not go to completion in scar tissue. We shall discuss this in more detail in a later chapter.

The Location of Cross-Links and the Action of Enzymes on Collagen

At first thought, it might seem of only academic interest to discuss where on the collagen molecule the cross-links may be located. However, the observation that cross-links may be destroyed by certain proteolytic enzymes without damage to the main body of the tropocollagen molecule suggests that advantage might be taken of this fact to remove unwanted scar tissue or fibrous adhesions. Also, such destruction of cross-links may be the first step in the catabolism of insoluble collagen in the body.

A number of years ago it was discovered that about 5 per cent of the tropocollagen molecule is susceptible to attack by pepsin and certain other proteases. Careful physical-chemical and electron microscope studies showed that collagen is not denatured by such treatment;

it still shows its characteristic structure under the electron microscope, but the molecule appears to be slightly shorter. Chemical studies showed that certain amino acids, notably tyrosine, but also some lysine, diminish markedly after such treatment. It was suggested that the enzymes split off a portion of one or more α chains at the amino terminal region. It was postulated, and later demonstrated by chemical isolation, that this end region, at least in the α1 chain, has a very different amino acid sequence from the remainder of the collagen molecule and, because of the absence of proline and hydroxyproline, is not involved in the helical structure of the rest of the molecule. These end regions were termed "telopeptides" and represent the residual portions of the "registration" peptides of procollagen. It was also shown that the helical coiled-coil structure of collagen prevents proteolytic enzymatic attack on the main body of the molecule. When collagen is denatured, and thus its tertiary structure is destroyed, it is quite susceptible to attack by trypsin, pepsin, and other proteases.

It will be recalled that the nonhelical peptide is removed by the action of procollagen peptidase after the triple helix formation is completed. Some evidence exists that among collagens there is a difference as to just how much of the nonhelical peptide is left after the action of procollagen peptidase. In type I collagen, a short 15 amino acid chain is left. However, in type III collagen there may be only one or two amino acids remaining in this region. This may be a significant difference since in type I collagen this is the region in which the intramolecular cross-link occurs and perhaps, later, where the histidine-merodesmosine cross-links form. If this region is lacking in some other types of collagen, it could make significant differences in solubility, stability, and strength of fibers that form.

Genetic Defects in Collagen Synthesis and Maturation

Several rare defects in collagen synthesis or maturation have been known for some time but only recently has the nature of these defects been elucidated. Dermatosparaxis occurring in cattle is a genetic disorder in which one of the procollagen peptidases is absent. This results in failure of conversion of procollagen to tropocollagen, and interferes with helix formation and with polymerization of tropocollagen to collagen and its subsequent cross-linking to form strong stable fibers. This causes fragility of all connective tissue structures, including bones and basement membranes. Severe deformities and cardiovascular disturbances are observed clinically.

In humans, a similar deficiency in one of the procollagen peptidases produces a form of Ehlers-Danlos syndrome known as type VII. The Ehlers-Danlos syndrome is characterized by hyperextensible skin, joint laxity, tissue fragility, and if severe, bleeding episodes and cardiovascular involvement, particularly affecting the heart valves. This syndrome includes at least seven different entities, of which the specific defect has been identified in four.

Type VI Ehlers-Danlos syndrome has been identified with a failure to hydroxylate lysine residues in collagen. In reported cases, the predominant clinical feature was kyphoscoliosis present from birth. In addition, patients exhibited joint laxity, hyperelastic skin, and a tendency to bruise easily. Analysis of connective tissue revealed collagen markedly deficient in hydroxylysine residues. It is assumed, without direct measurements, that there is a deficiency of the specific enzyme lysyl hydroxylase. It was notable in the reported cases that hydroxylation of proline was normal. The reduction of hydroxylysine residues concomitantly reduced the galactose and glucosyl-galactose normally coupled to hydroxylysine through an O-glycosidic linkage. The tendency to easy bruising (capillary hemorrhage) may be associated with this defect. Platelets contain glucosyl and galactosyl transferases and it has been suggested that platelet-collagen interactions somehow involve hydroxylysine residues in collagen and these transferase enzymes of platelets. Thus, with hydroxylysine-deficient collagen there may be a failure of this interaction resulting in failure of the release reaction of platelets.

Type V Ehlers-Danlos syndrome has been associated with a deficiency of lysyl oxidase. The collagen is excessively soluble and since allysine and hydroxyallysine fail to form, cross-linking and formation of strong stable collagen fibers are prevented. In this syndrome, hernias, short stature, poor lung compliance, and cardiovascular disease are prominent. The most serious defect appears to be in the heart valves; they are described as being "floppy." Mitral regurgitation and tricuspid regurgitation were present. In addition, patients present other features of Ehlers-Danlos syndrome such as dorsal kyphosis, stretchable skin, and joint hypermobility. The genetic defect of this type of Ehlers-Danlos syndrome is X-linked.

Type IV Ehlers-Danlos syndrome is associated with a failure to form type III collagen. Patients have fragile but inextensible connective tissues. Rupture of large arteries (which normally contain type III collagen) and of the bowel is the major defect in this type of disease. Patients show tight, thin skin over the face and ears, but oddly they have a tendency to form keloids and contractures despite their collagen deficiency.

STRUCTURE OF ELASTIN

The second major fibrous component of connective tissue is elastin. This fibrous protein is not readily replaced when removed and it plays practically no role in repair. However, its absence in repair tissue, particularly in skin and large arteries, has important consequences. It is thus of some interest to the surgeon. A brief description of its structure and synthesis will be given here; the implications of absence of elastic tissue will be discussed in a later chapter.

Elastic tissue has recently been demonstrated to contain two unique proteins. During development of elastic tissue in the embryo, microfibrillar material is laid down at the site of all future elastic fibers. This is followed by deposition of an amorphous material which gradually increases until in the adult it accounts for about 92 per cent of elastic fiber. This amorphous material is what we recognize as protein elastin. The microfibrillar material, which is always associated with elastic fiber, differs markedly from elastin in its amino acid composition. It has more polar, hydroxy- and sulfur-containing amino acids and less proline, valine, and glycine. This protein, as yet unnamed, may be an "organizer" for elastin which subsequently is laid down.

Elastic fibers occur in tissues which are subject to repeated distortional forces, such as skin, certain ligaments, and large arteries, and in certain fibrocartilaginous structures, such as the external ear. Their purpose is to restore the original contour after the distorting force ceases to act. Where the load that must be restored is great, as in some ligaments, elastic fiber content is high; where the load is low, as in skin, elastic fibers are sparse.

Elastin has a yellowish color, and is frequently referred to as yellow connective tissue, in contrast to collagen, or white connective tissue. Elastin is insoluble in all ordinary solvents and is resistant to acids and

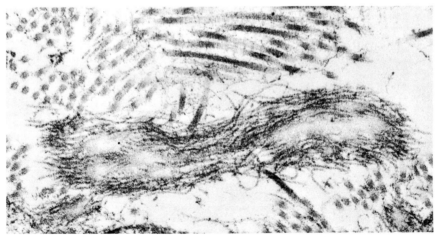

Figure 4–27.   Electron micrograph of an elastic fiber from fetal calf ligamentum nuchae. Although two components can be seen, densely staining, beaded microfibrils are predominant and surround two zones, at each end, which contain the amorphous component now identified as protein elastin. Collagen fibrils with their characteristic band pattern can be seen adjacent to the larger elastic fiber. × 35,000. (Illustration by courtesy of Prof. Russell Ross, University of Washington.)

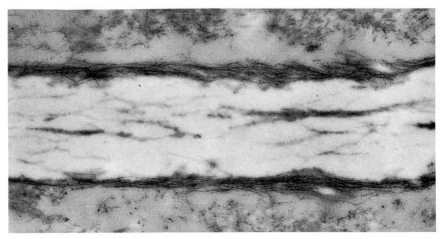

Figure 4–28. Electron micrograph of a maturing elastic fiber from a calf ligamentum nuchae. The amorphous component, elastin, is now predominant and microfibrils are arranged, for the most part, on the periphery of the fiber. A few, however, can be seen scattered within the amorphous component. × 30,000. (Illustration by courtesy of Prof. Russell Ross, University of Washington.)

alkalis. It is thus difficult to study, since there is no "soluble" form as is the case with collagen. It has a very low content of lysine and arginine and thus is not susceptible to the action of trypsin. Furthermore, since it contains only 4 per cent of tyrosine and phenylalanine residues, chymotrypsin is of limited value in structure studies.

Elastin also lacks the large number of polar amino acid residues of collagen, and as a consequence does not take up stains well. Orcein appears to be a selective stain for elastin and is widely used. The appearance of elastin varies considerably with the particular tissue in which it is found. In ligamentum nuchae, which has the highest elastin content of any tissue, it occurs in long thick parallel fibers. In arterial wall, on the other hand, it is found as longitudinally oriented fibers that show extensive branching. These are closely associated with collagen fibers and are embedded in a ground substance matrix. In other tissues, such as skin, the branching, net-like, character of elastin fibers is particularly apparent.

Elastin, like collagen, has nearly one-third of its amino acid residues as glycine. Proline accounts for 10 to 12 per cent of the residues, but hydroxyproline is present to the extent of about 1 per cent. Alanine and valine are also present in fairly large amounts. As we mentioned, the polar amino acids are notably deficient.

Elastin does not show a distinctive pattern, either by x-ray diffraction or by electron microscopy. It appears to exist as long, branched, randomly coiled chains. It does not exhibit denaturation, since it does not have crystalline regions in its structure.

Because of the observed branching of fine filaments of elastin, which serves to give it elastic properties, considerable attention has been devoted to determining the nature of the cross-linkages responsible for this type of structure. Elastin shows a characteristic fluorescence as well as a visible yellow color. It has been suggested that a yellow chromophore is at the site of cross-linked chains which form the branching network. Elastin was degraded with a specific enzyme, elastase, to obtain an H-shaped peptide. Further examination of this material suggested that the chromophore is at the center of a cross-linked structure involving three or four peptide chains.

The structures of two compounds were finally established and named "desmosine" and "isodesmosine."

Desmosine

Isodesmosine has the "m"
chain on the 6 position instead
of the 5 position.

It was later shown that in this structure $K = m = 1$ and $1 = 2$. It was found that in embryonic elastic tissue, desmosine and isodesmosine content is quite low after birth. The content of these substances increases with age. In embryonic elastin, the lysine content is high, and this decreases proportionately to the increase in desmosine and isodesmosine with age. Partridge has postulated that four lysine residues, each in a precursor peptide, are oxidatively deaminated at the ε-amino position and that aldehydes so formed then react to form the nitrogen-containing ring structure of desmosine and isodesmosine — thus uniting four peptide chains in a common cross-link.

This appears quite plausible, since lathyrogenic agents, when administered to embryos, appear to block the formation of these cross-links in elastin by a mechanism similar to that for collagen. There is also evidence that other types of cross-links, involving lysine residues, exist in elastin. These may also involve an aldehyde intermediate which represents condensation of two and three lysine residues.

It can be appreciated that cross-linking of elastin is very similar in mechanism to that which occurs in collagen. However, cross-linking in elastin is perhaps more widespread and involves many more lysine residues. Furthermore, most of the cross-links involve three or four peptide chains, thus forming a complex network. In collagen, probably owing to the triple helical conformation, fewer cross-links are formed and cross-links involving more than two or three peptide chains are comparatively rare. Thus collagen does not show the extensibility and elasticity seen in elastin.

It is the presence of these cross-links that gives elastin the property of being deformed under light loads and returning promptly to its original configuration when the load is removed. In skin, for example, collagen fibers exist as a network or mesh. When skin is stretched, the network becomes oriented in the direction of stretch, and when fully aligned, limits the amount of stretch. The elastic fibers restore the original network when the stretching force is released.

Elastic fibers decrease with age. Thus, aged skin becomes loose and baggy since the collagen network becomes oriented by gravity or by muscular pull, and there is little or no restoring force. In a scar, where there are few elastic fibers and where collagen fibers become oriented primarily along lines of tension, there is little "give," and stretching and relaxation are not possible. This accounts for the rigidity of scar tissue and its inability to undergo the repeated deformation and recovery needed in skin covering a joint or other moving part.

This failure to include new elastic fibers in the tissue of repair until long after the collagen fibers are formed is another example of the inferiority of scar tissue to the tissue it replaces. It has obvious implications in the repair of skin defects, of ligamentous structures, and of large arteries. These will be discussed in later chapters.

SUGGESTED READING

Bailey, A. J., and Peach, C. M. Isolation and Structural Identification of a Labile Intermolecular Cross-Link in Collagen. Biochem. Biophys. Res. Commun. *33*:812, 1968.

Balian, G. A., Bowes, J. H., and Cater, C. W. Stabilization of Cross-Links in Collagen by Borohydride Reduction. Biochim. Biophys. Acta *181*:331, 1969.

Barnes, M. J. Function of Ascorbic Acid in Collagen Metabolism. Ann. N.Y. Acad. Sci. *258*:264, 1975.

Blumenfeld, O. O., Rojkind, M., and Gallop, P. M. Subunits of Hydroxylamine-Treated Tropocollagen. Biochemistry *4*:1780, 1965.

Bornstein, P. Comparative Sequence Studies of Rat Skin and Tendon Collagen. I. Evidence for Incomplete Hydroxylation of Individual Prolyl Residues in the Normal Proteins. Biochemistry *6*:3082, 1967.

Bornstein, P., Kang, A. H., and Piez, K. A. The Nature and Location of Intramolecular Cross-Links in Collagen. Proc. Nat. Acad. Sci. *55*:417, 1966.

Brown, S. I. Collagenase and Corneal Ulcers. Invest. Ophthal. *10*:203, 1971.

Butler, W. T., and Cunningham, L. W. The Site of Attachment of Hexose in Tropocollagen. J. Biol. Chem. *240*:3449, 1965.

Chapman, J. A., Kellgren, J. H., and Steven, F. S. Assembly of Collagen Fibrils. Fed. Proc. 25:1811, 1966.

Chung, E., Keels, E. M., and Miller, E. J. Isolation and Characterization of the Cyanogen Bromide Peptides from the α(III) Chain of Human Collagen. Biochemistry 13:3459, 1974.

Chvapil, M., Hurych, J., Ehrlichova, E., and Cmuchalova, B. Effects of Various Chelating Agents, Quinones, Diazoheterocyclic Compounds and Other Substances on Proline Hydroxylation and Synthesis of Collagenous and Non-Collagenous Proteins. Biochim. Biophys. Acta 140:339, 1967.

Drake, M. P., and Davison, P. F. The Location of Cross-Links in γ Chains from Calf Skin Collagen. J. Biol. Chem. 243:2890, 1968.

Dunnington, J. H. Tissue Responses in Ocular Wounds. Amer. J. Ophthal. 43:667, 1959.

Dunnington, J. H., and Regan, E. F. The Effect of Sutures and of Thrombin upon Ocular Wound Healing. Amer. J. Ophthal. 35:167, 1952.

Dunnington, J. H., and Weimar, V. Influence of the Epithelium on the Healing of Corneal Incisions. Amer. J. Ophthal. 45:89, 1958.

Fairweather, R. B., Tanzer, M. L., and Gallop, P. M. Aldol-Histidine, a New Trifunctional Collagen Crosslink. Biochem. Biophys. Res. Commun. 48:1311, 1972.

Furthmayer, H., Timpl, R., Stark, M., Lapiere, C. M., and Kuhn, K. Chemical Properties of the Peptide Extension in the α-Chain of Dermatosparactic Skin Collagen. FEBS Letters 28: 247, 1972.

Goldberg, B., and Green, H. Collagen Synthesis on Polyribosomes of Cultured Mammalian Fibroblasts. J. Molec. Biol. 26:1, 1967.

Gross, J. Organization and Disorganization of Collagen. Biophys. J. 4:63, 1964.

Hodge, A. J., and Schmitt, F. O. The Charge Profile of the Tropocollagen Macromolecule and the Packing Arrangement in Native-Type Collagen Fibrils. Proc. Nat. Acad. Sci. 46:186, 1960.

Hutton, J. J., Tappel, A. L., and Udenfriend, S. Requirements for α-Ketoglutarate, Ferrous Ion and Ascorbate by Collagen Proline Hydroxylase. Biochem. Biophys. Res. Commun. 24:179, 1966.

Jackson, D. S., and Bentley, J. P. On the Significance of the Extractable Collagens. J. Biophys. Biochem. Cytol. 7:37, 1960.

Kefalides, N. A. Isolation of a Collagen from Basement Membrane Containing Three Identical α-Chains. Biochem. Biophys. Res. Commun. 45:226, 1971.

Kitano, S., and Goldman, J. N. Cytologic and Histochemical Changes in Corneal Wound Repair. Arch. Ophthal. 76:345, 1966.

Kivirikko, K. I., and Prockop, D. J. Enzymatic Hydroxylation of Proline and Lysine in Protocollagen. Proc. Nat. Acad. Sci. 57:782, 1967.

Lenaers, A., Ansay, M., Nusgens, B. V., and Lapiere, C. M. Collagen Made of Extended α-Chains, Procollagen, in Genetically Defective Dermatosparactic Calves. Europ. J. Biochem. 23:533, 1971.

Lichtenstein, J. R., Martin, G. R., Kohn, L. D., Byers, P. H., and McKusick, V. A. Defect in Conversion of Procollagen to Collagen in a Form of Ehlers-Danlos Syndrome. Science 182:298, 1973.

Manner, G., Kretsinger, R. H., Gould, B. S., and Rich, A. The Polyribosomal Synthesis of Collagen. Biochim. Biophys. Acta 134:411, 1967.

McDonald, J. E. Early Components of Corneal Wound Closure. Arch. Ophthal. 58:202, 1957.

Monson, J. M., and Bornstein, P. Identification of a Disulfide-Linked Procollagen as the Biosynthetic Precursor of Chick-Bone Collagen. Proc. Nat. Acad. Sci. 70:3521, 1973.

Newell, F. W. Some Aspects of Normal and Abnormal Corneal Wound Healing. Trans. Ophthal. Soc. U. K. 86:813, 1966.

Nimni, M. E., Gerth, N., and Bavetta, L. A. Reversibility of a Penicillamine-Induced Defect in Collagen Aggregation. Nature 213:921, 1967.

Page, R. C., and Benditt, E. P. A Molecular Defect in Lathyritic Collagen. Proc. Soc. Exp. Biol. Med. 124:459, 1967.

Page, R. C., Benditt, E. P., and Kirkwood, C. R. Schiff Base Formation by the Lysyl and Hydroxylysyl Side Chains of Collagen. Biochem. Biophys. Res. Commun. 33:752, 1968.

Priest, R. E., and Bublitz, C. The Influence of Ascorbic Acid and Tetrahydropteridine on the Synthesis of Hydroxyproline by Cultured Cells. Lab. Invest. 17:371, 1967.

Ramachandran, G. N., and Sasisekharan, V. Refinement of the Structure of Collagen. Biochim. Biophys. Acta 109:314, 1965.

Rhoads, R. E., and Udenfriend, S. Decarboxylation of α-Ketoglutarate Coupled to Collagen Proline Hydroxylase. Proc. Nat. Acad. Sci. 60:1473, 1968.

Robb, R. M., and Kuwabara, T. Corneal Wound Healing. I. The Movement of Polymorphonuclear Leukocytes into Corneal Wounds. Arch. Ophthal. *68*:636, 1962. II. An Autoradiographic Study of the Cellular Components. Arch. Ophthal. *72*:401, 1964.

Schmitt, F. O., Gross, J., and Highberger, J. H. States of Aggregation of Collagen. Soc. Sympos. Exp. Biol. *9*:148, 1955.

Speakman, P. T. Proposed Mechanism for the Biological Assembly of Collagen Triple Helix. Nature *229*:241, 1971.

Spiro, R. G. Studies on the Renal Glomerular Basement Membrane. Nature of the Carbohydrate Units and their Attachment to the Peptide Portion. J. Biol. Chem. *242*:1923, 1967.

Tanzer, M. L. Crosslinking of Collagen. Science *180*:561, 1973.

Tanzer, M. L. Intermolecular Cross-Links in Reconstituted Collagen Fibrils. Evidence for the Nature of the Covalent Bonds. J. Biol. Chem. *243*:4045, 1968.

Tanzer, M. L., Fairweather, R., and Gallop, P. H. Isolation of a Crosslink, Hydroxymerodesmosine, from Borohydride-Reduced Collagen. Biochim. Biophys. Acta *310*:130, 1973.

Trelstad, R. L., Kang, A. H., Igarashi, S., and Gross, J. Isolation of Two Distinct Collagens from Chick Cartilage. Biochemistry *9*:4993, 1970.

Van Winkle, W. The Fibroblast in Wound Healing. Surg. Gynec. Obstet. *124*:369, 1967.

Veis, A., and Anesey, J. Modes of Intermolecular Cross-Linking in Mature Insoluble Collagen. J. Biol. Chem. *240*:3899, 1965.

Weimar, V. L. The Sources of Fibroblasts in Corneal Wound Repair. Arch. Ophthal. *60*:93, 1958.

Chapter 5

THE BIOCHEMISTRY AND THE ENVIRONMENT OF WOUNDS AND THEIR RELATION TO WOUND STRENGTH

One of the most important aspects of wound healing is the rate at which an incised wound gains tensile strength. This chapter will deal with our knowledge of the mechanism by which a wound heals and the mechanical properties of the tissue of repair. The effects of variations in the internal and external environment on wound healing will be discussed. Many, if not most, of the environmental factors are under the control of the surgeon and an appreciation of their effects and their clinical significance can aid in the proper care of the surgical patient. These considerations will lead us to a correlation of the material in the previous chapters and to a consideration of the major biochemical events in wound healing.

Of necessity, most of the experimental data upon which this discussion is based were obtained in animals. It will be seen that there are differences, of a quantitative nature, in the healing of wounds in different species. Thus, one must be cautious in transferring the results obtained in animals to the problems of wound healing in human beings. Nevertheless, the basic mechanisms involved appear to be essentially the same in all species; only the rates differ and these, in many instances, can be accounted for by known metabolic or anatomical differences among animal species.

Since by far the great majority of surgical wounds involve skin, underlying fascia, and muscles, most of the studies have been concerned with tensile strength and biochemical changes in skin and fascia or in the full thickness of the abdominal wall. The measurement of tensile strength of a tissue such as skin or fascia is not a simple task and the literature is replete with data that, because of failure to appreciate the mechanical properties of these tissues or the meaning of tensile strength, are nearly worthless. Thus, it seems proper to discuss briefly what is known about the mechanical properties of skin and fascia.

MECHANICAL PROPERTIES OF SKIN

Skin is not a homogeneous substance. It contains cells, a fibrous network composed of collagen and elastin, and an amorphous ground substance which consists of protein-polysaccharides, glycoproteins, globular proteins, salts, and water. This heterogeneous composition, together with the physical arrangement of the components, is responsible for the mechanical properties of skin.

Skin exhibits tension and extensibility. Skin tension is one of the determining factors in the mechanical response to an incised wound. It also plays an important role in the course of wound contraction, as was discussed in Chapter 3. Tension varies with age and with site, and in some areas has a directional quality. The tension of skin is probably related to the content and direction of elastic fibers of the dermis. As these diminish with age, skin loses its elastic quality.

The extensibility of skin is the amount it will stretch before it breaks. This also varies with location and with age. Extensibility is made up of two parameters: elastic stretch and nonelastic stretch or plastic flow. Data for the extensibility, breaking strength and thickness of rat skin from rats of different ages have been published. The age range of the animals was 21 days to 601 days and the body weight varied from 26 grams to 467 grams. The extensibility increased to a maximum in rats 44 days old and then decreased to a very low level in the oldest rats. The breaking strength of skin, however, increased about fourfold (expressed as kilograms per square millimeter) with increasing age. The thickness of skin also increased steadily with age, reaching a maximum at about 270 days. This increase in skin thickness was paralleled by an increase in collagen content of the skin.

It has been shown that human skin behaves very much like rat

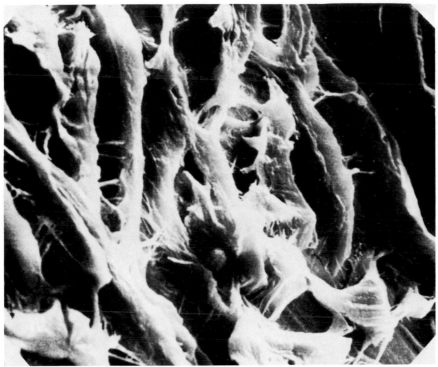

Figure 5–1.   Collagen fiber network in a 10μ section of normal rat skin, showing interlacing of fibers. Scanning electron micrograph. × 1000. (From J. C. Forrester, B. H. Zederfeldt, T. L. Hayes, and T. K. Hunt, in *Repair and Regeneration,* edited by J. E. Dunphy and W. Van Winkle, Jr. Copyright 1969, McGraw-Hill Book Company. Used with permission of McGraw-Hill Book Company.)

skin. Extensibility increases from infancy to about 40 years of age and then declines sharply with increasing age. However, collagen content of skin, contrary to what was observed in rats, does not change with age. The extensibility of skin in older persons declines less in skin from the forearm than in skin from the abdomen. It should also be noted that not all changes in mechanical properties of skin with age are due to the aging process *per se.* Ultraviolet radiation also produces changes in skin that are not confined to the epithelial layer. Long continued exposure to actinic rays produces changes in collagen. It is suggested that cross-linking may be increased. While cross-linking of any polymer, including collagen, increases its strength, a point is reached where the polymer becomes brittle and, although it can resist straight tensile forces, it is markedly weakened to shearing forces. Thus irradiated skin can become brittle and this is frequently seen in exposed skin of older persons who have led active outdoor lives. This is related to aging only in the sense that it takes prolonged exposure to sunlight to bring about these changes. Brittleness and fracture of collagen fibrils due to shearing forces may make these fractured fibers more susceptible to degradation and hence actually reduce the collagen content of skin.

In human skin the mechanical characteristics are dependent on the microarchitecture of the meshwork of collagen fibers. These are so arranged that, no matter in which direction skin is pulled, the fibers become aligned in that direction. The elastic fiber network also aligns itself in the direction of extension and serves as an energy storing device which, when the tension of pull is released, restores the collagen network to its original relaxed state.

Skin also shows a time-dependent viscoelastic behavior, which is of considerable significance in the measurement of tensile strength. During the stretching of skin, the interstitial fluid is displaced. This takes a finite time. Thus, if the rate of extension is too fast, breakage will occur before elongation can take place. On the other hand, if a rapid rate of extension is used, but the extension stopped before breakage, the tension required to maintain a given elongation will drop, owing to move-

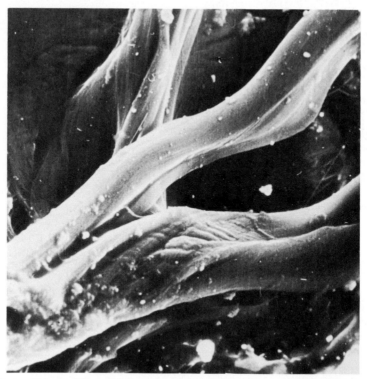

Figure 5–2.   Collagen fibers of dermis. Note the smooth appearance and great length as compared to diameter. Although fibers appear to branch, this is probably due to their close association and intertwining. Stereoscan electron micrograph. × 1500. (From T. Gibson and R. M. Kenedi, in *Repair and Regeneration,* edited by J. E. Dunphy and W. Van Winkle, Jr. Copyright 1969, McGraw-Hill Book Company. Used with permission of McGraw-Hill Book Company.)

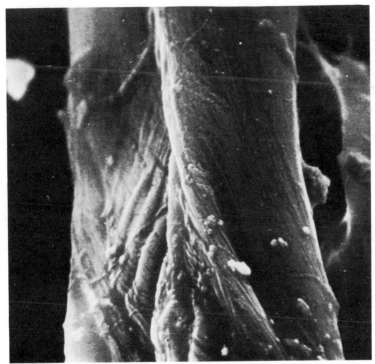

Figure 5–3. A higher magnification of dermal collagen fibers in which fine fibrils can be seen to course in parallel array in a slow helical twist along the fiber. Stereoscan electron micrograph. × 4400. (From T. Gibson and R. M. Kenedi, in *Repair and Regeneration,* edited by J. E. Dunphy and W. Van Winkle, Jr. Copyright 1969, McGraw-Hill Book Company. Used with permission of McGraw-Hill Book Company.)

ment of fluid out of the interstitial spaces. Thus, within certain limits, the breaking strength of skin depends upon the rate at which the force is applied. Highly cross-linked or brittle skin will disrupt if the rate of extension is too rapid. This is also true for other tissues such as tendon and bowel.

In summary, it can be stated that skin is a viscoelastic structure and that absolute values for the various parameters related to its mechanical properties depend on site, on direction of application of force, and on the rate of application of force. These properties at any one site change markedly with age as does skin thickness and, in some species, skin composition. All of these facts influence the measurement of the physical properties of healing wounds in skin.

TENSILE STRENGTH MEASUREMENT

The terms tensile strength and breaking strength must be defined. Tensile strength is measured in terms of load applied per unit of cross-

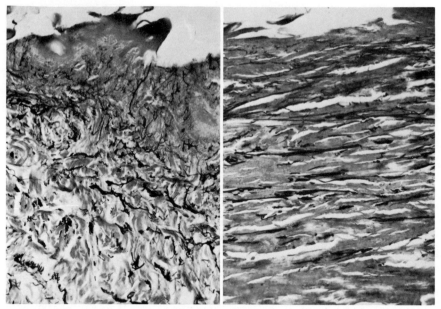

Fig. 5–4.   Fig. 5–5.

Figure 5–4. Normal skin showing arrangement of elastic fibers, stained black. These fibers run between collagen bundles; in superficial dermis they tend to be straight, but in middle dermis they are convoluted or spirillary, apparently looping around collagen. Elastica × 100. (Reproduced by permission from T. Gibson, R. M. Kenedi, and J. E. Craik, Brit. J. Surg. *52*:764, 1965.)

Figure 5–5. Fully stretched skin to show elastic fibers which, for the most part, have been straightened out and lie between collagen bundles. Elastica × 100. (Reproduced by permission from T. Gibson, R. M. Kenedi, and J. E. Craik, Brit. J. Surg. *52*:764, 1965.)

section area. It is given as pounds per square inch or kilograms per square centimeter (or square millimeter). Breaking strength, on the other hand, is the measure of force required to break a wound (or tissue) without regard to its dimensions. In different areas of the body, breaking strength can vary by several-fold for skin wounds of the same length, but tensile strength may remain constant. This can be due solely to variation in skin thickness. Furthermore, skin thickness may increase with age; thus breaking strength, but not tensile strength, can increase with age. Similarly, breaking strength of a wound can increase, but its tensile strength may stay constant or decrease, solely because of changes in thickness of wound tissue.

We must consider now some practical aspects of strength measurements. When comparing the strength of two homogeneous materials, i.e., wires of different metals of different diameters, tensile strength (force per unit area) is the preferred measurement. The diameter of the wire may be measured with a micrometer, and the force may be measured with a tensiometer. Accurate comparisons between two materials can be made. However, when nonhomogeneous materials are to be compared, the situation is not so simple. Skin is a good example. When we speak of the strength of skin, we speak of the strength of the composite of all the ingredients contained in skin—or do we? What we actually measure in the tensiometer is the strength of the strongest component. Does the presence of cells, water, amorphous ground substance, and so forth, contribute anything to the strength measurement? Consider two pieces of skin whose absolute content of all components, with the exception of water, is the same. One piece of skin is edematous, and one is not. The edematous skin has, let us assume, twice the cross-sectional area of normal skin. When we measure the breaking strength of the two pieces of skin in a tensiometer, we find the values equal, but when we calculate tensile strength, edematous skin has half the strength of normal skin. Which value should we use?

Here is a situation in which practical considerations must prevail. Is a surgeon interested in tensile strength or breaking strength? The surgeon wants to know how much force is required to disrupt skin. Thus he is interested in breaking strength. A scientist, on the other hand, may be interested in both measurements since comparison of breaking strength with tensile strength tells him that something was added to edematous skin which did not contribute to its strength.

While this comparison between edematous and normal skin is an oversimplification, since edema probably does weaken the breaking strength of skin by interfering with collagen fibril adhesion and in-

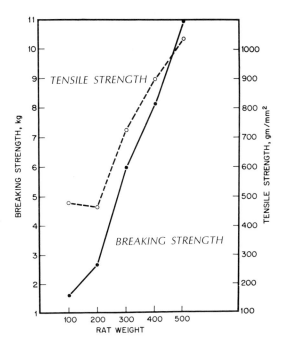

Figure 5–6. Breaking and tensile strength of unwounded rat skin as a function of rat weight. Note the lack of correlation between the two measurements in rats weighing 100 to 200 grams and the steep rise in both values with increasing age. The fact that both measurements rise indicates that the absolute strength of skin is increasing, as well as the thickness of skin. (Reproduced by permission from S. M. Levenson, E. F. Geever, L. V. Crowley, J. R. Oates, C. W. Berard, and H. Rosen, Ann. Surg. *161*:293, 1965.)

terlocking, the point to be made is that in most clinical situations, breaking strength provides information of importance to the surgeon.

When we consider tissues such as bowel wall, which is composed of distinct layers, we have an even more complicated situation. Usually only one layer determines breaking strength. Thus, to get a true reading of tensile strength, we should measure the cross-sectional area of this layer only. While this probably can be done with sophisticated optical micrometers, it is hardly worth the effort in terms of information to be gained.

Another problem is measurement of wound strength in hollow viscera such as stomach, bowel, and bladder. Some investigators have used "burst" strength and some have used breaking strength. The results obtained by the two methods are usually vastly different.

The usual method of measuring "burst" strength is to tie off two ends of the hollow viscus, insert a cannula into the lumen, and inflate the organ with air or liquid. The pressure at which rupture occurs is termed burst strength. It is argued that this method more closely approximates the clinical situation, since it is the force of distention that will rupture the anastomosis in a segment of intestine. Many workers, however, have neglected Laplace's law which defines the pressure-wall tension relationships in hollow organs. This law is a simple one:

$$T = P\left(\frac{1}{R_1} + \frac{1}{R_2}\right)$$

where T = wall tension (dynes/cm.), P = transmural pressure (dynes/cm.²), R_1, R_2 = principal radii of curvature (cm.).

In the case of a sphere (bladder, for instance), $R_1 = R_2$ and the formula becomes:

$$T = \frac{PR}{2}$$

In the case of a cylinder (intestine, for instance), we must distinguish between tension in the longitudinal direction and tension in the circular direction. In the longitudinal direction, the tension-pressure relationship is:

$$T_{long} = \frac{PR}{2}$$

and in the circular direction it is:

$$T_{circ} = PR$$

However, because of sutures, fibrosis, or other factors, the radius of curvature at an anastomotic site is not the same as the radius of curvature of the uninvolved bowel. Thus, if the radius of the uninvolved bowel is R, and the radius at the anastomosis is R_a, the ratio of the respective tensions at these sites will be:

$$\frac{T_{circ}}{T_{circ\ (anast)}} = \frac{R}{R_a}$$

It is obvious, therefore, that a simple measurement of pressure at the time of disruption does not measure the force (or strength) of the anastomosis since this will be equal to:

$$T_{circ\ (anast)} = \frac{R_a(T_{circ})}{R}$$

The two radii may be measured, but the tension on the uninvolved bowel is usually not measured. Even assuming this tension to be constant, it is generally impractical to measure both radii at the time of bursting. The only really practical way to study wound strength in viscera is to measure the breaking strength of excised strips of wall in a tensiometer.

The foregoing discussion may appear to be somewhat erudite and of interest only to laboratory scientists. This is not so; surgeons must evaluate laboratory data that bear on clinical problems. If they are unaware of the pitfalls of measurement, they may draw erroneous conclusions. Just because someone gives mathematical or numerical data does not necessarily mean that the data reflect reality. An understanding of methodology is a key to critical evaluation.

MECHANICAL ASPECTS OF HEALING INCISIONS

Most studies of the healing wound prior to 1929 were made on excised surface wounds and were concerned with the rate and extent of contraction and epithelization. In 1929 pioneering studies on the rate of gain of tensile strength of skin, fascial, muscle, and gastric wounds in the dog were reported. As with excised wounds, a so-called lag phase was observed extending from the time of wounding until postoperative day 4 to 6. During the lag phase, tensile strength did not increase and the wound appeared to be quiescent. Tensile strength then increased rapidly, reaching a maximal value around the fourteenth to sixteenth postoperative day. This phase of wound healing was identified as the period of fibroplasia. Restoration of mechanical integrity of the wound was attributed to the fibroplastic phase, which, as was subsequently shown, is not altogether correct. It was also shown that the rate of fibroplasia is the same in all common laboratory animal species. It was noted, however, that the time needed for scars to gain the original strength in tissue varies with the species. This was attributed to differences in ultimate strength to be attained.

During the lag phase or, more properly termed, the proliferative phase, wound debris must be disposed of, fibroblasts must be mobilized, and circulation must be restored. This sequence of events has been described in previous chapters. It should be noted, however, that it is during this phase that the wound is most susceptible to infection and this susceptibility is directly related to the extent of trauma and the amount of undebrided necrotic material remaining in the wound. In large open wounds, the necessity for debridement is readily recognized by the surgeon; it is equally important in clean incised wounds, but the need for it is usually unrecognized because the debris is microscopic. Nevertheless, tissue crushed by forceps or by heavy-handed retractor holders can form a pabulum for subsequent infection. Thus, gentle handling of tissue, meticulous hemostasis, and avoidance of dead space where tissue fluid may accumulate are important in the speedy healing of wounds.

Variations in Normal Healing Rate

The variability in healing rate among individual animals has been observed by a number of workers, and the fact that wound tensile strength never reaches that of the original tissue has been repeatedly demonstrated.

The rate of tensile strength gain of incisions made in the lumbo-dorsal aponeurosis of rabbits has been measured. Contrary to the reported rate for healing of skin wounds, it was found that the rate of gain of strength in fascia was slow, about 50 per cent of the original strength being regained at 50 days and only about 80 per cent at one year after operation. Similarly, the progress of healing in another predominantly fibrous tissue, tendon, has been measured, and the time required to achieve maximal tensile strength was found to be quite

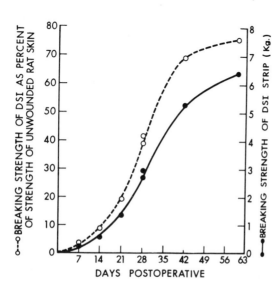

Figure 5–7. Increase in breaking strength of a healing wound shown absolutely and as a percentage of strength of comparable unwounded skin. Note that the strength of the wound levels off at about 80 per cent of the strength of unwounded skin. DSI = dermal skin incision. (Reproduced by permission from S. M. Levenson, E. F. Geever, L. V. Crowley, J. F. Oates, C. W. Berard, and H. Rosen, Ann. Surg. *161*:293, 1965.)

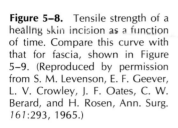
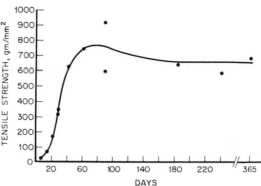

Figure 5–8. Tensile strength of a healing skin incision as a function of time. Compare this curve with that for fascia, shown in Figure 5–9. (Reproduced by permission from S. M. Levenson, E. F. Geever, L. V. Crowley, J. F. Oates, C. W. Berard, and H. Rosen, Ann. Surg. 161:293, 1965.)

prolonged. The usual lag period was observed, and this was followed by a period of very rapid gain in tensile strength which reached a plateau at about the fourteenth or sixteenth postoperative day. A small second increase in tensile strength was seen after three weeks, but if active motion was permitted, a rapid increase in strength occurred. If motion was permitted during the lag phase or fibroplastic phase of healing, either no effect or retardation of healing occurred, depending on whether separation of the wound occurred. However, motion during the third phase caused a marked acceleraion of healing. Tension also increases the tensile strength of aponeurotic wounds and the effect is evident from the seventh through the twenty-first day.

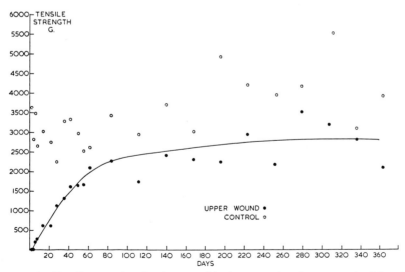

Figure 5–9. Tensile strength gain of a wound in the upper dorsal aponeurosis of the rabbit compared to the strength of unwounded fascia (*open circles*). Note the tendency for the unwounded fascia to gain strength with increasing age of the animal. Nevertheless, the wound at no time reaches the strength of the unwounded tissue. (Reproduced by permission from D. M. Douglas, Brit. J. Surg. 40:79, 1952.)

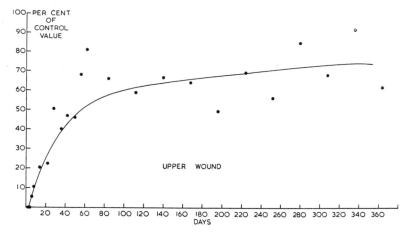

Figure 5–10. Tensile strength gain of a wound in the lower dorsal aponeurosis of the rabbit, expressed as a percentage of the tensile strength of unwounded fascia at the same time period. Note the exponential form of the curve and the fact that the wound reaches only about 80 per cent of the control value after one year. (Reproduced by permission from D. M. Douglas, Brit. J. Surg. *40*:79, 1952.)

The rate of healing varies not only among species but also among tissues in the same animal. Since data on mechanical properties of human wounds are not readily available, this discussion will have to concern itself with animal wounds. However, it has been observed that the differences among various tissues and organs in their pattern of healing are qualitatively the same among a wide variety of species. This gives us a little confidence in predicting that these observations probably hold for human wounds as well.

It has been observed that the rate at which all wounds gain strength is approximately the same during the first 14 to 21 days after wounding. However, the percentage of normal, unwounded strength that is gained by the wound varies markedly with the tissue. In general, there is an inverse ratio between normal breaking strength of the tissue and the percentage of that strength that the wound regains in 14 to 21 days. In the case of skin, only 20 to 30 per cent of "normal" strength is attained, whereas the bladder wound has achieved 100 per cent of strength of normal bladder wall. Stomach and colon wounds reach about 65 to 70 per cent of normal strength of these organs in 21 days. Fascia, on the other hand, has less than 20 per cent of strength of unwounded fascia at 14 to 21 days. This suggests that the absolute gain of strength in this early phase of wound healing is related to biochemical events occurring in the wound, which are the same in all tissues. The gain in strength is apparently limited by the rapidity with which these universal events occur.

The period from 3–5 to 14–21 days has been termed the fibroblastic phase of repair. It is during this period that fibroblasts multiply in the wound and lay down collagen. These fibroblasts do not know what tissue they are in. They carry on the process of wound repair irrespective of location of the wound. This is well illustrated by the healing of colon wounds.

Normal wall strength of the colon increases from the ileocecal valve to the rectosigmoid junction; at the latter location, breaking strength of colon is about twice that of cecum. A linear wound in the colon extending from the cecum to the sigmoid will have the same breaking strength at one end as at the other. However, the percentage of normal strength regained at 14 days in the sigmoid is only half of that regained in the cecum. In other words, the repair mechanism is oblivious to its location in the colon.

After this phase of fibroplasia, differences among wounds in different tissues and organs become apparent. Skin and fascial wounds continue to gain strength; the rate of gain becomes gradually less as time goes on, but even after a year there may be some slight gain in strength. Of more importance to the surgeon and the patient is the observation that even after a year wounds in skin and fascia are 15 to 20 per cent weaker than normal surrounding tissue.

Stomach and colon wounds show a markedly different behavior. After 14 to 21 days, the strength gain almost abruptly ceases. Very little gain in strength is measurable after the twenty-first day, up through the 120th day, the longest period such wounds have been followed. These wounds cease to gain strength at a time when they have achieved only 65 to 70 per cent of strength of normal tissue. There are also biochemical differences in these wounds as compared to skin and fascial wounds which will be discussed later in this chapter.

The observations just reported, made in dogs, appear to hold for all species of animal studied, with one exception. This exception has to do with the percentage of normal strength gained by the wound. In rabbits, visceral wounds appear to attain the strength of normal tissue, or exceed it within 14 to 21 days. Whether these differences among species are related to size, diet, or other factors is not known. Thus, the pattern of healing is similar but the extent to which the wound heals, as measured by breaking strength, appears to vary with species.

It is important to point out that although there are differences in healing among tissues, the end result of healing is identical: the formation of a fibrous scar. We must look more deeply into the biochemical mechanisms operating in the formation and maintenance of these scars if we are to understand what lies behind these differences.

BIOCHEMISTRY OF HEALING WOUNDS

Our knowledge of the biochemistry of wound healing is of fairly recent origin. Wound healing studies made prior to about 1940 were concerned with excised rather than incised wounds. Nevertheless, it was recognized that wounds do not have strength until fibrous tissue appears and bridges the area of the incision. However, most investigators were more concerned with the cells involved than their products. As we shall see, the products are what hold the wound together, and the cells are the factories that produce them.

Collagen and Wound Tensile Strength

It was mentioned before that early work emphasized the biochemical events in the healing wound that correlated with the changing mechanical properties. It was shown that during the so-called lag phase the major biochemical event is rapid production of ground substance. The measurement of ground substance production was the increase in hexosamine in the wound. It is now known that much of this hexosamine is derived from serum glycoprotein which leaks into the wound from the circulation in the early period immediately after injury.

During the fibroplastic phase of healing, increasing tensile strength parallels the rise in collagen content of the wound. The concentration of bound hexosamine in the wound immediately after infliction is the same as the plasma concentration, and decreases progressively thereafter. This must, therefore, represent serum glycoprotein and probably is not involved in the process of fibroplasia.

Collagen content and tensile strength of a wound may move in opposite directions. This may be more apparent than real because of the inherent error in tissue tensile strength measurements and because the wound in its early stages may have varying amounts of inflammatory tissue that does not contribute to its strength.

The biochemical studies that have been described so far point to two major components in the healing wound which appear to vary and with which some positive or negative correlation with tensile strength gain has been demonstrated. Since collagen is a fibrous protein and the hexosamine-containing component is amorphous, it is only logical to assume that the former contributes more to the total tensile strength of the wound. This, however, is not the whole story of wound tensile strength, as we shall see.

The problem of obtaining wound tissue, free of normal tissue, for biochemical analysis is a difficult one. An ingenious method of harvesting wound tissue and simultaneously correlating the biochemical studies with tensile strength changes has been described. Cellulose sponges were used to induce the formation of granulation tissue. One sponge was divided in half and then sewn together with cotton thread and implanted subcutaneously. At various times it was taken out, the thread was removed, and the force required to separate the two halves was measured. Since the two halves were held together only by newly synthesized wound tissue, an accurate tensile strength measurement of that tissue was obtained. The tissue in the sponge could then be submitted to biochemical analysis. A small amount of collagen appeared in the sponge within a few hours after implantation. The source of this collagen was not determined, and it could be either recently synthesized or recently depolymerized from damaged preexisting fibers. However, the gain in tensile strength of the new tissue roughly paralleled its amount—at least in the phase of active fibroplasia.

It should be remarked, however, that in every instance the gain in strength of a skin wound in the same animal was greater than that of granulation tissue in the sponge. Hexosamine increased slightly to day 7 and then decreased slowly. Uronic acid, a measure of glycoprotein, also increased slightly to day 7 and declined slowly thereafter. The changes in these substances appeared to be unrelated to tensile strength. Hydroxyproline, a measure of collagen concentration, increased rapidly beginning at day 4, with the highest rate seen between days 5 and 12, a lesser rate of increase between days 12 and 21 and a markedly lower rate from day 21 to day 60. The greatest part of the collagen was insoluble.

Many investigators have noted that tensile strength continues to increase for a considerable period after collagen content of the wound has stabilized. It is known that formaldehyde fixation of a wound increases its breaking strength and that this effect is more marked in young (up to six or seven weeks) than in old wounds. This finding is interpreted to indicate that the late gain of tensile strength of a wound is more closely related to cross-linking of the already formed collagen fibers than to the amount of collagen present. It should be noted, however, that there is increasing evidence that even an old scar is in a state of dynamic equilibrium and that some collagen is constantly being synthesized and broken down. This dynamic activity appears to be confined to a zone approximately 15 mm. around the wound. Studies of the rate of collagen synthesis in wounds have shown that although the rate is highest around the fourteenth day, it remains significantly higher than in unwounded skin up to 70 days. The gain in tensile strength correlates with the *rate* of collagen synthesis through the first ten weeks of healing.

The preceding discussion applies primarily to skin wounds on which most observations have been made. Visceral wounds apparently do not gain strength after the period of fibroplasia is over. As will be discussed later in this chapter, the rate of collagen synthesis remains markedly elevated subsequent to the fibroplastic phase, but collagen content decreases and strength remains unchanged. In skin, however, the rate of collagen synthesis remains elevated but gradually decreases to approach normal after four to six months, but strength gain still continues. We shall examine this in more detail when we consider wound strength in relation to cross-linking.

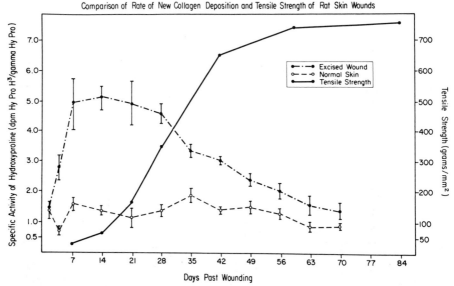

Figure 5–11. Relation of the rate of collagen synthesis to the tensile strength of rat skin wounds. (Reproduced by permission from J. W. Madden and E. E. Peacock, Jr., Surgery *64:* 288, 1968. Tensile strength curve taken from S. M. Levenson, et al., Ann. Surg. *161:*293, 1965.)

Mucopolysaccharides and Wound Tensile Strength

The lack of correlation of hexosamine or uronic acid content of wounds with the rate of tensile strength gain has been alluded to in the foregoing discussion. However, not all workers believe that these substances do not have an effect on wound healing. Histologic studies

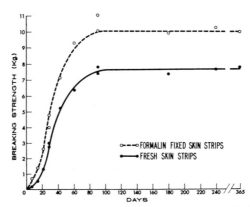

Figure 5–12. Breaking strength of skin strips taken from a rat wound, showing the effect of formaldehyde fixation on the breaking strength. (Reproduced by permission from S. M. Levenson, E. F. Geever, L. V. Crowley, J. F. Oates, C. W. Berard, and H. Rosen, Ann. Surg. *161:*293, 1965.)

at first appeared to indicate that in scurvy there is a failure to produce acid mucopolysaccharides. Staining methods to identify specific chemical substances are, however, notoriously unreliable. With chemical methods, it has been shown that wounds in scorbutic guinea pigs develop about five times as much mucopolysaccharide as do wounds in normal animals and that the predominant component is hyaluronic acid. Since the scorbutic wound has little or no tensile strength, but has adequate amounts of mucopolysaccharides, these cannot, of themselves, contribute directly to wound strength.

Using subcutaneously implanted steel mesh cylinders to harvest wound tissue, it has been found, by histochemical techniques, that there is a very rapid rise of acid mucopolysaccharides in the wound tissue within the cylinders during the first three weeks. Their level remains constant until the eighth week and then returns to control levels by the twelfth week. The neutral mucopolysaccharides do not show an increase until after the third week, and then increase steadily throughout the 32 week period that they have been observed. Glycoproteins predominate in the early phases of wound healing, and then acid mucopolysaccharides appear, first as hyaluronic acid and then as chondroitin sulfate. Some have postulated that these substances are in some way linked to collagen fiber formation.

At various times it has been suggested that different globular proteins or glycoproteins contribute significant strength to a wound. Definitive studies have shown, however, that only fibrous proteins have significant mechanical strength and, of these, collagen has by far the greatest strength. Observations of early wounds in which fibrin (a fibrous protein) is deposited have shown this material to be replaced by collagen. The suggestion was advanced that fibrin was chemically converted to collagen. Now that the sequential structure of these proteins is fairly well known, it is recognized that such a conversion is not possible. As was described in earlier chapters, fibroblasts migrate along fibrin fibers and secrete collagen. Capillaries forming behind advancing fibroblasts produce a fibrinolysin which removes fibrin. Thus there is a superficial appearance of fibrin being replaced by collagen.

In an attempt to define more precisely the role of mucopolysaccharides in wound healing, the effect of testicular hyaluronidase on wound collagen and on cell content as measured by deoxyribonucleic acid (DNA) was studied. Both collagen and DNA were depressed. The effect on collagen was most marked on the sixth day of healing. It was hypothesized that depolymerization of mucopolysaccharides delayed formation of collagen by one day and that mucopolysaccharides were essential for collagen formation. Unfortunately, examination of these data is not convincing that hyaluronidase produced any real effect. An anabolic steroid was also given to animals and it was reported that there was an increase in tensile strength of wounds over control animals. There was no difference in hydroxyproline content or in content of

DNA. There was, however, an increase in uptake of ^{35}S in the wound. This was alleged to be due to an increase in sulfated mucopolysaccharides. Examination of the data on tensile strength raises very serious doubts about the reality of the differences shown. The method used to measure strength was not well described but, as has been pointed out, there are numerous errors and variations that tend to make small differences meaningless. Furthermore, some statistical manipulations were performed which allegedly showed the differences to be significant. Actually, what was shown was that there was a significant difference between two *estimated* regression lines, but this does not necessarily mean that there was a significant difference between the sets of original data. Even if tensile strengths were different, the conclusion that "collagen . . . may not be an essential agent for healing" is completely unsupported. In fact, practically all the evidence discussed so far tends to prove that it is the single most important element in healing.

With chemical isolation procedures, the nature of mucopolysaccharide components of healing wounds has been established. Both chondroitin sulfate A and chondroitin sulfate B (dermatan sulfate) have been isolated. These two mucopolysaccharides account for less than 20 per cent of the hexosamine in wound granulation tissue. The remaining portion appears to be unidentified glycoproteins. Individual mucopolysaccharides have been followed quantitatively during healing and the chondroitin sulfates were found to increase steadily from the fifth to the seventeenth day of healing. Hyaluronic acid content, on the other hand, fell from the fifth to the tenth day and then remained relatively constant at a low concentration throughout the remainder of the healing process.

Mercuric chloride will increase tensile strength of wounds in a manner similar to that of formaldehyde. The effect of mercuric chloride could not be explained by cross-linking of collagen. In fact, the effect could be seen in three-day wounds when no discernible collagen was present. Thus, substances other than collagen can contribute to wound strength. The same conclusion has been reached by other workers, who studied the effects of sulfhydryl compounds, cyanide, thiols, and borohydride on tensile strength of skin. It was found that 10^{-3} M potassium cyanide increased tensile strength of rat tail skin strips by 50 to 100 per cent at pH 7.5, and at pH 6.0 the increase was threefold to fivefold. Thioglycollate, mercaptoethanol, cysteamine, cysteine, and reduced glutathione produced a marked reduction of tensile strength of rat tail skin strips at pH 6.0 to 7.5. These agents had no effect on strips of reconstituted, purified collagen. Sodium borohydride increased tensile strength of skin strips and prevented lowering of tensile strength upon the addition of thiols or increase of strength observed with cyanide. If tissue was previously treated with a thiol, sodium borohydride had no effect. These results are consonant with what we know about cross-linking in collagen. The cross-links composed of unreduced Schiff bases are susceptible to oxidizing agents and acid. Thus, any chemical that tends to disrupt these linkages will reduce the strength of collagen fibers. Treatment with borohydride is the standard method of stabilizing the Schiff base cross-links. Furthermore, cyanide ion will react with the double bond in the unreduced Schiff base and likewise stabilize the structure. Thus, the observed results with cyanide are in agreement with what we know about collagen cross-link chemistry.

Collagen Cross-Linking and Wound Tensile Strength

Most of the discussion regarding substances other than collagen which contribute to tensile strength of wounds has dealt with the early phase of healing. Certainly, within the first 24 hours after wounding, a properly coapted wound has an appreciable strength. This is not due to collagen, since appreciable amounts of collagen are not present until after the fourth or fifth day. Epidermal repair, where collagen is not involved, results in appreciable tensile strength. This suggests that epidermis is largely responsible for wound strength up to five days post incision. Most of this strength is derived from the adhesive forces existing among epithelial cells. However, until these cells have migrated across the wound, the only substance likely to contribute strength to the wound is the fibrin of the clot.

With formation of granulation tissue, capillaries grow into the wound space. Even capillaries and small blood vessels can contribute some strength to an early wound. This is particularly apparent in the "take" of skin grafts. As soon as capillaries from the graft bed invade the graft itself, the graft becomes fixed and appreciable force is required to dislodge it. At this time, collagen synthesis and deposition do not play a prominent part in healing and virtually the only connection between graft and host are the invading capillaries.

Turning our attention now to the later phases of healing, the question arises as to the role of noncollagenous substances in the ultimate mechanical properties of wounds. It has been pointed out already that tensile strength of a wound continues to increase for a considerable period when the collagen content of the wound is not increasing or is actually decreasing. This could be due to a further interaction of collagen with components of ground substance, or it could be due to a qualitative change in the collagen fiber itself, or both reactions might be occurring.

Qualitative alterations in collagen of the wound can bring about changes in mechanical properties. We have already mentioned the effects of formaldehyde. Deuterium oxide will increase the melt temperature of collagen. On the basis of reasoning that *in vivo* this should

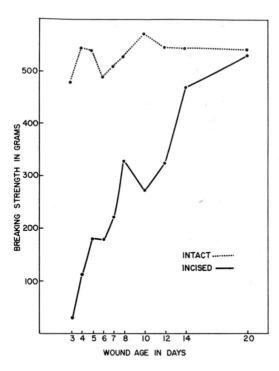

Figure 5–13. Breaking strength of epidermal incisions as a function of wound age. The upper curve represents the breaking strength of test strips, 4 mm. wide, of intact guinea pig skin. The bottom curve represents the breaking strength of similar strips of epidermis taken across an epidermal incision at various intervals after wounding. Note that the greatest increase in rate of strength gain is in the period three to five days after wounding. At this time little or no collagen synthesis will have occurred in a wound and, thus, nearly all of the strength will be due to the mutual adhesion of the newly migrated and proliferated epidermal cells. (Reproduced by permission from D. T. Rovee and C. A. Miller, Arch. Surg. 96:43, 1968.)

increase tensile strength of wounds, deuterium oxide has been fed to rats during the period of wound healing. Contrary to expectation, the animals fed heavy water showed a 40 per cent lower tensile strength than control animals. However, when wound tissue was fixed in formaldehyde, wounds from deuterium oxide-treated animals gained more strength than wounds from controls. This suggested that although deuterium may have stabilized the collagen helix, it interfered in some way with intermolecular cross-linking.

The importance of cross-links between collagen molecules and physical weave of collagen fibers in contributing to tensile strength of wounds has been emphasized by us. It has been suggested that these may be more important than the amount of collagen present between wound edges. It has been shown that by administering formaldehyde or 1-ethyl-3-(3-dimethylaminopropyl)carbodiimide directly to the wound, tensile strength could be increased and the effect could be produced at any time from the third to the forty-second day of healing. Both of these agents introduce cross-links into collagen, and it seems probable, therefore, that increased tensile strength was due solely to increased cross-linking. It has also been suggested that increases in tensile strength of skin with age are due to increasing cross-linking of collagen fibers.

On the basis of all of the evidence accumulated so far, it seems fair to say that during the lag phase of healing, the principal contributor of tensile strength is fibrin in the wound, and as it migrates and pro-liferates, epidermis can contribute substantially to strength. There is no evidence at all that glycoproteins, mucopolysaccharides, or other ele-ments of ground substance make any contribution to tensile strength at this stage. During the period from about day 5 to perhaps day 30, the evidence is overwhelming that almost all the tensile strength of the wound is due to its collagen content.

LATHYRISM, COLLAGEN CROSS-LINKING, AND WOUND STRENGTH. Perhaps the most convincing evidence of the importance of collagen, and particularly cross-linked collagen, in the tensile strength of wounds is derived from studies on lathyrism, which has been discussed in Chapter 4. This chemically induced disease affects connective tissue. The effects observed are related to a complete loss of structural stability of newly formed connective tissue including bones, tendons, and ligaments. Arteries may show aneurysmal dilatations and even rup-ture. Healing wounds in the lathyritic animal show markedly reduced tensile strength. Fiber formation is markedly decreased and those that are present fail to form large bundles. As was discussed in Chapter 4, the defect is due to a failure of cross-link formation in collagen due to blockage of an enzyme which oxidatively deaminates a lysine residue in collagen. The aldehyde that is normally formed at this site is essential for cross-linking.

The significance of these studies on lathyrism is that they show that interference with cross-linking of collagen has a profound, and even fatal, effect on the tensile strength of connective tissue including wound tissue. The effect is solely on collagen and hence it is obvious that the major contributor to the tensile strength of wounds is the cross-linked collagen fiber.

Having established that cross-linking is one of the major contribut-ing factors to the strength of collagen and that collagen is the compo-nent of wound and connective tissue that furnishes most of the strength, we can now ask the question. Do the cross-links in wound collagen differ from those in collagen of tissue in which the wound is located? Only preliminary work is currently available to answer this question, but the results are revealing.

Studies were made in guinea pigs. In one year old (adult) animals, open wounds were made and splinted. Granulation tissue that was har-vested and a piece of normal dermis from the same animal were both subjected to purification of their insoluble collagen by salt and EDTA extraction. The lyophilized insoluble collagen was reduced with sodium borotritide, which reduces the unstable cross-links and labels them with tritium. After hydrolysis, analytic chromatography of the labeled com-pounds was performed. This permits identification of the type of cross-link present and gives semiquantitative information regarding the rela-tive amounts of different types of cross-links.

Normal guinea pig dermis was found to have a large amount of hydroxylysinonorleucine and histidino-merodesmosine. The quantity of dihydroxylysinonorleucine was about one-fifth that of hydroxylysinonorleucine.

Guinea pig scar collagen, on the other hand, had large amounts of dihydroxylysinonorleucine and relatively small amounts of hydroxylysinonorleucine and histidino-merodesmosine. The type of collagen present in scar tissue was not identified, but it will be recalled that embryonic collagen is primarily type III whereas adult dermal collagen is primarily type I. One of the differences between type III and type I collagens is the large amount of hydroxylysine in the former and the presence of dihydroxylysinonorleucine as the principal cross-link. Thus, scar collagen resembles the embryonic type or type III. Subsequent to these studies, it was shown that collagen formed in turpentine or carrageenan granulomas was type III collagen. Studies made on normal human scars revealed that early in scar formation, type III collagen was deposited in the wound. During maturation of the scar, type III collagen was gradually replaced by type I collagen. Studies of hypertrophic scars in human beings showed that type III collagen was deposited but replacement by type I collagen did not occur.

These observations suggest that when a fibroblast is first activated, probably by modulation from an undifferentiated mesenchymal cell, the genes responsible for type III collagen synthesis are activated. As these cells mature, the gene for type III collagen is suppressed and that for type I is activated. Why, in the hypertrophic scar, the fibroblast fails to activate the type I gene and repress the type III gene is a fascinating subject for future study.

It is apparent, therefore, that repair, insofar as collagen is concerned, involves a recapitulation of ontogeny. In the wound, the fibroblast lays down embryonic-type collagen. However, as the wound matures this collagen is gradually replaced by the adult type. It is conceivable that the difference between maturation of visceral wounds as compared to that of skin wounds might be related to whether embryonic collagen persists in these wounds and was not replaced with adult-type collagen. Again, this is amenable to experimental investigation. In any event, it seems possible that biochemical studies of a quantitative nature on collagen types and cross-link types may explain many of the mechanical properties of wounds which make them different from normal tissue.

THE SECONDARY WOUND PHENOMENON

Although the observation that a wound inflicted within a week or so after an initial wound heals more rapidly had been made many times by many surgeons, this phenomenon was adequately and precisely demonstrated only relatively recently. An early investigation showed that if symmetrical incisions were made successively in skin of rabbits, the secondary ones healed more rapidly than the primary one. The effect appeared about five days after the primary injury and was maximal between the first and fourth week after that injury. It should be noted that secondary wounds were made on the opposite side of the body from the primary one. This fact led a number of investigators to postulate the existence of a wound hormone as the agent responsible for accelerating the healing of the secondary wound. This concept has been discussed in Chapter 2 in connection with epithelial healing and does not need further elaboration here.

During further investigations of the secondary wound phenomenon, it was discovered that previous observations were due not to an effect of the primary wound but rather to the effect of cold vasoconstriction on healing. In the earlier experiments, animals were depilated over the sites of the primary wound and secondary wounds just before the primary wound was made. However, if the site of the secondary wounds was depilated just before the wounds were inflicted, no difference in healing rate of primary and secondary wounds could be detected. In actual fact, in the original experiments the rate of healing of secondary wounds was not accelerated; the rate of healing in primary wounds was depressed.

However, the usual clinical observations on secondary wounds were made on wounds that for one reason or another had dehisced. If a primary wound was disrupted and then resutured, its rate of healing appeared to be greatly accelerated. This observation has been made

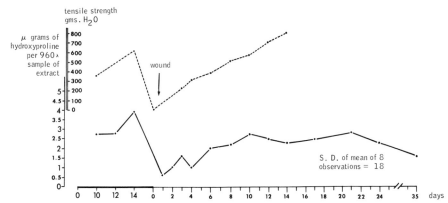

Figure 5–14. Saline-extractable collagen and rate of gain in tensile strength of scar tissue made by dehiscing and resuturing a 14 day old primary wound. *Top curve,* wound strength; *bottom curve,* hydroxyproline content. Note lack of a "lag" phase in the secondary wound and the lowered saline-extractable collagen content of the wound. Presumably, collagen formed during healing of the first wound has become insoluble. (Reproduced by permission from E. E. Peacock, Jr., Surg. Gynec. Obstet. *115*:408, 1962.)

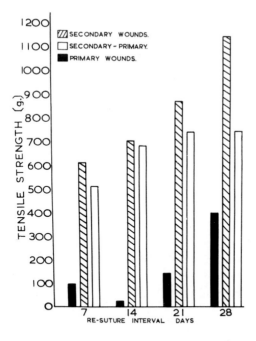

Figure 5–15. Tensile strength values in primary and secondary wounds in skin of rabbits. The clear columns indicate the difference in tensile strength between secondary and primary wounds. Secondary wounds were made by disrupting a primary wound after it had been allowed to heal for seven days. Values for the primary wound were obtained from new wounds made in the same animal at the time secondary wounds were created. (Reproduced by permission from R. R. Ogilvie and D. M. Douglas, Brit. J. Surg. 51:149, 1964.)

clinically by many surgeons, and has been demonstrated experimentally. It has been shown that secondary wounds on the abdomen heal no faster than primary wounds made on the back, but that resutured primary wounds do show a significantly greater tensile strength on the third day after resuture. The effect seems to be due to an immediate onset of fibroplasia, without the usual four to six day lag period. It is felt that there is a specific relation between the inflammatory response elicited by local trauma and subsequent connective tissue response. The response can be abolished by cortisone, provided inflammation is not established.

It cannot be emphasized too strongly that these observations on secondary wounds do not show that the rate of wound healing was increased. Examination of the rate of gain in breaking strength of secondary as compared to primary wounds shows that this rate is exactly the same in both wounds and the ultimate strength attained by secondary wounds is the same as that attained by primary wounds. The sole difference between primary and secondary wounds is the absence of a "lag phase" in the latter. The reason for this is that dehiscence or opening of the original wound did not destroy macrophages and fibroblasts that were present, and that on closure of the secondary wound, the healing process already under way in the original wound merely continued without alteration. No time was required to mobilize and activate cells.

Biochemical studies have been made on primary and secondary wounds in rats. It was found that total collagen, both soluble and insoluble, is decreased in secondary wounds as compared to primary wounds. It was suggested that the rapid gain in tensile strength of secondary wounds might be related more to organization and cross-linking of existing collagen than to its amount. It has also been shown that the secondary healing phenomenon can be abolished by excision of the primary wound as a 1 cm. strip. Thus, the secondary wound effect is a purely local phenomenon and does not involve humoral mechanisms.

One of the main events in the healing of any wound, whether primary or secondary, is the synthesis and deposition of collagen. As was mentioned previously, determination of the amount of collagen in a wound presents difficulties: Where does the wound begin and end? What is newly synthesized collagen and what is old collagen that was already at the wound margin? Collagen can be labeled with either ^{3}H-proline or ^{14}C-proline. During synthesis, part of the incorporated labeled proline is converted to labeled hydroxyproline, an amino acid peculiar to collagen. To obtain adequate labeling of newly synthesized collagen, sufficient labeled proline must be administered to overcome dilution by the body's pool of unlabeled proline. This can be accomplished only in small animals. It is unsuitable for large animals because of the size of the proline pool and the cost of labeled proline.

It is, however, possible to measure the rate of collagen synthesis. Advantage is taken of the fact that tissue removed from the body and placed in suitable buffers will continue metabolic activity for many hours. If labeled proline is added to such a tissue culture, the problem of the proline pool is obviated, and the amount of collagen synthesized during a set period of incubation can be determined by measuring the specific activity of labeled hydroxyproline. Usually four to six hours' incubation in the presence of label is sufficient to produce adequate amounts of labeled hydroxyproline.

The rate of collagen synthesis has been measured in a number of wounds in different organs. In skin wounds, the rate of collagen synthesis rises rapidly, reaching a peak around five to seven days post wounding. It then declines gradually, reaching the level of normal unwounded skin at about 120 days. The picture is much the same for other organs that have been studied, i.e., the peak rate of synthesis is seen early in healing at about 5 to 7 days. However, in the case of stomach and colon wounds, the decline in rate of synthesis is less than that observed with skin wound, and at 120 days the rate of collagen synthesis in stomach wounds is twice that of normal stomach wall. In colon wounds, at 120 days, the rate of collagen synthesis is five times that of uninjured colon wall.

It will be recalled that after 14 to 21 days, and during the period when the rate of collagen synthesis is markedly elevated, the strength of stomach and colon wounds remains essentially unchanged. During this period, inspection of the wounds reveals that they are becoming perceptibly smaller and, by 120 days, only a very thin scar is visible. Obviously, although collagen is being synthesized at a very high rate, it is being destroyed at an equally great rate. These wounds are, therefore, metabolically highly active.

The high metabolic activity of stomach and colon wounds can be demonstrated in another way. If, after incubation of wound tissue with labeled proline, collagen and noncollagenous proteins are separated by precipitation in hot trichloracetic acid, and the activity of protein-bound labeled proline is measured in the TCA precipitate, it is found that the rate of synthesis of noncollagenous protein is about twice that of normal stomach or colon wall. This increased rate of synthesis was seen throughout the 120-day observation period. In skin and bladder wounds, however, no increase in the rate of noncollagenous protein synthesis was observed at any time during healing.

Collagen synthesis in bladder wounds shows a slightly different pattern. It will be recalled that bladder wounds gained 100 per cent of the strength of normal bladder wall within about 14 days. The rate of collagen synthesis peaks at about seven days and then falls rapidly thereafter. Between 28 and 70 days, it reaches the level of normal bladder wall and, essentially, the events of healing are completed by 70 days.

In Chapter 2 we commented on the evidence for regeneration of the bladder, including smooth muscle and other elements of the organ. If true regeneration was occurring in a bladder, one would expect that the rate of synthesis of noncollagenous protein would be elevated in the wound. Actual measurements, however, reveal that this is not the case. Bladder wounds heal like other wounds, by formation of a fibrous scar.

REMODELING OF WOUND SCAR

The biochemical events leading to maturation of scars have already been discussed. To recapitulate: the main events are gradual intramolecular and intermolecular cross-linking which results in major gains in tensile strength and in stabilization of scar tissue through increasing insolubility of collagen. The weave, the way fibers are arranged in the scar, also has an effect on tensile strength. It has been shown by scanning electron microscopy that the arrangement of collagen fibers in scar tissue is disorganized and distinctly different from that in surrounding tissue. A scar is never as strong as tissue it replaces.

During remodeling of scar tissue, new collagen fibers are being laid down and others are being digested and removed. In general, fibers that remain in a scar are those that are oriented along lines of tension. However, some interweaving of fibers is seen, but the arrange-

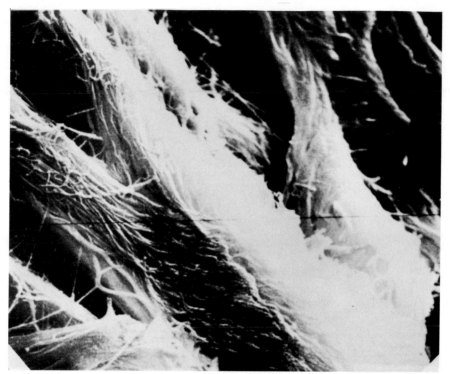

Figure 5–16. Collagen fiber network of normal, unwounded rat skin. Contrast this with Figure 5–18 which shows scar tissue in skin at the same magnification. Scanning electron micrograph. × 3000. (From J. C. Forrester, B. H. Zederfeldt, T. L. Hayes, and T. K. Hunt, in *Repair and Regeneration,* edited by J. E. Dunphy and W. Van Winkle, Jr. Copyright 1969, McGraw-Hill Book Company. Used with permission of McGraw-Hill Book Company.)

ment of fibers in a scar in dermis, for example, is quite different than that in uninjured dermis. As the scar ages, fibers and fiber bundles become more closely packed. This aids in positioning individual collagen polymer chains so that intermolecular cross-linking can take place. As cross-links are formed, collagen becomes more insoluble and more resistant to the action of collagenolytic enzymes.

It should be recognized that for a scar to hold wound edges together, newly formed collagen must be attached physically to old collagen in tissue surrounding the wound. If one observes how a wound ruptures when placed in a tensiometer, the importance of the wound-tissue attachment becomes obvious. This is best seen in testing breaking strength of intestinal wounds. In this organ the interface between wound and normal tissue is more readily visible than in other organs. At five days post healing, rupture occurs precisely at the location of the original incision. At days 14 to 21 rupture almost always occurs lateral to the line of incision, perhaps 2 to 3 mm. on either side

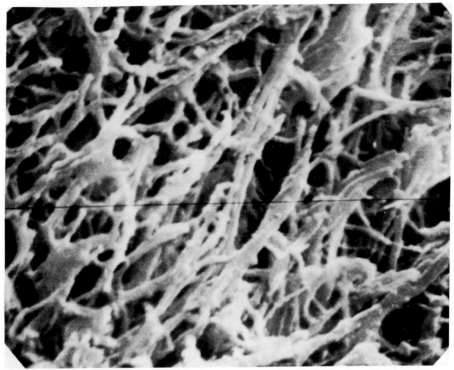

Figure 5–17. Collagen fibers in a ten day old sutured rat skin wound. Note the small fiber size, even at this magnification, and the random arrangement of the network. Scanning electron micrograph. × 10,000. (From J. C. Forrester, B. H. Zederfeldt, T. L. Hayes, and T. K. Hunt, in *Repair and Regeneration,* edited by J. E. Dunphy and W. Van Winkle, Jr. Copyright 1969, McGraw-Hill Book Company. Used with permission of McGraw-Hill Book Company.)

of the central scar, in a line differentiating the wound from normal tissue. Thus, it appears that at this stage of healing the point of greatest weakness is the junction between scar collagen and normal collagen.

Although there is no direct evidence to support this view, it would seem likely that interweaving of both old and newly formed collagen fibers can occur, and that under proper circumstances new collagen fibers can become covalently cross-linked to old, preexisting collagen fibers. That this process is inefficient at best is evidenced by the fact that most healed wounds are weaker than tissue surrounding them.

As water and mucopolysaccharides are lost from the wound, collagen fibers are compressed together. This permits closer approximation of cross-linking sites and thus promotes covalent cross-linking which is the primary event of wound maturation.

We have already commented on the prolonged increased metabolic activity of wounds. In scurvy, both that produced experimentally and that occurring naturally owing to dietary insufficiency, it has been

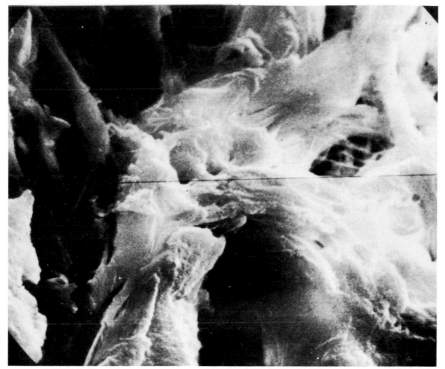

Figure 5–18. Collagen fibers in 100 day old sutured rat skin wound. Note the irregular collagen masses without obvious fibril structure. Compare this illustration with Figure 5–17, taken from a ten day old wound at much higher magnification, and with Figure 5–16, showing the arrangement of collagen fibers in normal rat skin taken at the same magnification. Scanning electron micrograph. × 3000. (From J. C. Forrester, B. H. Zederfeldt, T. L. Hayes, and T. K. Hunt, in *Repair and Regeneration,* edited by J. E. Dunphy and W. Van Winkle, Jr. Copyright 1969, McGraw-Hill Book Company. Used with permission of McGraw-Hill Book Company.)

observed that old wounds tend to weaken and break down. This tendency may well be a reflection of this increased metabolic activity. In a normal wound, synthesis of collagen is depressed but destruction proceeds normally. The result is eventual dissolution of the scar.

Tissue Collagenases

Studies on the remodeling of the tail fin in the metamorphosing amphibian suggested that there might be a specific collagenase responsible for breaking down collagen fibers. The fact that many people had looked for such an enzyme with no success suggested that it did not accumulate in tissues, if it existed at all, and that it might be rapidly inactivated or destroyed. A technique of culturing tissue on a purified, undenatured, collagen gel was developed by means of which the presence

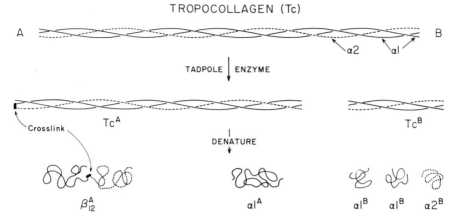

Figure 5–19. Diagrammatic representation of the collagen molecule and pieces resulting from digestion with an enzyme from tadpole. Similar enzymes, with identical actions, have been isolated from a variety of mammalian tissues, including the human. The minor helix of individual chains is not shown; the major helix is not to scale. The letters *A* and *B* refer to designations employed in electron microscopy to distinguish the ends of the molecule. In a sample of extractable collagen some molecules would be cross-linked between $\alpha 1$ and $\alpha 2$ as shown, others between two $\alpha 1$ chains, and some not at all. The denatured products would then include $\alpha 2^A$ and $\beta 11^A$ in addition to those shown. (Reproduced by permission from A. H. Kang, Y. Nagai, K. A. Piez, and J. Gross, Biochemistry 5:509, 1966. Copyright 1966 by the American Chemical Society.)

of the enzyme can be detected visually by noting a clear zone in the opaque gel, or chemically by analysis for soluble, dialyzable hydroxyproline-containing fragments or by release of radioactive tagged hydroxyproline from the gel. With this technique, it was demonstrated that a collagenase is produced by epithelial cells of the metamorphosing tadpole. It was shown that this enzyme is quite different from bacterial collagenase in that it splits the tropocollagen molecule in one place, across all three α chains, leaving two fragments representing one-third and two-thirds of the molecule, respectively. Electron micrographs showed that the triple helix structure is preserved in both fragments.

Since the pioneer work with collagenase of the metamorphosing tadpole, tissue collagenases have been isolated and identified in a variety of tissues and in both invertebrate and vertebrate species. Not all tissue collagenases are identical, as shown by immunochemical studies and differing responses to inhibitors. However, most of these collagenases attack the collagen molecule at a specific site, breaking a glycine-isoleucine bond in the peptide chain in $\alpha 1$-CB7 fragment, and at a comparable site in the $\alpha 2$ chain of type I collagen. Similar fragments have been isolated from the action of collagenase on type II collagen. Definitive studies have not been made on types III or IV collagen, but it seems likely that they are attacked similarly, particularly type III.

Another characteristic of these tissue collagenases is that they are active at neutral pH and, in fact, some of them are inactive at pH 6.0 or lower. Most of these collagenases are inhibited by EDTA and cysteine. A majority are inhibited by serum.

Initially it was believed that collagenase of skin was produced by epithelial cells. This is true in the tadpole and newt. In human skin, however, it is found in the upper layers of dermis and not in epithelium, whereas in open granulating wounds, collagenase is found in migrating epithelium as well as in underlying granulation tissue.

Collagenase has also been found in lysosomes of granulocytes. Unlike skin collagenase, this collagenase is not inhibited by serum.

Two distinct collagenases have been isolated from human rheumatoid synovial fluids. Collagenase B with a molecular weight of 20,000 to 25,000 appears to be identical to that obtained from cultures of synovial cells and, like skin collagenase, it is inhibited by serum. Collagenase A has a molecular weight twice that of enzyme B and is not inhibited by serum. Rheumatoid synovial cells, when cultured on human tendons, have been shown to release collagenases that will digest tendon. Similarly, these collagenases have been shown to attack cartilage. This would seem to explain the destructive effect of the rheumatoid pannus on joints and tendons which it invades.

Since bone is constantly being remodeled, with old collagen being destroyed and new collagen being laid down, it was logical to assume that collagen destruction was due to the presence of a collagenase. Such an enzyme was demonstrated in metaphyseal bone after treatment with parathyroid extract. The enzyme has been isolated and found to act on collagen in the same manner as does skin collagenase. It has been discovered that heparin increases production or release of bone collagenase, and use of this fact has been made in separating and purifying bone collagenase. A heparin-substituted sepharose, 4B gel has been

Table 5-1. *Collagenolytic Activity of Skin, Wound, Eschar, and Scars**
Note the uniformly positive response of the wound margin and granulation tissue. Normal skin shows only slightly more than a 58 per cent response whereas healed scars show a 72 per cent response.

Tissue	*Collagenolysis*	
	Positive	*Negative*
Normal skin	17	12
Wound margin	10	0
Granulation	8	0
Eschar	3	3
Healed scar (including 3 keloids which were positive)	23	9
	61	24

*From W. B. Riley and E. E. Peacock, Jr., Proc. Soc. Exp. Biol. Med. *124*:207, 1967, used by permission.

used for affinity chromatography of bone collagenase preparations. Collagenase is held to heparin by strong ionic bonds. Using this procedure for isolation of the enzyme, it has been shown that pretreatment of the animal with parathyroid hormone extract markedly increases collagenase activity of bone. There is a direct dose-response relationship.

Considerable destruction of collagen occurs in the postpartum uterus. Collagenase has been found in the endometrium and in postpartum uterine tissue cultures. This enzyme not only breaks collagen at the same site as do other tissue collagenases, but also is capable of further attack on the molecule, breaking it down into a number of smaller peptides. It is active at pH 7.0, but completely inactive at pH 6.0. It has also been found that if progesterone is added to cultures of postpartum rat uterus, collagenase activity is completely inhibited. This steroid has no direct effect on collagenase activity; thus, it is action of the hormone on cells producing collagenase that is responsible for the effect. Estradiol and testosterone do not affect collagenase activity.

Collagenase activity has been found in healing colon wounds. The greatest activity occurs shortly after wounding and is not confined to the area of trauma but appears to extend throughout the gastrointestinal tract. This seems to account for various reports that, following colon anastomosis, there is a generalized though temporary diminution in strength of the entire bowel wall with a concomitant lowering of collagen content.

With these observations of the ubiquitous presence of tissue collagenases in various tissues and in wounds, the probable mechanism of wound remodeling becomes clearer. Concomitant with the increased rate of collagen synthesis in the wound which was discussed earlier, there is also an increased collagenolytic activity. Presumably, collagen that is least cross-linked is more readily accessible to the enzyme and is preferentially destroyed. If mechanical tension plays any role in cross-linking, and at present there is only little indirect evidence that it does, then those fibers that are oriented in lines of tension and are performing a useful function in holding the wound together are more resistant to collagenase activity. In this way, the scar is remodeled to provide the best mechanical structure.

SYSTEMIC AND ENVIRONMENTAL FACTORS AFFECTING WOUNDS

Although a large number of factors, both within the patient and in his environment, have been alleged to alter the course of wound healing, only a few are of real clinical significance. The literature on this subject is confusing, owing largely to a plethora of uncontrolled observations and poorly designed experiments. Those factors which have been of most concern to the surgeon will be discussed briefly.

Infection

Infection by some organisms can be a serious deterrent to wound healing. At this point it is necessary to distinguish between infection and contamination. All wounds are contaminated in the sense that no amount of debridement, protection, sterile precautions, and so forth will prevent an occasional airborne or skin bacterium from finding its way into the wound. Fortunately, wound infection is not universal although in many places it is more common than it should be.

Infection occurs when the number of organisms exceeds the ability of local tissue defenses to handle them. The number of organisms that will produce an infection is known and, for most pathogens, is a concentration of 10^6 organisms per gram of tissue. With smaller numbers, local humoral and cellular defenses can dispose of invaders and this is what occurs in contaminated wounds.

Contaminated wounds can become infected wounds. This happens when there is a large amount of necrotic tissue present, when certain types of foreign bodies are in the wound or in its vicinity, or when something interferes with local tissue defenses, such as occurs in burns or in patients receiving immunosuppressant drugs.

In the presence of any of these factors, small quantities of organisms may multiply before adequate defense mechanisms are brought to bear. It does not take long for multiplying pathogenic organisms to reach a concentration of 10^6 per gram, thus converting a contamination to an infection. Obviously, the lower the initial concentration of organisms, the longer it takes to reach the point of infection and the better is the opportunity for local defenses to be mobilized and to attack invaders.

The best way to deal with infection is to prevent it. The best way to prevent infection is meticulous technique. In the traumatized patient this means wide and thorough debridement, meticulous hemostasis and elimination of dead spaces with the use of drains, if necessary. Use of antibiotics is a matter of judgment of whether (1) infection is already present, or (2) adequate wound care cannot, for one reason or another, be given. Blind use of antibiotics as a routine measure is to be condemned. When antibiotics are to be given, there must be a sound biologic reason for their use. This may involve the nature of the wound, the circumstances under which the wound was produced, the condition of the patient, and an assessment of the probable status of his defense mechanism. When all these factors are weighed, the decision can be made as to the appropriateness of antibiotic therapy. If the decision is in favor of giving antibiotics, the sooner they are started the better. It has been amply demonstrated that to be effective antibiotics should be started preoperatively or, at the latest, at the time of operation.

In elective surgery, except perhaps in bowel surgery, it is seldom necessary to give antibiotics. However, assessment of the status of the wound and of the patient should always be made in reaching this decision. It is important to recognize that the level of contamination in an operative wound rises steeply after about one and one-half hours' operative time. Thus, in very prolonged operations it may be advisable to use antibiotics, remembering, however, that they must be started prior to or at the time of surgery. Locally applied antibiotics have not been shown to be of any more value than those systemically administered, and local application of high concentrations of antibiotics may be detrimental by interfering with the healing process.

Protein Nutrition and Wound Tensile Strength

The feeding of a high-protein diet has been shown not to shorten the lag period, but to hasten the rate of tensile strength gain during the fibroblastic phase. Hypoproteinemia has been implicated as one cause of wound disruption by prolonging the lag phase and preventing onset of the fibroplastic phase. This defect can be corrected by administration of lyophilized plasma. However, the decreased rate of wound healing is not well correlated with plasma protein levels and it would seem that the lag phase is not prolonged; rather, fibroplasia is diminished. However, if the serum protein concentration is below 2 grams per 100 ml., wound healing is usually inhibited. The problem is

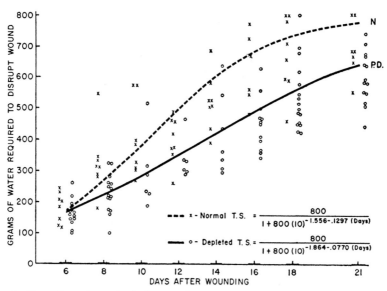

Within the figure:

$$x - \text{Normal T.S.} = \frac{800}{1 + 800 \, (10)^{-1.556 - .1297 \, (\text{Days})}}$$

$$o - \text{Depleted T.S.} = \frac{800}{1 + 800 \, (10)^{-1.864 - .0770 \, (\text{Days})}}$$

Figure 5–20. Effect of protein depletion (*PD*) on rate of gain in tensile strength of rat skin wounds as compared to that of wounds in normal rats (*N*). The abscissa represents days after wounding. (Reproduced by permission from E. E. Peacock, Jr., Proc. Soc. Exp. Biol. Med. *105*:380, 1960.)

complicated by the lack of a clear-cut end point for the lag phase or a definitive beginning of the fibroplastic phase. However, some investigators believe that protein depletion in fascia can lead to wound disruption. It is also reported that rats on a protein-free diet have a prolongation of the lag period of healing. The feeding of dl-methionine to protein-depleted animals has been shown to restore the lag period to its normal length and increase the rate of fibroplasia. This suggests that the effects of protein deficiency are due to the lack of a single specific amino acid. It would appear that an essential amino acid is necessary for the fibroblast to synthesize mucopolysaccharides and collagen and thus complete the fibroplastic phase of wound healing. Later work has shown that methionine is converted to cystine and that this amino acid is the critical one in healing the protein-deficient animal. The full explanation of the mechanism by which cystine brings about its beneficial effect is not known. It may be that cystine is needed as a component of one of the cellular enzymes concerned in the synthesis of collagen.

The recent discovery of the existence of procollagen, which contains nonhelical peptides attached to the amino and carboxyl terminus, and which may be required for assembly of the triple-helix structure, suggests that methionine or cystine supplementation may have a direct effect on collagen synthesis. These "registration" peptides contain several residues of cysteine. It has been suggested that formation of disulfide bonds between registration peptides provides for proper alignment of the chains to form a triple helix. Thus, sulfur-containing amino acids in the diet may contribute to collagen synthesis. This, of course, does not rule out the need for methionine or cystine as a component of one of the specific enzymes needed in collagen synthesis.

The fact that the first collagen deposited in healing wounds is type III collagen may be another reason why methionine and cystine are important nutritional factors in wound healing. Type III collagen contains cystine in contradistinction to other collagens. A severe deficiency of sulfur-containing amino acids might interfere with synthesis of type III collagen.

It is obvious that if the essential building blocks are not available a wound cannot be repaired. Likewise, a proper milieu is required. For instance, it has been shown that dehydration delays healing, but moderate edema has little or no effect on tensile strength gain. However, marked edema has a slight and temporary inhibiting effect on healing. This effect may be more mechanical than biochemical in nature. It should be noted, however, that wounds normally have an excess water content early in healing, and this should not be regarded as edema.

The recent availability of parenteral hyperalimentation has eliminated many postoperative nutritional deficiencies that can prolong or stop wound healing. However, long-continued use of hyperalimentation can also have untoward consequences and this form of nutrition cannot be relied upon for long periods of time. Failure of wounds to heal while the patient is receiving hyperalimentation is usually due not to nutritional problems but to mechanical problems, such as end fistulas, which may be a result of the condition for which hyperalimentation was deemed necessary. A fuller discussion of this subject is given in the chapter on visceral wounds.

Vitamin C and Wound Healing

Probably the first biochemical observation on wound healing was that of the relation of vitamin C to the healing process and to the integrity of wounds. It became evident that vitamin C is in some way connected with production of intercellular substances. This observation led some surgeons to attribute many deficiencies in wound healing to a suboptimal vitamin C intake. However, it was found that although tensile strength of wounds in guinea pigs varied with the daily dose of vitamin C, saturation with the vitamin was not essential to optimal healing. The primary defect in ascorbic acid deficiency was eventually recognized to be failure of fibroblasts to produce collagen. No diminution in tissue collagen can normally be found in scorbutic animals as compared to normal animals of the same weight. However, the metabolism of mature collagen is at such a low level, and animals with acute scurvy cannot be kept alive sufficiently long, that changes in normal structures are not seen.

With application of modern biochemical techniques to the study of scorbutic wounds, the changes in hexosamine and collagen in the wounds of normal and scorbutic guinea pigs were compared. In the normal animal, hexosamine increased up to day 4 and then decreased, leveling off at day 12 to 16. Collagen started to increase at day 4 and began to level off at day 16. In the scorbutic animal, however, hexosamine continued to increase after day 4 and did not show any downward trend until after day 12. Collagen rose only slightly over that seen at day 4 during the entire period of observation. It was concluded that the basic defect in scurvy was one of collagen synthesis. It was later shown that early increases in hexosamine were due to serum glycoproteins and were not related to fibroblastic activity. This has been discussed in Chapter 4.

Collagen formation in embryonic tissue cultures has been investigated and the conclusion was reached that synthesis of "normal" or "metabolic" collagen may not require ascorbic acid, but the requirement for rapid synthesis, as in a wound, may necessitate this vitamin. Even in the scorbutic animal a small degree of wound healing takes place; this fact agrees with these concepts. Wound scars in animals whose wounds have healed a long time previously lose strength and rupture easily when the animals are made scorbutic. It has been found that ascorbic acid accumulates in the scar and persists in this location

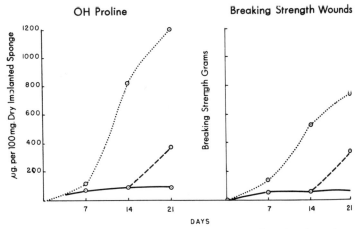

Figure 5–21. Relationship of hydroxyproline content of implanted polyvinyl sponge and breaking strength of wounds in same animal. Dotted lines represent animals fed 2 mg./day vitamin C; solid lines denote animals fed no vitamin C; dashed lines represent animals repleted with 2 mg./day vitamin C at the denoted time. (Reproduced by permission from S. M. Levenson, L. V. Crowley, E. F. Geever, H. Rosen, and C. W. Berard, J. Trauma 4:543, 1964. Copyright 1964, The Williams & Wilkins Co., Baltimore, Md. 21202, U.S.A.)

for long periods of time. Isotope studies indicate that there is a constant turnover of ascorbic acid in scar tissue since part of the vitamin is always derived from recently administered ascorbic acid. Fractionation of scar tissue reveals that ascorbic acid is concentrated in connective tissue and parallels high concentrations found in other connective tissues of the body. Until relatively recently, no satisfactory explanation for the effect of scurvy on old scars could be given. The role of vitamin C in collagen synthesis and the dynamics of scar maintenance have been discussed in Chapter 4, and these older observations can now be seen to fit very well into current concepts.

Anemia and Blood Loss

That severe anemia appears to interfere with wound healing has been observed and reported many times. Anemia has been produced by hemorrhage, and with blood volume restored with plasma, hematocrits were reduced to less than 50 per cent of the prehemorrhage level. No effect on wound tensile strength gain under these conditions is seen by one group of workers, whereas others have reported a sharp reduction in tensile strength of healing wounds. Progressive nutritional anemia in rats which results in hemoglobin levels of 5 to 7 grams per 100 ml. of blood did not cause any difference in healing rates between anemic and control animals for either incisional or open wounds.

It is now recognized that healing wounds depend upon the local microcirculation to furnish needed oxygen and nutriments. Anything that interferes with the microcirculation will inhibit wound healing. Thus, in anemia, particularly that due to blood loss, there will be varying degrees of hypovolemia. It has been well demonstrated that hypovolemia is the major deterrent to wound healing in anemia, hemorrhage, and shock. Wounds will heal in the presence of severe degrees of anemia provided the blood volume is adequate. In severe trauma, microvascular coagulation or sludging may contribute to interference with wound oxygenation and nutrition; thus, even though blood volume is restored, healing may be delayed.

Oxygen Tension

Oxygen is required for cell migration, cell multiplication, and protein synthesis. Additional oxygen is required by the fibroblast synthesizing collagen for hydroxylation of proline and lysine to form hydroxyproline and hydroxylysine, respectively. However, wound environment is characterized by low levels of pO_2. An oxygen gradient exists in wound tissue from the nearest functioning capillary to the wound edge, and the pO_2 falls rapidly as measurements are taken at increased distances from a functioning capillary. This decrease is due to two factors, the diffusion gradient and the oxygen consumption of cells in the margin of the wound. The measurements have led to the suggestion that the rate of wound healing may be limited by oxygen supply.

Direct observations of granulating wounds in rabbit ear chambers show that new capillary formation follows migration of fibroblasts. Measurements of oxygen tension in the vicinity of the leading fibroblast suggest that oxygen supply is always at the lower limit for migration: it is too low for replication or protein synthesis. Thus migration and synthetic activity of the wound fibroblast depend upon the rate at which new capillaries are formed. These, in turn, depend upon an adequate microcirculation from which these capillaries develop. Anything that interferes with this process will automatically interfere with wound healing.

The question naturally arises: Can one increase the rate of healing by furnishing a greater supply of oxygen? This possibility has been studied. Animals in which wounds had been made were kept in atmospheres of 10 per cent, 20 per cent (control), and 40 per cent oxygen. Temperature, humidity and carbon dioxide content were maintained constant. After seven days under these conditions, breaking strength of wounds was measured. In animals maintained in 10 per cent oxygen, there was a small but significant decrease in wound strength as compared to controls. Animals maintained in 40 per cent oxygen had wounds which were significantly stronger than controls, albeit the increase in strength was small. Increasing the carbon dioxide content of the environment from 0.5 per cent to 8.0 per cent had a markedly detrimental effect on healing. In these experiments, the pCO_2 of wound fluid increased from 70 to 85 and the pH increased from 7.25 to 7.35 in animals on high carbon dioxide inhalation. No effect on pO_2 of wound fluid was observed.

It has also been shown that as arterial pO_2 is increased, there is a concomitant increase in collagen synthesis in the wound. However, if wound pO_2 is measured, the increase is only about 3 mm.Hg in response to a 100 mm.Hg arterial increment. This suggests that most of the additional oxygen supplied was being consumed by wound tissue.

Turning now to the clinical implications of these observations, it can be categorically stated that anything that interferes with delivery of oxygen to the wound site will interfere with wound healing. The question whether giving patients additional oxygen will accelerate healing is not quite so clear. Obviously, if something is interfering with maintenance of a normal arterial pO_2, raising this by oxygen supplementation may aid healing significantly. On the other hand, although the experiments just described do indicate a statistically significant increase in wound strength in animals receiving 40 per cent oxygen, the differences were of no clinical significance. Thus it seems unlikely that, in the absence of factors interfering with tissue oxygen, administration of high concentrations of oxygen will significantly affect wound healing. Whether or not to use oxygen will depend upon arterial pO_2 and the presence of other factors that may be interfering with delivery of oxygen to tissues. Correction of these factors may be more important than administering high levels of oxygen.

Environmental Temperature

Hypothermia induced in animals by irrigation with cold water reduced tensile strength of wounds inflicted immediately after induction of hypothermia (below 28° C.) up to the fifth postoperative day. Blood sludging has been suggested as an important mediating factor.

Wounds have been reported to heal more quickly at an environmental temperature of 30° C. than at normal room temperature of 18 to 20° C. Dropping environmental temperature from 20° to 12° C. decreases tensile strength of wounds by about 20 per cent. This can largely be abolished by previous denervation of skin. This suggests that inhibition of wound healing is brought about by a reflex vasoconstriction.

Other studies in rabbits have shown that warm environments favor healing and cold or alternating cold and warm environments are detrimental to healing.

Zinc and Wound Healing

In recent years, a number of investigations on the effect of zinc on wound healing have appeared. It has been demonstrated that after trauma, surgical or otherwise, the amount of zinc in blood and tissues may fall to low levels. This is particularly noticeable in burned patients. Administration of zinc sufficient to restore normal levels of this trace element in blood and tissues increases rate of epithelization, rate of gain of wound strength, and synthesis of collagen and other proteins. However, it has never been shown that in patients with normal blood and tissue zinc levels, additional zinc will promote or accelerate healing. Uncomplicated surgical procedures rarely depress zinc levels markedly or for more than a few days.

A number of enzymes are zinc-dependent, notably DNA-polymerase and reverse-transcriptase. The effects of zinc depletion on wound healing are what one would expect if the amount or functions of these enzymes were depressed. Epithelial and fibroblast proliferation does not occur, since mitosis of these cells cannot take place without DNA-polymerase and reverse-transcriptase. Thus, although these cells may migrate normally, they do not multiply; hence adequate epithelization does not occur and collagen synthesis by the few fibroblasts migrating into the wound cannot supply the fibers needed to hold the wound together. In such a case, raising blood and tissue zinc concentrations to normal will restore normal progression of wound healing.

Zinc has other effects on cells which may be detrimental to healing. Zinc stabilizes lysosomal and cell membranes, probably by inhibition of lipid peroxidases. It has been observed that macrophages can be immobilized by high levels of zinc and phagocytosis is decreased or completely inhibited. As was discussed in Chapter I, macrophages are necessary for initiation of the healing process.

It has also been found that lysyl oxidase activity is significantly decreased both in animals on zinc-deficient diets and in animals on very high zinc diets. In the case of low zinc diets, it is possible that zinc is needed for enzymes involved in synthesis of lysyl oxidase. However, in the presence of high levels of zinc, the well known antagonism between zinc and copper may come into play. Lysyl oxidase is a copper-containing enzyme and copper is necessary for its synthesis and activity. The high level of zinc may make copper unavailable for the *de novo* synthesis of lysyl oxidase or it may actually displace copper from the enzyme.

What is important to the surgeon is that in patients in whom blood and tissue zinc levels are low, administration of zinc can restore normal healing. On the other hand, excess zinc can be detrimental (1) by inhibiting macrophage migration and phagocytosis and (2) by interfering with lysyl oxidase activity which can result in failure of collagen cross-linking. Finally, zinc administration to patients with normal zinc levels has no accelerating effect on wound healing, contrary to some claims in the literature.

Effect of Stress and Steroid Hormones on Wound Healing

The effects that have been discussed in the preceding paragraphs may be secondary to the well known stress syndrome. It is of interest, therefore, to examine the effects of stress on healing of wounds.

An adverse effect of ACTH on wound healing having been observed, investigations on the action of cortisone on experimental wounds were made. Both rats and rabbits were used and the two species were found to have different susceptibilities to cortisone. In the rabbit, from 5 to 10 mg. cortisone per kilogram per day completely inhibited formation of granulation tissue for 12 to 18 days. Smaller doses inhibited the appearance of granulations for shorter times. Fracture healing was also inhibited by cortisone. In rats tensile strength of wounds was drastically reduced by doses of 10 mg. of cortisone. The major effect of cortisone appeared to be the prevention of capillary proliferation and fibroplasia.

Local application of adrenocortical steroids to wounds also inhibits formation of granulation tissue. The action of cortisone and ACTH appeared to be due to retardation of production of all mesenchymal cellular elements of repair. Although relatively large doses of cortisone were needed to depress wound healing to a significant extent, it can be demonstrated that in conditions of mild starvation and protein depletion, which of themselves do not affect wound healing, the effect of cortisone is greatly enhanced so that relatively low doses have a markedly inhibiting effect on fibroplasia. Various degrees of stress also produce a depression of tensile strength of wounds, provided they are of a chronic nature. The effect of stress on tensile strength can be abolished by previous adrenalectomy. The healing of tendons in dogs can also be retarded by 10 mg. per kilogram of cortisone daily. Although tensile strength of healing tendon in the treated dog was 40 per cent less than that in the control, healing did go to completion and function was adequate. Epidermal regeneration, as well as connective tissue repair, has been shown to be inhibited by stress, by ACTH, and by cortisone, and the inhibition is abolished by adrenalectomy. Cortisone suppresses fibroplasia only when present before initiation of rapid growth by injury. It should also be noted that both collagen synthesis and mucopolysaccharide synthesis are inhibited by cortisone, and presumably by chronic stress. The cortisone effect cannot, in some circumstances, be offset by anabolic hormones.

Administration of these hormones to surgical patients, for a variety of reasons, is not uncommon and the literature contains a number of papers reporting adverse and beneficial effects of these substances on wound healing. Analysis of this literature is confusing and it is evident that such parameters as species, compound used, its dose, relation of drug administration to the time of operation, duration of treatment, and criteria used to assess the effect on wound healing have varied

Text continued on page 190

Table 5-2.   *Effect of Steroids on Wound Healing*

Animal	Daily Dose	Started	Maximum Duration	Type of Wound	Effect	Criteria	Reference
				A. CORTISONE			
Rabbits	8-10 mg./kg.	3d preop	8-11d	Excised	Delayed Healing	Histology	24
Mice	100 mg./kg.	1d preop	5d	Excised	Delayed Healing	Histology	27
Rats	12.5 mg./kg.	1d preop	6d	Turpentine Abscess	Inhibition of Granulation	Histology	28
Rats	0.1 mg. local	24d preop	36d	Excised	Inhibition of Granulation and Contraction	Wound Size	3
Rabbits	2-10 mg./kg.	2d preop	14d	Excised	Up to Complete Inhibition—According to Dose	Histology	15
Rabbits	8 mg./kg.	3d preop	11d	Fractures	Greatly Delayed Healing	Histology	5
Rats	40 mg./kg.	2d preop	14d	Incised	Low Tensile Strength—Disruption	Tensile Strength and Histology	1
Dogs	2 mg./kg.	1d preop	21d	Incised	No Effect	Histology	6
Rabbits	10-20 mg./kg.	Operation	21d	Fractures	Failure of Union—No Bone	X-Ray and Histology	26
Guinea Pigs	0.5-50 mg./kg.	Operation	22d	Corneal Wounds	Delayed Healing with Highest Dose	Histology	4
Rats	20 mg./kg.	7d preop	14d	Incised	No Effect	Tensile Strength and Histology	30
Rabbits	1-3 mg./kg.	2d preop	21d	Incised	Marked Inhibition	Histology	21
Rats	4-100 mg./kg.	3d preop Operation	24d 21d	Incised	Lower Tensile Strength—Dose Related. More Marked with Preop Treatment	Tensile Strength	19
Rats	4 mg./kg.	3d preop	8d	Incised	Slightly Lower Strength—No Different from Stressed Controls	Tensile Strength	18
Rats	12.5-25 mg./kg.	Operation	20d	Ivalon Sponge Implant	Less Collagen—Dose Related	Collagen Content	22
Rats	10 mg./kg.	Operation	10d	Incised	Low Strength at 5 Days, Normal at 10	Tensile Strength	20
Rabbits	12 mg./kg.	(1) Day of 2nd Wound	5d	Secondary Incised Wounds	(1) 39% Increase T.S. of 2nd Over 1st Wound	Tensile Strength	14
		(2) Day of 1st Wound	10d		(2) 21% Increase T.S. of 2nd Over 1st Wound		
		(3) 5d pre 1st Wound	15d		(3) No Difference in T.S. Both Very Low		

Animal	Dose	Time	Duration	Wound	Effect	Method	Ref
Rats	4.8-14.4 mg. Total	Operation	6d	Cotton Pledget Granuloma	Decreased Granuloma and Mucopolysaccharides	Biochemical	17
Rats	5-40 mg./kg. Locally	Operation	9d	Incised	No Effect Except at 20-40 mg./kg.	Tensile Strength	9
Humans	100 mg./day	12 mo. preop / 3 wk. preop	Not Stated	Total Colectomy	No Effect (2 Cases)	Inspection of Wound	13
Rats	6-150 mg./kg. Locally	Operation	Single Application	Incised	Low T.S. with Highest Dose Only	Tensile Strength	10
B. HYDROCORTISONE							
Dogs	5-10 mg./kg. Locally	At 2nd operation / At 3rd operation	2d / 2d	Jejunal Stripping / Blunt Dissection of Adhesions	Fewer Adhesions	Inspection	8
Rats	25 mg./kg.	5d Postop	6d	Skin Excision	Inhibited Contraction, Increased Protein and Nonprotein Components	Measurement and Biochemical	25
Rats	3.12 mg. Locally	(1) Operation or (2) 1-2d Postop	Single Application	Intestinal Stripping	Less Adhesions	Inspection and Measurement	11
Rats	6-150 mg./kg. Locally	Operation	Single Application	Incised	All Doses Lowered Tensile Strength	Tensile Strength	10
C. PREDNISOLONE							
Rats	0.15-2.5 mg. Locally	(1) Operation or (2) 1-2d Postop	Single Application	Intestinal Stripping	Fewer Adhesions	Inspection and Measurement	11
Rabbits	1 drop of 1% soln. Hourly Locally	At Operation	36 hr.	Epithelial and Stromal Corneal Wounds	Slight Retardation of Epithelization, Marked Reduction of T.S.	Measurement and Tensile Strength	2
Humans	2.5-200 mg. Daily	13 mo. to 4d Preoperatively	Not Stated	Splenectomy—14 pts. Colectomy—5 pts. Ileum Resection—1 pt.	8 pts. with Partial or Total Wound, Disruption Appears Dose Related	Inspection	13
Dogs	20-60 mg. Locally	Operation	Single Application	Intestinal Stripping or Anastomosis	No Effect	Amount of Adhesions	12
Rats	6-150 mg./kg. Locally	Operation	Single Application	Incised	All Doses Lowered Tensile Strength	Tensile Strength	10
D. DESOXYCORTICOSTERONE							
Rats	6 mg./kg.	1d preop	6d	Turpentine Abscess	No Effect	Histology	28
Guinea Pigs	9 mg./kg.	5d preop	19d	Incised	Excessive Granulation and Cell Proliferation	Histology	23
Rats	1 mg. Locally	Operation	Single Dose	Turpentine Abscess	No Effect	Histology	29

Table continued on following page.

Table 5-2. *Effect of Steroids on Wound Healing (Continued)*

Animal	Daily Dose	Started	Maximum Duration	Type of Wound	Effect	Criteria	Reference
Rats	20 mg/kg.	7d preop	14d	Incised	No Effect	Tensile Strength and Histology	30
Rabbits	1-3 mg./kg.	2d preop	21d	Incised	No Effect	Histology	21
Rats	10 mg./kg.	Operation	7d	Incised	No Effect	Tensile Strength and Histology	19
E. ESTRADIOL							
Rats	0.001-1 mg. Locally	Operation	Single Dose	Turpentine Abscess	Inhibition of Granulation at .01 mg. and Above	Histology	29
Rats	1 mg./kg.	7d preop	14d	Incised	No Effect	Tensile Strength and Histology	30
Rats	2.5 mg./kg. Twice a Week	Operation	4 wk.	Polyvinyl Sponge Implantation	Increased Granulation, Decreased Maturity	Histology	16
F. TESTOSTERONE							
Rats	8 mg/kg.	Operation	10d	Incised	Increased Collagen and Strength of Wounds	Tensile Strength and Histology	32
Rats	12.5 mg/kg.	5d postop	6d	Excised	Accelerated Contraction, Increased Protein and Non-Protein Nitrogen	Inspection and Biochemical	31
G. DIANABOL							
Rats	1-8 mg./kg.	7d preop	19d	Viscose Sponge Implantation	Increased Tensile Strength, Increased Collagen Formation	Tensile Strength and Biochemical	32
Rats	50 mg/kg. q 2d	Operation	5 wk.	Fractures	Increased Proliferation, Collagen, and Calcification	Histology and Biochemical	31
H. ACTH							
Humans	100 mg. d1 then 40 mg.	Preop	Not Stated	Excised	Collagen Synthesis Inhibited	Histology	7
Rats	14-28 mg./kg.	3d preop	15d	Incised	Moderate Inhibition at High Dose Only	Tensile Strength and Histology	1
Rabbits	2-6 mg./kg.	2d preop	21d	Incised	No Effect	Histology	21
Rats	40 mg./kg.	3d preop	17d	Incised	No Effect	Tensile Strength and Histology	19
Humans	20-100 units Daily	1 yr., 1d preop.	Not Stated	10 Splenectomy 6 Colectomy	2 Partial Disruptions 1 Prolonged Healing	Inspection	13

1. Alrich, E. M., Carter, J. P., and Lehman, E. P. The Effect of ACTH and Cortisone on Wound Healing. Ann. Surg. *133*:783, 1951.

2. Aquavella, J. V., Gasset, A. R., and Dohlman, C. H. Corticosteroids in Corneal Wound Healing. Amer. J. Ophthal. *58*:621, 1964.

3. Baker, B. L., ard Whitaker, W. L. Interference with Wound Healing by the Local Action of Adrenocortical Steroids. Endocrinology *46*:544, 1950.

4. Barber, A., and Nothacker, W. G. Effects of Cortisone on Nonperforating Wounds of Cornea in Normal and Scorbutic Guinea Pigs. Arch. Pathol. *54*:334, 1952.

5. Blunt, J. W., Plotz, C. M., Lattes, R., Howes, E. L., Meyer, K., and Ragan, C. Effect of Cortisone on Experimental Fractures in the Rabbit. Proc. Soc. Exp. Biol. Med. *73*:678, 1950.

6. Cole, J. W., Orbison, J. L., Holden, W. D., Hancock, T. J., and Lindsay, J. F. A Histologic Study of the Effect of Cortisone on Wound Healing per Primam. Surg. Gynec. Obstet. *93*:321, 1951.

7. Creditor, M. C., Bevans, M., Mundy, W. L., and Ragan, C. Effect of ACTH on Wound Healing in Adults. Proc. Soc. Exp. Biol. Med. *74*:245, 1950.

8. DeSanctis, A. L., Schatten, W. E., and Weckesser, E. C. The Effect of Hydrocortisone in the Prevention of Intraperitoneal Adhesions. Arch. Surg. *71*:523, 1955.

9. DiPasquale, G., and Steinetz, B. G. Relationship of Food Intake to the Effect of Cortisone Acetate on Skin Wound Healing. Proc. Soc. Biol. Med. *117*:118, 1964.

10. DiPasquale, G., Tripp, L. V., and Steinetz, B. G. Effect of Locally Applied Anti-inflammatory Substances on Rat Skin Wounds. Proc. Soc. Exp. Biol. Med. *124*:404, 1967.

11. Eskeland, G. Prevention of Experimental Peritoneal Adhesions in the Rat by Intraperitoneally Administered Corticosteroids. Acta. Chir. Scand. *125*:91, 1963.

12. Glucksman, D. L., and Warren, W. D. The Effect of Topically Applied Corticosteroids in the Prevention of Peritoneal Adhesions. An Experimental Approach with a Review of the Literature. Surgery *60*:352, 1966.

13. Green, J. P. Steroid Therapy and Wound Healing in Surgical Patients. Brit. J. Surg. *52*:523, 1965.

14. Hinshaw, D. B., Hughes, L. D., and Stafford, C. E. Effects of Cortisone on the Healing of Disrupted Abdominal Wounds. Amer. J. Surg. *101*:189, 1961.

15. Howes, E. L., Plotz, C. M., Blunt, J. W., and Ragan, C. Retardation of Wound Healing by Cortisone. Surgery *28*:177, 1950.

16. Kelly, E. W., Jr. Estrogen Effect on Sponge Implant Histology in Albino Rat. Arch. Pathol. *74*:550, 1962.

17. Likar, L. J., Mason, M. M., and Rosenkrantz, H. Response of the Level of Acid Mucopolysaccharides in Rat Granulation Tissue to Cortisol. Endocrinology *72*:393, 1963.

18. Localio, S. A., Chassin, J., and MacKay, M. The Effect of Stress, the Adrenal and the Pituitary on Healing. Amer. J. Surg. *92*:521, 1956.

19. Meadows, E. C., and Prudden, J. F. A Study of the Influence of Adrenal Steroids on the Strength of Healing Wounds. Surgery *33*:841, 1953.

20. Pearce, C. W., Foot, N. C., Jordan, G. L., Law, S. W., and Wantz, G. E. The Effect and Interrelation of Testosterone, Cortisone and Protein Nutrition on Wound Healing. Surg. Gynec. Obstet. *111*:274, 1960.

21. Perasalo, O., Wiljasalo, M. A., and Wiljasalo, S. Some Studies of Hormonal Influence on Wound Healing. Ann. Chir. Gyn. Fenn. *42*:168, 1953.

22. Pernokas, L. L., Edwards, L. C., and Dunphy, J. E. Hormonal Influence on Healing Wounds: The Effect of Adrenalectomy and Cortisone on the Quantity and Collagen Content of Granulation Tissue. Surg. Forum *8*:74, 1957.

23. Pirani, C. L., Stepto, R. C., and Sutherland, K. Desoxycorticosterone in Wound Healing. J. Exp. Med. *93*:217, 1951.

24. Ragan, C., Howes, E. L., Plotz, C. M., Meyer, K., and Blunt, J. W. Effect of Cortisone on Production of Granulation Tissue in the Rabbit. Proc. Soc. Exp. Biol. Med. *72*:718, 1949.

25. Reynolds, B. L., and Buxton, R. W. Aberrations Produced in Healing Regenerating Tissue by Exogenously Administered Testosterone, Hydrocortisone, and Methandrostenolone. Amer. Surg. *29*:859, 1963.

26. Sissons, H. A., and Hadfield, G. J. The Influence of Cortisone on the Repair of Experimental Fractures in the Rabbit. Brit. J. Surg. *39*:172, 1951.

27. Spain, D. M., Molomut, N., and Huber, A. The Effect of Cortisone on the Formation of Granulation Tissue in Mice. Amer. J. Path. *26*:710, 1950.

28. Taubenhaus, M., and Amromin, G. D. The Effects of the Hypophysis, Thyroid, Sex Steroids and the Adrenal Cortex on Granulation Tissue. J. Lab. Clin. Med. *36*:7, 1950.

29. Taubenhaus, M., Taylor, B., and Morton, J. V. Hormonal Interaction in the Regulation of Granulation Tissue Formation. Endocrinology *51*:183, 1952.

30. Taylor, F. W., Dittmer, T. L., and Porter, D. O. Wound Healing and the Steroids. Surgery *31*:683, 1952.

31. Udupa, K. N., and Singh, R. H. Certain Chemical Studies on the Effect of Anabolic Hormones in Healing of Fractures. Ind. J. Surg. *26*:849, 1964.

32. Viljanto, J., Isomaki, H., and Kulonen, E. Effect of an Anabolic Steroid on the Tensile Strength of Granulation Tissue in Various Nutritional States. Acta. Endocr. *41*:395, 1962.

widely among various investigations, including those discussed in the previous paragraphs.

Table 5–2 summarizes these factors for a representative group of investigations involving some of the most widely used steroid drugs. It would appear that the most commonly used corticosteroids whose effect on wound healing has been reported tend to inhibit wound healing in the doses used in laboratory animals. There are insufficient data to allow one to transfer these results to human surgical patients, however. In most instances the doses used in animals were considerably higher than those normally administered to patients. As was pointed out in the early investigations, there appears to be a marked species variation in the response to a given dose of any one of the corticosteroids.

The only conclusion that may be drawn is that the wound in any patient receiving corticosteroids of appreciable amount at the time of and following surgery should be watched carefully. Clinical experience, for what it is worth, would seem to indicate that only in exceptional circumstances does administration of these steroids affect the healing process significantly. Doses of steroids that affect wound healing usually slightly retard the rate of healing, but complete healing eventually occurs.

Low doses of cortisone may interfere with wound healing by inducing a mild anorexia, rather than by any direct action on the wound healing mechanism. However, large doses of the hormone may impair wound healing directly.

There seems, therefore, good evidence that chronic stress, or repeated administration of very large doses of corticosteroids, particularly if administered immediately prior to or at the time of wounding, may have an inhibitory effect on healing. Acute stress or single doses of cortisone have no effect on healing.

Desoxycorticosterone would appear to have no effect on wound healing. The evidence regarding an effect from administration of estrogens and androgens is less clear. It is known that these hormones have a slight anabolic effect and might be expected to aid the healing process. However, in women with breast carcinoma treated with these substances, no effects on surgical wound have been reported. It seems unlikely that estrogens or androgens in the doses ordinarily employed exert any favorable or unfavorable effect on wound healing.

Recently the so-called anabolic steroids have been alleged to increase the rate of wound healing, particularly of fractures. These substances do stimulate general protein synthesis in the body and thus might be expected to stimulate the repair process. Unfortunately, too few data are available, particularly in human subjects, to draw any such conclusions. Furthermore, until more is known about the long-term effects of these substances, the wise surgeon will not utilize them except under carefully controlled conditions.

Vitamins A and E and Wound Healing

One of the effects of vitamin A is the labilizing of ., through an action on lysosomal membranes. Thus excessive dose. tamin A have been reported to increase inflammatory reactions. Gl. corticoids have an opposite effect on lysosomal membranes, tending stabilize them. This is one of the mechanisms of the anti-inflammatory action of steroid hormones. It has been shown that inhibition of wound healing by high doses of glucocorticoids can be completely reversed by administration of high doses of vitamin A. Depressed collagen synthesis is elevated and wounds gain strength equivalent to that of control wounds in animals not receiving steroids.

Vitamin E, like steroids, stabilizes membranes. It has been shown that vitamin E in high doses significantly retards wound healing and collagen production. Vitamin A administration will overcome the vitamin E effect and the healing rate will return to normal.

There is no evidence that administration of vitamin A will alter the healing rate of wounds in animals not under the influence of steroids or vitamin E. It has been suggested that vitamin E could be used to modify scar formation since its side effects are less than those of comparable amounts of steroid hormones.

Histamine and Wound Strength

Histamine release has been known for a long time to be a part of the picture of inflammation and to occur early in trauma. This has been mentioned in Chapter 1. The major effects of histamine are on local microvasculature and, once released, histamine is rapidly destroyed. Thus it is not surprising that histamine has been found to play an important role in early stages of wound healing. Depletion of skin histamine retards wound healing and results in lowered tensile strength. Most of the histamine liberated and destroyed appears to be derived from granules of mast cells.

Although granulation and wound tissues contain little histamine, they produce the amine at high rates. This histamine is released and enters the tissue fluids and bloodstream. However, injected histamine does not appear to influence healing. If the histamine-forming capacity of tissues is increased by repeated injections of compound 48/80 or polymixin B, tensile strength of healing skin wounds is increased by about 22 per cent. Attempts to inhibit histamine formation by a polymyxin-deficient diet alone have produced no effect on wound healing. On the other hand, if semicarbazide is used to inhibit histamine formation further, a 40 per cent drop in tensile strength of wounds has been noted. But since semicarbazide interferes generally enzymes (including monamine oxidases), it cannot be concluded that effects on tensile strength were a result of depressed histamine formation.

Three days of treatment of rats with 48/80 has been reported as sufficient to increase collagen content of Ivalon sponge implants by 55 per cent. This increased collagen formation correlates well with an increased tensile strength of wounds in early phases of healing. Cortisone decreases the elevated rate of histamine formation in wound tissues when given before infliction of injury. It seems possible that this may be merely a general manifestation of its inhibitory action on inflammatory cells.

The histamine story has been further complicated by the observation that histamine depletion inhibits wound healing, but that heparin, which is also liberated from mast cells, enhances healing. Part of these discrepancies may be due to species differences. Immediately after wounding, the guinea pig shows a high histamine content whereas the rat, under the same conditions, shows a low histamine content. In the guinea pig, changes in vascular permeability appear to be mediated by histamine; in the rat, 5-hydroxytryptamine is the mediating agent. Both agents are released from mast cells, as is heparin, and anything that causes degranulation of mast cells will free these substances. However, the number of available mast cells and the concentration of the various agents in them can vary from time to time and this may explain, in part, some of the discordant results. It seems certain, however, that stimulation of production of histamine, provided the animal is capable of responding, enhances normal responses to injury in early phases of healing.

Serotonin has been shown to increase lysyl oxidase activity. This, of course, would be important once collagen has been laid down in the wound. A similar effect has not been reported for histamine, but the similarity in the actions of these two substances suggests that at least part of the histamine effect on wounds might be due to an effect on lysyl oxidase production.

The Effects of Anti-inflammatory Drugs

The importance of various inflammatory cells on wound healing was discussed in Chapter 1. In the absence of infection, anti-inflammatory agents whose principal effect is to diminish granulocytic inflammatory reaction would not be expected to influence wound healing. On the other hand, any agent that diminished blood monocytes or tissue macrophages or interfered with fibroblast migration or differentiation or with protein synthetic activity would be expected to inhibit wound healing.

Similarly, drugs that alter the circulatory response to trauma could have an effect on healing. Thus, a drug that would cause vasoconstriction and shunting of blood away from the wound area would diminish the inflammatory response and interfere with wound healing. Therefore, in attempting to analyze the possible effects of a particular anti-inflammatory agent, one must be aware of its pharmacology and, in particular, its mode of action.

Anti-inflammatory drugs may have actions other than a direct one on inflammation that may become evident when doses different from the dose for optimal anti-inflammatory response are given. Frequently, such side effects are not well understood, but some may have an effect on one or more steps of the wound healing mechanism.

The effect of aspirin and indomethacin on prostaglandins was discussed in Chapter 1. It seems probable that a major portion of the anti-inflammatory action of these drugs is mediated through their action on prostaglandins.

Figure 5–22 is a simplified schematic representation of the relation of inflammatory reactions to production of fibrosis or to scar formation. It can be seen here that any agent interfering with any of the various pathways shown may have an effect on one or more phases of wound healing.

In light of these observations the effects of such anti-inflammatory drugs as phenylbutazone and salicylate may be anticipated. Direct ex-

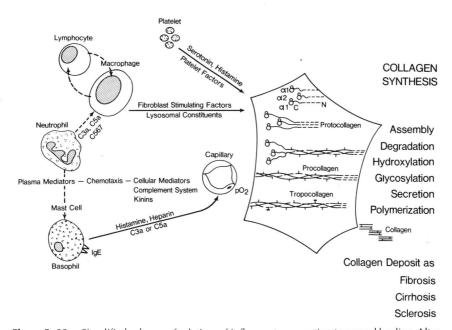

Figure 5–22. Simplified scheme of relation of inflammatory reaction to wound healing. Alteration or inhibition of any of the pathways shown may have an influence on the subsequent steps of the healing reaction. (Reproduced by courtesy of Prof. M. Chvapil.)

periments in animals indicate that in ordinary therapeutic doses these drugs have no effects on the course or quality of healing. Very large doses of aspirin, equivalent to 20 times the dose for a 70 kg. man, markedly diminish tensile strength of wounds in rats. The effect is strictly dose-dependent and no effect can be observed with the usually administered doses.

The Effect of Cytotoxic Drugs on Wound Healing

The recently introduced use in patients with cancer of cytotoxic drugs either alone or as an adjuvant to surgery raises important questions regarding the fate of wounds in surgically treated patients. Most of the cytotoxic drugs interfere in one way or another with cell proliferation. Cell proliferation is an important component of the healing process.

Mechlorethamine hydrochloride (nitrogen mustard) has been shown to decrease tensile strength of wounds in rats. However, these rats also lost weight and showed evidence of nutritional impairment. Pair-fed control animals showed a similar diminution in wound tensile strength; thus the effect of the drug may have been indirect. Thio-TEPA and chloroquine mustard have been shown not to affect wound healing when administered in therapeutic doses. Similarly, cyclophosphamide, which also has anti-inflammatory actions, adversely affected wound healing, but this appeared to be proportional to the debilitation produced in experimental animals. It is questionable, therefore, if the effect on wounds can be attributed directly to the drug.

Effects of Trauma on Wound Healing

Trauma is one form of stress. In today's society, multiple wounds are not infrequently seen. What influence does the presence of one wound have upon another? After injury a condition can develop which resembles scurvy and there may be a concomitant drop in urinary, blood and tissue ascorbic acid. Laparotomy wounds in burned animals heal abnormally and, although fibroplasia appears ample, collagen production is scanty and ground substance production is excessive. Vitamin C administration during the postoperative period can correct these abnormalities of healing.

In one extensive investigation, the effects of trauma of either femoral fracture or leg muscle contusion on wounds made on the backs of rabbits were studied. Tensile strength measurements were used as the index of healing. If wounds were made at the same time as the fracture was produced, the latent period was unchanged and tensile strength during the latent period was also unchanged. During the period 3 to 12 days after wounding, tensile strength was less than in control wounds in animals without fracture, but this difference disappeared at 15 days. If the wound was inflicted two days after the fracture, the wound was stronger during the latent period, but thereafter wound tensile strength was less than in controls. This was true for wounds made at any time up to 14 days after fracture. If the fracture was made two days after infliction of the wound, there followed a reduction in tensile strength of the wound equal to that observed when the wound and fracture were made simultaneously. The same type of result was seen if muscle trauma was substituted for femoral fracture, and the effects on the wound were proportional to the severity of trauma. Studies on intravascular aggregation, circulating blood volume, and erythrostasis following trauma led to the conclusion that retardation in the rate of healing following trauma is related to reduced suspension stability of blood, which leads to intravascular aggregation, erythrostasis in postcapillary venules, and impaired capillary flow. This work, taken in conjunction with that of others, again emphasizes the vital importance of local circulatory factors adjacent to the wound, particularly those which interfere with diffusion and oxygen tension, in the rate of healing and gain of tensile strength.

Effect of Denervation on Healing

In the discussion of the effects of environmental temperature on wound healing, it was observed that denervation could abolish the adverse effect of severe cold. Acute denervation has no effect on wound healing if the animal is not under stress. Denervation two months before wounding does not alter wound healing, but it does not protect against cold vasoconstriction as does acute denervation. A curious observation has been made that about half of the denervated animals develop spontaneous ulceration of skin even though tensile strength gain of their wounds is normal. Since neither wound contraction nor epithelization is affected by denervation, the explanation of this observation is that defense against mechanical injury was lessened in denervated animals.

Another explanation of the susceptibility of denervated skin to ulceration lies in observations of extensive necrosis and ulceration of skin and underlying tissue in paraplegics. These massive, rapidly destructive lesions can appear with minimal ischemia or pressure and are quite unlike usual pressure or bed sores seen in debilitated patients with intact nervous systems. Collagenase activity has been measured in these severe necrotic wounds and has been found to be exceedingly high. It is thought that for some unknown reason collagenase production in denervated dermis may be extremely high but that serum inhibitors prevent manifestation of this activity. However, even short periods of ischemia may remove the inhibitor and allow the high level of enzyme to exert its full effect.

Increase in collagenase production, though to a much lesser degree, has been observed in denervated dermis. Thus in the hand, if the ulnar nerve is severed, collagenase activity will be elevated in skin of the little and ring fingers as compared to the other fingers that are innervated by intact median nerves.

PHARMACOLOGY OF FIBROSIS

In the preceding chapters, a great deal of what is known regarding the basic biology of the repair process has been discussed. The clinically oriented surgeon may have found this knowledge difficult to relate to the everyday care of his patients. He will concede that such knowledge can be helpful in seeking the cause of and correcting problems in delayed healing, but he might ask whether all this detail is necessary or useful in the care of patients. It is hoped that the following discussion will indicate that this otherwise esoteric information may be applicable to clinical problems, some of which he may not have considered examples of wound healing. Some of the thoughts presented here will be discussed in greater detail in succeeding chapters. The material in this section will serve both as a summary of preceding chapters and as an introduction to chapters that follow.

There are many examples of wound repair in which the end results are disabling or even fatal to the patient. Repeated injury to the liver due to chronic abuse of alcohol, exposure to hepatotoxic chemicals, or infection with viruses leads to repair by fibrous scarring which we recognize as cirrhosis. Injury to the esophagus by strong acids or alkalis leads to repair by a circumferential scar which, when remodeled into a shortened position, produces stricture. Chronic infection combined with complex immune responses in the bowel can cause ulceration, with healing by extensive scar formation that ultimately destroys intestinal function. Repeated infection or trauma to the urinary tract, particularly in the urethra, leads to repair by circumferential scarring that results in stricture. The process by which tendons heal results, in many instances, in scarring and loss of gliding function. Exposure to silica dusts or other irritant or toxic inhalants produces injury of the fine structures of the lungs. Repair is accomplished by synthesis of a fibrous scar which interferes with pulmonary function. Scar tissue interposed between cut ends of a nerve prevents functional axonal regeneration. These are a few examples of the unwanted and detrimental effects of healing that depends upon synthesis and deposition of collagen to form a dense fibrous scar. Many of the clinical problems which confront the surgeon result from undesirable consequences of the healing process. We propose to discuss some possible approaches to the prevention or solution of these problems by application of the basic biologic information discussed in the preceding chapters.

The essence of the problem lies in the control or direction of fibrosis, which ultimately involves interfering with or altering some aspect of the synthesis, deposition, or remodeling of collagen. This can be approached from two major aspects: (1) the specific, which involves a direct attack on collagen itself by altering or inhibiting its synthesis or deposition or by removing it using direct and specific means; or (2) nonspecific, which involves processes that lead to migration and modulation of mesenchymal cells, or processes that alter the environment in which both the early and late stages of wound repair occur.

Specific Control of Collagen in the Healing Process

First let us look at the possibilities of controlling collagen synthesis. At the outset it is necessary to discard such approaches as the use of actinomycin D, puromycin, or other drugs that act on general pathways of protein synthesis. While they may effectively inhibit collagen synthesis, they also inhibit synthesis of all other proteins, resulting in severe morbidity or even death of the patient. Fortunately, there are several steps in synthesis of collagen that are unique to this protein. Hydroxylation of proline and lysine is an essential step that occurs only in collagen synthesis. The responsible enzyme requires four co-factors—iron, oxygen, ascorbic acid, and α-ketoglutarate. Iron can be removed by iron chelators such as α,α-dipyridyl. However, iron is needed for other enzymes and for other body processes. This approach has been tried experimentally and, as might be expected, was ineffective due to toxic effects.

It has been known for more than 200 years that scurvy causes weakening and disruption of scar tissue. Vitamin C, an activator of both prolyl hydroxylase and lysyl hydroxylase, is necessary for synthesis of wound collagen. Lack of vitamin C has been shown many times to prevent synthesis and deposition of collagen, but it produces many effects other than the specific action on collagen synthesis. However, before discarding the idea of utilizing deliberately induced scurvy in control of fibrosis, one needs to examine the possibility that short periods of scurvy under controlled conditions may not produce significant morbidity, particularly if the condition could be induced and ended quickly. Experimental work to explore this concept is already under way.

Another approach to interfering with collagen synthesis or, more correctly, to interfering with the functional integrity of newly synthesized collagen is to alter the building blocks of the molecule. Substitution of an analog of proline which cannot be hydroxylated or which will alter helix formation is one such approach. Two such analogs are 3,4-

dehydroproline and cis-hydroxyproline. In tissue culture, these appeared to interfere with collagen secretion. However, when fed to intact animals, both proved ineffective and toxic. The ineffectiveness was probably due to inability to feed sufficient quantities of the analogs to swamp the body's pool of normal proline. The toxicity was probably related to incorporation of the analog into other proteins in which even small amounts could seriously interfere with function. Of course, a direct toxic effect may also have occurred. 3,4-Dehydroproline produces cytotoxic effects involving smooth endoplasmic reticulum, mitochondria, and rough endoplasmic reticulum. cis-Hydroxyproline is much less toxic, and only after chronic administration are effects on the metabolism of other proteins seen. At present, the approach to control of fibrosis through use of proline analogs does not seem promising.

One can attempt to interfere with secretion of collagen from cells by tampering with microtubular function. Colchicine has been used for this purpose. Contrary to expectations, a marked increase in rate of collagen synthesis has been observed following colchicine administration. In spite of increased collagen synthesis, the collagen content of wounds was depressed and breaking strength of wounds was significantly decreased. The mechanism of this action of colchicine will be discussed later in this section.

Regarding the possibility of controlling extracellular events in collagen fiber formation, we have observed that failure to convert procollagen to collagen prevents proper aggregation of tropocollagen molecules into fibrils and inhibits cross-linking reactions. This is evidenced in two genetic abnormalities: dermatosparaxis and type V Ehlers-Danlos syndrome. Conversion of procollagen to collagen is accomplished by one or more enzymes known as procollagen peptidases. Whether or not the action of these enzymes is limited to collagen and how they may be inhibited are not yet known. The possibility of altering or inhibiting the action of these enzymes must, however, be kept in mind as a possible mechanism for control of collagen fiber deposition.

Control of collagen cross-linking has so far proved to be the most feasible method of altering scar formation. The specific action of amino nitriles, particularly β-aminopropionitrile, on lysyl oxidase, inhibiting the oxidative deamination of the ε-amino group of lysine, leads to failure of cross-linking. Uncross-linked collagen is soluble and more readily attacked by tissue collagenases. It is weak and fibers are readily disrupted. Clinical studies involving prevention of urethral strictures and tendon adhesions are already under way. Experimentally, β-aminopropionitrile has been shown to be effective in prevention of dimethylnitrosamine-induced liver cirrhosis and lye-burn induced esophageal stricture. All of these are preliminary studies and much experimental and clinical work remains to be done before it can be said that this specific chemical or even this method of approach is a solution to the clinical problem of unwanted fibrosis. Results so far have been encouraging since it has clearly been demonstrated that beneficial, even life-saving results can be obtained by applying our knowledge of the biology of collagen.

The fact that cells in and around wounds produce a specific collagenase provides another possible means of attack on scar tissue formation. We have already mentioned that colchicine appears to decrease wound strength, not by inhibition of collagen synthesis or secretion but by increasing collagen destruction. Direct measurement of collagenase activity in these wounds reveals a several-fold increase in collagenase production. In colchicine-treated animals, even though collagen production is increased, the excess amount of collagenase degrades newly formed collagen as fast as it is produced. Unfortunately, prolonged use of colchicine can lead to other, undesirable effects and this may prevent clinical application of this finding. Nevertheless, the demonstration that it is possible to increase collagenase activity in wounds offers the exciting possibility that agents will be found that produce this effect more selectively. It is conceivable that local application of such agents will enable one to confine the effect to the particular tissue or wound that one wishes to control.

Finally there exists the possibility of inhibiting or destroying the cell responsible for collagen synthesis. Glucocorticoids do this in a rather nonspecific way and at doses that produce a number of undesirable side effects. Nevertheless, steroid hormones are used in treatment of keloids and esophageal stricture. Recently a specific antifibroblast serum has been produced. This has a high degree of specificity and is currently being studied for its possible effects on preventing pathological scarring. It is much too early to predict the ultimate outcome of these investigations, but from a strictly biological point of view, the approach is logical and may prove rewarding.

Obviously, for various reasons, a single approach to the problem of controlling fibrosis may not ultimately prove desirable. Since there are so many points of attack along the pathway of collagen synthesis, deposition, maturation, and destruction, a combination of inhibitory or destructive agents may prove to be advantageous from the standpoint of precise control with minimal side effects. Exploration and study of such combinations of agents will be time-consuming and difficult. It is hoped, however, that from these there will become available new tools that are useful to the surgeon in controlling a large variety of conditions characterized by unwanted fibrosis.

Nonspecific Control of Collagen Synthesis

By nonspecific control of fibrosis we refer to manipulation of the environment or of processes involved in repair that have an indirect effect on collagen synthesis and deposition. Almost all of the methods suggested are aimed at one or more aspects of the inflammatory phase of wound healing.

There is evidence that invasion of granulocytes into the wound area results in humoral messages to macrophages. However, this cannot be the only signal, since macrophages appear when granulocytes are absent, such as after treatment with anti-leukocytic serum. It is possible that other cells such as platelets release humoral chemotactic materials. In any event, it has been demonstrated that the absence of macrophages inhibits the subsequent events of wound healing. Unfortunately, to be effective anti-macrophage serum must be administered with steroids. Steroids in high doses also inhibit the cellular response to injury, but they produce many other undesirable effects and their use cannot be recommended except in certain cases of life-threatening fibrosis.

High levels of zinc have been shown to inactivate functioning of macrophages, most cells, and platelets. More work needs to be done to define the possible role of zinc in wound healing. It can accelerate healing when the process is depressed in individuals with low tissue zinc levels, but it can also depress healing when zinc levels are significantly above normal.

High levels of lipid peroxides have been demonstrated in activated macrophages, aggregated platelets, and subcellular particles isolated from injured tissue. Strong oxidants, drugs metabolized to free radicals, and ionizing radiation all induce lipid peroxidative changes. These increased lipid peroxides may be one cause of tissue damage or necrosis and of the increase in the inflammatory reaction. The trial of anti-oxidants and free radical scavengers may prove useful in lung, liver, or radiation-induced injury in which fibrosis is a prominent consequence of prolonged or repeated injury.

It seems likely that in the future the surgeon will have available to him tools which will enable him to alter or affect every step of the healing process from initial inflammatory reaction to final maturation of the fibrous scar. His skill in managing the repair process will depend upon his knowledge of the fundamental biological and biochemical processes in each stage of repair, and his ability to manipulate pharmacologically each process at the right time and in the right direction. By this means he can make the healing process work *for* the patient and not *against* him.

SUMMARY

Tensile strength is the most important parameter of an incisional wound, both to the patient and to the surgeon. In experimental observations on changes in the strength of wounds, failure to appreciate a number of technical factors associated with measurement of tensile strength can lead to erroneous conclusions.

The healing of the normal incisional wound can conveniently be divided into three phases: lag, latent, productive, or substrate phase of healing; fibroplastic phase; and phase of maturation.

The lag or latent phase extends from the time of wounding until the fourth to sixth day in humans and may be shorter in some species such as the rat or guinea pig. During this phase, the inflammatory reaction prepares the wound for subsequent healing by removal of debris, necrotic tissue, and bacteria. At the same time, there is mobilization and migration of fibroblasts and epithelial cells and accumulation of noncollagenous proteins and glycoproteins from the general circulation. During the lag phase, only the gluing action of fibrin and subsequently the adhesion of migrating epidermal cells hold wound edges together.

About day 4 to 6, proliferating fibroblasts begin to synthesize collagen, mucopolysaccharides, and glycoproteins. Collagen is secreted from cells in monomeric form but quickly aggregates into fibers. From this point on there is a rapid gain in tensile strength. There is no sharp demarcation between the end of the fibroplastic phase and the beginning of the phase of maturation. In fact they probably overlap each other. Collagen increase in the wound ceases some time after the fifteenth day. The precise time is difficult to determine because of sampling difficulties.

Although collagen content of the wound remains constant, or decreases, after the phase of fibroplasia, there is a steady gain in tensile strength of the wound, although not at the rate seen during the fibroplastic phase. This strength gain is due to two factors: intramolecular and intermolecular cross-linking of collagen fibers, and remodeling by dissolution and reforming of collagen fibers to give a stronger, more efficient weave. This cross-linking and remodeling may require six months to a year for completion, the longer time being observed in essentially fibrous tissues such as fascia.

Wounds in visceral organs such as stomach, colon, and bladder complete their strength gain in about two to three weeks; in the case of stomach and colon, the ultimate strength gain is only about 70 per cent of normal unwounded tissue, but in the case of bladder, full strength is regained. All organs have a prolonged period of increased metabolic activity in their wounds characterized by greatly accelerated rates of collagen synthesis and destruction and, in the case of colon and stomach, increased rate of noncollagenous protein synthesis.

Although collagen fibers are the principal components responsible for tensile strength of wounds, as evidenced by experiments in scorbutic and in lathyritic animals, some of the late gain in strength may also be due to interactions of collagen with components of ground substance, such as mucopolysaccharides and glycoproteins. Furthermore, there is evidence that mucopolysaccharides stabilize collagen fibers and possibly control their ultimate and characteristic size.

Various tissue collagenases participate in remodeling of scars. Nonfunctional and unneeded collagen fibers are removed and functionally oriented fibers are preserved. This process occurs over fairly prolonged periods of time. Collagenases also appear in pathological processes such as rheumatoid arthritis where they cause destruction of joint cartilage and nearby tendons.

Tensile strength of wounds can be adversely affected by severe protein depletion, by prolonged hypovolemia, by increased blood viscosity or intravascular coagulation brought about by remote trauma, by cold vasoconstriction, and by chronic stress, to mention a few of the systemic and environmental factors that must be considered. There are, of course, many other factors that can alter wound tensile strength that are outside the scope of this discussion. Among these are the effects of other drugs, hormones, and irradiation. However, an understanding of the process of normal healing and the mechanism by which a wound gains strength provides a basis for predicting the probable effects of altering the environment of a wound upon its subsequent course.

SUGGESTED READING

Adamsons, R. J., Musco, F., and Enquist, I. F. The Chemical Dimensions of a Healing Incision. Surg. Gynec. Obstet. *123*:515, 1966.

Bailey, A. J., Bazin, S., Sims, T. J., LeLous, M., Nicoletis, C., and Delaunay, A. Characterization of the Collagen of Human Hypertrophic and Normal Scars. Biochim. Biophys. Acta *405*:412, 1975.

Bailey, A. J., Sims, T. J., LeLous, M., and Bazin, S. Collagen Polymorphism in Experimental Granulation Tissue. Biochem. Biophys. Res. Commun. 66:1160, 1975.

Bauer, E. A., Eisen, A. Z., and Jeffrey, J. J. Regulation of Vertebrate Collagenase Activity *in Vitro* and *in Vivo.* J. Invest. Dermat. *59*:50, 1972.

Bentley, J. P. Rate of Chondroitin Sulfate Formation in Wound Healing Ann. Surg. *165*:186, 1967.

Chvapil, M. Pharmacology of Fibrosis: Definitions, Limits and Perspectives. Life Sciences *16*:1345, 1975.

Chvapil, M. Zinc and Wound Healing. In: *Symposium on Zinc.* Edited by B. Zederfeldt. Lund, Sweden, A. B. Tika, 1974.

Chvapil, M., Elias, S. L., Ryan, J. N., and Zukoski, C. F. Pathophysiology of Zinc. Int. Rev. Neurobiol. Suppl. 1, 1972, p. 105.

Douglas, D. M. The Healing of Aponeurotic Incisions. Brit. J. Surg. *40*:79, 1952.

Dunphy, J. E. The Effect of Local Trauma on Repair by Connective Tissue. Bull. Soc. Int. Chir. *22*:121, 1963.

Dunphy, J. E., and Udupa, K. N. Chemical and Histochemical Sequences in the Normal Healing of Wounds. New Eng. J. Med. *253*:847, 1955.

Dunphy, J. E., Udupa, K. N., and Edwards, L. C. Wound Healing. A New Perspective with Particular Reference to Ascorbic Acid Deficiency. Ann. Surg. *144*:304, 1956.

Ehrlich, H. P., and Hunt, T. K. Effects of Cortisone and Vitamin A on Wound Healing. Ann. Surg. *167*:324, 1968.

Ehrlich, H. P., and Tarver, H. Effects of BetaCarotene, Vitamin A and Glucocorticoids on Collagen Synthesis in Wounds. Proc. Soc. Exp. Biol. Med. *137*:936, 1971.

Eisen, A. Z., Bauer, E. A., and Jeffrey, J. J. Animal and Human Collagenases. J. Invest. Dermat. *55*:359, 1970.

Forrester, J. C., Zederfeldt, B., Hayes, T. L., and Hunt, T. K. Mechanical, Biochemical and Architectural Factors in Repair. In: *Repair and Regeneration. The Scientific Basis for Surgical Practice.* Edited by J. E. Dunphy and W. Van Winkle, Jr. New York, McGraw-Hill Book Co., 1969, p. 71.

Gibson, T., and Kenedi, R. M. Factors Affecting the Mechanical Characteristics of Human Skin. In: *Repair and Regeneration. The Scientific Basis for Surgical Practice.* Edited by J. E. Dunphy and W. Van Winkle, Jr. New York, McGraw-Hill Book Co., 1969, p. 87.

Gross, J., and Lapiere, C. M. Collagenolytic Activity in Amphibian Tissues: a Tissue Culture Assay. Proc. Nat. Acad. Sci. *48*:1014, 1962.

Harkness, M. L. R., and Harkness, R. D. Mechanism of Action of Thiols on the Mechanical Properties of Connective Tissues. Biochim. Biophys. Acta *154*:553, 1968.

Hastings, J. C., Van Winkle, W., Barker, E., Hines, D., and Nichols, W. The Effect of Suture Material on Healing Wounds of the Stomach and Colon. Surg. Gynec. Obstet. *140*:701, 1975.

Hastings, J. C., Van Winkle, W., Barker, E., Hines, D., and Nichols, W. The Effect of Suture Materials on Healing Bladder Wounds. Surg. Gynec. Obstet. *140*:933, 1975.

Hawley, P. R., Faulk, W. P., Hunt, T. K., and Dunphy, J. E. Collagenase Activity in the Gastrointestinal Tract. Brit. J. Surg. *57*:896, 1970.

Howes, E. L., Sooy, J. W., and Harvey, S. C. The Healing of Wounds as Determined by Their Tensile Strength. J.A.M.A. *92*:42, 1929.

Hunt, T. K., and Pai, M. P. The Effect of Varying Ambient Oxygen Tensions on Wound Metabolism and Collagen Synthesis. Surg. Gynec. Obstet. *135*:561, 1972.

Hunt, T. K., and Zederfeldt, B. Nutritional and Environmental Aspects in Wound Healing. In: *Repair and Regeneration. The Scientific Basis for Surgical Practice.* Edited by J. E. Dunphy and W. Van Winkle, Jr. New York, McGraw-Hill Book Co., 1969, p. 217.

Jackson, D. S. Some Biochemical Aspects of Fibrogenesis and Wound Healing. New Eng. J. Med. *259*:814, 1958.

Jeffrey, J. J., Coffey, R. J., and Eisen, A. Z. Studies on Uterine Collagenase in Tissue Culture. II. Effect of Steroid Hormones on Enzyme Productions. Biochim. Biophys. Acta *252*:143, 1971.

Kahlson, G., Nilsson, K., Rosengren, E., and Zederfeldt, B. Wound Healing as Dependent on Rate of Histamine Formation. Lancet *2*:230, 1960.

Levenson, S. M., Birkhill, F. R., and Waterman, D. F. The Healing of Soft Tissue Wounds; the Effects of Nutrition, Anemia and Age. Surgery *28*:905, 1950.

Levenson, S. M., Geever, E. F., Crowley, L. V., Oates, J. F., Berard, C. W., and Rosen, H. The Healing of Rat Skin Wounds. Ann. Surg. *161*:293, 1965.

Madden, J. W., and Peacock, E. E., Jr. Studies on the Biology of Collagen during Wound Healing. I. Rate of Collagen Synthesis and Deposition in Cutaneous Wounds of the Rat. Surgery *64*:288, 1968.

Niinikoski, J. Oxygen and Trauma. Europ. Res. Office, U.S. Army, London, 1972.

Niinikoski, J., Hunt, T. K., and Dunphy, J. E. Oxygen Supply in Healing Tissue. Amer. J. Surg. *123*:247, 1972.

Peacock, E. E., Jr. Some Aspects of Fibrogenesis during the Healing of Primary and Secondary Wounds. Surg. Gynec. Obstet. *115*:408, 1962.

Peacock, E. E., Jr. and Biggers, P. W. Measurement and Significance of Heat-Labile and Urea-Sensitive Cross-Linking Mechanisms in Collagen of Healing Wounds. Surgery *54*:144, 1963.

Sandblom, P. The Effect of Injury on Wound Healing. Ann. Surg. *129*:305, 1949.

Sandblom, P., and Muren, A. Differences between the Rate of Healing of Wounds Inflicted with Short Time Interval. Ann. Surg. *140*:449, 1954.

Savlov, E. D., and Dunphy, J. E. Mechanisms of Wound Healing. Comparison of Preliminary Local and Distant Incisions. New Eng. J. Med. *250*:1062, 1954.

Stephens, F. O., and Hunt, T. K. Effect of Changes in Inspired Oxygen and Carbon Dioxide Tensions on Wound Tensile Strength. Ann. Surg. *173*:515, 1971.

Van Winkle, W., Hastings, J. C., Barker, E., Hines, E., and Nichols, W. The Effect of Suture Materials on Healing Skin Wounds. Surg. Gynec. Obstet. *140*:7, 1975.

Van Winkle, W., Hastings, J. C., Barker, E., and Wohland, W. Role of Fibroblast in Controlling Rate and Extent of Repair in Wounds in Various Tissues. In: *Biology of Fibroblast.* Edited by E. Kulonen and J. Pikkarainen. London, Academic Press, 1973, p. 559.

Viljanto, J. Biochemical Basis of Tensile Strength in Wound Healing. Acta Chir. Scand. Suppl. 333, 1964.

Watts, G. T., Baddeley, M. R., Crawford, N., and Wellings, R. Wound Healing. Biochemical Methods for Observation of the Cellular and Intercellular Phases. Brit. J. Clin. Pract. *16*:733, 1962.

Williamson, M. B., and Fromm, H. J. Effect of Cystine and Methionine on Healing of Experimental Wounds. Proc. Soc. Exp. Biol. Med. *80*:623, 1957.

Woessner, J. F., and Gould, B. S. Collagen Biosynthesis. Tissue Culture Experiments to Ascertain the Role of Ascorbic Acid in Collagen Formation. J. Biophys. Biochem. Cytol. *3*:685, 1957.

Zederfeldt, B. Studies on Wound Healing and Trauma. With Special Reference to Intravascular Aggregation of Erythrocytes. Acta Chir. Scand. Suppl. 224, 1957.

Chapter 6

REPAIR OF SKIN WOUNDS

The most important consideration in a treatise on healing of skin wounds can be summarized by a single statement: skin is not a simple tissue such as epithelium, fascia, or fat; it is a highly complex organ containing multiple structures derived from multiple germ layers. More mistakes in the management of surface wounds can be attributed to failure to understand fully the significance of this basic fact than to any other factor. Realizing that skin is a compound organ is important because, with the possible exception of liver parenchyma, organs do not regenerate. Injured organs heal by means of a relatively simple mechanism—formation of a predominantly fibrous tissue scar. Although simple tissues such as fat, connective tissue, and epithelium regenerate superbly, and some lower forms of life regenerate compound tissues or organs with amazing efficiency, the evolution of man is marked by loss of regenerative powers in compound organs and appendages. Although it is undoubtedly important in evolution by natural selection, healing by scar formation now appears to be a poor substitute for pristine regenerative powers.

That the fibrous nature and nonspecificity of the healing process actually replaces or chokes out regenerative potential in some tissues is suggested by two biological observations. First is the reaction to injury by a coelenterate; another is prolongation of regenerative potential by pharmacological methods during maturation of a newt. When the hydra, tubularia, loses a hydranth it will either regenerate a new one or heal the wound by developing simple scar tissue. Both never occur, however; formation of a scar apparently prevents any regenerative activity. In the case of the newt, there is a period when regeneration of a new limb will occur following amputation. After this period has passed, however, regeneration does not occur, and only fibrous tissue in the form of a dense scar will be synthesized.

204

If a powerful lathyrogen such as β-aminopropionitrile (see Chapters 4 and 5) is administered during the transition period when regeneration ceases and scar tissue develops, rigid scar tissue cannot be assembled and regenerative activity is prolonged. Because β-aminopropionitrile is believed to act primarily by interfering with intermolecular and intramolecular cross-linking, one might speculate that assembly of structurally stable collagen actually affects regenerative efforts by relatively delicate totipotent cells. The possibility that regenerative capacity is present in some compound tissues and might be exploited by controlling fibrous tissue formation following wounding is interesting.

If natural processes are not interfered with, a compound organ such as skin will restore surface continuity by contraction, epithelization, and synthesis of dense connective tissue. But rarely does healing by these processes produce an acceptable clinical result. The shortcomings of a lump of disorganized collagen holding stretched skin in an abnormal position and covered only with one or two layers of easily abraded epithelium are so obvious that it is usually worthwhile to interfere with natural phenomena so that a scar with superior physical and esthetic characteristics will be produced. Physical and chemical manipulations which can be performed on wounded skin and the biological basis for their success when selected and performed correctly are discussed in the following sections.

WOUNDS IN WHICH CONTINUITY OF SKIN HAS BEEN INTERRUPTED BUT FULL-THICKNESS DERMIS HAS NOT BEEN LOST

The most important difference in healing which affects treatment of lacerations or superficial burns not resulting in loss of dermis, compared to avulsions or deep burns in which full-thickness dermis is lost, is that the natural phenomenon of contraction plays a more significant role when dermis is lost. Contraction of linear scars following healing of a simple laceration usually does not result in significant movement of uninjured skin, for such a contracture usually is caused by a rigid scar traversing areas of changing dimension where elasticity is needed for normal function and appearance. Thus a linear scar crossing a flexion crease on the volar surface of a finger or around the lip or eyelid can produce a serious relative contracture; dense connective tissue in the scar does not lengthen and shorten (stretch or recoil) as smoothly and extensively as uninjured skin. If healing and secondary remodeling of the scar occur with the tissue in a short position (finger flexed), the final contracture will appear to have been caused by active wound or scar contraction. Actually, contracture produced in such wounds is not the result of active wound contraction; contracture occurred because secondary remodeling of the scar produced a rigid internal splint while

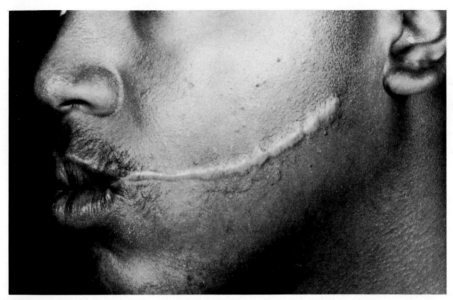

Figure 6-1. Linear scar crossing lines of changing dimension. This type of scar may cause a contracture by splinting tissue in a shortened position. Movement of tissue by wound contraction is not a prominent feature of this type of scar.

the affected tissue remained in a recoiled or shortened position. Contracture under these circumstances is distinctly different from a contraction produced by healing in a wound where skin is missing. When skin is absent, the healing process produces a significant change in length (or width) by active movement of skin edges which may pull a finger or the chin into a severely flexed position.

The tendency for short scars to widen is much more predictable than the tendency for long scars to shorten. Undoubtedly some scars do shorten a little when they occur in areas such as the lips or eyelids where redundant skin is easy to move. When dermis has not been lost, loss of redundancy and elasticity usually is more important in development of deformity than the mechanical shift of uninjured tissue which occurs when dermis has been lost. The term contraction has been applied rather loosely to both conditions because of the similarity in the final appearance of the scar. This is unfortunate, because similarity is only in the final appearance; the mechanism by which each deformity is produced and the steps which an experienced surgeon will take to prevent or alter contour deformity may be entirely different, depending upon whether skin has been lost or only lacerated.

The major biological processes involved in restoration of physical integrity following simple laceration of skin are synthesis of fibrous protein and epithelization. Of the two, epithelization is the less important to the surgeon because it involves only a small area and occurs relatively quickly without need of an external catalyst. Exactly the opposite is true, however, for fibrous protein synthesis and ultimate remodeling of scar tissue. Almost everything that is important to the patient is dependent upon the manner, speed, and extent of these processes. They are processes which extend over a relatively long period of time and about which we know enough now to take positive steps to make the outcome more predictable in terms of cosmetic and functional success. Thus, active treatment of skin lacerations is primarily manipulation and control of fundamental processes involving connective tissue metabolism.

Initial considerations in the care of a skin laceration involve cleaning or preparing the wound and making a decision about whether it should be closed mechanically or allowed to heal by natural processes. The technique of preparation and the judgment involved in making a decision about coapting skin edges demand sounder biological understanding than was possible only a few decades ago. Both involve clear recognition of the important difference between contamination and infection. As a general rule, contaminated wounds can be converted to surgically clean wounds and surgically clean wounds can be closed almost routinely. Infected wounds cannot be prepared or converted by simple quick procedures to surgically clean ones; therefore, they cannot be closed by mechanical methods designed to produce minimal scars. The key to accurate diagnosis and successful management of lacerations at this stage rests largely upon diagnostic ability in distinguishing between contamination and infection.

Immediate Wound Management

In the extremely important differentiation between infection and contamination, both history and physical examination provide data for judgment. The most important considerations in the history are length of time between injury and treatment and the strength and type of foreign inoculum. In the history of wound management, it is notable that search for a safe number of hours between injury and closure which could serve as a rule by which the decision to close all wounds could be made has shown that no such reliable numerical indicator exists. During World War I, an intensive search by French military surgeons to determine the number of hours under which primary closure was permissible was made by studying the bacterial content of open contaminated wounds. By performing serial cultures and bacterial counts it was noted that, around 12 hours after injury, the number of colonies of bacteria on a wound surface often doubled. This finding suggested that, by 12 hours, bacteria had established a firm right of domain and could proliferate in an unimpeded manner. Closure of a wound at this stage seemed foolhardy, and so 10 to 12 hours was unofficially established as the longest period a wound should remain open if primary closure was to be attempted.

The fallacy of such reasoning is indicated by the consistent shortening of the safe time in each new edition of surgical textbooks on wound management. Some recent texts have even implied that after two hours primary closure should not be used. Obviously, each generation of surgeons has found that some wounds which were closed according to the safe period or a time rule became infected or developed other serious complications. Each such experience suggested that the time rule for closure of wounds was too lenient, and so a shorter time before closure must be recommended. Thus, the time interval rule became more and more stringent—another example of the never ending fallacy of trying to develop simple rules for complicated problems in surgical sciences. Actually, the surgeon with modern biological training realizes almost intuitively that the length of time the wound had been open is not nearly so important as accuracy in assessing the natural defenses in the area; the known or suspected strength and type of inoculum introduced; and the treatment the patient has received during the interim between injury and definitive surgical care.

Nothing is more valuable in making the final judgment between contamination (which can be converted to surgical cleanliness) and infection (which cannot be completely removed) than the cardinal signs of inflammation. Calor, rubor, tumor, and dolor following bacterial invasion are positive contraindications to mechanical closure of a wound, regardless of the length of time the wound has been open. When these signs are not present, however, the true state of affairs has to be estimated by piecing together bits of data obtained from the history and physical examination. That a lag in time occurs between bacterial invasion of tissue and the development of clinical signs of inflammation also must be remembered. Locally effective blood supply is probably the most important natural defense mechanism. Lower extremities have less efficient normal circulation than upper extremities, and the face and scalp contain the richest capillary network found anywhere on the surface of the body. Extent of injury to surrounding tissues also is important. Local defense mechanisms such as lymphatic obstruction, vascular supply, and other less well understood phenomena are rendered significantly less effective if soft tissue surrounding the wound has been contused or damaged in some other way. The shape and dimensions of the wound, the importance of structures lying within or close to the defect, and the general condition of the patient all must be considered when a positive contraindication to closure such as inflammation is not present. Deep penetrating wounds, lying between important nerves and tendons, can be less easily and effectively debrided than superficial defects in redundant tissue. Equally important is the size of the wound, especially in the hands or face of young people where there is no extra skin. In these areas, sacrifice of even a small amount of normal skin may result in functional or cosmetic impairment. Thus, a deep penetrating wound or laceration of a foot incurred in a recently fertilized garden wisely might be deemed unsatisfactory for primary closure minutes after the injury. On the other hand, a clean laceration of the face caused by clean fragments of glass might be closed safely several days after the injury was sustained.

Debridement

Selection of a local or general anesthetic does not influence significantly the biology of wound healing, and techniques for instilling anesthetic agents have little to do with the healing process except for occasional technical errors which affect circulation to wounded tissue. In this regard, the vasoconstrictive effect of some anesthetic agents (and such additives as epinephrine which prolong their effect) should be remembered while anesthetizing areas where segmental blood supply is critical. Damage to digital circulation by injection of procaine and epinephrine into relatively rigidly enclosed phalangeal compartments is an example of a preventable technical error which may not only inhibit

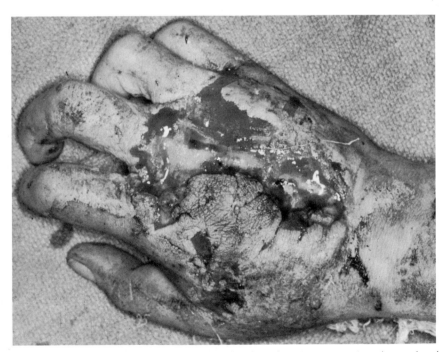

Figure 6–2. Avulsion of skin from dorsum of hand resulting in a contaminated wound and severely contused and fractured skin. After debridement, a primary abdominal pedicle flap was applied (see Chapter 7). (Reproduced by permission from E. E. Peacock, Jr., Southern Med. J. 56:56, 1963.)

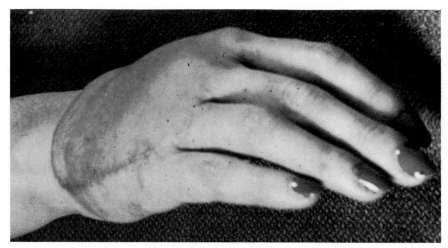

Figure 6–3.   Appearance of hand after primary debridement and application of abdominal pedicle flap. (Reproduced by permission from E. E. Peacock, Jr., Southern Med. J. 56:56, 1963.)

healing but occasionally will result in loss of an entire digit. Performing regional metacarpal nerve blocks in loose areolar tissue and avoiding use of anesthetics with added vasoconstrictors will prevent such complications.

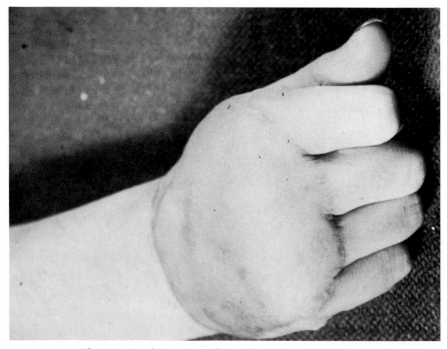

Figure 6–4.   Flexion view of same hand shown in Figure 6–3.

Once a decision to close a wound has been made and the area has been properly anesthetized, a technique for converting the wound to a surgically clean one must be selected. The simplest way is to excise the wound completely. In areas such as the trunk or an extremity, where excess tissue is present, complete excision is by far the simplest and most certain way to assure elimination of damaged and contaminated tissues. During excision of a deep, serpiginous defect, converting the wound to a unilocular cystic cavity by forcibly packing it with gauze and then placing several sutures in overlying skin to hold the gauze conformer inside the wound has been a useful technical adjuvant. The entire wound can then be treated as a tumor (imagining the gauze to be the tumor mass) by completely excising the tumor mass with a margin of normal tissue so that the gauze is never exposed.

When complete excision of a wound is not feasible, hydraulic cleansing by forceful irrigation, followed by specific excision of all fragments of dead tissue, is the best method for making the surface surgically clean. Again, however, judgment is essential and too much of a good thing can be detrimental to the fundamental cellular processes in healing of soft tissue wounds. A recently introduced instrument designed to cleanse crevices between teeth by hydraulic force is being used in emergency rooms to cleanse soft tissue wounds. It should be remembered that a stream of water can be ejected and pulsed sufficiently hard and often to damage tissue, kill cells, and actually drive bacteria into soft tissue. More gentle debridement by gravity flow or syringe ejection probably is safer than pump force from the standpoint of wound healing biology. By similar reasoning, a biologically oriented surgeon would never select a solution to irrigate a wound which he would not be willing, for instance, to instill into his own conjunctival sac. Chemical antiseptics and antimetabolites effective in killing bacteria also kill cells which either contribute to the local defense mechanism or participate in other ways in the healing process. The effectiveness of wound irrigation, therefore, should be primarily that of ejection of surface contaminants by a turbulent swirl of some liquid. Hydrogen peroxide is occasionally added to irrigating solutions with the mistaken notion that oxidizing properties might be of some value in poisoning anaerobic organisms. Such a brief exposure obviously does not significantly affect tough anaerobes, however; if any benefit is derived from adding hydrogen peroxide to irrigating solutions, it is from mechanical foaming, which is of particular value in removing recently clotted blood. Forceful irrigation of a wound by manually operated syringe or by holding a finger or extremity under an open tap (followed by sterile saline or water irrigation) is effective only in removing bacteria and tissue debris which are lying free on the surface. Devitalized tissue may remain attached to the wound by small strands of collagen or fat; these nonviable fragments may provide a dangerous pabulum for bacteria as well as produce a physical impediment to healing. It is imperative, therefore, that all fragments of tissue which are not clearly viable be excised after hydraulic irrigation has been accomplished. In a compound wound of the hand, such selective debridement will be tedious and exacting compared to more simple excision of an entire wound in an area such as the buttocks.

A specific exception to the general principle of removing all devitalized tissue involves the handling of special tissue which performs important physical functions regardless of whether cells within it are dead or alive. Such tissues can be transplanted as free grafts without living cells, with the anticipation that recipient cells from the new wound will invade the graft as part of the healing process. Most such grafts, of course, are fibrous tissue grafts, such as dura, fascia, and tendon. Although it would be unthinkable to leave any portions of these structures in a wound if there was reasonable doubt that they could be rendered surgically clean, tenuous fragments of dura or tendon, obviously devitalized by disconnection from their blood supply, could and should be used in repairing a wound if their surfaces have not been damaged so badly that irrigation and surgical preparation cannot render them surgically clean.

An example of such a mistake in surgical judgment involves unnecessary removal of exposed or partially avulsed tendons in the distal extremities. It is known that even trypsin-cleared tendon allografts (in which every single viable cell has been removed by enzyme activity) make excellent tendon replacements by virtue of the stability of the collagen framework during a period of approximately four weeks required for host cells to migrate into the graft. Hence, a surgeon would not be acting on sound biological grounds if he removed tendons from an extremity just because the cells within them were suspected of being devitalized. On the volar surface of the hand, where long amplitudes of tendon motion are required, it is likely that damaged tendons might not glide even though retained by surgical reconstruction and host cell replacement. Nothing is lost by treating them as free grafts at the initial surgical manipulation, however. Whether or not gliding function is restored is a problem of secondary remodeling of newly synthesized connective tissue (see Chapter 8).

On the dorsum of the hand, when only a small amplitude of extension is needed, a structurally stable scar may extend the fingers completely even though an anatomically separate tendon is not discernible. Following deep burns on the dorsum of the hand, the extensor tendons in the depth of the wound may be brown in color and obviously seriously damaged by thermal injury. Even though not one viable cell remains, such tendons contain tightly packed longitudinally oriented bundles of heat-denatured collagen which are exactly the right length and in an ideal location to transmit power from the forearm muscles. To excise these collagenous structures during debridement would make it necessary later to perform complex secondary restorative procedures. If the wound can be prepared for closure in all other respects, burned tendons should be protected and allowed to remain beneath adequate skin and fat coverage; ultimately they will be recellularized and will be as good as any free extensor tendon graft.

During extensive debridement of extremity wounds, the tourniquet test is useful in distinguishing viable from nonviable structures. This test is based on Sir Thomas Lewis' "triple response to injury," and is sometimes referred to as the tourniquet blush effect. As every reconstructive surgeon knows, producing ischemia in an extremity by applying a proximal arterial tourniquet results in release of various tissue amines almost instantly after arterial flow has been reestablished. The release of these substances causes immediate temporary closure of precapillary shunts, opening of capillary networks, or both. The tissue literally blushes for three to five minutes, after which it may become slightly cyanotic. Apparently sphincters on the venous side of the capillary network exert constrictive action before preischemic tone on the precapillary side is regained. Because capillary perfusion is dramatic immediately after release of the tourniquet, unjustified confidence may be placed in the potential vitality of tissues which show a blush reaction. The tourniquet blush test is of value only in that it shows the potential of the tissue at that moment to respond to circulating amines, but a sound understanding of the physiology of post-tourniquet hyperemia is needed to interpret the blush test correctly. Hyperemia is only temporary, and is usually followed by a short phase of venous congestion, which in itself may promote thrombus formation. Thus, tissues retained because they "blush" following removal of a proximal tourniquet do not always remain viable. In judging the viability of skin margins, it is helpful to remember that studies of vascular supply to dermis reveal a relatively rich arterial input. Clinical experience has shown that venous return, not arterial input, is the critical factor in survival of skin flaps. When damaged skin is lost because of vascular insufficiency, it usually becomes turgid in consistency and dark in color. Blood obviously is being trapped, and restoration of venous drainage is the key to successful reversal. The blush test in skin with embarrassed circulation is not nearly so meaningful, therefore, as the appearance of a permanent dusky discoloration after hyperemia and initial venous congestion have passed.

Understandably, search continues for a test of tissue viability which can be used by the surgeon as a guide to wound debridement. One should remember, however, that a test of viability for tissue is really of no more value than a test of viability for the whole body. What is really needed is a forecast of whether tissue will survive during the healing process. A few minutes' reflection leads the surgeon to the inescapable conclusion that such a test is impossible. Because one cannot forecast what conditions will affect viability in the hours and days ahead, there is no possibility of forecasting whether tissue will survive except to give it a "sporting chance."

In testing the skin flap for potential viability, a sharp line of color demarcation is the single most important clinical observation. A flap which is a little dusky on one end but in which there is no single point or clear line where the surgeon can say that circulation is normal on one side and abnormal on the other probably has adequate venous return. A sharp line or clean demarcation, however, so that there is normal color on one side and cyanosis on the other, is a dangerous sign; and unless the sharpness of the line can be modified by removal of a few sutures, performing a proximal relaxing incision, or adjusting the overall tension, the discolored part of the flap should be excised and a replacement procedure performed.

Primary Closure

As soon as debridement has been accomplished, the wound is ready for closure. The surgeon's objective is to place various layers in close apposition so that a minimal amount of new connective tissue will be required to restore structural integrity in the shortest possible time.

A thorough understanding of the composition of various layers of skin and subcutaneous tissue (particularly as regards their relative natural fiber content) and a thorough understanding of the physical and chemical properties of currently available artificial fibers are fundamental to the proper selection and placement of sutures in a skin wound. Even the selection and placement of a suture can be based upon sound biological principles. Selecting sutures out of habit and passing them through all layers of the wound in routine, mechanistic fashion may lead to unnecessary wound complications or produce a scar of less than optimal physical and esthetic characteristics. A more desirable approach is to select thoughtfully and analytically the best artificial fiber (suture) to maintain the edges coapted until a natural fiber (collagen) is synthesized.

In these introductory statements, the word fiber has been frequently used, intentionally. A skin wound results in a loss of strength in that area. The objective of both surgical treatment and natural healing is to restore physical strength; the key process for both is insertion, utilization, and synthesis of fibers. Of all of the elements involved in the healing process, many of which contribute strength to the finished product, fibers are the most important as far as strength is concerned. Cells, blood vessels, ground substance, and fibrin contribute to the development of tensile strength — particularly in the early period (day 2 to 5). In fact, in some wounds, sutures are removed at a time when these substances or structures account for most of the strength of the wound. Wounds held together only by nonfibrous material, however, are relatively fragile and often undergo considerable changes in size and appearance during the two to three week period following removal of artificial fibers, as well as during the synthesis and before the effective remodeling of natural fibers.

The objectives of using sutures are to obliterate space, stop hemorrhage, and impart physical strength to a discontinuous surface. The position which a suture occupies in a multilayered wound is governed by a clear analysis of the task the suture is expected to accomplish. For example, a suture placed through cells (which are approximately 90 per cent water) could not be expected to impart very much in the way of physical strength no matter how strong the suture material might be. For providing strength, placing sutures in fat or epithelium is comparable to suturing such tissues as liver or spleen. Placing sutures in fascia and dermis, however, is a different matter, provided the sutures are left in place until the natural fiber has been synthesized and assembled and the end product remodeled until it is as strong as the suture. This process may require many months. Sutures which hold dermal edges together, but are tied on the outside of the skin, cannot be left in place for months without producing epithelium-lined pits and sinus tracts. Such tracts often become infected and leave unsightly scars. To remove stitches before suture marks develop, yet before natural fibers effectively replace them leaves the immature scar at the mercy of deforming physical forces. The only glue to oppose these forces is the relatively inefficient combination of cells, blood vessels, and fibrin.

Sutures and Suturing

Suture materials are of two general types: absorbable and nonabsorbable. These classifications may be broken down into two additional types: monfilament and multifilament. Other classifications have been proposed, such as natural fibers and synthetic fibers, but studies have shown that such classifications serve no useful purpose from a biological point of view.

ABSORBABLE SUTURES.   Four types of absorbable sutures are currently available: catgut, collagen, polyglycolic acid, and a co-polymer of glycolic and lactic acids in the ratio of 90:10. Catgut is derived from the submucosa of sheep intestines or the serosa of beef intestines. The jejunum and ileum of these animals are slit into two or more longitudinal ribbons. The mucosa, muscularis, and other unwanted layers are removed by a combination of mechanical and chemical treatments. These cleaned ribbons are treated with a dilute solution of formaldehyde which blocks hydroxyl and amino groups on collagen that is the major component of the suture material and increases its strength and resistance to enzymatic attack in the body. If more resistance is required, an additional treatment with basic chromium salts is given. Thus two types of catgut are produced: plain and chromic.

Depending upon the size of suture desired, one, two, or more ribbons are twisted together and the twisted strands are dried under tension, on frames. When dry, they are polished by centerless grinders to the correct size, cut into required lengths, have needles attached to them, are packaged and are sterilized by cobalt-60 irradiation.

Collagen sutures are prepared from the long flexor tendons of steers. After cleaning, the tendons are frozen, sliced, treated with ficin, washed, and swollen in dilute cyanoacetic acid, and the viscous gel so produced is extruded through a spinerette into an acetone bath, formed into a ribbon which is stretched, treated with formaldehyde or chromic salts or both, twisted, and dried. These sutures are currently made only in fine sizes and are used almost exclusively in ophthalmological surgery. Polyglycolic acid and the co-polymer of glycolic and lactic acids, termed polyglactin-910, are prepared from monomers, and polymerization is catalyzed by organometallic compounds. The polymers are extruded from a hot melt and undergo stretching and annealing. The fine fibers so produced are braided into strands of various sizes.

Catgut when implanted into the body undergoes digestion by acid proteases produced by inflammatory cells. This process of digestion is usually slightly slower for chrome-treated catgut than for plain catgut. The rate of digestion, however, is highly variable. In some sites and under certain conditions, digestion may be rapid, and both plain and chromic catgut may disappear within two or three weeks. On the other hand, both types of catgut may be found in tissues as long as two years after implantation.

The fact that catgut sutures are digested by proteolytic enzymes derived from inflammatory cells has important biological implications. The most rapidly absorbed suture, plain catgut, incites a greater inflammatory reaction than chromic catgut. Thus use of plain catgut in skin or dermis close to the surface produces so great an inflammatory reaction that the overlying tissue may be red and inflamed for a long period. Chromic catgut usually produces a much milder reaction.

Polyglycolic acid and polyglactin-910 do not depend upon enzymatic action for absorption. These polymers are slowly hydrolyzed by water. Hydrolysis will proceed more rapidly in alkaline media than in neutral or acid media. The principal cellular reaction to these sutures is invasion of the interstices by macrophages. The disappearance of these sutures is quite constant and occurs in about 80 days in the the case of polyglactin-910 and in about 100 to 120 days in the case of polyglycolic acid.

It is an interesting and biologically important fact that both catgut and synthetic absorbable sutures lose strength more rapidly than they disappear. It is not uncommon to retrieve one of these sutures which appears intact, but which has absolutely no strength. This suggests that several points along the polymer chain have been attacked and the backbone broken. This would destroy the strength, but would not cause the suture to disappear. Consider a rope: if one cuts it, the entire length of the rope has no strength, but the rope has lost no mass. In general it can be said that catgut has lost about 50 per cent of its strength in 20 to 30 days. This is true also for polyglactin-910. Polyglycolic acid loses strength slightly faster; it is more hydrophilic than polyglactin-910 since the latter material has methyl groups projecting from portions of the polymer chain which make it somewhat hydrophobic and thus more resistant to hydrolysis.

NONABSORBABLE SUTURES.   The principal nonabsorbable sutures are silk, cotton, nylon, polyester (Dacron), polypropylene, and steel. Nylon and steel exist in both monofilament and multifilament form. Polypropylene is provided only as a monofilament and the other sutures only in multifilament form.

Although silk is usually classed as a nonabsorbable suture, it has been demonstrated that silk gradually loses tensile strength in tissue so that after about a year it has no strength and will usually have disappeared by two years. It should, therefore, be classed as a slowly absorbable suture.

With the exception of nylon, none of the truly nonabsorbable sutures changes in strength in tissue after implantation. Nylon will swell in tissue and lose about 20 per cent of its initial strength after a year. No further diminution of strength has been observed.

Braided multifilament sutures present an abrasive surface to tissues as the suture is drawn through. In an attempt to provide a smoother and more "slippery" surface, various substances have been used to coat multifilament sutures. Some 75 years ago, beeswax was used on silk, usually in the operating room, to "lubricate" silk sutures; later suture manufacturers applied it at the time of production. For a while, some silk sutures were coated with silicone oil and now this treatment has been applied to polyester sutures. Polyester sutures have been impregnated with emulsions of polytetrafluoroethane (Teflon). These coatings have reduced the coefficient of friction of the suture materials and thus reduced "drag" through tissue. Unfortunately, the coating materials used tend to detach from the suture and be deposited as globules or flakes in tissue. Macrophages engulf the particles, but since they cannot dispose of them, a small chronic granulomatous reaction may occur. Very recently, a new coating material, 1,4-polybutanediol adipate, has been used to coat polyester sutures. This material appears to be firmly bonded to the suture, provides good lubrication, and may prove to be an acceptable and superior substitute for older bonding or lubricating agents.

All nonabsorbable sutures induce a cellular reaction around them. Silk and cotton produce the greatest reaction. Polyester, whether or not it is coated, produces a distinctly less cellular reaction than silk or cotton. Nylon is less reactive than polyester, and polypropylene and steel are the least reactive suture materials. In the case of silk and cotton, the initial reaction may be truly inflammatory with polymorphonuclear cells, lymphocytes, and macrophages. This usually passes to a strictly macrophage reaction and these cells attract fibroblasts which produce a fibrous collagenous capsule around the suture. The other suture materials differ only in the extent of the macrophage reaction produced and in the density of the fibrous capsule which eventually surrounds them. In noninfected wounds, all of these cellular reactions are microscopic and seldom encompass an area more than twice the diameter of the suture. The reactivity of the suture material is really only of importance in areas close to the body surface.

In the presence of bacterial contamination or infection, the construction and biological properties of suture material become important. Catgut will be absorbed rapidly in an infected wound since the presence of large numbers of inflammatory cells increases the concentration of proteolytic enzymes which can attack catgut. The synthetic absorbable sutures are not affected by inflammation since they are not attacked by enzymes. All sutures, however, are foreign bodies and, as such, tend to prolong an existing infection. From the standpoint of the surgeon and the patient, the choice of suture material in a potentially contaminated wound is very important. The construction of multifilament sutures is such that bacteria and tissue fluids can penetrate the interstices of the strand, but inflammatory cells cannot. Thus, bacteria are sequestered in a nutrient environment away from the body's first line of defense, the polymorphonuclear cells and the macrophages. These bacteria can multiply and convert a contamination to an infection. Monofilament sutures, on the other hand, provide no place for bacteria to hide and are thus less likely to convert contamination into infection.

Finally, another aspect of suture materials must be considered—their handling qualities. In general, multifilament sutures are easier to handle than monofilament sutures. They are more pliable, are easier to tie, and lie flatter, without stiff projecting ends where cut. Because of their braided construction, multifilament sutures are slightly more difficult to remove from skin wounds than monofilament sutures. Sutures made from synthetic polymers such as polyester and nylon require more knots to hold them in place than do natural fibers such as silk and cotton. Synthetic polymer fibers possess "memory," the strain and orientation introduced during the extrusion and stretching process that results in their resisting bending forces and attempting to return to a straight configuration. In monofilament nylon, for instance, this tendency for knots to untie and the suture to return to a straight fiber is so pronounced that some surgeons jokingly place one knot for each day they wish the suture to stay in place. Polypropylene is less likely to untie because it is a softer, more plastic material than the other synthetic materials and, if the knots are set firmly, a flattening occurs where strands cross each other, providing a "locking" action. The synthetic absorbable sutures handle much like silk, which has the best handling qualities of all sutures, and knot holding has not been a problem with these materials.

SELECTION OF SUTURES.   With the large number of different suture materials available, many surgeons in the past have chosen their suture material on the basis of what they became accustomed to during their period of training or what "felt" best to them. Now that we know more about the biological and mechanical properties of sutures and the process of wound healing in various tissues and organs, suture selection can be made on a more rational basis.

A principle to bear in mind is that a suture is not needed after a wound has healed. Unfortunately we do not have sutures that retain strength for varying but known periods of time and then disappear. Furthermore, wounds in different tissues achieve their maximal strength at widely different times. For some tissues the available absorbable suture materials are adequate and, indeed, preferred. In others, the time to achieve maximal healing is so long that a nonabsorbable material should be used since none of the available absorbable sutures retain useful strength long enough.

Visceral wounds heal rapidly, attaining maximal strength within 14 to 21 days. In such organs as stomach, intestine, bladder, and bile duct, absorbable sutures are adequate and are probably preferable since some, the colon, for example, are potentially contaminated areas. Another reason for using absorbable sutures in organs such as the bile duct and urinary tract is that these organs contain crystalloids that are in a nearly saturated solution, and the presence of a foreign body such as sutures can cause precipitation or crystallization of these relatively insoluble materials, leading to stone formation. Thus, a suture that disappears quickly after healing has occurred is a necessity.

Fascia heals very slowly; ultimate strength is not attained for nearly a year. Although some surgeons use absorbable sutures for fascial closure, consideration of the biological properties of suture materials and the rate of wound healing argues strongly for closure with nonabsorbable suture materials.

In cardiovascular surgery, the insertion of a synthetic material to replace a section of a major artery, or the replacement of a damaged heart valve with a synthetic substitute, dictates the use of a nonabsorbable suture. The suture will have to hold the vascular prosthesis or heart valve in place for the rest of the patient's life, as these synthetic substitutes are never incorporated into living tissue. It was the use of silk sutures in the early days of vascular prosthesis and heart valve substitution that led to the discovery that silk was not a permanent suture material. Late failure of the suture line led to several fatalities.

Many surgeons fail to appreciate that skin heals slowly. Late remodeling of scars in skin after early suture removal results in widening of the scar and a cosmetically undesirable result. Skin wounds of the face heal more rapidly than skin wounds in the abdomen, probably because the blood supply in facial skin is better. Nevertheless, widening of the scar can occur unless the wound is held in the coapted position for a considerable period of time.

Another consideration in the use of sutures in skin is the propensity for epithelial migration along the suture tract. As discussed in Chapter 2, epithelium migrates down a wound surface and the placing of a suture creates a wound. When the suture is removed, a scar is formed in the wound and migrating epithelium meets and crosses over this scar, creating a small pit or dimple at each suture site. The only way to prevent this unsightly pitting is to remove the suture early before epithelization has progressed deeply into the suture tract. As will be discussed later, one of several maneuvers is required to keep wound edges closely apposed during the healing process that is still in progress following early suture removal.

The basic principles in suture selection involve a knowledge of the biological and mechanical properties of suture materials and the rate at which wounds of various tissues heal, as well as an assessment of local conditions in the particular wound. Consideration of these three factors will enable the surgeon to select the material best suited to a given clinical situation.

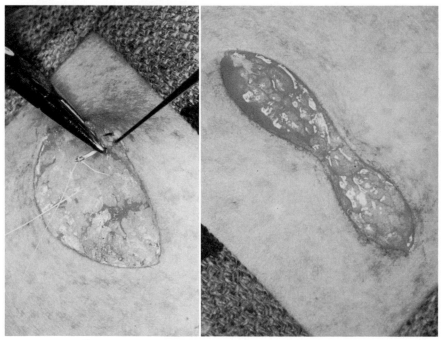

Fig. 6–5   Fig. 6–6

Figure 6–5. Insertion of subcutaneous suture to close dead space and control capillary oozing.
Figure 6–6. Appearance of wound following insertion of subcutaneous suture.

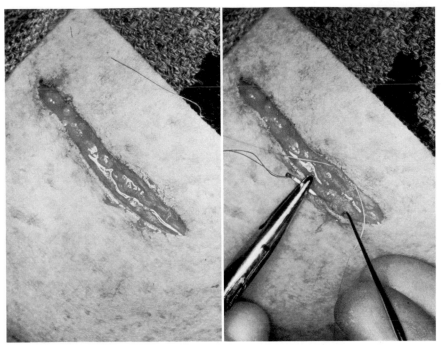

Fig. 6–7   Fig. 6–8

Figure 6–7. After insertion of multiple subcutaneous sutures, skin edges still are not in approximation. If a scar of this width is acceptable, skin sutures can be inserted. Otherwise, a permanent suture must be used to bring fibrous protein (dermal) layers together.

Figure 6–8. Insertion of subcuticular suture into deep layers of dermis.

SUTURING. In addition to consideration of the proper suture material, selection of the plane or layer of the wound which will receive the sutures has biological importance. Essentially, sutures which are expected to provide temporary strength have to be placed in fibrous structures. Sutures which are used to obliterate dead space, discourage capillary hemorrhage, or make fine adjustments in tissue surfaces can be put in any layer. The selection of sutures and the position they will occupy in a typical wound of skin and subcutaneous fat can be worked out in terms of modern wound biology as follows:

The main objective of placing sutures in subcutaneous fat is to control capillary hemorrhage and obliterate a space which would be caused by pulling skin edges together over the top of a subcutaneous defect. Blood, liquefied fat, serum, and other wound contents form a perfect culture medium for bacteria. A subcutaneous space acts as a reservoir for such material which, even if infection does not occur, can cause complications such as dehiscence or excessive deep scar formation. A few loosely tied sutures in subcutaneous fat will obliterate space beneath skin; it makes no difference in most instances whether the sutures are absorbable or nonabsorbable. If there is no reason to fear infection, nonabsorbable sutures usually are selected because of ease of handling and minimal tissue reaction.

After subcutaneous tissue has been closed and before skin sutures are inserted, a decision should be made about the type of surface scar desired. The reason for such consideration is that, if skin sutures are put in next, the resulting scar usually will be about the same size and shape as the defect, following closure of subcutaneous tissue. At this time there usually is about a 0.5 cm. gap between skin edges and, if this is the case, a 0.5 cm. width scar will develop approximately four weeks after skin sutures have been removed. Fundamental collagen biochemistry can be held accountable for enlargement of the scar; therefore, there is no reason to accept such an occurrence as inevitable if collagen synthesis and remodeling are considered. Most skin sutures should be removed after five to ten days if the likelihood of stitch abscesses and suture marks is to be minimal. Although there is some biochemical evidence of collagen synthesis as early as the end of the second day following injury, collagen fibrils and fibers cannot be recognized in human wounds at light microscopic magnifications before the seventh to ninth day. New collagen that is recognizable at this time, however, appears

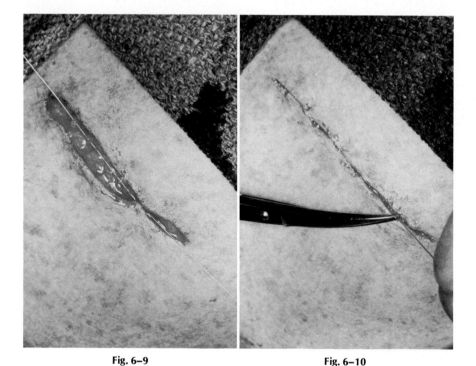

Fig. 6–9   Fig. 6–10

Figure 6–9.   Accurate approximation of dermis by tying subcuticular suture. A dark suture will show through overlying epithelium; a light-colored suture should always be used.
Figure 6–10.   Fine-pointed scissors are introduced between overlying epithelial edges to cut subcuticular sutures so short that tails do not extrude.

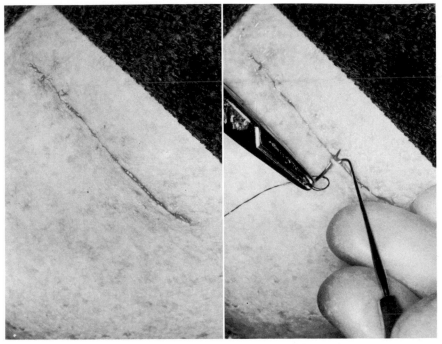

Fig. 6–11   Fig. 6–12

Figure 6–11. Appearance of wound after subcuticular sutures have been inserted. Note that although skin edges are in relatively close approximation, a vertical unevenness persists.
Figure 6–12. Insertion of No. 6-0 silk epithelial sutures. Note that the distance from wound edge to insertion of suture is no more than the width of the needle. This suture is primarily an epithelial stitch.

completely devoid of purposeful organization and probably contributes surprisingly little to the strength of the wound. The amount of total collagen which can be measured by hydroxyproline analysis in healing incised and sutured wounds does not reach maximal levels until about the forty-second day. Then although total collagen in the scar does not increase after the forty-second day, there is measurable increase in tensile strength for at least 24 months and elevated collagenolytic enzyme activity for an equally long period of time. These findings suggest that continual collagen remodeling occurs and that the result of this remodeling is a more efficient, yet smaller, scar. At six days, the wound has not accrued enough collagen to assemble a scar with strength comparable to that of artificial sutures, much less assemble that collagen into an efficiently woven scar. Therefore, removal of sutures at that time subjects coapted skin edges to a deforming force which is resisted only by fibrin and cells. The wound rarely breaks open at this stage, but the width of the scar will increase gradually over the next three weeks because there is little to resist deformation other than a gelatinous in-

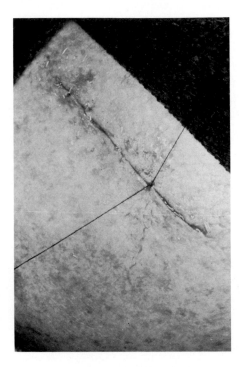

Figure 6–13. Epithelial edges are leveled. Note that suture marks are impossible because of proximity of suture to wound edge.

tradermal matrix. Theoretically, sutures should stay in wound edges for at least three to four months if appearance is not a concern.

An interesting question relates to whether collagen would remodel effectively and whether the total amount of collagen synthesized would be as great if sutures were allowed to remain for an extended period of time. One laboratory experiment and several clinical observations suggest that both quantity and quality of scar would be affected if sutures remained a long period of time. In normal skin and in healing incised and sutured wounds of rats, saline-extractable collagen is significantly elevated if normal skin or new scar is subjected to elastic traction. The size of cutaneous scars which characteristically develop around the pectoral, deltoid, and knee regions is usually out of proportion to scars which result from healing of similar wounds elsewhere on the body. Both clinical and laboratory observations, therefore, lend support to the notion that both the amount and organization of scar tissue are influenced by physical forces acting across the wound. Such data provide a sound biological basis for the use of subcuticular sutures to maintain coapted cutaneous edges and thus reduce the amount of new scar tissue.

A subcuticular suture is usually a nonabsorbable suture placed in a primarily fibrous structure (dermis), but beneath epidermis, so that it can remain, at least during the four to six months when scar remodel-

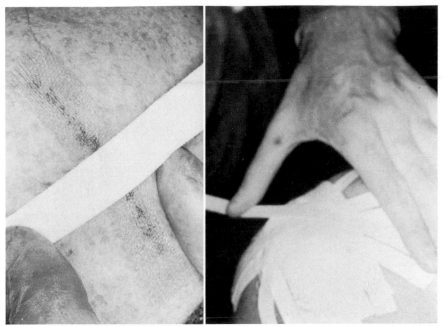

Fig. 6–14   Fig. 6–15

Figure 6–14. Application of fine-mesh gauze to suture line and relief of tension across wound by adhesive tape splinting.
Figure 6–15. In areas where skin tension is likely to be great, skin may be splinted with multiple strips of narrow adhesive tape extending in radial directions.

ing is in progress. Actually, although some subcuticular sutures are extruded (presumably because of mechanical irritation or excess foreign body reaction), most of these sutures remain within dermis forever. In selecting materials for subcuticular sutures, nonabsorbable characteristics are desirable. Soft, natural fibers such as cotton or silk are better than stiff wire or synthetic substances. Even cotton and silk lose tensile strength progressively, however, after being embedded in tissue.

Proper placement of subcuticular sutures requires some practice, for the long-term function of the suture is dependent upon the suture's being superficial enough to hold skin edges in close approximation but deep enough so that a healthy layer of epithelium will cover it. A common error in placing a subcuticular suture is to pierce the under surface of epithelium so that the suture passes through it before it passes through underlying dermis. Any foreign fiber passing through epithelium, producing interruption of intercellular bridges and cell surfaces, provides both the initiating stimulus and the physical template for mitosis and migration. This is particularly true when germinative layers of epithelium are involved. The result is that epithelium migrates along the suture, following it through dermis and up to the opposite epithelial surface. Only when like cells are encountered on the opposite side does contact inhibition put an end to such migratory activity. The wound will then be traversed by both a suture and an epithelium-lined tract. Such a tract may not always cause serious abnormalities in the final appearance or function of the scar but, from a biological standpoint, closed epithelial sinuses, cysts, or internal tracts are unnecessary hazards.

It is normal for epithelium to die, shed its corporeal remains, and renew itself in cyclical fashion. The pulsing or stimulating factors which govern epithelial cycles are apparently general in their action, and intradermal tracts are subject to the same type of cyclical responses as surface cells. Because skin epithelium normally undergoes pronounced keratinization, keratin embedded within dermal layers or subcutaneous tissue produces cysts which have a propensity to become secondarily infected. Occasionally subcuticular sutures which pass through epithelial tissue are extruded without inflammatory reaction; more often they serve as a nidus for a sterile or bacterial inflammation and produce more scar on the surface than if the suture had not been extruded. A simple and effective technical maneuver to prevent extrusion of subcuticular sutures involves proper preparation of skin edges during debridement and elective excision of surface lesions. The trick is to bevel the edges under the epithelial surface so that an overhanging epithelial edge is produced. The epithelial layer is then clearly defined and can be retracted with a hook while intradermal sutures are being inserted. After the sutures have been tied, the overlying wound shelf can be adjusted to cover the sutures in dermis.

There probably is not any real advantage to using a subcuticular suture of absorbable material unless a chromicized suture is selected. Actually, the most important need from a biological standpoint for a subcuticular suture is during the period following removal of cutaneous sutures and the remodeling of newly synthesized collagen. If the suture is significantly weakened or absorbed during this critical period, widening of the scar will occur. The relatively severe inflammatory reaction to untanned collagen and the short period of time it remains structurally stable makes a suture of plain gut unacceptable in the subcuticular region. The biological basis for using subcuticular sutures is best realized by selecting a small, strong, light-colored material with low-intensity tissue reaction. A popular suture is number 5–0 white silk; various new synthetic materials also appear promising.

Following insertion of a row of subcuticular sutures, epithelial edges should be in such close approximation that use of additional sutures appears unnecessary. However, further adjustment of epithelial edges with a fine suture or surface adhesive has a sound biological basis. It is important to remember that the tensile strength requisites during all stages of healing have been satisfied by placing a permanent nonabsorbable suture in a superficial, predominantly fibrous, protein structure. It is not only unnecessary to pass a subcutaneous suture

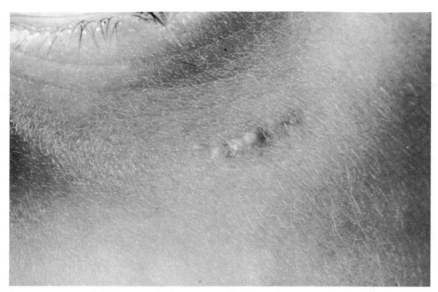

Figure 6–16. Epithelial cysts which occasionally form along skin suture tracts. Such cysts are not seen when skin is taped together without using sutures.

through the dermal layer of skin; it is essential for a surface suture not to pass into dermis if epithelial tracts, sinuses, and pits are to be avoided. Actually, the only reason for putting in epithelial sutures or applying tapes to the surface is to provide a fine adjustment or leveling device for epidermis. This can be very important in facial wounds, as it is almost impossible to put in a row of subcuticular sutures without making unrecognizable errors in the level of dermal approximation. If such errors are not corrected on the surface, a scar with an uneven vertical plane will occur. Such a scar can produce troublesome, ill defined shadows when the face is illuminated from a unilateral source. Shadows produce a sort of hardness in the countenance, and revision of vertically uneven scars makes an amazing difference in overall facial appearance. Correcting surface unevenness is sometimes appropriately referred to as "softening the expression."

Because epithelial sutures in a properly repaired wound contribute virtually nothing to the overall strength of the wound, there is no reason to place them more than one cell away from the wound edge. If such sutures are placed widely, or are allowed to penetrate dermis, suture marks are inevitable and plastic tape would have been preferable. When epithelial sutures are used, considerable accuracy in placing them is necessary. Actually, a properly placed epithelial suture of number 6–0 or number 7–0 silk may not even have to be cut for removal. The normal desquamating process causes the suture to be extruded so that most of these sutures can be gently picked off the surface after a few days, with only desquamated epithelium attached to them.

If a scar of approximately the same width as the defect before cutaneous sutures are inserted is acceptable (which is usual in sites other than the face), cutaneous sutures can be used to approximate the entire thickness of skin. Nonabsorbable material usually is selected to keep the surface skin reaction minimal. It should be remembered, however, that chromicized collagen sutures produce relatively little skin reaction, and fine chromic gut sutures are useful sometimes in closing wounds in small children or in areas where removal of the sutures will be troublesome. Even absorbable sutures inaccurately selected and inserted without regard to the reaction of skin to penetration, compression, and ischemia, however, may produce suture marks, cross-striations, uneven scars, and other familiar but usually unnecessary complications. Such is the price of a mechanical approach to a sensitive biological system.

Postoperative Care and Complications

All of the complications from mere mechanical handling of skin wounds are not instantaneous in production or appearance. A wound of skin which has been closed by widely placed, too tightly tied, or tissue necrosing sutures often can be partially salvaged. A surgeon with sensitivity to the delicacy of cellular and fibrous protein stages in wound healing can make a big difference in the final appearance of a scar even as late as four days after skin edges have been roughly approximated. Certainly during the first 36 hours, an opportunity exists to prevent epithelial tracts from forming, relieve tension that may lead to ischemia, and prevent wide suture marks. Even if it is necessary to separate wound edges to insert a subcuticular suture or correct a vertical misalignment, the healing process is not significantly delayed. The well known secondary healing effect will result in such accelerated healing in these wounds that the overall time for healing will be scarcely altered.

Here it should be mentioned that the secondary healing phenomenon, in addition to being of tremendous importance in the study of experimental healing and in managing a complete dehiscence of surgical wounds, also can be utilized to considerable advantage when elective incisions are being made. When a scar from a previous skin wound is present in the area where another incision is required, many surgeons either avoid the scarred area completely or excise the scar with an ellipse of surrounding skin. Such practice eliminates the potential usefulness of the secondary healing phenomenon. Not only does a wound made through a previous scar heal faster and with greater burst strength than scars of similar age in unwounded skin, but interestingly, the amount of collagen in the final scar is less and the appearance of the scar usually is better than in primary wounds of the same age. The surgeon who is knowledgeable about recent investigations of the mechanism of secondary healing will make every effort commensurate with good surgical exposure to place an incision through an old scar. Even if the scar is hypertrophic, no scar tissue should be excised. The final secondary scar almost invariably will have less collagen and appear less hypertrophic than the first, even though no collagenous tissue was removed. Although the important factors which affect collagen metabolism in scar tissue and thus affect the final appearance are not understood completely, such phenomena as natural collagenolytic enzyme production and proliferation of cells containing acid hydrolases follow a second opening of a wound—even if years have elapsed since the first wound healed. Reopening an old wound starts a different set of events than occurred when previously uninjured skin was incised. The scar which results from a second wound, therefore, is different both in physical characteristics and in appearance from the scar which developed after the initial wound.

DRESSING OF WOUNDS.   Many surgeons feel that skin wounds need not be covered by any dressing, provided skin is protected from additional trauma or inordinate bacterial contamination. In skin wounds which involve facial features, such as a cleft lip repair, the sutures require more care than in other areas of the body, for surface scarring can be held to a minimum by insuring that stitch abscesses do not develop beneath tiny blood clots or other surface debris. Because a surface suture produces a small indentation or well where it enters skin, if a drop of blood or plasma forms a small clot over this pit a tiny space for infection beneath the clot may be produced. The surrounding skin may give little hint that low-grade infection is occurring along the suture tract but when the suture is removed the clot also comes off, and it is very distressing sometimes to find a small crater caused by destruction of epithelium by bacteria. Healing of stitch abscesses usually is rapid, but a small increase in width of the scar or development of punctate suture marks may provide a permanent record of the events which took place beneath the blood clot. The obvious solution is to prevent micro stitch abscesses by providing continuous surface drainage. Continual removal of any blood which collects around sutures during the first 24 hours and application of a water-soluble emollient after oozing ceases (either free or on a fine-mesh gauze) is all that is necessary.

In addition to protecting the suture line, a dressing contributes to the healing process by partially immobilizing skin surrounding the wound. Similar biological reasoning can be used in the decision to use a splint, as was recommended in the selection and placement of sutures. An injured area of skin can be immobilized very effectively by applying numerous narrow strips of adhesive tape in as many different directions as possible. There is little scientific justification for applying such splints, however, unless they can be maintained almost continually during the active part of collagen synthesis and remodeling. If surface splints are used to reduce mechanical stress during collagen synthesis and alignment, the time they are needed most is between the seventh and forty-second days. Splints removed at the same time cutaneous sutures are taken out (when surface healing is primarily by fibrin and epithelium) serve no useful purpose so far as the final appearance of the scar is concerned. Even when subcuticular sutures have been used, external splinting to relieve tension across the wound is desirable provided it is continued through the period of active collagen turnover. While simple adhesive strips (which can and should be removed and replaced daily to protect the skin from adhesive irritation) will usually suffice, stronger measures are required for wounds around the knee, below the mandible, or around the shoulders of young individuals. Movement of skin in these areas produces such strong tension of skin that more rigid immobilization techniques may be required. Following revision of an extensive soft tissue scar in the vicinity of the mandibular symphysis, interdental wiring may be required to maintain immobility and reduce skin tension. A walking cylinder cast can be used for immobilization of the knee, although the length of time required to make any lasting effect on the final appearance of scars in this area is so great that such measures are hardly worthwhile except in special cases.

REMOVAL OF SUTURES. "When do you remove the sutures?" is frequently asked by people studying the practical aspects of wound management. Such a question suggests ignorance of the basic principle of rate variation which characterizes most biological processes. The answer to the question is, "The sutures are removed when the specific job they have been asked to do has been completed." To remove sutures earlier invites complications such as dehiscence and widening of the scar. To leave sutures in longer than necessary increases the likelihood of epithelial tracts, infection, and unsightly scars. Such an assertion sounds simple; that healing occurs in varying periods of time according to age, body area, type of wound, and general condition of the patient, however, is often overlooked. Even in a simple problem such as estimating the best time to remove cutaneous sutures, a rule cannot be formulated to eliminate the need for scientific reasoning. Just as patients have to be quizzed and examined until a diagnosis is certain, so wounds have to be quizzed and examined in order that a proper diagnosis or appreciation of the state of healing at that moment can be recognized. The history is important in that we know certain areas of the body heal slowly, such as the back of the hand, while others heal rapidly, such as the face or scalp. We know that patients with advanced neoplasms or who are under the influence of certain drugs heal slowly, while wounds made in old scars show accelerated healing. Examination of the wound contributes additional valuable information; for example, a continual leak of serum is an ominous sign of failure to heal. When blood tinged fluid escapes from between the skin edges of an abdominal wound, the likelihood of deep layer dehiscence is great. Removal of skin sutures in these patients usually results in prolapse of bowel. Necrosis of skin edges or palpation of deep collections of blood or serum usually means that removal of skin sutures will be followed by dehiscence. As a last resort, an experiment can be conducted if the history and physical examination are not diagnostic. A few sutures can be taken out and skin edges carefully tested to see whether healing is only the result of epithelization or whether significant fibrous protein synthesis has occurred between dermal edges. When it is advisable to get a patient into a more substantial dressing, such as a cast, sutures can be removed early and adhesive tapes applied to keep wound edges coapted even though collagen synthesis and remodeling have not occurred.

Failure to heal usually is a manifestation of some local complication. The most common factors interfering with healing are undue tension on skin edges, necrosis and ischemia of tissue, hematoma, infection, or retention of foreign material. Overhealing with production of hypertrophic scars and keloids seems to be the result of both local and systemic factors.

Hypertrophic Scars and Keloids

Although many attempts have been made and various signs advanced to distinguish hypertrophic scars from keloids, conclusive tests have not been developed to separate these two clinical terms. Even on a clinical basis, in the view of many observers, keloids seem to differ from severe hypertrophic scarring only in the amount of scar production. There seems to be a tendency to call the largest deposits of scar keloids, and the not so large (yet more than the surgeon expected) deposits of scar hypertrophic scars. More discerning criteria have been advocated on the basis of changes which occur in the shape of the enlarged scar. On the basis of these criteria, the scar which showed moderate hypertrophic tendencies and then either regressed or remained stable might be called a hypertrophic scar. Deposits of collagen which continue to enlarge beyond the original size and shape of the wound can be labeled keloid. The authors are not convinced that any such clinical discrimination is necessary; in all probability, all classifications are arbitrary, with their only biological basis being that of quantity. Nevertheless, differences in degree of abnormal scar formation can be considerable, and if different semantic terms are needed to describe these differences, the additional feature of "overflow" may serve some useful purpose.

The term overflow refers to the suggestion in some scars that newly synthesized collagen has developed so rapidly that the resulting scar is pedunculated. The term pedunculation refers only to the fact that in some of these scars the mass of scar tissue is many times the size of its base. All attempts to find some histochemical, morphological, or any other biological or behavioral differences between these two types of abnormal scars have, in the authors' opinion, been unconvincing. Expressed differently, similarities, except in amounts of collagen, are more striking than differences some investigators have claimed to be able to show. Similarities between the two types of scars include solubility of collagen, increased proportion of mucopolysaccharides to collagen, and a striking lack of purposeful organization of fibers and small fiber bundles. The appearance of both types of scars is delayed for four or five weeks after apparent normal wound healing has occurred. All degrees of excess scar formation can produce discomfort because of itching or inability of their external surfaces to remain epithelized when exposed to trauma.

The cause of keloids and hypertrophic scars is unknown. Certain races, such as Negroes and Orientals, are more susceptible than Caucasians; young individuals are affected much more severely than adults. The finding of a bad hypertrophic scar or keloid in an elderly person is a medical rarity. The face and the pectoral and deltoid regions are most commonly affected, but no region of the body is immune. Some-

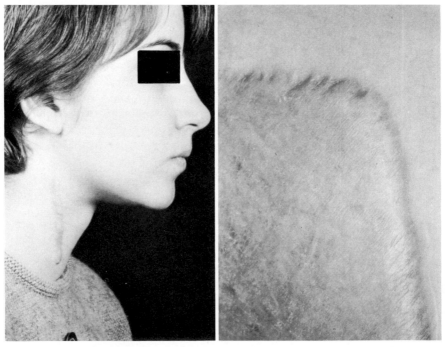

Fig. 6–17   Fig. 6–18

Figure 6–17. Hypertrophic scar which is not producing any functional disability and which follows the outline of the wound accurately.
Figure 6–18. Hypertrophic scar in skin graft donor site.

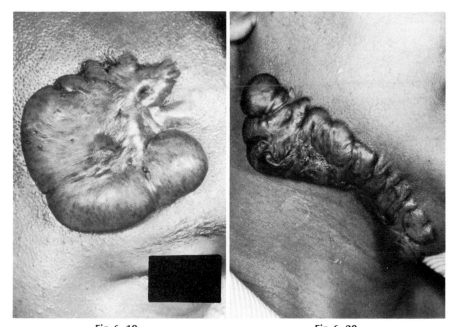

Fig. 6–19   Fig. 6–20

Figure 6–19. Typical keloid. The original wound was a linear laceration. Note that the keloid does not show any relation to the original size or shape of the wound.
Figure 6–20. Typical keloid following a simple laceration of the anterior neck. Scar tissue does not follow the outline of the wound and is out of proportion to the severity of the injury.

times a hypertrophic scar and a normal scar appear close to each other in the same region. Rarely, hypertrophic scar formation and normal healing occur in the same hypertrophic wound. A tendency to excess scar formation in some patients seems to be hereditary, but no good studies have been performed which show conclusively that overhealing is a genetically induced condition. One of the most striking observations is that individuals do not form excess scar tissue at the same rate or frequency over their entire life span. Patients who form severe keloids or hypertrophic scars during childhood or teenage years may not show these tendencies during adult years. This latter fact is an important biological characteristic of overhealing which serves as a basis for one good approach to treatment.

Recent studies on the nature and type of collagen in hypertrophic scars and keloids have revealed the presence of type III collagen in both lesions. Apparently type III collagen is more likely to be found if immunological techniques are utilized than if biochemical analysis of CBr fractions is the method of identification. Adequate studies have not been performed on "normal healing" to state whether type III collagen in hypertrophic scars has any significance in the etiology or treatment of these lesions. Although the presence of type III collagen represents a significant variance in scar tissue and other normal tissues, it is not

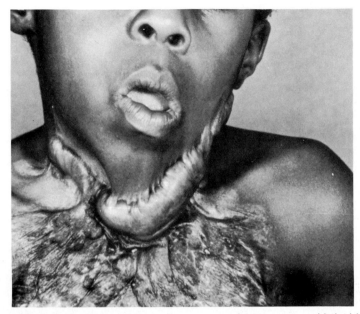

Figure 6–21. A combination of hypertrophic scar, wound contraction, and keloid formation in a thermal burn of the anterior neck and chest.

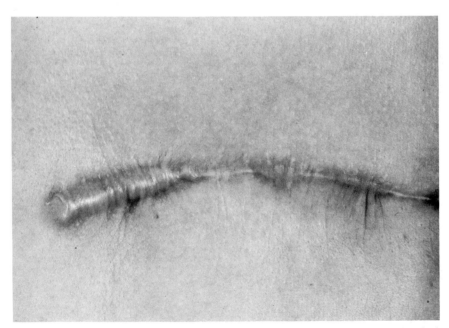

Figure 6–22. A transverse scar on anterior chest wall following a simple mastectomy which healed without complications. Note alternate areas of "normal" healing and hypertrophic scarring within the same wound.

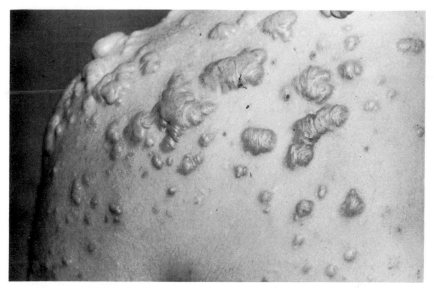

Figure 6–23. Hypertrophic scar formation following healing of acne pustules on the shoulder and anterior neck of a 17 year old patient. Two siblings and his mother exhibited similar hypertrophic scar reaction to any surface injury.

clear at this time whether type III collagen in scar tissue is characteristic of hypertrophic scarring as compared to normal healing. There is increasing evidence that many areas where rapid synthesis and deposition of collagen are occurring may contain some type III collagen. Prolyl hydroxylase activity and collagenolytic enzyme activity have been

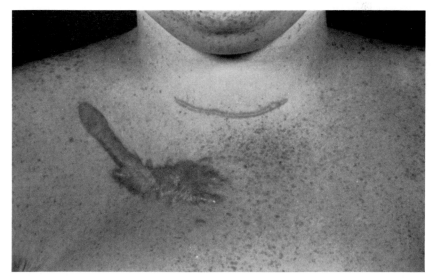

Figure 6–24. Lower scar was the result of an angular laceration of the anterior chest. Upper scar is a surgical incision. Both scars are exactly the same age and in almost the same location. Upper scar shows mild proliferation of collagenous tissue while lower scar borders on frank keloid formation.

reported to be elevated in hypertrophic scar and keloid as compared to normal deposits of scar tissue. These findings support the hypothesis that abnormalities responsible for hypertrophic scar and keloid formation primarily are quantitative and not qualitative in nature.

Because the cause of keloids is unknown and probably is not the same for all people, treatment cannot be planned on a sound biological basis. The best hypothesis for the cause of those complications presently classified as overhealing relates to recent knowledge and interest in the dynamic nature of collagen metabolism. Perhaps this can best be illustrated by identifying a "normal" scar around seven weeks of age as one which has reached equilibrium between collagen synthesis and collagenolytic activity. The increased extractable collagen which such a scar will show for as long as two years obviously cannot all be due to monomeric collagen passing into the scar. Some collagen must be coming out of the scar by virtue of increased collagenolytic activity, a process which also can be measured for a number of years. Although many important physical characteristics of scar are changing constantly, the scar does not vary a great deal in size after the first excess collagen has been absorbed. Mature scar tissue, therefore, appears to be a product of opposing forces of collagen synthesis and collagen destruction, and the result of these forces will vary according to the relative rate and effectiveness of each.

The concept that all collagen to some extent—and healing wound collagen particularly—is undergoing simultaneous construction and destruction can serve as a basis for speculation concerning some of the previously unexplainable findings in the healing process. One such enigma is the behavior of wounds during ascorbic acid depletion. In the classic description of scurvy, it is important to remember that sailors' wounds did not fail to heal—they actually disrupted months after apparent perfect healing. This observation has been verified in animals, and raises the question of whether collagen is dependent upon ascorbic acid for structural integrity. Because we know that collagen can be depolymerized and reconstituted in the laboratory repeatedly without contact with ascorbic acid, and because artificially reconstituted collagen does not lose tensile strength progressively, the notion that vitamin C has anything to do with strength of mature scar is untenable. Because synthesis of new collagen is blocked during ascorbic acid deficiency, and because collagenolytic activity probably proceeds normally, a possible explanation for old scar dehiscence would seem to be that tissue previously in equilibrium becomes unbalanced by having synthesis depressed and lysis continue. Inexorably, such a scar would become weaker until a point was reached at which normal tissue tension produced complete disruption.

If, because of some genetic or other presently unknown factor, a slight deficiency in collagenolytic activity existed, normal collagen synthesis might exceed collagenolytic activity. The result would be a typical hypertrophic scar or keloid. Between these two extremes all variations of external scars could be produced by temporary or permanent imbalances in the synthesis and destruction equilibrium.

The many and varied treatments which have been recommended for excess scar reflect a cyclical expression of overhealing and the natural tendency for the surgeon to advocate to others a treatment which appeared to work best for him in the last case he attended. Such efforts have included the use of ionizing radiation before and after surgical excision of scars, complete excision followed by skin grafting, partial excision, direct instillation of cortisone, and application of mild surface pressure by the use of elastic bandages. All of these procedures have been reported at one time or another as having been successful, partially successful, or complete failures. The relative success and failure of each can, at least partially, be explained by the known changes which occur in collagen metabolism following surgical, radiological, and pharmacological interference. The fact that some manipulations seem to work in certain patients at specific times and do not work in the same or other patients at other times indicates that a single cause of hypertrophic scarring probably does not exist even within a single individual. As far as is known, severe hypertrophic scars or keloids do not occur in domestic or laboratory animals; the only data we have are scattered observations on human patients. Obviously we do not have adequate controls; so the validity of each remains suspect.

Basic wound healing biology has demonstrated fairly consistently that tissues are endowed locally with cells which have the potential to synthesize collagen, that these cells can be destroyed by ionizing radiation, and that they are not replaced by bloodstream delivery of distant cells with similar capacity. Theoretically, therefore, it might be possible to destroy just enough cells to strike a balance or correct an unequal metabolic equilibrium between collagen synthesis and degradation. The possibility that externally administered radiation is able selectively to affect collagen maturation in this way, however, seems unlikely. But there is no evidence to prove that such an effect is impossible, and the fact that in occasional patients keloids do not re-form after excision and soft radiation may mean that in these patients a previously unbalanced equilibrium was restored to a more favorable balance. The possibility also exists that these individuals happen to have been operated upon and irradiated at a time when the tendency to overheal was not present. Under these conditions, postoperative or preoperative radiation would appear to affect overhealing.

Relief of soft tissue tension has been thought for ages to be mandatory in the correction of keloids; surgical treatment must include, therefore, release of wound tension by the addition of more skin or change in direction of the scar. Probably relief of tension (with or without radiation or with partial or complete excision of the scar) has been the most consistently successful approach to excess scar formation, regardless of the degree. One of the reasons partial excision (in which a rim of scar is retained like a picture frame and the central denuded area is resurfaced with a skin graft) may work is that the peripheral picture frame of scar tissue acts as a circumferential splint. Such a splint can prevent retraction of wound edges or transmission of external deforming forces to the central area where new collagen synthesis and remodeling will occur. Another biologically sound factor which could explain the results of partial excision is the secondary wound healing effect which would be encountered if the new wound was confined completely to the center of the old one. Recent enthusiasm for injecting cortisone, or cortisone derivatives such as triamcinolone, into keloids also has been shown to be based on a measurable alteration in collagen in *in vitro* systems. Although the solubility and the susceptibility of collagen to attack by collagenolytic enzymes has been reported to be affected by prolonged exposure to corticosteroids, it is more likely that these steroids inhibit protein synthesis. Thus, according to one investigator, injection of cortisone into a keloid repeatedly over long periods might exert a depolymerizing action, thereby rendering pre-

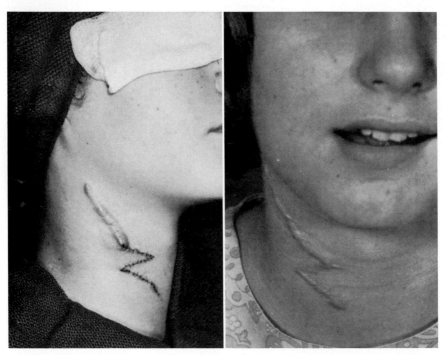

Fig. 6–25   Fig. 6–26

Figure 6–25. An attempt to reduce hypertrophic scar formation in a linear scar by revising the lower half with a Z-plasty to change tension across the scar. Patient is the same patient shown in Figure 6–17.

Figure 6–26. Same patient shown in Figure 6–25 three months after revision of lower half of scar. Recurrence of hypertrophic scar suggests that tension had little influence on formation of the scar.

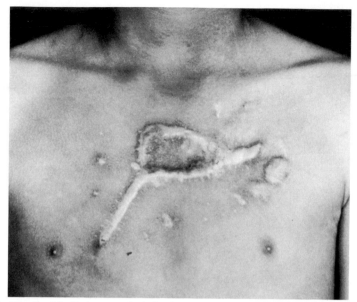

Figure 6–27. Partial elimination of a keloid of the chest by excision of only the central half and resurfacing of the defect with a split-thickness skin graft. Circumferential scar which was allowed to remain may have had a beneficial effect by splinting the wound against the effect of surface tension.

viously insoluble scar more susceptible to tissue collagenases. If this hypothesis is correct, other, more active depolymerizing procedures, such as exposure of collagen to papain or ficin, might be effective in reducing collagen excess without the need for making another surgical wound. Although injection of Kenalog solution with a pressure injector apparatus has produced significant and sometimes even dramatic reduction in the size of hypertrophic scars and keloids, experience in recent years strongly suggests that the effect is more dependent upon use of pressure than the particular substance injected. The end result appears to be one of internal necrosis, perhaps produced by violent elevation of tissue pressure within the lesion, followed by ischemia and necrosis. Inhibition of further collagen synthesis would allow the normal collagenolytic activity to remove excess collagen. Certainly, the biological approach to overhealing is more exciting now than the pure mechanical approach of the past.

The most recent claim for clinical control of hypertrophic scar tissue has been that constant pressure exerted by external elastic dressings will reduce the size of surface accumulations of collagen. Because there is a significant amount of water in hypertrophic scar, particularly during early stages of development, it is theoretically possible to reduce the size of scar by steady unrelenting external pressure. That pressure of the order of that produced by elastic dressings currently being manufactured and sold for this purpose is sufficient to remove water or that removal of water in this way would produce permanent dehydration and loss of scar bulk has not been shown to the satisfaction of the authors. There are no biochemical or enzymatic studies suggesting any measurable alteration of collagen metabolism caused by elastic dressings. A few ultra-structured differences in the weave of collagen fibrils and fibers following application of external pressure have not been convincing as being related necessarily to application of external force. Basic measurement of some parameters of collagen synthesis and deposition is needed to evaluate objectively some of the claims which presently are being made by clinical observers.

Scar Revision

The concept that any plastic surgeon (presumably because of attention to and mastery of fine surgical technique) can improve any scar at any time just because the original scar is the result of wound closure by another surgeon is, of course, completely unsound. Although fine surgical technique often can produce a superior scar or secondarily improve an old scar caused by inaccurate approximation of wound edges, many unsightly scars are not the result of poor surgical technique and can be improved only if the surgeon thinks in terms of the specific biological phenomena or techniques within his control which seem to have gone awry.

When surgical manipulation of an imperfect scar seems indicated, the following technical points, which are based on sound biological phenomena, have been helpful: Excision and revision of the skin edges obviously are needed when surrounding tissue has been distorted by an error in approximating undulating skin edges in the horizontal plane. If vertical unevenness is present, opening the scar is necessary only if dermal layers are grossly mismatched. When epithelial sutures either have been omitted or have been lost because of infection or necrosis, epithelium may be all that is uneven. Tiny pits and linear depressions which characterize epithelial errors can be corrected by simply abrading epithelium over a wide area and allowing new epithelium to migrate over an even surface. When dermal vertical mismatch has occurred in a scar that is sufficiently narrow and in an area where tension is considerable, the common practice of excising a scar with an ellipse of normal tissue should be avoided. Everything we know about the biology of primary and secondary wound healing points to the advantages of going through an old scar rather than removing it and starting all over with a primary wound. Scars which are not too wide but have inverted trough-like depressions below the surrounding skin surface usually need only insertion of dermal subcuticular sutures. Where width of the scar also is objectionable, however, the question of whether skin has been lost is of paramount importance; slightly unsatis-

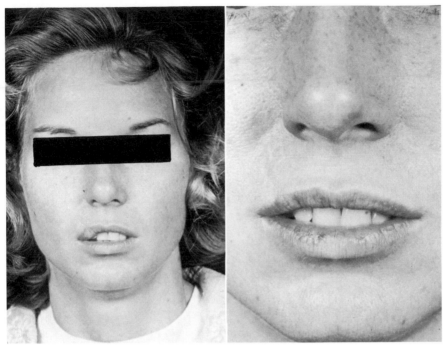

Fig. 6–28   Fig. 6–29

Figure 6–28. Uneven vermilion of upper lip is the result of inaccurate approximation of deep and epithelial tissues at the time a laceration of the upper lip was repaired.
Figure 6–29. Secondary revision of lip in patient shown in Figure 6–28 has resulted in accurate approximation of vermilion and reduction of lip fullness.

factory scars can be made infinitely worse by repeated excision and resuturing skin edges when the fundamental defect was always a lack of tissue. The situation which most commonly leads to unsatisfactory scars is a chemical or thermal burn—particularly around the face and neck in young people where no extra skin is present. Management of these injuries will be considered in depth in another chapter, but a word of caution should be inserted here: one must be sure that linear scars (or scars of any shape for that matter) are not the result of tissue loss before attempting secondary revision by any measure other than one which brings new tissue into the defect.

The examination of a scar, like the examination of a wound, can be an intriguing diagnostic problem. As soon as all data have been obtained and the best possible definition of the essence of the problem has been formed, one can turn to meager but rapidly accumulating basic knowledge of the various biological processes which are involved. When epithelization has not been as satisfactory as one had a right to expect, abrasion affords a new opportunity for cell movement to resurface the area. If contraction or other mechanical distortion is involved, revision, with or without addition of more skin, specifically is indicated. If a technical mistake in matching tissues on either side of the wound occurred, revision by surgery should be performed at an appropriate time. If collagen-mucopolysaccharide metabolism is unbalanced, time is perhaps the most important adjuvant with a sound biological foundation. Certainly, no good scientist in the midst of observing a series of antagonistic reactions which had some possibility of coming into satisfactory equilibrium would interrupt the experiment before the reaction was complete. With the knowledge available today relating to temporal aspects of the healing processes, plunging a knife into the center of a collagen synthesis-collagen degradation reaction while it is still undergoing measurable change illustrates the worst of the purely mechanical approach. To allow fundamental changes to proceed to a natural conclusion and then to search for a time when there is some evidence that the same reactions would not occur again is mandatory before repeating mechanical adjustment. The authors feel strongly that surgical manipulation of scars should be done only when the surgeon can clearly define the course of the undesirable effect in relation to time. Then, if his hypothesis is correct, and on the basis of sound wound healing biology, he may be able to propose a mechanical maneuver which has a measurable expectation of producing a different result. Certainly, gratifying changes can be wrought in surface scars when skilled mechanical intervention is based on sound biological reasoning. The key to successful revision of surface scars, however, is diagnosis, diagnosis, diagnosis! If the surgeon can define accurately and clearly what went wrong before and how he proposes to avoid or correct the phenomena during a second try, secondary revision of scars usually will be predictably good. The type of vanity which says "I can do it better" without defining "it" and how "it" can be done better often leads to disappointment following secondary revision of a scar.

Another type of injury which does not result in loss of full-thickness skin but which may result in unsatisfactory scarring can be described as a fracture of skin. Severe blunt trauma is the usual cause of such injuries, and the appearance of skin is one of multiple stellate cracks without producing gaping wounds. Because the full thickness of dermis usually has not been interrupted, these wounds are comparable to a hypothetical wound in which there were multiple radially oriented, partial-thickness lacerations, all of which contain perfectly placed subcuticular sutures. Consequently, a vertical mismatch of the dermal edge would not occur. Surface irregularities following injuries of this type can be troublesome, however, and they usually are the result of slight irregularities or indentations of epithelium. Although occasionally these indentations may actually be dirt tattoos which will have to be excised, the gray color of the striations can be due more to the effect of shadow than to retained foreign bodies. Epithelium can be driven into dermis in such injuries, producing small keratin cysts or inclusions which appear darker than surrounding healthy epithelium. In addition, the collagen content of skin is elevated; intradermal fibrosis occurs for some distance from the injury. Skin so affected may have both the collagen content and the physical properties of scar, even though a full-thickness break in dermis did not occur. To improve the shadowy appearance, abrasion with a rotatory brush, sandpaper, or knife edge can be used effectively as both primary or secondary treatment. Intradermal scarring, of course, is not improved by abrasive surgery. A word of caution should be expressed about abrading skin in patients with olive complexion, particularly those of Latin extraction. Denuding the surface is in some respects similar to exposing epithelium to solar energy. Epithelium which remains usually will respond by producing excess melanin, which may last for several years. If abrasion is contemplated in patients with a tendency to form excess pigment, a small area in a nonexposed place should be selected for a test abrasion. All patients should be protected from exposure to solar radiation for several months after abrasion; even individuals with fair complexions will form some excess pigment if exposed to solar radiation following dermabrasion.

WOUNDS CHARACTERIZED BY LOSS OF FULL-THICKNESS DERMIS

Loss of all layers of skin produces a wound in which many of the phenomena described in Chapters 1 and 3 will play a role. Moreover, the final functional and cosmetic result will be determined to a great extent by the relative prominence of epithelization, contraction, and connective tissue synthesis. Treatment of wounds in which full-thickness skin has been destroyed is planned to alter the relative contributions of each process and thus influence, as much as possible, the appearance or physical characteristics of the scar. The single most important biological consideration in planning of treatment for full-thickness skin wounds is the principle stated earlier in this and several other chapters: skin is a complex multigerm layer-derived organ, not a simple tissue. Regeneration of skin, as of most organs, does not occur in human beings.

Treatment of full-thickness skin defects begins with consideration of whether permanent loss of skin can be afforded in the area without causing unacceptable cosmetic or functional deformities. Answering this question immediately places treatment in one of two treatment categories: closure of the wound by mechanical or natural means, or addition of new skin. Surgical wounds, or contaminated wounds which can be made surgically clean, can be closed directly or new skin can be added as a primary procedure (see previous section on wound closure). Infected wounds must be treated by allowing contraction and epithelization to occur or by applying thin grafts as a sort of temporary dressing after eliminating soft tissue infection. The relative advantages and disadvantages of both forms of treatment will be considered in detail in this section.

Full-thickness dermal wounds can be divided arbitrarily into those induced by mechanical injury and those induced by radiant injury. At first, the main difference between the two is that one exposes subcutaneous or deeper structures immediately while the other results in a "naturally dressed" wound in which the irradiated skin is converted to a collagen dressing affording some protection for underlying tissue. In wounds caused by a mechanical avulsion of dermis, a surface scab can perform the same function as irradiated tissue for a short period of time. Radiant energy-damaged skin, however, can provide a stable dressing for remarkably long periods. The main difference between a scab and an eschar, however, is that a scab contains dead cells and flimsy fibrin whereas an eschar does not contain viable cells and consists almost entirely of tough collagen fibers in various states of radiant energy denaturation. Collagen, even though damaged severely by radiant energy, may still be extremely tough. Dehydrated, thermally denatured collagen can be so extensively cross-linked that it is almost leathery in consistency. This type of transformation by radiant energy is almost always the result of long-wave radiation from thermal sources. Instantaneous conversion of normally pliable, soft, elastic skin to brittle eschar usually is the result of flame, which dehydrates the skin rapidly and severely. Thermal burns which are incurred in a high-humidity environment, such as those caused by water and steam, usually do not produce leathery transformation of skin. The water content of skin actually increases following injury of this type; the same is often true following short-wave radiation injury. In these injuries, instead of becoming fused or glazed into a brittle, leathery condition, the skin becomes boggy and granular and literally fragments when enzyme activity occurs. Under these circumstances, dehydration of the eschar by therapeutic methods can convert one type of eschar (high-humidity destruction) into another type of eschar (produced by dehydration with subsequent increase in cross-linking). Alteration of physical properties in heat-denatured collagen to make dead skin serve as a better natural dressing is a practical example of applied collagen biology.

As far as the defect in skin is concerned, the physical condition of the eschar or, for that matter, complete absence of an eschar makes little difference. In untreated wounds, the basic processes of contraction and epithelization can be greatly delayed by formation of an eschar, but restoration of function and final appearance will be the same whether an eschar is present or not. In wounds in which an eschar is not present, one can obtain an excellent idea of what the final result of healing will be by simply grasping skin edges and mechanically pulling them together. This is precisely what the contraction process does. The only difference between mechanically coapting skin edges and allowing natural healing to occur is that, during wound contraction, fibrous protein synthesis also will occur. Depending upon how long the wound remains open, a variable amount of central scar tissue will be produced.

Thus, a large mass of central scar tissue may actually keep skin edges from migrating as effectively as they would if scar was not present. Excess scar formation, therefore, will prevent distortion which would have occurred if the edges had been mechanically coapted. The price that must be paid for lack of contraction and distortion, however, is high. The difference between physical properties of central scar and physical properties of normal skin which could have been moved into the area (even though maximal streching was required) is considerable. From the standpoint of physical properties of the scar, it often would be desirable to produce temporary lathyrism or scurvy so that no collagen could be synthesized until wound contraction had brought normal dermis into contact with normal dermis. Under these circumstances there would not be an unsightly central mound of scar covered only by a thin layer of epithelium. This is precisely the result that can be prevented by suturing skin edges together in a noninfected wound.

Wounds in areas where skin is not redundant enough to permit direct approximation of the edges will heal by contraction and simultaneous synthesis of epithelium-covered scar. In these wounds, formation of central scar is mandatory if the wound is to be closed entirely. The

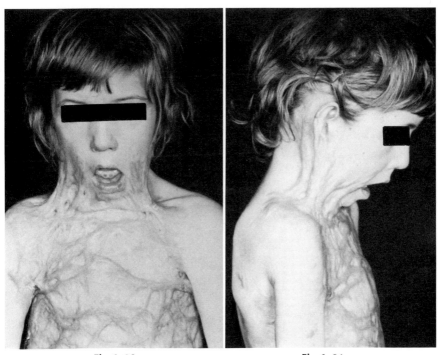

Fig. 6–30   Fig. 6–31

Figure 6–30. Full-thickness skin loss of the anterior chest which was allowed to heal by wound contraction. Wound contraction resulted in an anterior flexion deformity of the neck and distortion of facial features.
Figure 6–31. Lateral view of same patient shown in Figure 6–30.

combination of maximal wound contraction and replacement of the remaining defect with epithelium-covered scar should not be confused with regeneration. Regeneration, of course, is the ideal solution to full-thickness loss of skin; many mistakes in management of compound wounds of skin are attributable to the notion or hope that some regeneration of skin will occur.

The biological characteristics of scar tissue which make it inferior to unwounded skin are familiar. The lower leg ulcer is an example of a defect of skin in an area where effective movement of surrounding skin is impossible. To begin with, enough extra skin simply is not present in this area. What little extra skin is present seldom can be moved after years of chronic inflammation have made it inelastic because of deep scar replacement. For some reason, large plaques of new scar tissue do not fill gaps in this area, and the only hope for an intact surface lies in epithelization. Most conventional means of treating lower leg ulcers are protective and immobilization programs designed to allow a relatively delicate process such as epithelization to proceed in a relatively indelicate area. Accurate dressings, bed rest, and elevation provide this sort of protection. Excision of excess granulation tissue, elastic wraps, and

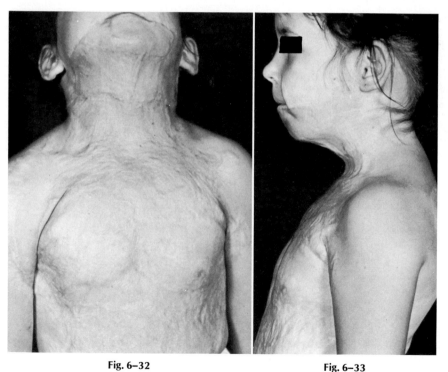

Fig. 6–32   Fig. 6–33

Figure 6–32.   Relief of deformity by excision of products of wound healing and resurfacing of the defect with large split-thickness skin grafts.
Figure 6–33.   Lateral view of same patient shown in Figure 6–32.

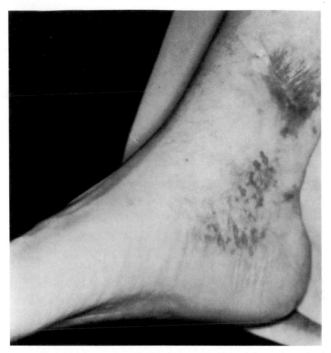

Figure 6–34. Typical appearance of medial malleolus ulcer of lower leg which has healed by epithelization. Subcutaneous pigment is clearly visible through extremely thin epithelial cover. Wound contraction has played little part in healing process.

elevation reduce edema and improve the contour of the surface over which epithelial cells must migrate. As soon as other epithelial cells have been met and contact inhibition stops the migratory process, the wound is considered to be healed. Almost no force is required, however, to abrade the new epithelial surface; highly specialized rete pegs, keratin, and self-renewing mechanisms found in normal epithelium do not develop in the absence of underlying dermis to act as an inductor. With the exception of highly specialized epithelium, such as that covering the tongue, the physical characteristics of epithelium are controlled by inductive influence from dermis. Epithelium which does not overlie dermis apparently is not induced to develop specialized functions, is poorly attached to the underlying tissue, and is unable to cope with environmental hazards. The result is a constant removal of cells, leaving exposed mesenchymal tissues. Secondary infection, more scar formation, and reepithelization over and over again demonstrate vividly in these patients that epithelization without wound contraction or scar synthesis can provide only a temporary seal.

Wounds on the back, where skin is thicker and somewhat more elastic than on the leg, also may not close completely by wound contraction. Epithelization in these wounds occurs but, for some unexplained reason, more fibrous tissue is synthesized so that a thin layer of epithelium may cover a relatively large wound which is filled by a deep fibrous cicatrix. A similar situation may occur in the hands and feet. Surface epithelium in such scars is fragile, and the level of the scar (usually above surrounding tissue) may make epithelium even more vulnerable by placing it on a rigid, raised platform of scar tissue. In these scars, loss of epithelium usually is not followed by ulcer formation. The mass of collagen is relatively stable even after it has been denuded. Instead of ulcers, deep cracks or furrows may develop, which can become secondarily infected and harbor organisms of low virulence for relatively long periods. Such fissures often are painful and persistent.

Thus, epithelium-covered scars with either low collagen content or high collagen content are vastly inferior to normal skin. Neither type provides adequate coverage unless the size of the defect is small or the scar is found in a relatively protected area. Management of wounds in

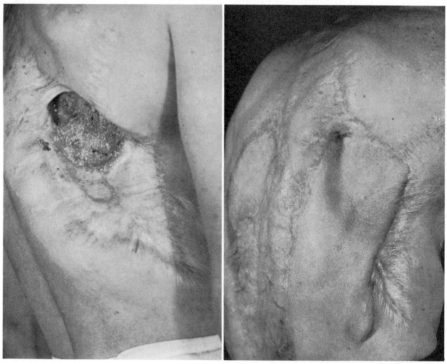

Fig. 6–35   Fig. 6–36

Figure 6–35. Soft tissue defect in subscapular area of the posterior chest which healed primarily by epithelization. Wound contracture is impossible because of adherence of tissue to immovable structures. Bronchopleural fistula is present because of inadequate soft tissue coverage.

Figure 6–36. Resurfacing of defect shown in Figure 6–35 with a full-thickness rotation skin flap. Donor site is on the left side of the vertebral column (see Chapter 7).

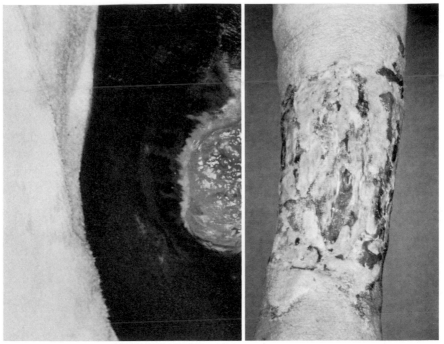

Fig. 6–37   Fig. 6–38

Figure 6–37. Migrating epithelium shown as clear advancing margin of wound. The epithelial margin is delicate and can be easily damaged by application of noxious agents or dressing changes.
Figure 6–38. Epithelization on dorsum of the wrist which does not cover exposed tendons. Advancing epithelial edges are repelled by dense connective tissue such as fascia, tendons, or organized scar.

which a decision has been made to allow healing by epithelization and contraction is only slightly different from that described under management of abrasion injuries. When epithelium only is missing, a smooth dermal bed remains and epithelization can occur over a surface that is nearly perfectly contoured. In a full-thickness wound where no dermal scaffold remains, however, an irregular contour caused by lobules of fat, edematous granulation tissue, or other uneven debris may present quite a formidable terrain for delicate cells to negotiate. In addition, certain tissues, such as tendon, seem to exert a repelling action on epithelial cell migration. This phenomenon is more striking in wounds where tendon is exposed than where fascia must be covered. Rapidly moving epithelium will cover exposed fascia at a slow rate; for all practical purposes, epithelium will never migrate over exposed tendon. Any wound in which healing by epithelization is desired must be cleared of exposed tendon or fascia. Granulation tissue, although apparently not biologically antagonistic to epithelial migration, can present a rather serious physical impediment which is markedly increased by secondary infection. The term granulation, of course, means granular appearance. Purple, boggy tissue which rises above the surface of surrounding skin, although frequently referred to as granulation tissue by physicians, is really more accurately described by patients who often refer to it as "proud flesh."

Alteration of the physical shape and water content of granulation tissue so that the least physical impediment to epithelial movement is produced can be accomplished by surgical excision of excess granulation tissue and by skillful application of dressings. Whether the wound is being prepared for optimal epithelization for contraction, or to receive a free graft, the objective is to reduce proliferating blood vessels and mesenchymal tissue to a relatively even surface, marred only by the fine granular nature of capillary loops. Thus, the ideal surface is finely granular in consistency and bright red in color. Boggy, purple masses of spongy vascular tissue which protrude in an uneven shape above the wound surface should be excised, particularly when they are infected. They should be prevented from re-forming by application of an accurate occlusive dressing. The depth of excision is a critical point, and whether the granulation tissue should be merely scraped off, or the en-

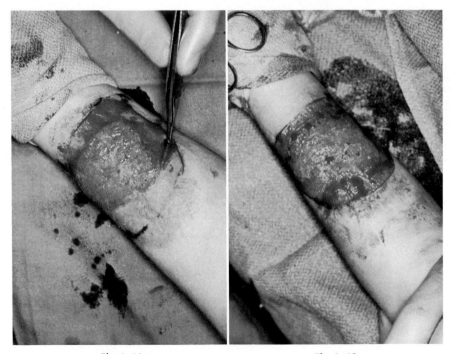

Fig. 6–39   Fig. 6–40

Figure 6–39.   Advancing epithelial edge on a lower leg ulcer elevated by forceps. Although it is extremely delicate, epithelial edge can be identified and manipulated.
Figure 6–40.   Same wound as shown in Figure 6–39 after excision of advancing epithelial edge in preparation for skin grafting.

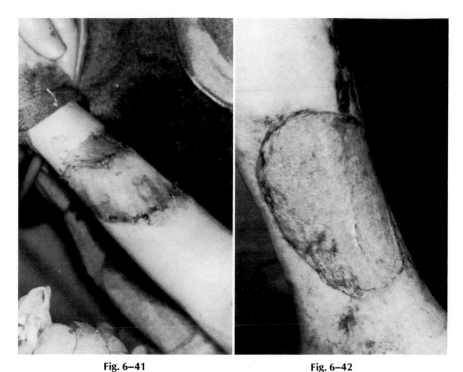

Fig. 6–41   Fig. 6–42

Figure 6–41. Application of split-thickness skin graft to lower leg.
Figure 6–42. Appearance of skin graft three months after excision of wound and resurfacing. Note apparent change in thickness and shape of graft due to secondary remodeling effect.

tire wound, including skin margins, excised, is crucial in controlling the appearance and function of the subsequent scar. In this decision, several biological considerations are fundamental. These include the presence or absence of infection, the amount of contraction which already has occurred, the amount of contracture which is permissible in the final result, and finally, the general condition of the patient, including the extent of all open wounds which have to be covered. Consideration of these factors will usually lead one to the following conclusions: if contraction is permissible or desirable, the base of the wound should not be excised, particularly the circumference of the base where presently available evidence indicates that a major force in wound contraction is located. If the defect is large and epithelization is going to be needed in addition to contraction to achieve a healed wound, granulation tissue should not be scraped but should be treated with an accurately applied occlusive dressing to adjust the surface as smoothly as possible. If contraction is desirable and a skin graft will be needed because the defect is too large to close by contraction and epithelization (as in extensive burns), proliferating edematous vascular loops should be scraped off so that the contracting process is not interfered with and the gain achieved from past contraction is not lost.

Although many surgeons remove excess granulation tissue at least one day prior to application of skin grafts to insure hemostasis, such precautions are not always necessary, particularly in small wounds. Even the slightest trauma to excess granulation tissue produces profuse hemorrhage, but the blood pressure in granulation tissue is low, and such hemorrhage is usually easy to control with epinephrine sponges, pressure, and elevation. By rapidly scraping excess granulation tissues down to a fibrous tissue bed but not making incisions through dense connective tissue, 20 to 30 per cent of the body surface can be prepared for grafting in a few minutes. Rapid application of compression dressings within seconds after removing granulation tissue makes it possible to perform such an extensive procedure with negligible blood loss. In large wounds, the occlusive dressing can be removed gently in 10 to 15 minutes. Usually all oozing will have ceased and extensive grafting can be done. If capillary oozing persists after a reasonable length of time, a more permanent occlusive dressing should be applied and grafting postponed until the field is dry.

The choice of dressing used to prepare a freshly denuded wound for subsequent grafting or to condition a granulating base for wound contraction and epithelization also is based on sound biological foundations. The first layer of the dressing is selected on the basis of the principles outlined in detail in other sections on treatment of abrasions or donor split-thickness skin graft wounds. A difference between these wounds and wounds which have no dermis, however, is that more material must be used for full-thickness wounds to make up for the absence of normal skin tension in the wound crater. Circumferential narrowing of the actively moving wound perimeter tends to cause underlying tissue in the center of the wound to be squeezed up out of the wound. Counterpressure is needed to hold the wound contents below the surface; all surface healing phenomena are enhanced by adding a corset effect to the denuded area. The most fundamental principle in construction of dressings designed to "hold a wound surface down" is that it is impossible to produce effective pressure without some sort of counterpressure. Actually, the term pressure dressing probably should be discarded, as studies carried out by placing pressure sensitive transducers in gauze or cotton dressings reveal that, regardless of how the dressing is applied, pressure is dissipated within 30 minutes. Cotton and other similar materials become packed, and unless an elastic material is used to add tension continually, it is impossible to maintain pressure on a wound surface with cotton or linen dressings. The term occlusive dressing is more accurate when cotton has been used, as the dressing material plays an important role both as external protection against surface contamination and trauma and as an internal conformer to maintain the configuration of the wound. Conformer effect is possible only when an extremity, torso, or head is wrapped in a circular fashion. Conformer effect is seldom adequate when adhesive tape is used alone to fix a dressing on the side of the face or some other area.

Selection of material for the bulk of the dressing usually is dictated by the economic advantage of cotton waste. Various synthetic substances, such as rubber and sea sponge, make excellent conformers but are not used as extensively as cotton waste because of expense or difficulty in obtaining them. A few layers of gauze sponges (without cotton in the interstices) usually are placed over the medicated, fine-mesh, gauze layer to prevent cotton lint from adhering to the wound surface. A bolus of cotton waste or some similar material is then carded into a loose arrangement and placed in the wound on top of the sponges. A loosely woven roll of gauze can then be used to wrap the bolus of cotton waste in position. When this material is loosely woven, it has little more resistance to stress than cotton waste and cannot, therefore, be utilized as the final strength-providing outside layer. A finely woven nonyielding cotton gauze roll should be used to tighten the dressing into final size and shape. This material can make the entire structure compact and relatively solid. Finally, adhesive tape is added to provide a degree of permanent stability. Such dressings seldom should be used midway in an extremity, for distal edema will be inevitable if early pressure and nonyielding conformation are produced. Dressings for mid-extremity wounds should extend from the top of the toes or fingers to well above the wound. Tips of the digits always should be left exposed so that sensation and microcirculation can be monitored. It is important to place gauze sponges loosely between fingers so that pressure is not exerted against the web. This is particularly true if there has been any injury to neurovascular structures. Special attention is required around the eyes and ears if good occlusive dressings are to be tolerated for long periods of time. Removal of a dressing covering an eye becomes an emergency if the patient reports that something is in the eye; 30 to 40 minutes of corneal abrasion by cotton fibers can result in permanent scarring. In addition, patients with massive dressings of this type should never be sedated without adequate examination; restlessness may be an early, important sign of anoxia.

Treatment of Infected Full-Thickness Wounds

Wounds in which full-thickness loss of skin has occurred and in which the complication of infection has intervened present special problems: Epithelization is practically impossible while major infection is uncontrolled; delicate cells are no match for the potent enzymes elaborated by bacteria and cells which are involved in trying to destroy bacteria. Contraction can occur during infection, but it does not progress to final closure until the main issue between bacteria and host defenses has been settled. The management of an open, infected wound, therefore, involves therapeutic measures in addition to those outlined for noninfected wounds.

The time-honored treatment of wet dressings for infected wounds has a sound biological basis; but, like so many time-honored remedies, lack of understanding of the fundamental biology involved is often responsible for the use of wet dressings in ways which are not in the best interest of healing as we understand it today. To begin with, there is nothing miraculous or mystical about water as an agent to destroy bacteria or catalyze the healing of a wound. A wet environment does not enhance the success of any of the basic phenomena described in the first six chapters. Moreover, successful treatment of a noninfected wound often involves development of a dry scab or eschar. There is no evidence that bacteria can be drowned and, as every patient knows, infected wounds usually produce enough moisture of their own to saturate dressings without the addition of any more fluid. From a physical standpoint, however, water can make a sound contribution to the control of infection, and if used properly, these physical principles may be of value in accelerating the healing process. If physical alterations which water produces are not specifically needed in a given wound, however, wet dressings can actually be harmful. They macerate tissues and often are uncomfortable. Water can accomplish two desirable physical changes: transport of heat and enhancement of capillary attraction, thus promoting drainage. Both effects are beneficial and both are based on sound biological principles.

Whether externally produced heat has any effect on control of infection other than to cause capillary dilatation is unknown. Although the healing process can be reduced dramatically by lowering temperature (such as occurs in hibernating animals, whose wounds do not heal during periods of low temperature), whether healing can be enhanced by raising the temperature has not been established. Whether elevated local temperatures selectively attract specialized cells or affect lymphatic function in other beneficial ways also is not known. But there are very few wounds, closed or open, which are not made to feel better by the application of moderate wet heat, and thus testimonials are abundant even though accurately analyzed data are scarce. The factor of capillary attraction is a sound one, however, which can be extremely helpful in promoting drainage. It should be remembered, though, that more adequate drainage often can be obtained by other methods. A wound which has only a small amount of viscous drainage that coagulates readily and thus partially seals the wound can be benefited greatly by preventing such a coagulum from forming. A wet dressing will insure dilution and removal of thick exudate by reducing the viscosity of the secretions. Wounds which are discharging copious amounts of low-viscosity exudate with no tendency to aggregate are actually better drained by applying a bulky dry dressing; a dry mop will absorb more water than a wet one.

The effectiveness of heat in increasing the inflammatory response and producing local anesthesia is undeniable. Wet heat is far more effective than dry heat. Cold wet dressings not only do not increase the inflammatory response but may be uncomfortable until body heat brings them to a higher temperature. Another misuse of wet dressings is their application and repeated removal for debridement purposes. The surgeon often labels this procedure "cleaning up" the wound for a few days with wet compresses. If the material to be cleaned up is water-soluble, use of wet compresses to rid the wound of surface debris is biologically sound. If the debris is not water soluble or if it is attached mechanically to the surface (such as strands of collagen, necrotic fat, or dead muscle), debridement by repeated washing could be classified as medical debridement. Sooner or later such measures will result in cleansing of the wound but not in much less time than if wet dressings were not used. Necrotic attached tissues that are not water soluble are best removed with a knife. If, for some reason, a surgical procedure is unsafe, or if tiny fragments of tissue are so numerous that surgical excision is not practical, a dry dressing, removed as often as it becomes adherent to the wound, will be more effective. Enzymes have been used to speed digestion of dead tissues, but the expense and time required to obtain and activate them has kept the use of enzymes from being practical in many cases. Attempts to encourage natural enzyme activity or discourage bacterial growth by changing the pH of the wound surface also have been used with some success. An acid pH produced by weak acetic acid appears particularly helpful when urea-splitting organisms are prevalent. Salicylic acid and Dakin's solution also have been used to speed up digestion and separation of necrotic dermis and fascia.

As has been suggested, many large open wounds can be closed satisfactorily only by replacing the missing tissue with similar tissue derived from some other area of the body, where such tissue can be spared. This is such an important procedure that it deserves separate consideration from the handling of skin wounds which can be closed by suture, wound contraction, or epithelization. Skin grafting together with the problems of burn treatment will be discussed in the next chapter.

LOWER LEG ULCERS

One of the best known patients in surgical clinics is the one with chronic ulceration of the medial surface of the lower leg. Quite often ulceration appears after many years of symptoms thought to be the result of inadequate venous return. Certainly inadequate vascular dynamics can be demonstrated in many ulcerated extremities—particularly when a large segment of the venous system has been obliterated by thrombophlebitis. Cause and effect relationship between obliteration of a venous channel and loss of skin on the medial surface of the lower leg is not clear, however. Ulceration does not always occur following severe thrombophlebitis and many ulcers are seen without evidence of obstructive thrombosis. A frequent association with chronic ulcerations is varicose tortuosity of the superficial venous system but, again, a cause-and-effect relationship between tortuosity and dilatation of superficial veins and loss of full-thickness skin over the medial surface of the lower leg is difficult to sustain. The simple explanation frequently advanced that a static column of blood in a dilated superficial system embarrasses nutrition and diffusion to skin is not supported by fundamental direct observations on blood flow and oxygenation of blood in varicose veins. Absolutely accurate measurement of venous oxygenation is so technically difficult that most of the reported values must remain suspect, but there is some evidence that the blood in tortuous superficial varices often approaches arterial saturation. Although the external appearance of a varicose vein suggests venous stasis, the possibility that flow is actually increased has not been disproved. The possibility that increased flow and high oxygenation are a result of numerous arteriovenous fistulas has been suggested and, if this hypothesis can be supported by accurate direct measurements, many older concepts of the cause and effect of varicose veins and accompanying ulcers will have to be revised.

An enormously complex system of capillary beds and direct shunts in skin is controlled by formations of smooth muscle under complex neurohumoral control. Although it is certain that the greatest portion of the capillary bed is not perfused under normal circumstances, the exact location and controlling influences for the smooth muscle valves have not been defined. Just as the microcirculation to many other organs may hold the answers to questions of function and maintenance, the intricate microcirculation of skin undoubtedly is of fundamental functional importance in addition to the better known cosmetic effect of blushing and blanching.

That the fundamental process in production of a medial lower leg ulcer is as simple as insufficient oxygenation or skin nutrition, however, seems somewhat unlikely in that the sequence of events seen in skin following occlusion of arteries or veins is well known and follows a pattern quite different from that observed along the medial surface of the lower leg. When arterial insufficiency occurs, skin develops a characteristic yellow, leathery appearance—often with remarkably little surrounding inflammation. Occlusion of major veins produces a typical dark eschar—often with sharply demarcated margins and always engorged with erythrocytes which impart a dark color to the affected area. Neither condition is characteristically found in the development of a medial leg ulcer. Eschar formation is occasionally seen in the more infrequent lateral leg ulcer and this observation may lend support to the old clinical axiom that lateral leg ulcers are more often the result of arterial insufficiency while medial ulcers are caused by venous obstruction.

The most characteristic signs and history accompanying a medial leg ulcer are a history of longstanding venous incompetency represented by varicose veins, edema, thrombophlebitis, or some combination of the three. Skin over the lower leg is often deeply discolored by hemosiderin deposition which may follow a known contusion or simply appear without the patient's being aware of injury. Relatively small injuries may have required an inordinate period to heal—particularly if edema is unremitting and prominent. With the exception of the occasional patient who reports that the ulcer was caused by a traumatic wound which did not heal, most ulcers begin so insidiously that the patient cannot relate accurately exactly how they began. The most common early sign of ulceration when patients are under medical observation is either a small clear vesicle without inflammatory components or a tiny inflamed spot which subsequently develops a small amount of purulent exudate and then widens in diameter, instead of becoming smaller as healing occurs by contraction and epithelization. Although a scab may form at any time in the genesis of a chronic ulcer, eschar formation indicating that a segment of skin has suddenly become ischemic or inadequately drained is not typical. The process seems most likely to be one of very gradual loss of ability of skin to maintain itself, either in the presence of normal "wear and tear" or in response to a more severe injury or bacterial invasion. The result is that collagenolytic activity apparently overpowers collagen synthesis so that skin is literally lysed by its own metabolic mechanisms. The disappearance of skin in the manner just described is associated with high levels of measurable collagenolytic activity as determined by tissue culture techniques. The actual cause of increased collagenolytic activity is, of course, only speculative but enough direct measurements of tissue collagenase in normal skin, eschar, and medial leg ulcers have been made that we are reasonably certain that the mechanism by which skin disappears is lysis due to tissue collagenase. Although decreased blood flow, including venous stasis, may be an initiating or only promoting factor in upsetting the balance between collagen synthesis and degradation, the sequence of events in development of a typical ulcer suggests that the reaction is of a different order than that seen in acute severe vascular insufficiency, which not only produces an eschar but also stops collagenolytic activity temporarily. Tissue collagenase is produced by living cells and measurement of collagenolytic activity in an area of vascular insufficiency is not possible until bacterial contamination produces bacterial collagenase or epithelial cells migrate into and beneath the eschar, elaborating tissue collagenase as they go. Further studies on the factors which control the microcirculation of skin and the primary or secondary effects on collagen synthesis and degradation have great promise in providing practical information concerning the course and prevention of medial leg ulcers.

Once a medial leg ulcer has developed, however, the problem is clearly one of loss of full-thickness skin in an area where wound contraction is virtually impossible and epithelization is unsatisfactory. Almost no extra skin exists in this area before injury; the chronic injury has produced abnormal amounts of collagen, so that skin is very inelastic; and there are no joints which can participate in formation of a contracture. This combination of factors means that epithelization is the only known healing phenomenon which can be effective in restoring the surface. Thus healing, if it occurs at all, provides only a filmy, cellular cover for one of the most constantly traumatized and exposed areas in the body. Whatever the initiating cause may have been, this explains why large ulcers which have been treated by any measure (not including transplantation of composite layers of skin) almost invariably recur. The multitudinous treatments of lower leg ulcers, including topical drugs, dressings, boots, and so forth, have been successful or unsuccessful in direct proportion to their beneficial or rehabilitating effect on the fundamental process—epithelization.

Principles of treatment for wounds in which epithelization is desired, or various thicknesses of skin transfer are needed, have been covered in detail. The principles outlined in this chapter and in Chapter 7 should be applied to the treatment of leg ulcers just as in other wounds. The reason for going into the biology of the development of leg ulcers in detail and considering their treatment apart from that of other ulcers is the need for a biologically oriented plan of preoperative and postoperative care. Such a plan is imperative for success. It is no great feat to follow the general principles of wound preparation, surgical excision, and application of a graft as outlined in Chapter 7 to produce a healed ulcer. Healing of the wound is almost always achieved if the principles outlined earlier are carried out. As nearly every surgeon knows, however, the real challenge in patients with these ulcers lies in making split-thickness skin coverage persist so that a new ulcer does not develop. The relatively high incidence of recurrent ulceration in a superbly grafted wound attests to the hypothesis that, unlike other wounds such as simple avulsion, the medial leg ulcers are not a problem of simple loss of tissue. Loss of skin is merely a symptom of an abnormality that is not well understood, and the possibility exists that associated venous abnormalities may also be only symptoms and not causative in nature. Correction of symptoms by obliterating a few dilated veins (sometimes erroneously referred to as feeder veins) and replacing skin which was lost in all probability has nothing whatsoever to do with the fundamental pathological process—it only prepared the area for repeat development of an ulcer. Thus until the fundamental abnormality is understood and corrected, empirical treatment in addition to successful grafting must be followed if anything more than temporary coverage is to be achieved.

An approach to the fundamental pathological process, which must be classified now as purely hypothetical since the pathogenesis of ulcers is obscure, is interruption of the sympathetic nervous system by performing a lumbar sympathectomy. This approach has not been based on recognition of signs of sympathetic overactivity, however. Sympathectomy has been advocated for relief of pain and for any possible beneficial effect it might exert on blood flow to skin. The finding that the venous blood in tortuous superficial veins has a high oxygen saturation has suggested the possibility that some varicose veins might be due to abnormal shunting of arterial blood across dermal capillaries directly into the venous system. If this is true, short-circuiting the microcapillary beds of skin could diminish the ability of skin to repair itself after minor trauma or repeated infection. Critical in the judgment of whether a sympathectomy might influence abnormal shunting of arterial blood into venous networks is the position and innervation of smooth muscle sphincters. Although these important microcirculatory valves have been identified histologically and their overall functional significance appreciated, the important details of how they are controlled under normal and abnormal situations simply are not available. The known ability of sympathetic stimulation to increase peripheral flow in some tissues and diminish it in others may be explained by the finding that precapillary smooth muscle valves are located on the shunt in some tissues and on the main feeder vessel to a segment of capillary network in other tissues. Even without this information, however, sympathectomies have been performed in conjunction with skin replacement and removal of tortuous veins as definitive treatment for chronic lower leg ulcers. Relief of pain is usually given as the reason for performing sympathectomy, even if vascular dynamics are not improved. There is no doubt that sympathectomy and skin coverage have been relatively successful in controlling ulceration in some patients, but the effect of sympathectomy alone is not clear. Even considered as an empirical treatment, sympathectomy has not been properly studied by modern scientific methods. From a biological standpoint, the basis upon which it is advocated is only theoretical in that direct measurement of microcirculatory dynamics has not been made. Perhaps the single most valuable measurement that could be made at this time—both in helping to understand pathological physiology responsible for chronic ulceration and in evaluating the various methods for correcting it—would be a direct measurement of tissue oxygen tension. Although such a measurement is scientifically possible with an oxygen electrode, the oxygen electrode is not a practically useful instrument because it is too unstable for widespread utilization by relatively untrained individuals.

In summary, although sympathectomy has been found to be a useful procedure for patients with ulcers who have considerable pain related to pathological changes of blood vessels (inflammation, distention, spasm), and the theoretical physiological alterations which might be achieved are intriguing, it can only be stated now that we simply do not have either controlled clinical observations or direct scientific measurements upon which to base a statement that sympathectomy is of any real value other than as a symptomatic treatment for pain.

Several other phases and modalities of treatment have been more thoroughly evaluated, and treatment based on clinical experience of this type can be gratifying. Successful management of lower leg ulcer requires mastery of the fundamentals of preoperative and postoperative preparation of chronic ulcers followed by a few operative maneuvers especially applicable to the problem of lower leg ulcer. Details of postoperative care are more important in treating medial lower leg ulcers than in almost any other coverage problem.

The first operative principle which seems to make a difference in obtaining permanent closure of a wound is to excise completely all the products of previous attempts at wound closure either by natural healing or operative intervention. This often involves a rather radical excision of skin, ulcer base, and deep scar tissue. During such excision periosteum should be carefully preserved and precaution should be taken not to remove the last film of vascular tissue over large tendons. If tendons are inadvertently exposed so that no vascular tissue covers them, excision of tendon in that area should be done. The only exception to this is if the exposed area is very small (less than 5 mm. in diameter) or the exposed tendon is so close to a normal skin edge or layer of subcutaneous tissue that a small local adjustment can provide adequate soft tissue coverage.

The second principle is meticulous hemostasis. The key to the type of meticulous hemostasis required in resurfacing a large lower extremity defect is patience. After every recognizable bleeding vessel has been ligated, an occlusive dressing should be applied and the extremity elevated for 48 hours before a graft is applied. It is imperative that every millimeter of transplanted skin survive. The tiny ulcerations or vesicles which develop over small hematomas in other large surface grafts, and sometimes produce skin loss which later heals by epithelization or contraction without significantly detracting from the appearance or function of the graft, cannot be tolerated on the inside of the lower leg. The only solution to this problem, in our experience, is to dress the leg, using a layer of plastic or rubber (cut from a rubber glove) next to the wound so that adherence does not occur and so that removal several days later will not produce capillary oozing. After 48 hours, such a dressing can be removed carefully with the leg still elevated. A relatively thick (18/1000 inch) split-thickness graft is then applied cautiously, and this is followed by application of a typical occlusive dressing reinforced with a posterior plaster of Paris splint which extends from the tip of the toes to midthigh. If any hematoma (no matter how small it may be) is seen five days later, the segment of the graft overlying the hematoma should be carefully excised and a spot replacement of split-thickness skin performed. Even the tiniest area of scar and epithelium can serve as a nidus for subsequent vesicle formation or eroding infection. Uncompromising demand for complete skin replacement is the sine qua non at this stage in restoration of the lower leg.

The next stage is based on the histological changes which occur following transplantation of skin. The most important of such changes is the almost complete turnover of collagen which is believed to occur during the first six weeks. Collagen turnover studies recently performed by sophisticated techniques and histological studies strongly suggest that a great deal of transplanted collagen is rapidly absorbed and replaced during the first few weeks after transfer. The process is a sort of remodeling process which results in temporary thinning and weakening of the graft and may result in a graft which ultimately is either thicker or thinner than the one initially transplanted. Collagenolytic activity is measurably higher in split-thickness skin grafts after transplantation than it was in normal skin. Increased collagenolytic activity probably indicates a state of rapid collagen turnover during which time the graft appears to be more susceptible to physical stress than it will be after fibrous tissue becomes more stable. Thus grafts on the lower leg, which are more susceptible to trauma than grafts elsewhere in the body, must be protected more carefully and for a longer period of time.

Another biological change in grafted skin which should be considered in outlining the postoperative care for a grafted lower extremity is temporary atrophy and inactivity of skin appendages such as exocrine glands. Skin grafts may become quite dry for three or four weeks if left unprotected; the susceptibility of grafts of the lower leg to cracking and subsequent bacterial invasion is greater than in some other areas of the body.

Finally, the destructive effect of edema must be taken into consideration for the rest of the patient's life. Edema caused or contributed to by local vascular abnormalities will continue to be a problem after the wound has been resurfaced. How much edema actually contributes to degeneration of skin is not known, but a universal clinical observation which cannot be disregarded is that a grafted extremity must not be permitted to develop severe unremitting edema. If the extremity is kept free of edema the possibilities of permanently preventing recurrence of the ulcer are vastly improved. If edema is not controlled, secondary breakdown of the grafted area is almost certain. The postoperative care of a grafted lower extremity after the sutures have been removed should be planned as follows.

A water-soluble medicated fine-mesh gauze should be used against the graft for four weeks. One of the combinations of Neosporin and cortisone has been useful for maintaining proper moisture and discouraging bacterial proliferation. The cortisone fraction, again, is empirical and has appeared useful in reducing inflammatory vesicle reaction. Although almost no work on this aspect of ulcer formation in the lower leg has been done, the possibility of allergic reaction has been raised and is supported by the fact that vesicle formation and subsequent degeneration occur without obvious trauma or bacterial infection. The possibility of allergic reaction to contact allergens (bacteria, clothing, drugs, dressing material, and so forth) or an autoimmune reaction to skin or skin breakdown products is worthy of consideration. The use of local cortisone has been advocated as a preventive measure during the first four or five weeks and as a therapeutic measure whenever vesicles appear. After the dressing has been removed, patients should use such an ointment daily for an additional four weeks and whenever inflammation or vesicle formation threatens the integrity of the graft.

Patients should be kept on strict bed rest for three weeks and then permitted non-weight-bearing crutch walking with an Ace bandage support from toes to upper calf for an additional four weeks. A total of seven weeks without weight bearing and with extraordinary protection is barely sufficient to permit remodeling and maturation of the graft before the rigors and trauma of normal leg function are permitted. After seven weeks, the patient should be furnished with a high-quality custom-fitted elastic stocking. The stocking should be fitted by appointment after a 12 hour period of bed rest followed by wrapping the leg with an Ace bandage and transportation with the leg in an elevated position. Elastic stockings furnished out of stock or fitted without taking exacting precautions to insure that the extremity is completely free of edema do not protect the foot sufficiently and may even promote formation of edema. If the stocking is not as comfortable as it is possible to make it by exacting custom fitting, it will not be worn or, even worse, it may be worn in an incorrect manner.

The last consideration is probably the most important and generally the least appreciated. This is best described as the conduct of a scientific experiment in which doctor and patient set out to determine what level of activity and time of dependent function it is possible to permit so that edema does not develop. A small amount of transient swelling which disappears after two to three hours' elevation, although not desirable, is not likely to be injurious. Whatever the cost in adjustment of the patient's activities may be, however, a level of activity must be determined and adhered to which will insure that prolonged or massive edema will not occur again in the affected extremity. For some patients, wearing an elastic support may be all that is required; for others intermittent elevation of the extremity or sharp curtailment of ambulatory function may be necessary. Some combination of elastic support, intermittent or sustained elevation, crutch walking, and curtailment of activities must be found for every patient if the permanent beneficial effect of skin grafting is to be realized. Perhaps more than anything else at this time, it is important for the surgeon to realize that the ulcer is only a symptom of a pathological condition which is not understood and probably has not been corrected. As in the case of every disease process which we do not understand at present, there is an empirical treatment which can be followed even though the basic pathological physiology is not clear. To assume, however, that medial leg ulcer is the result of a "stagnant" column of blood in a dilated vein "feeding" the base of an ulcer, perhaps all caused by a "congenital lack of a valve" in a vein, is to do little more than apply a sort of anesthetic balm to the irritation which application of the scientific method based on sound biological facts is bound to produce. The type of therapy which such reasoning inexorably leads to—stripping of a vein and grafting the ulcer—is in some ways similar to advocating an opiate for pain and Dicumarol to lower the clotting time in a patient with thrombophlebitis secondary to carcinoma of the pancreas. The symptoms may be relieved but the main pathological process is unaffected. Until the fundamental process (most likely to be found in the physiology of microcirculation of the skin) has been fully elucidated, the major contribution of the surgeon, after symptoms have been controlled, is to realize that a major abnormality still exists and that prevention of further symptoms is dependent upon making major changes in the patient's life to conform to his altered physiology. In the case of leg ulcers, prevention of edema is the intermediate step in the direction of treating the fundamental problem; in most patients, the symptoms of ulceration can be controlled permanently by taking whatever steps are necessary to prevent the lower leg from becoming significantly edematous.

All of the foregoing plan obviously is predicated on the assumption that patients are willing to alter their habits to meet the requirements imposed by abnormal microcirculation of the lower leg. However, as in so many problems in medicine (particularly those in which specific "lock and key" diagnosis and treatment are not available), success depends upon skill in selection of patients. Skill in selection of patients is of enormous importance in the successful practice of surgery; this statement has nothing to do with protection or establishment of the reputation of the physician. Occasionally a study is disparaged on the basis that the patients were not representative because they were carefully selected; this criticism is not warranted, in our judgment. No example serves more clearly to illustrate the point of view than the patient with an ulcer of the lower leg. To inflict an expensive, often prolonged hospital admission and procedure on a patient who either does not understand or is unable to follow a complete program of postoperative care and rehabilitation is not justifiable in view of the risk of such care. The alternative to applying the skin graft is to teach patients to care for an open wound until such time as pain and extensive exposure make amputation advisable. In an understandable zeal to produce a healed wound surgeons have overlooked the fact that even a leg with extensive ulceration can be used for limited painless weight bearing for an amazingly long period of time. Healthy granulation tissue provides a second-best coverage and one which can be kept serviceable if cared for properly. Our approach to chronic lower leg ulceration, therefore, has been to accept for extensive skin grafting only those patients who understand and agree to cooperate completely with a full program of postoperative rehabilitation including, if necessary, severe curtailment of their former activities. At the earliest sign of vesicle formation or inflammatory change, complete bed rest followed by crutch walking and gradual resumption of activity is insisted upon. If patients are unable, refuse, or are judged incapable of participating in a prolonged rehabilitation program based on the time-consuming maturation of transplanted skin, they should not be accepted for skin grafting even though it is likely that a healed wound could be obtained with only a few weeks' investment of time and cooperation. Such patients, with even minor care of their wounds, may be able to ambulate better on an ulcerated leg than they can on a prosthesis for a long period of time. If, however, major deep structures such as joints, extensive areas of bone and tendon, or any tissues which will not be covered by healthy granulation tissue become involved, or if pain becomes uncontrollable, amputation is advisable to prevent life-threatening complications.

TROPHIC ULCERS IN ANESTHETIC AREAS

The classic explanation for the paraplegic or tetraplegic patient's tendency to develop extensive ulceration of skin is that skin (particularly over bony prominences) is deprived of circulation by being compressed between bony prominences and an external surface. Although this explanation has provided an excellent basis for teaching preventive nursing care, it leaves a good bit to be desired as a complete explanation of the biology of tissue necrosis. There is no doubt that ischemia of skin is usually not appreciated in a paralyzed patient and that extraordinary nursing precautions which eliminate any possibility of ischemia will usually prevent ulceration of skin. Ischemia is very likely an initiating cause of skin loss. The picture becomes cloudy at this point, however, because the length of time skin needs to become ischemic before changes leading to ulceration become irreversible, the sequence of events between ischemia and skin loss, and the susceptibility of anesthetic skin to disintegration when subjected to ischemia are not explained by the simple statement that skin without blood supply becomes necrotic and disappears.

Skin in normally innervated areas can be kept ischemic for five hours without becoming irreversibly damaged. As short a time as two hours of ischemia in a tetraplegic patient can produce vesicle formation which progresses to complete destruction of skin even though the compressive effect is relieved. The tendency for a compressed area of skin to form vesicles varies among patients and in the same patient. Some patients go through periods when skin is so fragile that even the smallest error in positioning for an almost insignificant period of time produces a rapid loss of skin in that area. Such extreme dermal fragility is not seen immediately after transection of the spinal cord and usually does not last forever after it appears. Skin in anesthetic areas may become quite resistant to ischemia-induced degradation only to become extremely susceptible as long as years after the initial episode. Finally, the morbid anatomy of development of a trophic ulcer in anesthetic skin is not similar to that observed when skin is rendered ischemic by simple obliteration of an arterial or venous channel. Eschar formation is rare but the time between first compression and degeneration of subcutaneous tissue is considerably shorter than after occlusion of a vessel.

The inescapable conclusion would seem to be that although we can accept compressive ischemia as an initiating stimulus, the elimination of which will prevent trophic ulceration, the sequence of events beginning with erythemic reaction and progressing rapidly through vesicle formation and disappearance of skin is a more complex biological phenomenon than the production of an eschar by vascular insufficiency. One simple yet provocative reflection is that the development of typical trophic ulcers requires living cells. Skin detached from a living body does not go through the familiar stages of disintegration when subjected to compression. Cadavers can lie on a bony prominence for several days without trophic disintegration of skin. The facts that living cells are needed, that an eschar is not usually a prominent part of the pathological physiology, and that complete dissolution of skin is so rapid suggest that an imbalance of collagen metabolism may be induced or promoted by the combination of deficient innervation and ischemia. The removal of collagen is so rapid that skin collagenolytic activity must be a paramount part of the pathological process, and indeed measurement of collagenolytic activity in trophic ulcers of paraplegic patients has produced some of the highest levels of collagenolytic activity ever measured in human tissues by the tissue culture technique. Unwounded skin in anesthetic areas of tetraplegic patients also has seemed to have a higher rate of collagenolytic activity than innervated skin. Recent demonstration that progesterone inhibits the effect of tissue collagenase may provide another therapeutic approach to the rapidly developing trophic ulcer. Although data on unwounded skin are incomplete, exacerbations and remissions of the tendency to form trophic ulcers strongly suggest that collagen metabolism is under the influence of biological controls other than ischemia and innervation, which remain constant, whereas the tendency to ulcerate is quite variable.

Treatment of trophic ulceration of anesthetic skin is most like that of the local treatment of cancer. Although temporary or biological dressing types of coverage can be obtained by a free graft, complete excision of the wound, alteration of the contour of underlying bony prominences, and restoration of the surface with large composite tissue flaps is needed if permanent healing is to be obtained. The treatment still sometimes utilized in debriding a soft tissue wound—distending the wound with gauze, and excising the contents of the area, much as one would excise a tumor—is a useful one. No more skin than necessary should be removed but any deep tissue such as fascia or muscle, and particularly bone which is present in the wound surface, must be removed. In addition, a bony prominence such as the sacral promontory or ischial tuberosity should be reduced in size and protrusiveness whether it is exposed in the depth of the wound or not.

Small, conservatively designed, and accurately fitting flaps which are frequently used to resurface facial and hand defects cannot be used to cover a defect in the sacrum or hip of a paraplegic patient. Such flaps have a high incidence of circulatory failure and usually result only in a larger soft tissue defect. The biological basis for this clinical observation is not clear but it is probably a combination of normally modest blood supply which is further altered by lack of peripheral innervation. The latter factor may not have any importance in the survival or death of the skin flap except as it influences the stability of skin through other mechanisms such as inflammation or regulation of collagen metabolism. Even though fundamental alterations in microcirculation and soft tissue metabolism caused by central denervation are far from clear, clinical experience has shown that small rotation flaps which can be utilized quite successfully in normally innervated areas simply do not survive transplantation in paraplegic or tetraplegic patients. Restoration of soft tissue coverage usually must be accomplished by moving large areas of the body wall on broadly based pedicles. Skin over both flanks or buttocks can be undermined and rotated inferomedially to resurface a large sacral defect, but the superolateral incision to mobilize skin must be placed so that the entire flank on both sides is mobilized and most of the lateral abdominal and gluteal vessels are maintained to nourish the mobilized tissue. Another application of the same principle is to turn a large flap of gluteus maximus muscle medially on its origin and blood supply to fill a central sacral defect. The muscle can then be grafted with a split-thickness skin graft.

In the trochanteric region, the removal of a trochanter and excision of soft tissue on each side should make it possible to close the wound as a linear incision without back cutting in a direction to produce a rotation flap. Attempts to close lateral defects by making parallel incisions so the lateral flaps can be moved medially should not be utilized in this area. For all practical purposes, if enough bone and soft tissue cannot be removed so skin can be brought together as a straight line closure, other attempts to close the wound by local shift of tissue should be abandoned.

Ischial ulcers are the easiest to close; usually the removal of the ischial tuberosity and extension of the thigh on the buttocks will make closure relatively easy without radical mobilization of surrounding tissue. If transfer of tissue is required, mobilization of most of the posterior thigh should be done by making a long lateral incision and an inferior transverse incision in the middle of the thigh. These incisions produce a large flap nourished by all the vessels on the medial surface of the thigh. The relative thinness of skin on the medial surface of the thigh and the movability of skin in that area make it possible to shift a posterior thigh flap based on the medial surface into the ischial area. A small donor site wound may be produced in the center or lower third of the thigh which is easily resurfaced with a split-thickness skin graft. A split-thickness skin graft will provide adequate coverage in the lower portion of the posterior thigh since bony prominences are not present.

Prevention of hematoma and protection from mechanical stress are the most important postoperative objectives. Fibrotic denervated muscle and subcutaneous scar tissue have a propensity for bleeding slowly during the first few days after surgery, even though the wound appears completely dry at the time of wound closure. Before various devices for continual wound suction were readily available, drains and difficult occlusive dressings were mandatory. Strategically placed catheters attached to appropriate suction will prevent hematomas provided they are properly placed and cared for so that a small negative pressure is maintained until the wound surfaces become agglutinated. Nothing demonstrates so vividly the fragility of anesthetic skin as the use of multiple sutures under tension to close a trophic defect. Skin edges literally must fall together if primary healing is to be assured.

It is usually difficult and sometimes impossible to obtain healing by first intention when reflex spasm is pronounced. Small defects in the ischial tuberosity area sometimes can be repaired even though spasm is present but large defects in patients who are subject to violent reflex spasms are not amenable to restorative surgery. The first step in these individuals is to try to control the spasms by alcohol or electrical destruction of the lower cord. If patients refuse to have the lower cord destroyed, they probably should not be subjected to extensive resurfacing procedures. An even larger denuded area several weeks after attempts to close the wound by flap transposition is the usual reward for attempting to close a wound in a hyperactive patient.

Amputation of the extremity may be the best approach to extensive defects in difficult patients. A long anterior thigh flap containing the entire femoral circulatory system makes a good flap to turn into a posterior defect in the gluteal or sacral region. Amputation of both legs has been practiced and is recommended by some surgeons for extremely large posterior defects complicated by lower leg and patellar soft tissue ulceration. Bilateral amputation produces a severe mutilation and only an unusual person can lose the lower third of his body and still be rehabilitated to any gratifying degree. It is particularly true if disarticulation at the hip is performed. Although it is possible to prop patients with bilateral disarticulation in a sitting position, the cosmetic and functional disability is so severe that such procedures should be performed only as a last resort and after considerable planning and preparation. Finally, just as the best design and planning for treatment of lower leg ulcers in some patients may be to take care of the defect without attempting further surgical closure, a similar decision for trophic ulcers may be wise. There are patients with trophic ulcers who have such intractable contractures, extensive loss of skin, and uncontrollable spasms that surgical closure is not possible — no matter how much the patient and the surgeon would like to have closure as an objective. Some such patients either will not accept or should not have an amputation. Provision of adequate drainage and protection against further skin necrosis can often be produced by conservative management of the wound. Recognition of this state of affairs can save patients interminable hospitalization and expense. Stubborn persistence in trying to obtain a completely closed wound by surgical manipulation of tissue may, in addition to wasting a great deal of time and money, tie up hospital beds for months with almost no chance of beneficial returns. Again, realization that some wounds simply are not amenable to surgical closure can be an important service to patients which should not be disregarded.

When it is not certain whether surgical manipulation can provide wound closure, the experiment must be performed so that one can be certain that the best has been attempted. Sound biological reasoning and willingness to admit failure to achieve definitive coverage will keep such attempts from extending over prolonged periods of time. The realization that failure to succeed in closing a trophic ulcer on the first attempt may mean that months of secondary wound care often discourages a surgical service from admitting paralyzed patients who have extensive or trophic ulcers. Such an attitude is not necessary if doctor and patient agree at the beginning that the test will be attempted and that both will be able to accept failure if soft tissue coverage cannot be obtained. Because the same tissue may vary from time to time in this response to stress and transplantation, unsuccessful attempts to close the trophic ulcer should be terminated relatively soon with the idea that another attempt can be made if conditions warrant it. Once a patient is admitted with a trophic ulcer he does not necessarily have to remain on the service until his skin is completely healed. Long periods of hospitalization are justified only when success is continually measurable. Failure to achieve success by means which can be performed only in a hospital should be a signal to abandon the initial objective and set an objective which can be reached even if it is only good nursing care to prevent further complications.

SUGGESTED READING

Baier, R. E., Shafrin, E. G., and Zisman, W. A. Adhesions: Mechanisms That Assist or Impede It. Science *162*:1360, 1968.

Bentley, J. P. Rate of Chondroitin Sulfate Formation in Wound Healing. Ann. Surg. *165*:186, 1967.

Bernstein, H. Treatment of Keloids by Steroids with Biochemical Tests for Diagnosis and Prognosis. Angiology *15*:253, 1964.

Calnan, J. S., and Copenhagen, H. J. Autotransplantation of Keloid in Man. Brit. J. Surg. *54*:330, 1967.

Calnan, J., Fry, H. J. H., and Saad, N. Wound Healing and Wound Hormones. A Study of Tensile Strength in Rats. Brit. J. Surg. *51*:448, 1964.

Conolly, W. B., Hunt, T. K., Sonne, M., and Dunphy, J. E. Influence of Distant Trauma on Local Wound Infection. Surg. Gynec. Obstet. *128*:713, 1969.

Conolly, W. B., Hunt, T. K., Zederfeldt, B., Cafferata, H. T., and Dunphy, J. E. Clinical Comparison of Surgical Wounds Closed by Suture and Adhesive Tapes. Amer. J. Surg. *117*:318, 1969.

Ebert, P. S., and Prockop, D. J. Influence of Cortisol on the Synthesis of Sulfated Mucopolysaccharides and Collagen in Chick Embryos. Biochim. Biophys. Acta *136*:45, 1967.

Ehrlich, H. P., and Hunt, T. K. The Effect of Cortisone and Anabolic Steroids on the Tensile Strength of Healing Wounds. Ann. Surg. *170*:203, 1969.

Forrester, J. C., Hayes, T. L., Pease, R. F. W., and Hunt, T. K. Scanning Electron Microscopy of Healing Wounds. Nature *221*:373, 1969.

Forrester, J. C., Zederfeldt, B. H., Hayes, T. L., and Hunt, T. K. Wolff's Law in Relation to the Healing Skin Wound. J. Trauma *10*:770, 1970.

Goldin, E. G., and Joseph, N. R. Responses of Connective Tissue Ground Substance in Wound Healing. Arch. Surg. *97*:753, 1968.

Grillo, H. C. Origin of Fibroblasts in Wound Healing: An Autoradiographic Study of Inhibition of Cellular Proliferation by Local X-Irradiation. Ann. Surg. *157*:453, 1963.

Harris, E. D., and Krane, S. M. Collagenases. New Eng. J. Med. *291*:651, 1974.

Holmstrand, K., Longacre, J. J., and DeStefano, G. A. The Ultrastructure of Collagen in Skin, Scars and Keloids. Surgery *27*:597, 1961.

Ketchum, L. D., Cohen, I. K., and Master, F. W. Hypertrophic Scars and Keloids. Plast. Reconstr. Surg. *53*:140, 1974.

Kischer, C. W., and Shetlar, M. R. Collagen and Mucopolysaccharides in the Hypertrophic Scar. Connective Tissue Research *2*:205, 1974.

Klein, L., and Rudolph, R. Turnover of Soluble and Insoluble ^{3}H Collagens in Skin Grafts. Surg. Gynec. Obstet. *139*:883, 1974.

Leibovich, S. J., and Ross, R. The Role of the Macrophage in Wound Repair. A Study with Hydrocortisone and Antimacrophage Serum. Amer. J. Pathol. *78*:71, 1975.

Leveen, H. H., et al. Chemical Acidification of Wounds. An Adjuvant to Healing and the Unfavorable Action of Alkalinity and Ammonia. Ann. Surg. *157*:745, 1973.

Levenson, S. M., Geever, E. F., Crowley, L. V., Oates, J. F., III, Berard, C. W., and Rosen, H. The Healing of Rat Skin Wounds. Ann. Surg. *161*:293, 1965.

Madden, J. W., and Peacock, E. E., Jr. Studies on the Biology of Collagen During Wound Healing. I. Rate of Collagen Synthesis and Deposition in Cutaneous Wounds of the Rat. Surgery *64*:288, 1968.

Mathews, M. B., and Decker, L. The Effect of Acid Mucopolysaccharides and Acid Mucopolysaccharide-Proteins on Fibril Formation from Collagen Solutions. Biochem. J. *109*:517, 1968.

Milch, R. A. Tensile Strength of Surgical Wounds. J. Surg. Res. 5:377, 1965.

Myers, M. B., Cherry, G., and Heimburger, S. Augmentation of Wound Tensile Strength by Early Removal of Sutures. Amer. J. Surg. 117:338, 1969.

Peacock, E. E., Jr. Inter- and Intramolecular Bonding in Collagen of Healing Wounds by Insertion of Methylene and Amide Cross-Links into Scar Tissue: Tensile Strength and Terminal Shrinkage in Rats. Ann. Surg. 163:1, 1966.

Peacock, E. E., Jr. Production and Polymerization of Collagen in Healing Wounds of Rats: Some Rate-Regulating Factors. Ann. Surg. 155:251, 1962.

Peacock, E. E., Jr., and Biggers, P. W. Measurement and Significance of Heat-Labile and Urea-Sensitive Cross-Linking Mechanisms in Collagen of Healing Wounds. Surgery 54:144, 1963.

Pennell, T. C., and Hightower, F. Malignant Changes in Postphlebitic Ulcers. Southern Med. J. 58:779, 1965.

Ross, R. Wound Healing. Sci. Amer. 220:40, 1969.

Rovee, D. T., and Miller, C. A. Epidermal Role in the Breaking Strength of Wounds. Arch. Surg. 96:43, 1968.

Salthouse, T. N., and Williams, J. A. Histochemical Observations of Enzyme Activity at Suture Implant Sites. J. Surg. Res. 9:481, 1969.

Singer, M. The Regeneration of Body Parts. Sci. Amer. 199:79, 1958.

Weiss, P. The Biological Foundation of Wound Repair. Harvey Lect. 55:13–42, 1961.

White, B. N., Shetlar, M. R., and Schilling, J. A. The Glycoproteins and Their Relationship to the Healing of Wounds. Ann. N.Y. Acad. Sci. 94:297, 1961.

Chapter 7

SKIN GRAFTING AND TREATMENT OF BURNS

The two most common types of radiant energy-induced wounds of skin are those caused by long-wave or thermal radiation and those caused by short-wave or x-radiation. When full-thickness dermis has not been destroyed, wounds are classified as first and second degree burns; in third or fourth degree injuries the full thickness of dermis has been destroyed. Although heat and short-wave radiation produce much the same type of reaction when only the superficial layers of skin are involved, the biological connotations (especially those regarding prognosis) are vastly different. These differences are reflected primarily in the epithelial layer, where cell growth and turnover are most rapid. Although we badly need more subcellular measurements to confirm present hypotheses based on clinical observations, a useful approach to understanding the major difference between thermal and x-radiated wounds is to think in terms of production of mutant cells. Any wound which is prevented from healing, or any scar which is repeatedly injured, is a likely site for epidermoid carcinoma to occur. Although this undoubtedly is an oversimplified approach, the point can be emphasized by restating the principles outlined in Chapter 2, where it was pointed out that loss of contact inhibition in epithelial cells produces powerful, predictable, and unrelenting forces leading to dedifferentiation and ameboid motion. Epithelial cells in a wound too large and irregular to be traversed by epithelial migration, or wounds covered only by epithelial cells which are constantly abraded by repeated mechanical trauma, may be subjected to biological stimulation for years. What finally happens to the various rate-regulating processes

271

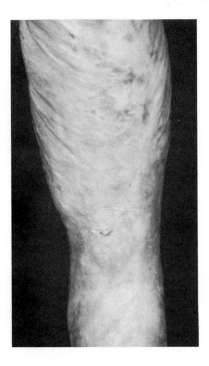

Figure 7–1. Deep second and third degree burn wound of posterior popliteal area healed by wound contraction and epithelization. Note superficial ulcer in popliteal space where subcutaneous tissue was covered only by thin epithelium which was denuded by contact with clothes.

in such stimulated cells is, at present, unknown, but, if the process continues long enough, controlled dedifferentiation, mitosis, and movement become uncontrolled growth and invasion. Bereft of their abilities to do anything useful for the organism, such cells then embark on a mad course of unimpeded growth and destruction of surrounding tissues. Ultimately they may develop autonomy so that they are able to grow wherever the blood or lymph deposits them. At this point, cancer usually is incurable by present methods of treatment. Recent demonstration that vascular penetration of epithelial tumors seems to occur simultaneously or just before invasion and metastasis strongly suggests a cause-and-effect relation between vascularization and changes leading to incurability.

With the exception of a few nonspecific measurements of small quantitative and kinetic differences in enzymes, there is a puzzling lack of morphological, chemical, or biophysical difference between epithelial cells which behave normally and epithelial cells which can be recognized as epidermoid carcinoma. The changes which cause such behavioral differences and the external forces which direct these changes obviously are important to both wound healing and experimental oncology. Considered in this light, a cancer is really a healing wound which somehow never responded to normally acting forces which dampen or suppress an embryonic potential. If the exact nature of these forces could be determined, we might have in one magnificent coup the answer to a number of problems in the wound healing field as

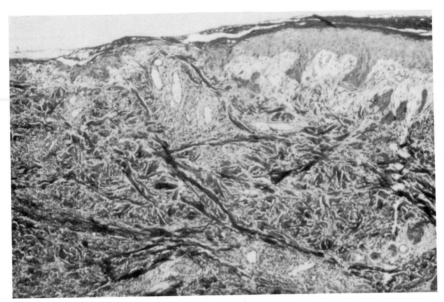

Figure 7–2. Characteristic thinning of leading edge of epithelium migrating across an open wound. (From E. E. Peacock, Jr., in *Principles of Surgery*, edited by S. I. Schwartz. Copyright 1969, McGraw-Hill Book Company. Used with permission of McGraw-Hill Book Company.)

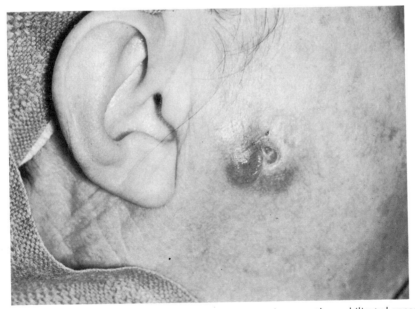

Figure 7–3. Epidermoid carcinoma of skin. Note contrast between the umbilicated appearance of this lesion and lesion shown in Figure 7–1. (Reproduced by permission from E. E. Peacock, Jr., in *Surgery: Principles and Practice,* 3rd edition, edited by C. A. Moyer, J. E. Rhoads, J. G. Allen, and H. N. Harkins, Philadelphia, J. B. Lippincott Co., 1965.)

well as the control of neoplastic cells. Actually, the histological appearance of a four or five day old healing wound has many of the aspects of surface neoplasms, such as increased number of mitoses, disorganization, and lack of polarity of all elements. In most wounds, however, something brings order out of disorder, provides controlled cell proliferation out of rapid division and, in general, exerts a sort of maturing or calming effect over a process which is almost embryonic in intensity. It has been suggested that one such control is the specific tissue chalone discussed in Chapter 2.

Epithelial discontinuity produced by mechanical means, although relatively dangerous compared to uninjured epithelium, is less likely to result in production of invasive cancer during the life span of human beings than epithelial damage due to radiant injury. Thermal or long-wave radiation is less likely to result in carcinoma than is an injury produced by short-wave radiation. Moreover, the length of time between injury and development of invasive cancer seems directly proportional to the wave length of the damaging radiation. Most thermal burns are caused by radiant energy with wave lengths long enough to be almost within the visible spectrum; 20 years may elapse before carcinoma develops in the scar from such a wound (Marjolin's ulcer). Invasive cancer can develop in short-wave (x or gamma) wounds in only a

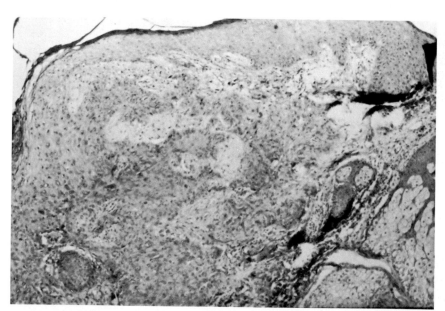

Figure 7–4. Microscopic view of epithelial edge in carcinoma shown in Figure 7–3. Note piling up of cells at the margin which gives the characteristic umbilicated appearance of carcinoma as contrasted to the thin advancing margin of a healing wound. (From E. E. Peacock, Jr., in *Principles of Surgery*, edited by S. I. Schwartz. Copyright 1969, McGraw-Hill Book Company. Used with permission of McGraw-Hill Book Company.)

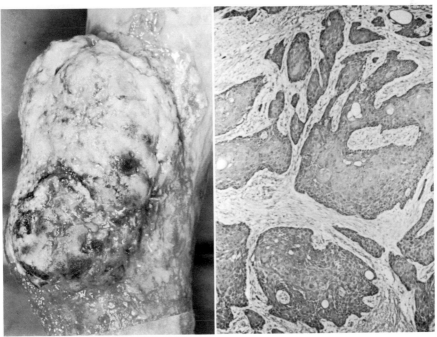

Fig. 7–5   Fig. 7–6

Figure 7–5. Epidermoid carcinoma in an unhealed burn wound of the thigh. Wound was 18 years old. (From E. E. Peacock, Jr., in *Principles of Surgery,* edited by S. I. Schwartz. Copyright 1969, McGraw-Hill Book Company. Used with permission of McGraw-Hill Book Company.)

Figure 7–6. Microscopic appearance of lesion shown in Figure 7–5. (From E. E. Peacock, Jr., in *Principles of Surgery,* edited by S. I. Schwartz. Copyright 1969, McGraw-Hill Book Company. Used with permission of McGraw-Hill Book Company.)

few months. Chronically exposed skin, such as facial skin of farmers and sailors, may require 30 or 40 years to develop multiple skin cancers, but the ultra-short-wave cosmic and solar radiation responsible for these changes has been filtered through relatively dense atmosphere so that the dose factor becomes more important than the wave length. The biological basis for most clinical observations, although not certain, seems related to the production of mutants with varying potential, requiring a varying length of time for external recognition. Production of a mutant following mechanical trauma is probably dependent upon chance development, during many thousands of mitoses, of a cell which has lost controlling systems. The possible effect, whether promoting or initiating, of viruses must not be forgotten. It is possible to produce transformation of benign to malignant cells by viruses. What is not known, however, is whether viruses involved in transformation of human epithelial cells are specific and thus initiating factors or whether they are ubiquitous and fall more in the realm of promoting influences on preconditioned substrates.

In cells exposed to radiant energy, the chromosomes are actually struck by primary or secondary radiation of sufficient strength to cause either immediate or delayed chromosomal aberrations. A basic biological understanding of tissue response to radiant energy erases or reduces to the point of insignificance the popular lay classification of safe or dangerous radiation. Such terms hardly do anything more than define a sort of LD_{50} measurement of an amount of radiation which will or will not result in measurable clinical damage. The radiation biologist seldom uses or relies upon such terms, however, as they carry the connotation that there is a dose of radiation which is not harmful. It is very important for physicians to see clearly that all radiant energy of short enough wave length or sufficient external force to change nuclear deoxyribonucleic acid (DNA) and ribonucleic acid (RNA) is destructive. From a therapeutic standpoint, radiation should never be used except to destroy something; an informed physician will always consider radiation as a damaging force regardless of the dose or form. Admittedly, no other form of energy has been of more therapeutic value when cells go berserk and must be destroyed. Nevertheless, destruction of even a single undesirable cell involves the risk of producing damage to other cells, which, though less severe, may become uncontrolled. As a general rule, most physicians who understand the sobering ramifications of radiation biology will not intentionally expose living tissue to short-wave radiation except to destroy or inhibit a condition which is at least as bad as epidermoid carcinoma. Technical innovations and increased professional skill continually decrease risk of inducing carcinoma in normal tissues; the principle that radiant energy

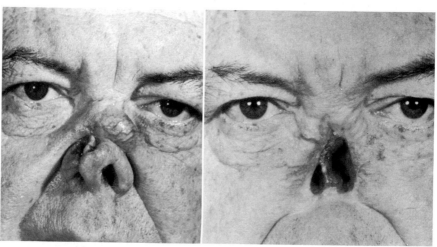

Fig. 7–7   **Fig. 7–8**

Figure 7–7. Epidermoid carcinoma developing in skin of the nose secondary to radiation for basal cell carcinoma three years ago.
Figure 7–8. Total excision of the nose and exenteration of paranasal sinuses was needed to eradicate the carcinoma shown in Figure 7–7.

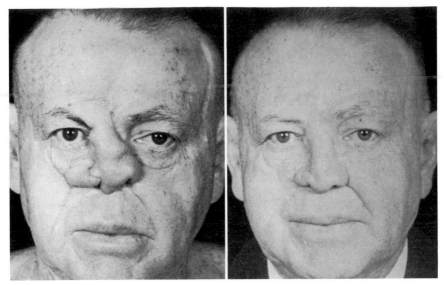

Fig. 7–9   **Fig. 7–10**

Figure 7–9.   Use of nasolabial flap to replace tissue lost during a forehead flap reconstruction of the nose in patient shown in Figure 7–8. A portion of the forehead flap was lost owing to a severe topical drug reaction.

Figure 7–10.   Final view of patient shown in Figure 7–7. The donor site on the forehead has been resurfaced with a thick split-thickness skin graft with freckle pattern similar to skin on the remaining part of the forehead.

in any amount is destructive to some degree, however, is an important concept in human biology which cannot be overemphasized.

Symptoms and related pathophysiology of radiation-induced wounds vary with the wave length and intensity of the damaging ray. The classic first degree wound or radiation effect (radiation effect administered from an external source by a physician for therapeutic reasons should never be referred to as a burn) is characterized by redness, tenderness, and edema of skin. All of these signs and symptoms probably relate to release of various amines from damaged cells, such as mast cells. The effect on the surrounding tissue is one of closure of precapillary shunts, flooding of the vascular bed, and change in capillary permeability. The magnitude and potential dangerous effect on the whole body should never be underestimated; a first degree thermal burn of a large portion of the body surface can be a lethal injury.

Second degree burns are characterized by vesicle formation; the degree of thermal injury and escape of fluid is enough to detach epidermis in large areas. In extensive burns, vesicle formation may be a good sign; epidermis which is structurally intact and waterproof enough to contain sequestered fluid usually overlies dermis that has not been damaged beyond natural repair. This is not always true, however,

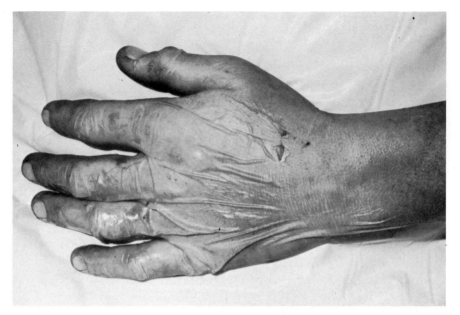

Figure 7–11. Typical second degree burn of the hand with massive vesicle formation.

particularly in steam burns. In flame or hot air burns the presence of an intact blister is a good sign that circulation in the deeper areas of dermis has been preserved and that repair by reepithelization from undamaged cells in deep recesses of hair follicles and dermal glands is possible.

After a first or second degree injury, the most important difference in the biological changes wrought by thermal radiation as compared to x- or gamma wave radiation is reflected in the prognosis. Thermal injury is, in many respects, similar to an abrasion or contusion in that destructive events are maximal at the completion of the injury. All subsequent events are reparative, and the end result may be indistinguishable from normal tissue because only cellular regeneration is required. Such is certainly not the case in a wound caused by shortwave radiation. The initial first or second degree effect of hyperemia, edema, and vesicle formation is really a relatively unimportant prelude to more serious events. The key to understanding these long-term destructive processes is the known susceptibility of dividing cells to radiant energy damage. Cells in prophase stage of mitosis are relatively susceptible. Thus, after general body radiation, tissues such as gastrointestinal tract epithelium, bone marrow, and neoplasm and embryonic tissue are damaged more than dermis, fascia, and other less actively regenerating tissues. Within a composite organ such as skin, epithelium is the most actively germinating layer. Therefore, germinating epithelium will be damaged more severely than other cells. Moreover, the long-term effect of these injuries, such as unpredictable behavior of mutant cells and delayed occlusion of damaged capillaries,

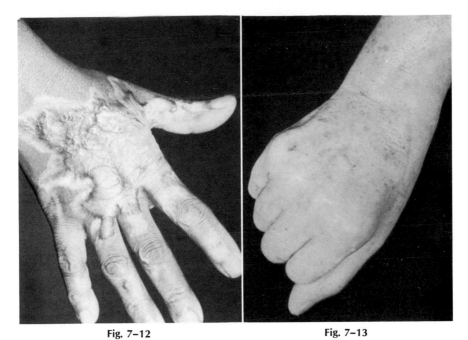

Fig. 7–12   **Fig. 7–13**

Figure 7–12. Hypertrophic scarring typical of a thermal burn.
Figure 7–13. Atrophic skin of the hand typical of a short-wave radiation burn which destroyed cells with collagen-synthesizing potential.

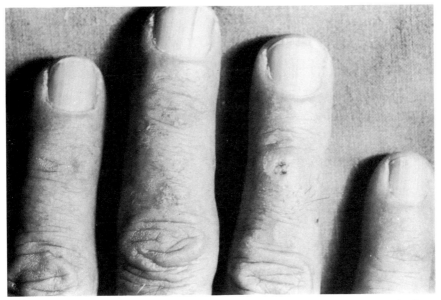

Figure 7–14. Typical radiation coal spots on hands of a physician who performed a large number of fluoroscopic examinations. Note early epidermoid carcinoma on dorsum of ring finger.

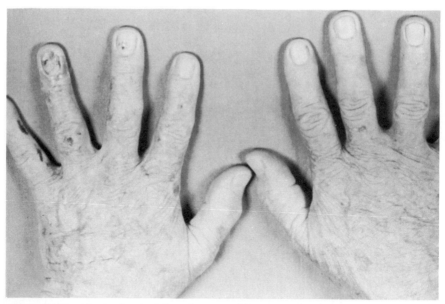

Figure 7–15. Hands of a physician who reduced fractures under direct fluoroscopic vision.

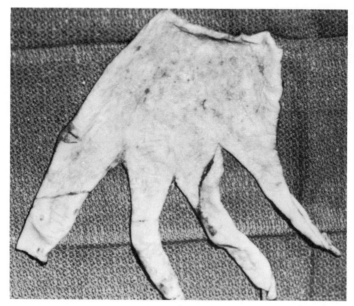

Figure 7–16. Specimen of skin excised from one hand of patient shown in Figure 7–15. Carcinoma was not present.

increascs the overall damage with passage of time. Long after erythema and edema have subsided, more ominous signs of short-wave radiation damage may develop. One such sign commonly is called a "coal spot." These dark specks are areas in skin where a tiny thrombus in a superficial capillary has formed. Other dark spots in skin may be caused by keratin formation, which can be either excessive or unnoticeable according to the type of radiation injury. Dermis may take on a thin, glazed, or waxed appearance because of destruction and fragmentation of collagen bundles; new collagen synthesis is decreased by radiation destruction of fibroblasts. Tiny new capillaries will make abortive attempts to revascularize partially ischemic skin; these new vessels have a characteristic venous appearance which is caused by some resistance in the outflow tract. Groups of these small vessels are often called telangiectases. Pigment formation can be disturbed in varying ways to give different appearances. If melanin-producing cells are not destroyed, they will react by producing increased pigment, thus giving the skin a characteristic tanned appearance. If melanin-producing cells are destroyed completely, skin can appear unnaturally light. If epithelial cells are only partially damaged, surface keratinization will be increased to give skin a spotty, brown tinge in contrast to the pale, waxy appearance if keratinization is diminished over partially damaged dermis. In a word, the appearance of skin at any one time following short-wave radiation damage reflects the degree of ischemia and the abortive attempts of skin to repair the damage.

One of the most important concepts in radiation biology is the inability of any reparative process to go to a logical conclusion—presuma-

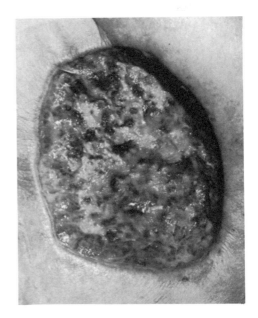

Figure 7–17. Radiation-induced ulcer of the sacrum in a patient who was treated for carcinoma of the cervix. Ulcer is six months old. Note complete absence of collagen synthesis and wound contraction.

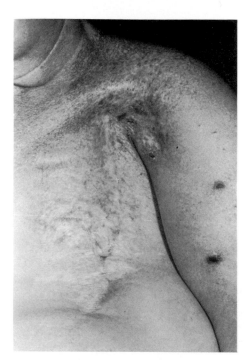

Figure 7–18. Typical radiation effect following extensive radiation of the axilla and chest wall.

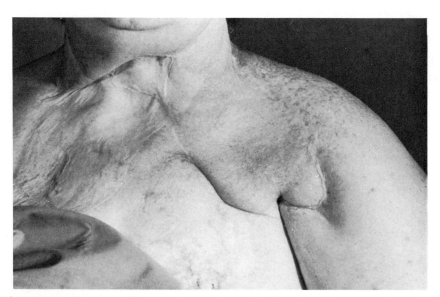

Figure 7–19. Permanent blood-carrying rotation pedicle flap from right anterior chest to left anterior thorax and axilla. Note improvement of surrounding tissue because of increased blood supply. This type of flap is best considered as a permanent transfer of blood vessels into an area of diminished vascularity.

bly because of inadequate blood supply. Thus, radiant energy wounds frequently show three zones of involvement: There may be a central necrotic zone, a midzone of mild inflammation and partial ischemia, and a marked inflammatory zone on the periphery which apparently is unable to extend into the midzone and central zone where scavenger and healing processes are needed.

In a thermal burn, regenerative processes are relatively unimpeded so that remarkable healing can be achieved. In a short radiation-induced wound, however, reparative processes are slow, often are seriously impeded by ischemia, and may exert a dangerous influence on the rest of the body for many years. The biologically oriented surgeon views irradiated skin, therefore, regardless of degree, as an area where invasive cancer is likely to develop throughout a patient's life.

MANAGEMENT OF FIRST DEGREE THERMAL BURNS

Management of first and second degree thermal burns is not complex. The objectives are relief of pain and protection from further injury so that epithelization can occur. No catalyst presently is available which will speed or improve the series of events described in Chapter 2. An interesting chapter in the history of our attempts to speed wound healing, however, includes discovery during the early 1900's of various chemicals which are true carcinogens in that they can, alone, produce epithelial neoplasms. One of the most powerful of such agents is 20-methylcholanthrene, but other agents (many of which are in the general group of cyclic hydrocarbons) also are able to induce epithelial cancer. The azo dye industries have produced several such compounds, and it was hoped that a substance could be found which would be slightly different in some side chain or other structural way from dangerous carcinogens but would still have significant epithelium-stimulating properties. Such a substance (which was popularly endorsed without supporting data) is scarlet red ointment—a by-product of the azo dye industry. Epithelium-stimulating reactions, however, seem to be an all-or-nothing phenomenon, for no chemical agent is known at present which will stimulate epithelization without producing neoplastic changes. All that can be done to promote epithelization falls in the general category of protecting the denuded surface and preventing further injury or complications which will interfere with natural proliferation and migration of dedifferentiating cells. Mechanical injury, chemical injury, or infection will delay epithelization; any measure which protects a healing surface from these destructive influences is worthwhile.

A protective umbrella for epithelization can be artificial or natural. Artificial protection can be afforded by a dressing, but unskilled application or careless selection of dressing materials can retard epithelization. Adverse effects from unskilled application of artificial dressings include both mechanical interference with cell migration and promotion of bacterial proliferation. Selection of a substance for an artificial cover beneath which epithelization can proceed at the fastest possible rate can be done on a scientific basis. To begin with, the actual application of a second surface or cover to a healing wound is biologically sound in that the rate of epithelial movement on a glass slide is literally doubled by addition of a second surface in the form of a glass cover slip. The type of second surface is important, however, and whether fabric or some other substance is chosen, the most important physical characteristic is tightness of weave. The cheapest available material is fine-mesh (less than No. 44) gauze. If larger mesh is substituted, capillary or cellular growth into the interstices is invited, and removal of such a dressing usually causes hemorrhage and detachment of delicate surface cells. Similar reasoning supports the use of new tightly woven synthetics, such as nylon, and older materials, such as Telfa, silver foil, or charged gold leaf. Metallic dressings are esthetically appealing, but are so expensive that practical considerations have loomed larger than theoretical advantages.

Since most dressings have to be changed before healing is complete, preparation should be made for removing the layer of dressing directly against the denuded surface and new epithelium as atraumatically as possible. Thinking in these terms, one usually impregnates the gauze with some type of water-soluble emollient so that coagulating exudate will not seal the dressing to the wound surface. Vaseline and other greasy preparations have been used successfully with this in mind, but water-soluble substances such as polyethylene glycol are superior; maceration of the wound surface is not as likely to occur with water-soluble preparations. A few layers of coarse gauze sponge can be added for additional protection, but there is no biological basis for applying pressure to an artificial dressing designed to protect a surface undergoing epithelization.

Patients who should stay in bed because of some other condition or for whom an artificial dressing is desired because of age or inability to tolerate mild pain are best treated by applying a few strips of fine-mesh, emollient-impregnated gauze only. The gauze becomes a sort of artificial scab as it dries and becomes attached to the wound surface. Once a gauze dressing attached to a wound surface which is undergoing epithelization becomes dry, it should not be removed until epithelization is complete. If infection should develop beneath the dressing, enzyme digestion of the plasma clot will occur and the dressing literally will float away. If epithelization proceeds without infection, however, the dressing will become gradually detached so that it can be trimmed circumferentially. The interface between dedifferentiated, migrating epithelium and the underlying dermal edge is extremely fragile. This is the plane where separation will occur whenever manual force is applied to any portion of the multilayer dressing-wound complex. Collagenolytic enzyme activity is more pronounced here than in other areas. In addition, rete pegs and intracellular bridges do not develop until epithelium returns to a more normal resting condition. There is little or no resistance, therefore, to mechanical deformation of an advancing epithelial edge.

Epithelization can progress at a maximal rate beneath a natural dressing (scab). There is no biological reason, therefore, for applying an artificial dressing to a first or second degree skin wound, provided a natural dressing can be maintained long enough for epithelization to occur. Actually, present data suggest that epithelization does not proceed along the surface, but that advancing epithelial cells literally cut through an irregular dermal surface by producing powerful fibrinolytic and collagenolytic enzymes. Delicate as the advancing epithelial edge may appear, it carries a powerful weapon in the form of ability to stimulate production of enzymes which actively prepare a road ahead. Compared to an eschar or artificial dressing (both of which contain fibers), however, a scab (mostly cells and fibrin) is not very strong. It soon becomes so dry and brittle that it must be protected from physical deformation. Allowing a scab to form and then protecting the scab from physical deformation, as is done with donor sites and abrasive injuries, is called exposure treatment. The popular term *open treatment* should be discarded, as it implies that the wound is not covered by anything, thus eliminating professional responsibility for maintaining an accurate dressing. Nothing could be further from the truth. Exposure treatment of all degrees of thermal wounds means only that a natural dressing of blood clot or heat-denatured fibrous protein is being skillfully utilized to dress the wound.

Natural dressings may require more attention than artificial ones although care is of a different type. As will be discussed in detail in the next section, a natural dressing contains fibrous protein to make it stronger than one which contains only fibrin, serum proteins, and dehydrated cells. Scabs, though they require careful protection from mechanical deformation and contact with liquids, are safer than artificial dressings in prevention of infection; they form a tighter biological seal as long as they are kept dehydrated. A major disadvantage is the length of time required for scabs to become adequately dehydrated, and the length of time they can be kept in a satisfactory dehydrated condition. The relatively short life of a scab militates against its use in a full-thickness wound, therefore, and the length of time required to dehydrate a scab makes their use in small children or emotionally unstable patients less desirable than an artificial dressing. Approximately 24 hours is required for an average scab to seal a wound effectively; until all oozing of blood and plasma has ceased, the surface clot does not become completely dehydrated. During the time the clot is gelatinous, patients often complain of a burning sensation. By the end of 24 hours, however, the clot usually is completely dehydrated and the patient is free of pain. During this time, the affected area should be immobilized and bed linen should be suspended above the wound so that mechanical deformation by liquid soilage does not occur.

In summary, selection of an appropriate dressing for wounds in which epithelization only is needed involves both mechanical and biological considerations. By far the most important of these is the biological factor of prevention of infection. Infection in a subdermal wound, particularly if unrecognized, may convert a relatively simple wound which will heal without perceptible scar into an extremely complex one which may heal only with considerable scarring. Complications of this magnitude in the donor sites of patients with extensive burns have meant the difference between survival and death. Care of donor sites in such individuals obviously is as important as any other aspect of the patient's care. Whenever infection in a donor site carries such a danger, all other considerations such as pain and soiling of bed linen fade into insignificance. In these cases, the decision to treat all donor sites by the exposure method is easy. In patients who should remain in bed because of the nature of their recipient wound or for some other reason, the exposure method still may be preferable, particularly if the donor site is large and the patient is oriented and able to cooperate. Small donor sites in ambulatory patients or in very young or disoriented individuals are best treated by an occlusive dressing of medicated fine-mesh gauze and an external covering to absorb drainage during the first 48 hours. After 36 to 48 hours all of the outer layers of the dressing can be removed. The innermost layer of fine-mesh gauze forms a temporary fiber graft providing structural stability for the cellular aggregate. It should be allowed to remain until it separates spontaneously, leaving a newly epithelized surface below. A blood-impregnated layer of fine-mesh gauze provides a dry, fairly rigid dressing utilizing both natural and artificial materials which will allow patients to be ambulatory under most conditions.

SECOND DEGREE BURNS

A burn wound which can cause special difficulty is a deep second degree burn in relatively thick skin. Particularly after a high-humidity burn involving hair-bearing portions of the face or the back and buttocks where skin is very thick, epithelium and superficial dermis may be destroyed without complete destruction of deep capillary networks. Such a wound may have little or no hemorrhage, but will leak almost pure plasma for five or six days. Skin is too tender to shave easily, and in thick hair-bearing areas the combination of beard and fibrin clot is difficult to manage. Shaving such a patient under anesthesia or deep sedation interferes with epithelization and promotes escape of plasma. A fibrin clot tenaciously surrounding facial hair provides a good pabulum for secondary infection. The essential problem is to establish continued drainage without interfering with epithelization; usually this can be accomplished by use of intermittent warm saline compresses and by shaving with an electric razor. Between application of compresses and shaving, a light film of some water-soluble emollient such as ophthalmic-strength boric acid will prevent drying of plasma transudate. Dressings covering the face are difficult to maintain accurately and often are not tolerated well by the patient. Failure to achieve epithelization within a week or ten days almost always means that dermal infection is present and that the end result will be less than optimal because of deep or superficial scarring.

Infection is the most dreaded complication in second degree burns, regardless of where they occur. Investigation by phage typing reveals that the source of secondary infection may be the patient (i.e., organisms the patient carries elsewhere on his body). Infection from attendants and other patients is more frequent, however, and usually is the result of errors in aseptic technique. Recently, exposure under controlled environmental conditions and application of surface antibacterial or antibiotic agents have received considerable attention. Effective in preventing serious infection in second degree burns, both of these methods will be covered in detail in a subsequent section; but during a discussion of second degree burns some consideration should be given to these methods as they apply to management of large blisters. Whether to protect and preserve blisters or rupture them by excising detached epithelium is the question. The answer, like most problems in wound management, does not come from a simple directive from an authoritative source. The problem is best met by thinking in terms of skin morphology and pathology and how the eventual goal of repairing deep capillary damage and restoring surface epithelium can be achieved without supervening infection. The essence of the question is: Will detached epithelium and plasma filtrate acting as a natural dressing over injured dermis be preferable to any other natural or artificial dressing? Theoretically, the fluid in a blister should provide an optimal covering for epithelization, against which further fluid sequestration would not occur. Also, during the first 24 hours, blisters are more comfortable than open second degree burn surfaces although this is usually of only minor importance. But it is not normal for the outer surface of skin to be bathed continually in a liquid medium. Moreover, it is almost impossible to keep a blister intact during the time required for epithelization to cover a large second degree burn.

The question usually is resolved by allowing blisters to remain intact for 24 to 36 hours, and then excising partially detached epithelium so that the surface can be treated with an antibacterial protective dressing or allowed to remain dry. If drying is permitted, a surface plasma

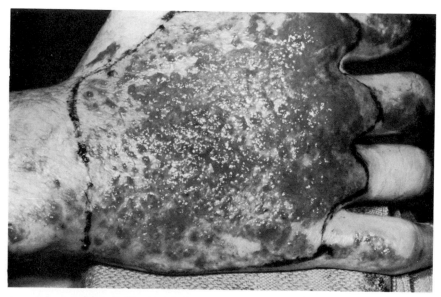

Figure 7–27. Detailed view of hand shown in Figure 7–26.

the burn, whereas the capillary proliferation associated with granulation tissue commences after several days.

This vascular proliferation in perigranulation tissue is not associated with fibrosis as is the vascular proliferation in granulation tissue.

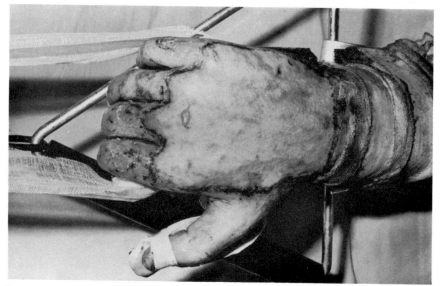

Figure 7–28. Same hand as shown in Figure 7–27 following partial resurfacing of wound with thick split-thickness skin graft.

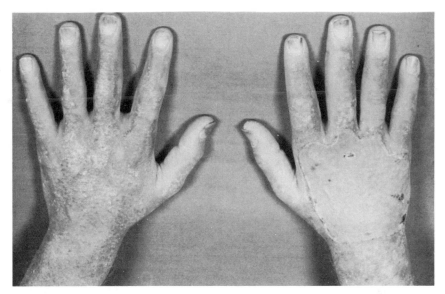

Figure 7–29.   Same hands as shown in Figure 7–28. Right hand has been treated with a skin graft and left hand has been allowed to heal by epithelization.

These new blood vessels increase in numbers up to two to five days after burning and then begin to regress after one or two weeks. They are gone after a month. These vessels do not appear to revascularize the injured area and hence their function is unexplained. However, the

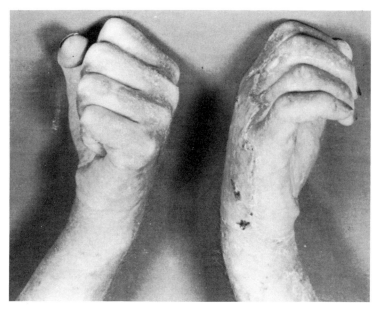

Figure 7–30.   Same hands shown in Figure 7–24 two days after removal of dressing from skin graft placed on the right hand. Note stiffness of metacarpophalangeal and interphalangeal joints caused by two weeks of immobilization.

presence of these vessels may be of importance in augmenting the heat loss in burned patients and in changing the vascular dynamics.

When faced with a structurally intact area of skin which has been damaged severely by radiant energy, a surgeon must determine first whether skin has been irretrievably converted into nonliving eschar or whether enough viable cells remain so that it can be classified as deep second degree injury not requiring replacement. Although some injuries pose an insoluble problem in this regard, so that only the passage of time permits diagnosis, most radiation injuries can be classified accurately. The history is helpful; flame burns are almost always full-thickness burns whereas short exposure to steam usually does not kill all cells in a thick dermis. Damaged skin in which capillary function is not destroyed will usually show marked effects of change in capillary permeability. Thus edema of skin is often a favorable sign. Heat-fused and dehydrated collagen is smaller in volume than before exposure to radiant energy. Thus, if the examiner palpates a burned area and is able to demonstrate sudden change in contour between burned and unburned skin, he gains a valuable bit of information. Burned skin elevated above the level of normal skin most likely is not damaged beyond repair as it can still react physiologically to what must have been a less than lethal injury. Eschar which is unquestionably lower than the level of less severely burned or normal skin is usually damaged through all thicknesses and should be classified as third degree eschar. In this instance, the ability to react to injury by sequestration of fluid has been eliminated and some degree of dehydration and denaturation has occurred. A form of treatment of deep second degree and some third degree burns known as tangential excision and grafting is based upon the fact that few burns destroy every living element in the full thickness of skin. A patient almost has to lie in flames as epileptic patients sometimes do or be exposed to extremely high temperatures such as produced by an electric arc to have a uniform, complete destruction of skin. In areas such as the back, this almost never occurs. Thus in most areas following exposure to moderate heat, it is possible to excise 50 to 70 per cent of the thickness of burned skin or eschar in a uniform manner such as when taking a skin graft. Such a procedure produces a surface that can support a thin split-thickness skin graft. Such surfaces have several advantages over those produced by excising all of the skin, eschar, and subcutaneous fat followed by application of a graft. The thin remaining eschar following tangential excision is really a filmy collagen network that does not interfere with diffusion of gases and nutrients or with revascularization; it prevents wound contraction and produces a smooth surface as contrasted to lumpy subcutaneous fat or uneven fascia.

Carbonization, or severe heat denaturation, forming a typical charred appearance, is an obvious sign of deep fourth degree damage. A small test incision to see if hemorrhage will occur is indicated in some cases. Interpreting anesthesia in a burned area as an unfavorable sign may be misleading; it is probably the least reliable test in common use. Edema, particularly if a layer of keratinized or heat-fused epidermis is present, can markedly reduce sensory perception even though the deep layer of dermis is viable and capable of repairing skin. Full-thickness eschar can transmit pressure mechanically to hypersensitive peripheral or deep sensors, thus causing a patient to respond to touch or pin prick even though skin that was stimulated directly is damaged beyond possibility of regenerative repair. False-positive and false-negative impressions can be elicited from sensory examination of burned areas. Circulation of vital dyes and clearance of radioactive substances have enjoyed spurts of enthusiasm as tests for skin viability. Sustained reliance on such tests has never developed, however, because the very nature of the burn injury is such that tests of circulation cannot predict what is happening to cells outside the circulatory system. Blood volume determinations are almost unobtainable during stages of vascular leakage, and any test which depends upon an intact circulation is fraught with so many inaccuracies that it yields little useful information.

Even if an accurate test of skin viability were available, the biologically oriented surgeon would not feel any great elation; the problem is not just one of knowing the present state of cell viability. More impor-

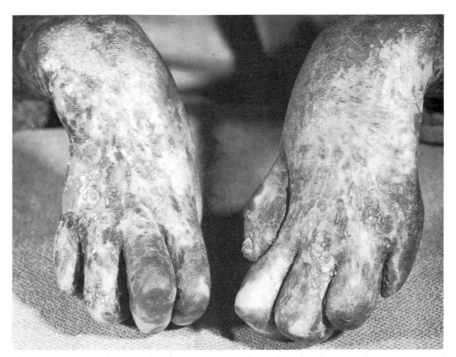

Figure 7–31. Mutilation of hands caused by prolonged healing by wound contraction and epithelization. (From E. E. Peacock, Jr., in *Reconstructive Plastic Surgery,* vol. IV, edited by J. M. Converse, Philadelphia, W. B. Saunders Co., 1964.)

tant is: What is happening to the cells and how long will they remain viable? If everything is cooked, the diagnosis is usually clear. When there is some chance that all cells have not been destroyed, important questions need to be answered: Can life be sustained? Can complications such as infection be prevented? And will regenerative and healing efforts produce new covering which will be better than that which could be obtained by immediate removal of the eschar and application of a free skin graft? No simple, single test of viability can answer all these questions. So we are faced again with the inescapable conclusion that treatment of wounds is an exercise in applied cellular biology. It cannot be relegated to reading a dial and applying a remedy.

The choice of type of coverage needed in specialized areas weighs heavily in some decisions to preserve damaged skin and allow it to heal, or to excise islands of viable skin and resurface the entire area with a free graft. For instance, in the hand, coverage alone simply is not enough. The back of the hand, even though entirely healed following a deep burn, can be inadequately covered for normal function. In this instance, complete excision of the the naturally healed wound will be required for full flexion of the fingers. Even though skin on the dorsum of the hand may not be destroyed through all layers and would ultimately heal if treated carefully, most surgeons recommend early ex-

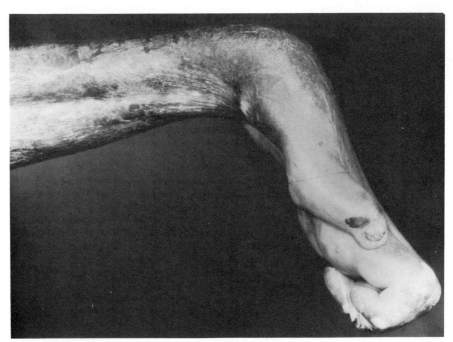

Figure 7–32.   Lateral view of same hand shown in Figure 7–31. (From E. E. Peacock, Jr., in *Surgery: Principles and Practice,* 4th edition, edited by C. A. Moyer, J. E. Rhoads, H. N. Harkins, and J. G. Allen, Philadelphia, J. B. Lippincott Co., 1970.)

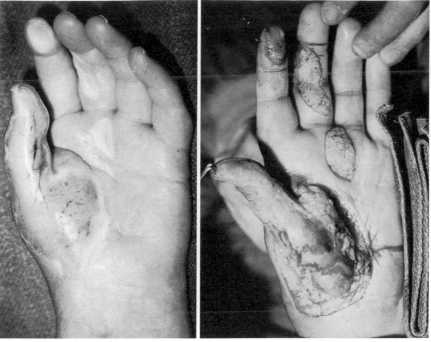

Fig. 7–33   Fig. 7–34

Figure 7–33. Deep third degree burn of thumb, palm, and index and long fingers caused by hot iron.
Figure 7–34. Excision of all burned areas, converting the thermal wound into a surgically clean one within hours of the injury.

cision and replacement of skin which is burned so deeply that it is impossible to be sure whether deep second degree or a third degree injury has occurred. The rationale behind this approach is that skin so badly damaged that the diagnosis is in doubt will, even if allowed to heal by scar formation and epithelization, be inadequate and will have to be replaced at some future date. Moreover, if the diagnosis of a deep second degree burn should be wrong, or if a complicating infection converts a second degree into a third degree injury, grafting will have to be done on a hand which already has been immobilized for several weeks. Moreover, if infection has developed, grafting will have to be done on a bed of granulation tissue. Both courses are undesirable and should be avoided if possible.

When skin obviously is burned through all layers, two courses of action are open. The first is to excise the eschar (debride the wound) and close the wound immediately; the other is to allow the eschar to serve as a bandage for some period of time. If the latter course is chosen, two additional alternatives are available: to take care of the eschar by exposing it, or to apply a dressing in conjunction with

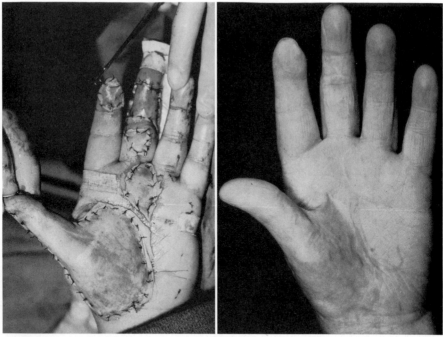

Fig. 7–35   Fig. 7–36

Figure 7–35.   Closure of wounds with split-thickness skin graft immediately after debridement of burned tissue.
Figure 7–36.   Appearance of hand three weeks after skin graft. Small web contracture between thumb and index finger will require secondary revision.

application of a local antibiotic or antiseptic. Selection of a method for treating third degree wounds covered with eschar can be based on knowledge of the biology of eschar formation and by comparing the way a wound will heal with or without eschar.

The most important concept and one often overlooked in management of wounds temporarily covered with eschar is the concept of a burn as a wound. One often needs to be reminded that, regardless of what type of agent (mechanical or radiant) destroyed skin, the situation is basically a defect produced by loss of skin. All of the basic processes described in Chapters 1 to 4 are involved in healing. This is true whether the wound is temporarily dressed with biological ashes, temporarily dressed with a synthetic substance, or left open. Inability of skin to regenerate is fundamental no matter how the wound is treated. If eschar is selected as a temporary dressing, it will require care if it is to be utilized as long as possible; ultimately it will have to be changed. As soon as this has been done, the burn wound is exactly the same as any other wound characterized by full-thickness loss of skin.

Ideal treatment of a burn can best be described in the highly selected case of a soldering iron burn of the slightly redundant soft tissue of the thigh. Ideal management of such a wound would include immediate excision of the burned area and closure of the defect by suturing as described in Chapter 6. If the wound was caused by a flat iron, the defect following excision cannot be closed with sutures but requires either a graft or prolonged care while contraction, fibrous protein synthesis, and epithelization produce a relatively unsatisfactory cosmetic and functional result. No matter which method is utilized, there is no need to preserve the heat-denatured collagen. The sooner it is removed, the faster grafting can be accomplished or secondary healing will take place. Consideration of such relatively small burns is worthwhile, as it emphasizes the concept of the burn as a wound, the eschar as an impediment to healing, and early closure as the most certain method of avoiding undesirable scars.

A burn caused by exposure to flame or steam resulting in destruction of 25 to 60 per cent of the body surface creates a problem more serious than the soldering iron or flat iron from every standpoint. It is in these situations that a surgeon may become so overwhelmed by other factors that he loses appreciation of the burn as a wound and makes decisions involving treatment which are not based on sound principles of wound healing biology. Confronted with a massive wound, the biologically oriented surgeon considers the condition of the natural dressing and analyzes the likelihood of injuring the patient further by removing it. These possibilities can then be compared with advantages (local and general) of preserving the eschar. Removal of the eschar, like any other extirpative surgical procedure, involves risks which include converting early localized infection into generalized bacteremia and septicemic shock. In addition, if the wound produced by removing nat-

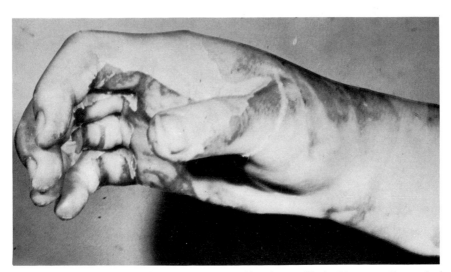

Figure 7–37.   Circumferential third degree burn of hand caused by igniting a gasoline-soaked glove.

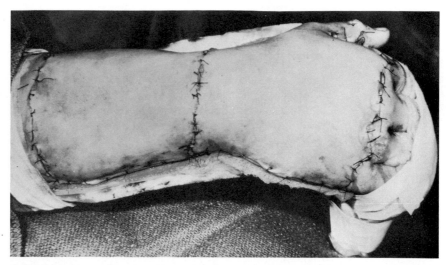

Figure 7–38. Immediate resurfacing of dorsum of the hand with a thick split-thickness skin graft. Five days later volar surface of the hand was excised and similar grafts were applied.

ural dressing is too large to cover with grafts, artificial material, not as desirable as natural eschar, might have to be used to provide cover. In these cases, utilization of the eschar as a biological dressing might be lifesaving, whereas excision could be rapidly fatal. The puzzle is usually resolved by considering the size of the eschar and the amount of donor skin which is available. Of the two, available skin is, by far, the more important. Most surgeons would agree that if the denuded area does

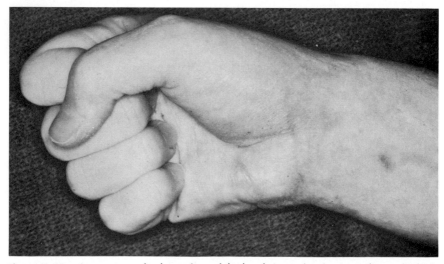

Figure 7–39. Appearance of volar surface of the hand six weeks after immediate split-thickness skin grafting.

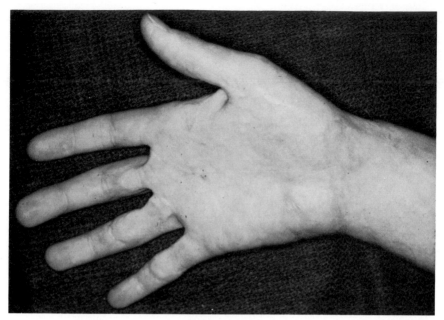

Figure 7–40. Flexion view showing normal active and passive motion in all digits in same hand shown in Figure 7–37.

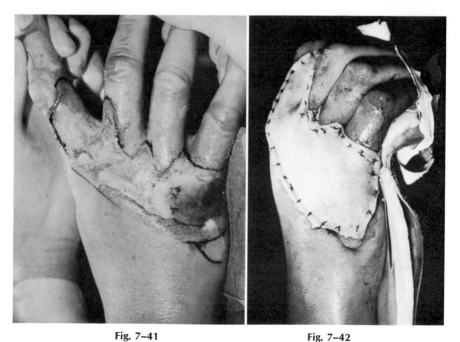

| **Fig. 7–41** | **Fig. 7–42** |

Figure 7–41. Deep electrical burn of dorsum of the hand. (Reproduced by permission from E. E. Peacock, Jr., Southern Med. J., 56:1094, 1963.)

Figure 7–42. Appearance following excision of burned tissue and immediate application of thick split-thickness skin graft. (Reproduced by permission from E. E. Peacock, Jr., Southern Med. J., 56:1094, 1963.)

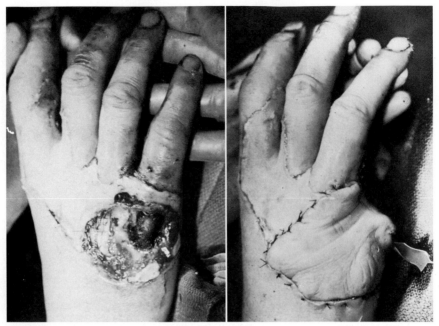

Fig. 7–43   Fig. 7–44

Figure 7–43. Appearance of hand at first dressing showing loss of graft over ulnar side. This is characteristic of electrical burns; the depth of burn tissue was not fully appreciated. Note, however, that the remainder of the hand is covered satisfactorily. (Reproduced by permission from E. E. Peacock, Jr., Southern Med. J., 56:1094, 1963.)

Figure 7–44. Utilization of skin flap from amputated small finger to resurface the wound shown in Figure 7–43. (Reproduced by permission from E. E. Peacock, Jr., Southern Med. J., 56:1094, 1963.)

not exceed available donor skin, early excision and replacement of the eschar should be done. In an extremely sick patient, or when excision and grafting will be tedious and time-consuming (hands or face), the process should be done in stages. When the burned area exceeds the donor surface by no more than two or three times, a delay will be unavoidable between excision of the eschar and healing and maturation of donor sites. The time required for healing and maturation after a second set of grafts has been removed is longer, and the process is fraught with more complications than when only one graft has been removed. Thus, at least part of the eschar in large burns may need to be utilized as a dressing for as long as three or four weeks.

Whether eschar is preserved as a natural dressing or some biological or nonbiological artificial dressing is substituted depends upon many factors. If the burned area exceeds by more than three times the total area of skin available for grafts, the eschar will have to be used to dress the burn, for it offers the only possible chance for patient survival. Particularly on the back, where skin is relatively thick, it is rare to find uniform full-thickness destruction of every living cell. Scattered islands of living cells may have been spared; if they are not destroyed by subsequent infection or excised by radical debridement, these islands of viable cells could serve as a source of epithelial regeneration. Admittedly, a wound covered only by epithelium is in a precarious condition. Combined with wound contraction and what skin grafting can be done, however, the proliferation of islands of epithelium can be the key to obtaining a healed wound of some type so that life can be sustained. In such patients a biological dressing unquestionably can be life-saving. Consideration of these principles has been responsible for recent emphasis on preserving and utilizing eschar as a temporary dressing for thermal injuries.

Prevention of Infection under the Eschar

At present, three methods for taking care of eschar are popular: dry exposure, addition of topical agents such as Sulfamylon, silver sulfadiazine (Silvadene) or gentamicin, and dressing with 0.5 per cent silver nitrate saturated dressings. The biological basis for each and the practical advantages and disadvantages which have become apparent with rather extensive clinical trials are as follows.

DRY EXPOSURE. The exposure method of burn treatment has been recognized and evaluated periodically for many years. The history of periodic enthusiasm for its use correlates with the military history of a country. This is particularly true during the last part of a war when large numbers of casualties exceed hospital capacity and also during the immediate postwar period when military surgeons have time to study what they have done. This sort of analysis brings out an important point in the exposure principle—it has repeatedly proved superior to any other method when medical facilities are overtaxed and trained personnel are limited. The fundamental biology is readily apparent, bringing into light the time-honored surgical observations that bacteria do not thrive on a dry surface. Expressed differently, a well drained wound does not become an abscess leading to internal drainage or bacteremia. Particularly during handling of large numbers of casualties or during other less than optimal circumstances, it is impossible to prevent surface contamination of an eschar. If the eschar, which is a perfect pabulum containing bacterial nutrients, is placed in a warm, enclosed, gauze dressing where moisture and body heat are retained, putrefaction is almost inevitable. The biological basis for the exposure technique is that by preventing moisture from accumulating and lowering the temperature slightly, the ideal incubator conditions of a closed dressing can be altered. In addition, the potential culture plate can be kept under direct observation. This is important, as early infection can be spotted and either drained or sequestered from the rest of the body. The therapeutic measures used in this approach are primarily those of keeping the external surface dry and protected from mechanical trauma and excessive bacterial inoculation. More mundane advantages are that expensive dressing materials are not required and substantially less time of physicians is required in changing dressings or administering anesthetics. The disadvantages of the exposure method are that more nursing time may be required to keep patients comfortable when they cannot turn freely or lie on all surfaces. External heat is needed to keep practically naked patients from shivering and additional heat may be needed to evaporate transudate from the surface. This is particularly true during early stages of reaction to a high-humidity burn. The most serious disadvantage to the exposure method of eschar treatment, however, is that energy requirements are dangerously escalated. The basic biology involved may not be obvious, but the danger is real and may go unrecognized until too late. The surface of an eschar should be bone dry when it is adequately prepared to resist bacteriological inoculation. Actually, however, the eschar, even in a dry condition, offers no resistance to the passage of water to the surface—and pass it does, particularly in air-conditioned rooms or when external heat has been used to achieve a dry surface. The amount of water passing through an area of eschar in a specified time interval has been measured. The loss of heat through evaporation from a burn of 50 per cent of the body surface may raise the body's total caloric requirement to astronomical heights: 5000 to 10,000 calories per day. The required increase in cardiac output to keep this quantity of liquid moving can be the equivalent required for strenuous exercise. In the severely burned patient, the heart is no match for the combination of a heat lamp and efficient air conditioner. In a death struggle the biological pump will lose. Unfortunately we now have data which strongly suggest that heat loss from convection, conduction, radiation, evaporation, and so forth, is not the only or even the prime cause of energy depletion and exhaustion in burned patients.

Additional contraindications to the exposure treatment are eschar involving hands, genitalia, or face, circumferential eschar on the torso preventing adequate exposure of all burned areas, and burns in small children who will pick at the eschar or soil it continually. The main advantages to the exposure method are that it requires less time and attention of physicians (although more nursing care) and it is the most practical method of treating large numbers of burned patients under less than ideal situations. Its main disadvantages are the impracticality of treating certain areas and the danger of adding significantly to the work of the cardiovascular system. When ideal treatment of small numbers of casualties is possible, the exposure treatment is seldom called upon. During emergencies or military crises, however, it is an extremely useful method of treating large numbers of casualties.

TOPICAL APPLICATION OF SILVER NITRATE. Approximately ten years ago, the possibility of solving the bacteriological complications of

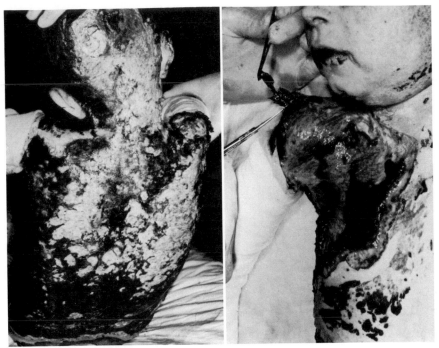

Fig. 7-45   **Fig. 7-46**

Figure 7-45. Typical appearance of burn eschar treated with silver nitrate. Note deposition of silver chloride on burned and unburned skin alike.

Figure 7-46. Technique of performing small debridements without anesthesia in silver nitrate-treated burn wound.

preserved eschar while simultaneously overcoming the metabolic hazards of a dry surface was investigated. Such studies evaluated the use of many topical antibiotics and antiseptics to control infection while maintaining a moist surface from which evaporation would not produce dangerous cooling. Two substances appeared promising: 0.5 per cent silver nitrate, applied as a wet dressing; and Sulfamylon acetate, applied as a topical gel or paste. Early success in preventing surface infection was significant enough to alter overall mortality of burns in some institutions. Failure to control infection completely with topical agents, however, suggested that preservation of a sterile eschar by topical medication was not the final answer to the problem of infection. At this time it seems that, although extremely valuable in the management of burns of all degrees of severity, topical agents probably are not going to alter the mortality of burns significantly except in a relatively small group of patients. Studies on the use of topical agents have made monumental contributions to burn therapy, however, because they have pointed out so clearly that it is the burn eschar that harbors lethal organisms. The relatively enormous number (as many as 5 million bacteria per cubic centimeter of burned fat or skin) of bacteria in eschar apparently is the source of fatal bacteremia. To prevent transient bacteremia in patients harboring this number of organisms is, of course, impossible. To prevent a lethal septicemia as long as a source of organisms of this magnitude remains is a major task for both natural and therapeutic processes. Thus the attempt, by pharmacological means, to prevent inoculation and proliferation of bacteria is a sound biological endeavor.

After exhaustive tests to find the most effective antiseptic that would still not affect adversely epithelial cell proliferation, Moyer, in 1964, determined that 0.5 per cent silver nitrate was the topical agent of choice to control surface contamination and prevent deep infection of burned fat and skin. To be effective, silver nitrate must be applied as a continuous wet dressing, and the deleterious effects of rapid evaporation must be overcome by using a dry, occlusive dressing over the wet compresses. Dressings of this type should be changed by specially trained personnel at least once a day. In this routine, no radical debridement is performed; only tissue which can be teased away with minimal traction and without producing pain or hemorrhage is removed. Obviously, debridement of dead tissue requires a long time; the absence of bacterial action means that only natural collagenolytic or acid hydrolase activity, plus the rather minuscule picking away of tissue by attendants, can rid the wound of dead tissue. This, of course, is the biological basis for this form of treatment — to perform debridement so slowly and gently that only completely necrotic tissue is removed and viable islands of epithelium or connective tissues are preserved. As stated before, however, the hypothesis that skin is not destroyed uniformly and that small islands of living tissue remain is the only basis for advocating treatment of this sort. If skin is uniformly burned and no viable cells remain, debridement over a long period of time only extends interminably the debridement process, thus delaying dangerously any healing or replacement procedures. Such an approach to carbonized skin would be useful only while waiting for donor sites to heal so that a second crop of skin grafts could be taken.

Another important advantage to the use of topical silver nitrate is that minuscule debridement during silver nitrate therapy can be done without general anesthetics. Patients are relatively comfortable and able to move freely when they are properly dressed. They usually eat normally and maintain their weight much better than when the exposure method is used or after excision and skin grafting begins.

The major disadvantages to the use of topical silver nitrate are the time required and the excessive removal of both sodium and chloride from the body by exchange with silver nitrate to produce silver chloride and sodium nitrate. In addition, the staining of the patient's skin as well as of attendants and equipment with silver is of some importance. The soiling of attendants and environment is only annoying, but deposition of silver salts in the keratinizing and superficial layers of

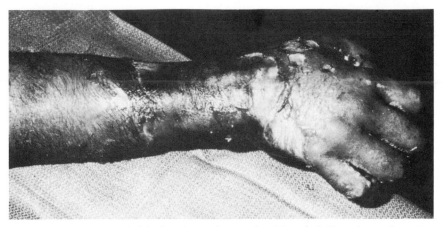

Figure 7–47. Burn wound of the hand treated six weeks with topical silver nitrate. The patient became severely septic.

epithelium of burned skin and new grafts is considerably more serious. It is impossible to tell in skin discolored with silver nitrate precisely what is going on beneath the surface. Silver nitrate does not always protect the deeper tissues from bacterial contamination; deep infection covered with darkly stained keratin may be masked until systemic signs signify that septicemia is occurring. Patients have been lost who might have been saved if deep subeschar infection had been suspected and aggressive debridement performed. Such complications can best be prevented by careful inspection of the eschar and frequent cleansing by immersion in a tank. Patients in whom silver nitrate is successfully preventing infection in the eschar should not have fever, leukocytosis,

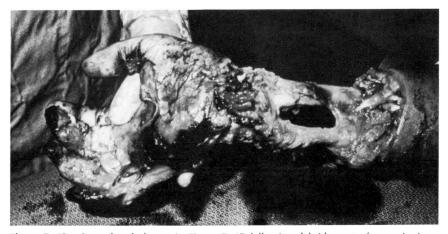

Figure 7–48. Same hand shown in Figure 7–47 following debridement of necrotic tissue beneath silver chloride-stained eschar. The entire hand and forearm were destroyed by a deep abscess which was not appreciated during the period of silver nitrate treatment of the surface.

rapid pulse, or other signs of systemic toxemia. Patients who show general deterioration while under silver nitrate therapy should be suspected of harboring deep sepsis. When clinical signs of infection persist, subcutaneous abscess formation should be assumed and a surgical investigation of the deep tissues must be done. If infection is found, the inescapable conclusion is that preventive treatment did not work; extensive debridement usually must be undertaken if dangerous risks are to be avoided.

In assessing the value of topical agents on the overall mortality and morbidity of burns, several factors should be remembered. First, most hospitals which have adopted new forms of topical treatment have, for obvious practical reasons, also sequestered burn patients in one area, thus developing a burn unit. Personnel assigned to these patients are usually assigned on a restricted or permanent basis. Such attendants are given special training in burn care along with specific instructions in the preparation and application of silver nitrate dressings. Often some of the best nurses in an institution will be assigned to the "new burn unit" and the overall quality of nursing care invariably rises. The value of wet dressings is demonstrated by increased interest in the technique of applying and changing the dressings. Thus, some improvement would occur even if the dressings were moistened only with saline. Most hospitals, which in the past treated burns in many areas simultaneously, or relegated treatment of burns to inexperienced or often disinterested house officers, have been able to show rather spectacular improvements in many aspects of burn treatment following establishment of a burn unit featuring a new, dramatic approach. That all of such improvement was the result only of bringing a topical agent into the treatment plan, however, is far from convincing. The fact that satisfactory antisepsis may be completely missed even under the most ideal circumstances strongly suggests that other factors such as those mentioned above may play a substantial role in the overall results. At the moment, about all that can be said is that Moyer, in particular, has made a fundamental contribution to the burn problem by calling attention to the importance of burned skin as reservoir for bacteria. In addition, 0.5 per cent silver nitrate appeared several years ago to be the topical antiseptic of choice to prevent infection of burned skin and subcutaneous tissue via external contamination. Application of these contributions also brought out, however, the value of expertly applied wet dressings and the importance of attentive and skilled nursing care. Properly used, silver nitrate dressings can substantially reduce infection of the eschar for relatively long periods of time; for this reason, it has been a valuable contribution to the treatment of some burned patients.

Perhaps even more important than what topical agents applied to burns will do is what they most certainly will not do. The student who is not aware of the biological principles of healing, in his quest for a miracle that will make complex reasoning unnecessary, is likely to seize any innovation as a solution to all aspects of a difficult problem. But complex problems such as burns are usually not reduced to single mechanical or pharmacological manipulations by any one discovery, and the multiple problems connected with thermal injury to skin certainly have not been solved by the use of a topical agent. To begin with, the main objective, prevention of infection, is not always achieved. When it is achieved, a doctor still may be confronted months later with a patient who has come through aseptic and atraumatic debridement only to be confronted with exactly the same problem he would have been confronted with following immediate surgical debridement — more open wound than the combination of contraction, epithelization, and utilization of all available skin can cover. The premise upon which prevention of infection without surgical removal of all burned tissue is based is that within the burned area there must be viable cells which, if preserved, ultimately will participate in the healing process. If the burn destroyed all cells in skin, all one will have to show for four or five months of aseptic debridement is a thoroughly debrided wound without bacteria. This is a noteworthy achievement, but far from enough to solve the real essence of the problem — lack of skin. In the final analysis, it is the lack of skin that will cause death of the patient, whether superficial infection occurs early or late. Even if full-thickness death of skin has not occurred and infection is prevented, regeneration of epithelium may not produce either a safe or a useful scar. Life may have been saved temporarily by closure of the wound with epithelium (a remarkable achievement which would not have been possible in some patients had not infection and surgical removal of germinal centers been prevented), but a body covered only with epithelium and distorted by grotesque contractions hardly can be exhibited as evidence of having solved the burn problem. For some reason, the notion has become prevalent that topical agents, by preventing infection, also have prevented severe scar formation and wound contracture. By this reasoning, regeneration of epithelium becomes equivalent to regeneration of skin. We do not know how many burned patients have been lost or subjected to unnecessary delay or complications because fundamental, hard-earned, biological knowledge was discarded in the exciting search for a single solution to all problems. It is embarrassing to remember that contracture and hypertrophic scarring occur predictably in the absence of infection, and that none of the fundamental processes described in the first five chapters of this book are influenced by bacterial invasion except to produce a transient delay when tissue necrosis occurs. A scar crossing lines of changing dimension will restrict motion regardless of whether the wound which produced it was infected or not. The fundamental fact that scar tissue — so different from normal skin — contains mainly nonyielding collagenous fiber bundles separates it directly from normal skin. Biological differences between scar tissue and uninjured skin are not changed by bacterial infection;

thus they are not altered by the effect of a topical antiseptic. Similar reasoning holds for wound contraction, cross-linking, epithelization, and so forth.

In considering the usefulness of topical agents to prevent infection of an eschar, a clear distinction should be made between contamination and infection. That silver nitrate is unquestionably an effective agent in preventing contamination of eschar does not necessarily mean that it is of equal effectiveness in treating infection. The casual observer, entranced with the cleanliness of wounds successfully managed by silver nitrate dressing, may assume that any infected wound also can be made sterile by similar techniques. Silver nitrate dressings do reduce the number of bacteria in infected wounds, and some studies strongly suggest that such limited control of infection plays a significant role in the take of a graft. It is important to remember, however, that the primary role of silver ions is to become covalently linked with protein. In all probability, all free carboxyl groups enter into the reaction and the silver proteinate so produced liberates only a relatively few silver ions. The reaction is rapid and, in effect, competes with formation of insoluble silver chloride. This is why silver nitrate dressings must be changed frequently and why application of silver nitrate does not eliminate completely all deep or subeschar infection. Topical silver nitrate does not produce the same effect upon infection as introducing a highly soluble antibiotic which can penetrate all vascularized tissue and selectively affect living organisms. The gross appearance of infected wounds treated with silver nitrate may be deceiving, as the clean surface produced by wet dressings and a topical antiseptic does not portray accurately what often lurks in deeper layers. Application of a free skin graft to such a wound often demonstrates the failure of a surface antiseptic to eliminate infection. A combination of excision of all infected issue followed by application of silver nitrate to prevent further contamination or destroy bacteria accidentally spilled on the surface may utilize the best of surgery and a topical antiseptic.

In summary, eschars too extensive to be replaced by free grafts can be protected from bacterial contamination for extended periods by surface antiseptics. About ten years ago 0.5 per cent silver nitrate appeared to be the most effective surface antiseptic. Neither silver nitrate nor infection, however, has anything to do with the fundamental processes of wound healing. Repair, although occasionally retarded by infection, will proceed to a natural conclusion whether the wound is kept sterile or successfully treated after infection develops. The main disadvantages to silver nitrate antisepsis are the selective removal of sodium and chloride ions from the body and the deposition of silver chloride salts which prevent deep infection from being recognized.

TOPICAL APPLICATION OF SULFAMYLON. The disadvantages of silver nitrate topical antisepsis stimulated search for other topical agents which might control bacterial growth. Of course, such agents should not interfere with epithelial proliferation, should not cause profound alterations in body metabolism, and ideally should not produce staining of the burned or normal surface. A promising agent in this search appeared to be an old by-product of the azo dye industry — para-aminomethylbenzene sulfonamide hydrochloride (commonly called Sulfamylon). Sulfamylon was issued rather widely to the German Army on the eastern front during World War II to control clostridial infections. Although, in one of the blackest chapters of investigative medicine, numerous tests of the effectiveness of this substance were made in human wounds deliberately produced at Ravensbruck and other concentration camps, virtually no useful data were obtained. The Allies also were stocking other sulfonamides and using them sporadically as topical agents, but for some reason Sulfamylon was not considered as having important use until the search for topical agents to control eschar contamination commenced. At present, other sulfonamides such as silver sulfadiazine appear more promising than Sulfamylon; most are inhibited by para-aminobenzoic acid, which is plentiful in necrotic tissue. Para-aminobenzoic acid does not inhibit or inactivate Sulfamylon, and thus it has, at last, come under close study for use in burned patients. Sulfamylon appears even more attractive with the realization that it is water-soluble, diffuses easily through the eschar, and can be easily applied or removed as a hydrophilic cream. The drug is a strong carbonic anhydrase inhibitor which results in an alkaline urine, thus obviating the problem of crystalluria seen with other sulfonamides which have been used previously for topical thera-

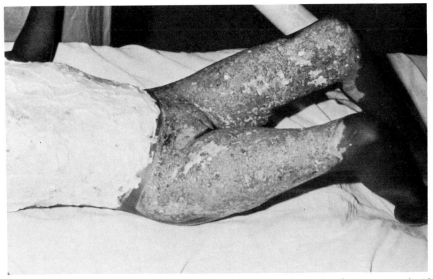

Figure 7–49.   Third degree burn of the anterior chest and thighs. The chest is covered with Sulfamylon cream. The thighs are ready for grafting.

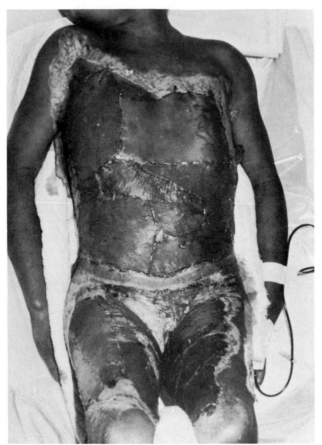

Figure 7–50.   Same patient shown in Figure 7–49. The burn wounds have been covered in stages by split-thickness skin grafts.

py. Early use of Sulfamylon in the form of Sulfamylon hydrochloride caused severe acidosis, which required administration of large amounts of fixed base. This problem, reminiscent of sodium withdrawal by silver nitrate, has not been completely eliminated by switching the preparation to Sulfamylon acetate. Occasional acidosis has been reported with Sulfamylon acetate, but the degree and frequency are not as serious as with the hydrochloride preparation. Another problem with the use of Sulfamylon has been keeping the material on the eschar. The manufacturer has changed the base several times to try to make it adhere to eschar more satisfactorily, but the problem of keeping a satisfactory layer of Sulfamylon on a burned surface still exists. Mild burning pain is frequently experienced by patients at the time the drug is applied. Finally, successful use of Sulfamylon results in a sterile eschar which will last for months and thus delay skin grafting unless aggressive surgical therapy also is utilized. Sulfamylon and silver sulfadiazine are the topi-

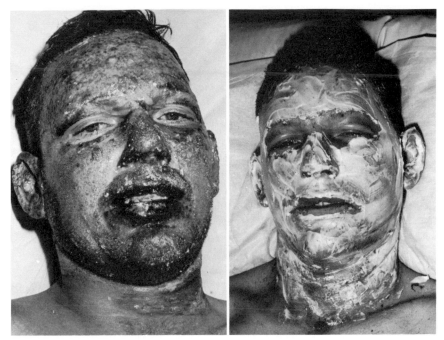

Fig. 7–51   Fig. 7–52

Figure 7–51.   Deep second degree burn of face.
Figure 7–52.   Treatment of patient shown in Figure 7–51 with Sulfamylon.

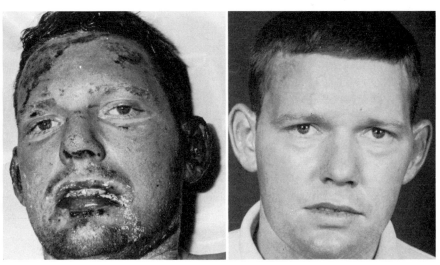

Fig. 7–53   Fig. 7–54

Figure 7–53.   Same patient shown in Figure 7–51 after one week of topical Sulfamylon therapy.
Figure 7–54.   Same patient shown in Figure 7–51 six months after treatment with Sulfamylon.

cal agents of choice to prevent eschar infection at this time. As with silver nitrate, however, they are not the answer to the whole problem of burns and, when used in place of, instead of as an adjunct to, modern surgical therapy, they can prolong and complicate the healing of a burn unnecessarily.

In summary, a third degree burn eschar can be treated by exposure, by silver nitrate dressings, or by topical application of Sulfamylon or silver sulfadiazine. The exposure technique finds greatest application during catastrophic times but has disadvantages in the loss of water and the need to protect and later remove eschar, just as any other artificial dressing has to be protected and changed. After eschar has been removed, exposure is no longer desirable, for a scab without underlying dermis is not satisfactory wound coverage and exposure of fat, muscle, or granulation tissue only leads to more serious complications. Protection of an eschar by topical antibiotic agents has been a definite step forward in the prevention of infection and preservation of general health during convalescence from a burn. Utilization of this principle does not always produce success, however, and if it is injudiciously used, it may draw out interminably the convalescent period of a burn or contribute to deforming contractures which would not have occurred had the eschar been removed and the wound resurfaced as soon as possible. Unless a burn is so extensive that preservation of every island of incompletely destroyed epithelium is desirable, antibiotic or antiseptic protection for eschar should be used only as an adjunct in helping to prepare a patient for the earliest possible debridement and skin grafting. Used in this manner, these agents have exerted a measurable, beneficial result on the mortality and morbidity of burned patients. Used injudiciously, as if these agents were the definitive answer for all burn problems, topical antiseptics and antibiotics have actually caused the death of patients who might otherwise have been salvaged. Moreover, the convalescent stage has been prolonged and the deformity increased in patients who have been denied surgical therapy for relatively small burns. The same can be said for exposure techniques. A life may be lost while the wound is being properly exposed or a wound may be made infinitely worse by exposure for too long a time or when exposure is not positively indicated, such as after eschar has been removed. Fortunately, enough is known about the biology of normal healing and both local and general reactions to thermal injury so that the decision of what type of wound treatment and for how long it should be carried out can be placed on a sound scientific basis.

SKIN REPLACEMENT

Consideration of skin as a compound organ without capacity to regenerate and a study of the biology of the healing process (and how it can be altered) provide the basis for consideration of skin replacement. Skin deficits are corrected by transferring skin from one area to another. Essentially, two methods are available for accomplishing this: free grafts and pedicle grafts. Free grafts are completely detached from all connections with the donor site and thus must reconstitute new connections with the vascular system. Pedicle grafts are never completely detached from all of their vascular connections; they continue to be nourished by some donor site vessels even after they have been transferred to a recipient area. Obviously, there are a great many more restrictions in the use of pedicle grafts than when skin can be cleanly detached and moved as a free graft.

Preparation of a wound for grafting involves, among other things, consideration of the amount of contraction that has occurred and the amount of contraction that is going to occur after a skin graft has been applied. These considerations raise the question of whether skin grafts contract. Even superficial examination of the fundamental biological processes which reduce the size of a wound or scar brings one to the realization that active contraction of a skin graft in the same sense that a muscle contracts is not possible. There simply are not cells within a skin graft which have this capability. The fact has been established, however, that a graft measuring 100 sq. cm. at the time it is applied to a wound can be found some months later to measure less than 50 sq. cm. The obvious question of how reduction in size of the graft occurs can be answered now only by saying that at least two mechanisms are

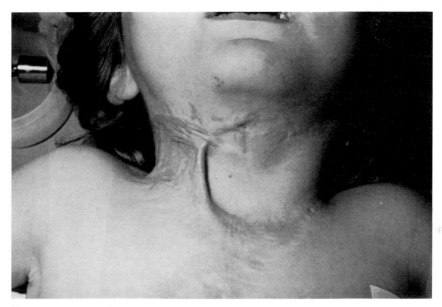

Figure 7–55. Wound contracture caused by a combination of wound contracting process (note wrinkled graft) and allowing scar tissue to form along lines of changing dimension.

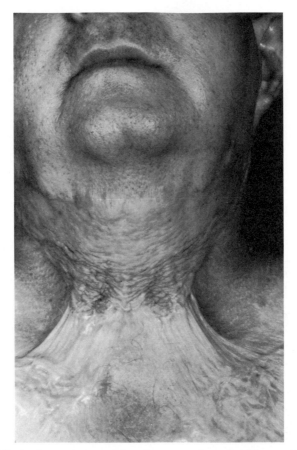

Figure 7–56. Contracture not stopped by placement of a split-thickness skin graft on an actively contracting wound. Note that the wound continued to contract, resulting in movement of surrounding tissue and a wrinkled appearance of the skin graft.

known to be possible, and that either or both may exert separate or simultaneous forces in a single wound. That different mechanisms are involved has been suspected from observations that some grafts appear folded or corrugated several months after they have been transferred while others appear tightly stretched even though their circumference is 50 per cent less than when they were placed upon the wound. In the case of the wrinkled or corrugated graft, it is natural to postulate that the wound contracted and the graft became wrinkled as circumference was reduced. In the case of a smooth, tight graft, one is forced to conclude that some of the graft is missing; a rather remarkable remodeling in which collagenolytic activity exceeded collagen synthesis must have occurred. There are considerable data to support both hypotheses. Once wound contraction begins, it is not stopped suddenly by application of a skin graft. Contraction eventually stops once dermal edges touch other dermal edges, but cessation of peripheral wound edge migration is not instantaneous, particularly between the eighth and eleventh days when the contracting forces are maximal. Grafted wounds seldom contract as severely as ungrafted ones, but once contraction is under way, it is only modified or retarded by application of a free skin graft. Thus, a wound in which an ideal surface free of significant infection has been obtained must also be prepared from the standpoint of controlling the contracting mechanism, if peripheral distortion is to be avoided. This can be accomplished in two ways: If contraction which has already occurred is desirable but no further contraction is wanted, the entire contents of the wound, including granulation tissue, scarred base, and a millimeter ring of normal dermis, should be excised. In essence, the "picture frame" area and the central granulation tissue mechanisms should be

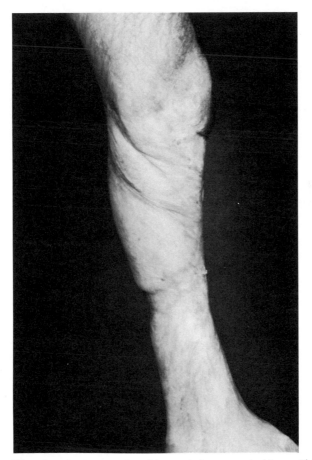

Figure 7–57.   Wound contracture produced by a spiral movement of tissue. This wound was characterized by loss of full-thickness skin, and deformity is the result of movement of skin by the contracting process.

removed (see Chapter 3). The picture frame area must be delicately excised without detaching dermis from underlying scar; otherwise the wound will retract to its original dimensions. A wound prepared as described in the discussion in Chapter 6 on subtotal excision of keloids, is virtually free of tension. If a thick skin graft is applied immediately, subsequent contraction will be minimal.

If no contraction is acceptable, and some centripetal movement has already occurred, complete excision of the wound including a wide margin of normal skin is demanded. Obviously, infection must be eliminated before so radical a procedure is performed, or bacteria may be introduced into the circulatory system when local tissue defenses are cut through. If it is impossible to control infection satisfactorily, a temporary, thin, split-thickness skin graft should be applied; after the wound has remained closed and free of infection for several weeks, the entire scar and graft can be reexcised. This re-creates the original defect and allows distorted uninfected skin to return to its normal prewound position. Application of a thick split-thickness graft or pedicle flap immediately after re-creation of the defect will prevent secondary contraction from occurring. It should be remembered that the secondary healing effect does not apply to wound contraction but only to the gain of tensile strength in healing incised wounds.

Another indication for excising the entire bed of an open wound is when the healing process has been progressing for such a long time, without epithelization or contraction having closed the wound, that an

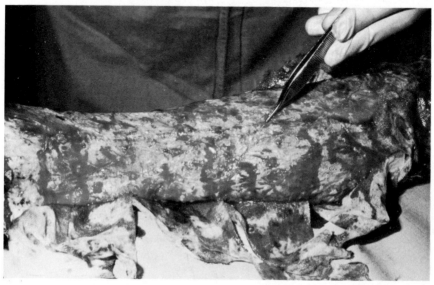

Figure 7–58. Extensive debridement of burn of thigh. Note that all subcutaneous tissue and burned skin have been removed down to fascia. Saphenous vein has been preserved.

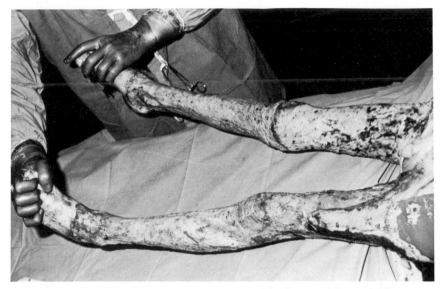

Figure 7–59. Lower extremities following extensive debridement of skin and subcutaneous tissue in preparation for grafting. This is about the largest area of skin that can be grafted safely in one procedure.

enormous amount of collagenous tissue has accumulated. Chronic leg ulcers are examples of how the entire base of such a wound can be converted into a relatively avascular sheet of dense connective tissue. There are two reasons why this tissue should be excised before a skin graft is applied. The first is that adequate blood supply may be prevented from reaching the graft by the physical barrier of thick fibrous cicatrix. The second, and usually more important, reason is that take of a graft on such a base means that new skin will be relatively immovable, thus unable to yield with external trauma. Movability of skin is important in that it means that the external surface of the body can shift in response to deforming forces. Skin firmly attached to an immovable surface is damaged more severely by even moderate trauma than is movable skin.

In summary, the decision to maintain and prepare, scrape, partially excise, or completely excise granulation tissue is not an easy problem which can be solved by learning an operation and applying it to an open wound. Selection of a preparation procedure should be based upon accurate knowledge of epithelization and mechanisms of wound contraction. Such knowledge must be utilized only as it applies to specific requirements or objectives for a specific wound. This sort of biological reasoning assures that the end result will be at least predictable, if not optimal. There is, however, still a great deal we need to know in this area. Particularly, we would like to learn why some grafts become wrinkled as their bed is reduced in size and why others seem to respond superbly by remodeling collagenous tissue to fit the size of the bed. Perhaps remodeling of the graft is actually fundamental in the process of wound contraction. There is some evidence that a new graft is rapidly replaced by cells from the recipient area and that these cells then replace collagenous tissue. If this is true, transplanted skin is an extremely active tissue where many remarkable changes could be accounted for. The induction and control of various wound healing phenomena by transplanted dermis also is a fertile field for study. Certainly a wound reacts differently to thick dermal grafts than it does to thin ones. Whether this merely represents the type of wound upon which the grafts were applied or whether the transplanted dermis exerts some controlling force over wound contraction presently is unknown. The work of Medawar suggests the latter in rabbit skin. Measurements will have to be made in human beings or pigs, as healing in human skin is quite different from that in most hairbearing animals.

Free Skin Grafts

Free grafts are of two main types: split-thickness and full-thickness. The difference relates only to the amount of dermis removed with the graft. Transfer of a full-thickness graft can be looked upon as merely transferring a skin dressing from one area of the body to the other. If the entire thickness of dermis is transferred, and subcutaneous fat is exposed in the donor area, some provision must be made to resurface the donor wound. If the donor site is one in which skin is redundant, such as the groin or submammary fold, a full-thickness skin graft donor site does not pose any serious problem. Simple closure with sutures is all that is needed. If the donor defect is larger than can be closed by coaptation of skin edges, a graft from still another donor site will be needed. Complicated as this principle may sound, it has numerous applications in the closure of human wounds. Split-thickness skin graft donor sites retain enough elements of dermis with regenerative capacity so that restoration without contraction occurs as in other areas of skin denuded only of epithelium.

One of the most important biological considerations in deciding what type of graft should be used for any wound is the mechanism by which a free graft survives following detachment from its blood supply. When circulation is reestablished in the graft in its new position, the phenomenon is spoken of affectionately as "take" of the graft. The word *take* is used frequently and so it is important to have a clear understanding of the fundamentals involved in *take* or *failure to take*. Clinically, there usually is no question about whether or not a graft has taken, and the term is applied most often to a graft which has become stuck to its new surface, is not deformed by underlying hematoma or serum, and, most important of all, is pink in color and will blush immediately following application of digital pressure. In summary, take

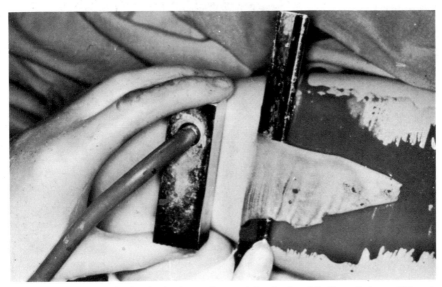

Figure 7–60. Removal of split-thickness skin graft by freehand knife technique. Although mechanical dermatomes are more satisfactory for small grafts of cosmetic importance, large sheets of skin often can be obtained most satisfactorily with a knife. (From E. E. Peacock, Jr., in *Principles of Surgery*, edited by S. I. Schwartz. Copyright 1969, McGraw-Hill Book Company. Used with permission of McGraw-Hill Book Company.)

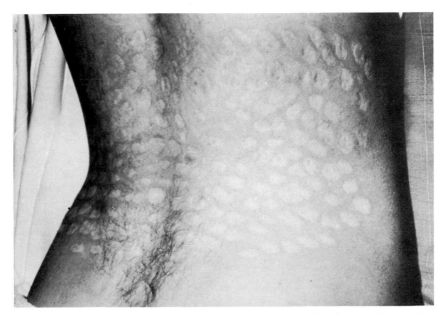

Figure 7–61. Mutilated donor site caused by removal of pinch grafts. There is little or no place for pinch grafts in modern reconstructive surgery.

means that arterial connections have been reestablished and venous drainage is adequate. Until the time that signs of reestablishment of circulation are obvious, the take of a graft is in question; after circulation has been reestablished, the fate of the graft is secure unless something untoward, such as severe mechanical trauma or infection, intervenes.

It is still not certain, however, whether take means merely a connection of a preexisting capillary network in the graft with blood vessels in the recipient area or whether an entirely new vascular network within the graft must be developed. Most studies indicate that the capillary network of transplanted skin is made functional again when blood vessels in the recipient area develop afferent and efferent connections. Whatever the process is, however, it requires about four days to show clinical evidence of successful function.

The question of what initiates capillary proliferation has not been definitively answered. What evidence there is suggests that low tissue oxygen tension may play a significant role. Certainly there seems to be some relationship between tissue growth and the extent of capillary proliferation. When granulation tissue is being formed actively, it is richly endowed with capillaries. However, as scar tissue matures, i.e., as the synthetic aspect gives way to remodeling, the absolute number of capillary loops diminishes markedly, and the mature scar is relatively avascular.

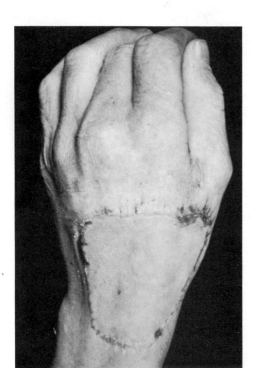

Figure 7–62. Typical appearance of a skin graft at five days when take has been complete. Plasmic circulation has been replaced by capillary filling.

In newly forming granulation tissue, the new capillaries appear to be formed by "budding" of existing capillaries. Actually, endothelial cells, proximal to the "bud," undergo mitosis. The distal cells either do not have a basement membrane, or detach themselves from such a membrane and move out by thrusting pseudopodia, or ruffled membranes, in the direction of motion. Endothelial cells do not move as individuals; rather, contact is maintained among them and they follow the advancing fibroblasts, forming true capillaries as they go. Leukocytes and macrophages have been identified as the "spear" leading a capillary phalanx into ischemic tissue. Because the formation of new capillaries is occurring simultaneously in many different regions of a wound, growing capillaries frequently come in contact with each other and form anastomoses.

A question of both biological and practical importance is: How do cells survive in a graft without exposure to circulating red cells for four days? The first answer is that a great number of transplanted cells do not survive. From the time a free graft is detached from its donor site until revascularization has provided sufficient metabolic support for cell renewal, a measurable number of cells die. At what stage the number of viable cells drop below that which is compatible with the phenomenon of take is unknown. It may be that position of cells is more critical than the actual number that survive, and that take depends primarily upon survival of a few strategically located cells with germinative potential. The fate of cells already clogged with keratin and too far along their path of differentiation to participate in renewal of cell population is probably not important in the overall phenomenon of take. That this is at least partially true seems supported by the fact that all skin grafts go through a period of desquamation of superficial layers which may be so severe that actual blister formation exists. In all probability, the most important cells are those in the stratum germinativum of epithelium; thus full-thickness grafts are more treacherous than split-thickness skin grafts because a thick layer of dermis separates these cells from the vital surface-graft interface where revascularization must occur. It also explains why the early recommendations of pioneers in the art of skin grafting were wrong in recommending that the thinnest possible graft should be taken—preferably through epithelium alone to assure take of the graft and healing of the donor site. It was first thought that split-thickness grafts should be cut through the rete ridges so that some germinative epithelium would be left to resurface the donor site. Actually, technical success in taking a graft through rete ridges would probably assure biological failure, for a majority of the cells transferred would be dead. If a few cells in the upper strata of the rete ridges did survive, the newly resurfaced area would be covered only with epithelium. There can be little doubt that this is what actually happens in many wounds grafted by masters of the art of taking extremely thin grafts. The dead keratin transferred to the wound serves

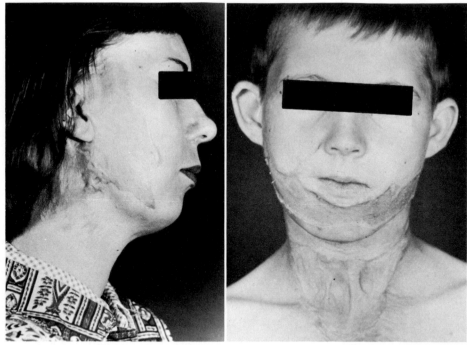

Fig. 7–63   **Fig. 7–64**

Figure 7–63. Anterior cheek, infraorbital area, and side of the nose has been resurfaced with a near-full-thickness skin graft. Posterior cheek and subauricular area will be resurfaced as a second stage. (From E. E. Peacock, Jr., in *Principles of Surgery*, edited by S. I. Schwartz. Copyright 1969, McGraw-Hill Book Company. Used with permission of McGraw-Hill Book Company.)

Figure 7–64. Typical appearance of a thin split-thickness skin graft on the face. Note excess pigmentation and thin appearance of skin in grafted area. Thin split-thickness skin graft on the face should be avoided whenever possible.

as an excellent biological dressing beneath which normal epithelization occurs. The best indication we have that a critical level of cell survival is mandatory in the take of a graft is that free skin grafts can remain detached from the body before successful transplantation for varying lengths of time, depending on the temperature at which they are stored. Grafts can be refrigerated for as long as 17 days and still be transplanted successfully, but the rate of success falls precipitously after three or four days of refrigeration. It seems likely, therefore, that death of cells begins immediately after detachment from blood supply and that a critical number of strategically located cells of a specific type must remain viable for the phenomenon of take to occur.

The next question to be considered in the biology of take of a graft is whether anything other than formation of vascular flow has been re-established. The answer, again, is that we do not have direct measurements which make it possible to answer this question. Indirect evidence and deductive reasoning strongly suggest that diffusion of gases and nutrients occurs through a semipermeable area and that creation of an efficient diffusion gradient is extremely important during the period of vascular insufficiency. A critical gradient also may have much to do with whether proliferating blood vessels will find viable cells to nourish. Certainly it is clinically helpful to picture the undersurface of a skin graft and the wall of a capillary loop in the wound as a single interface or semipermeable membrane. From the moment a graft is detached, oxygen becomes depleted and waste products such as carbon dioxide begin to accumulate. The same reasoning holds for metabolites such as sugar and urea; a detached skin graft invariably becomes acidotic. Thus, separation from the general circulation means that the graft will have a high level of waste products and a low level of basic raw materials as compared to the body from which it came. Until circulation is developed to correct these imbalances efficiently, there does not seem to be any reason why diffusion through cells and capillary walls could not occur. Undoubtedly diffusion is occurring, but how much it affects take cannot be stated at this time. We can say, however, that diffusion alone cannot assure survival for an indefinite time. It seems almost equally certain, however, that diffusion can make a difference in survival,

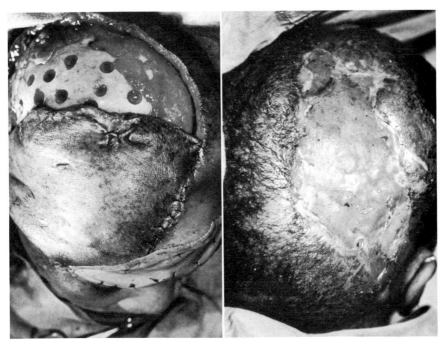

Fig. 7–65   Fig. 7–66

Figure 7–65. Preparation of exposed calvaria for split-thickness skin graft. Holes in outer table allow granulation tissue to form on the surface of exposed bone. Many surgeons prefer to remove the entire outer table.

Figure 7–66. Successful split-thickness skin grafting of same patient shown in Figure 7–65.

because situations which interfere with diffusion (such as formation of hematomas or collections of serum or pus) usually result in complete loss of full-thickness or composite tissue grafts. Similar accumulations beneath thin split-thickness grafts may not result in complete loss of the graft; take is still possible four or five days after a hematoma has been evacuated. Thus, thickness of a graft also has a great deal to do with survival, especially when conditions for revascularization are not optimal. Although we simply do not know to what extent, if at all, diffusion affects the take of a graft, it seems likely that diffusion is involved, for a graft stored at body temperature for four days without contact with any viable base will not be revascularized and survive as well as one which is kept against a living wound even though vascularization does not occur immediately. In all probability a small amount of gases and nutrients is exchanged between graft cells and recipient bed circulation. Such exchange may play a role in preserving a critical number of cells until vascular connections are established. In this regard, the surgeon can bank excess skin for a few days following a grafting procedure on the original donor site better than at low temperature or under any other artificial conditions.

The hypothesis of early preservation of living cells by diffusion of gases and nutrients provides a model for analysis of failure of grafts to survive and for planning of the type of graft and the means of immobilization of the graft during restorative procedures. Expressed simply, the take of a graft may depend for at least three or four days on the development of some sort of semipermeable membrane effect constructed by placing the under surface of the graft accurately against the recipient wound surface so that gas and nutrients will diffuse across the interface. Failure of a graft to take usually is the result of something happening in this interface or membrane to render it nonpermeable either to diffusible products or to penetration by small blood vessels.

Blood and pus are two commonly encountered substances which destroy the semipermeable membrane effect. In addition, motion will prevent penetration of the graft by recipient area capillaries. Thus, most of what the surgeon does to insure take of a graft is directed toward maintaining a semipermeable state at the interface of the graft and bed and stabilizing both so that proliferating blood vessels will be able to penetrate the transplant. In very thin grafts, requirements for diffusion may be less strict, for diffusible substances will have a shorter distance to traverse. Small collections of blood or serum are not as serious beneath thin as beneath thick grafts where diffusion must occur over a greater distance.

A time-honored and reliable method for obtaining stability as well as an accurate interface between graft and wound is the stent fixation. The principle of the stent is not always understood, however, and as a result it may be used needlessly or under conditions where it cannot be of much benefit in assisting diffusion and revascularization. The stent fixation technique involves leaving the ends of sutures that attach the graft to the wound edge long and tying them over a bolus of cotton waste at the end of the procedure. The surgeon may have the impression (as he ties the bolus down with a firmly adjusted surgeon's knot) that he is putting pressure on the graft by forcing the cotton bolus against the wound surface. This is true, however, only if surrounding skin is both movable and somewhat elastic. As described in the section on the use of cotton waste in other types of dressings, a cotton bolus becomes packed very quickly, and pressure applied in this manner is usually gone within 30 minutes. A cotton bolus can serve as a conformer after all pressure effect is gone, but, in trying to develop a semipermeable membrane effect between the graft and underlying wound surface, sustained mild pressure also is desirable. Sustained pressure and conformer effect can be accomplished by a stent if one realizes that the elasticity or resilience of skin can provide continued force if it is movable and elastic. In a properly conceived and applied stent, the sutures actually draw skin edges up and around the dressing. Thus, the elasticity of skin acts continuously to transmit mild pressure to the graft surface. A slight concavity is created where a level plane or even slight convexity existed before the sutures were tied.

Very little is gained by using a stent dressing in an area such as a chronically scarred lower leg ulcer. In this situation, the surface is markedly convex, skin is attached to underlying bone and fascia, and both skin and subcutaneous tissues are rigid because of partial replacement by fibrous tissue. Understanding the stent principle also makes one reluctant to use this technique of immobilization in wounds where a free skin graft is adjacent to a flap. The object of a properly designed and constructed stent is to elevate surrounding skin edges over and above a split-thickness skin graft. The object of most dressings applied to a flap is to hold the flap in juxtaposition to the wound surface to prevent hematoma or bursa formation. Thus, the junction of a free graft and a pedicle flap is a difficult site for a stent dressing. Some surgeons, apparently determined to use a stent for all grafts, attempt to get around this problem by inserting a number of subcuticular or subcutaneous stitches in the flap to hold it down before applying a stent dressing to the split-thickness graft. If hemostasis has been satisfactory and the wound and flap are favorable, satisfactory take of a graft and adherence of the flap may result. In other instances, the stent and the subcutaneous stitches merely neutralize each other, and very little is gained from either a mechanical or a biological standpoint.

A much simpler and more reliable technique which does not set up oppositely acting forces is to develop a fairly noncompressible conformer, which extends above the level of the flap, for the free grafted wound. A good way to accomplish this is to saturate and wring out flat cotton sponges until they are relatively noncompressible. An exact outline of the wound is traced on the sponges, which are then cut to fit the shape of the wound exactly. Additional layers are added until a firm, noncompressible mold of damp cotton sponges rises above the level of the flap. Compressible cotton, or sponge, or whatever would have been used to dress the flap if a free graft was not present, is then added over both graft and flap. A circular gauze and tape bandage completes the dressing. Such a dressing transmits most of its temporary pressure effect to the graft without putting dangerous pressure on the surface of the flap.

Although it is not usually appreciated, it is possible to put too much pressure on a free graft as well as on a flap. Regardless of whether diffusion plays an important early role in the take of a graft, the fundamental process required for permanent survival is the establishment of vascular channels. Fragile, proliferating capillaries can be closed by external pressure; the place this is most likely to occur is where grafts are placed over nonyielding surfaces such as bone or cartilage. A graft will take nicely on periosteum or on viable bone without periosteum. If the new blood supply connecting host with graft blood supply is compressed by an external force, however, take will not occur for obvious reasons. This phenomenon is most often seen when skin grafts are placed on the forehead or anterior lower leg. It is so easy to put on a tight circular dressing in these areas that too much pressure easily is applied. Even the packing effect of cotton waste may not relieve the pressure enough during the first few hours. The usual appearance of the graft when too much pressure has been applied is one of adequate revascularization around the periphery (particularly if the graft covers a convex surface) with a white nonvascularized area in the center. The technical error frequently responsible is that of winding tape directly off a roll and onto the head or extremity. Storage conditions alter the adhesive qualities of tape, and the force required to pull it from a roll may be too great if it is transmitted to a dressing by rolling tape directly onto the afflicted part. Tape should be stripped from the roll and then applied to the dressing under controlled tension.

Open Grafting

One of the most useful techniques for grafting difficult wounds is open grafting. For a number of reasons it may be impossible in some wounds to achieve an ideal surface to receive grafts. Usually this is because a chronic infection persists in areas where further excision or debridement is imprudent because of the certainty of exposing bone, tendon, or some other important structure which will not accept a free graft. Very large wounds, such as burns, also may become chronically infected and are too large for extensive excision or debridement of granulation tissue. In these wounds, open grafting is a superb method of obtaining wound closure. It has as its most important advantage the ability to provide constant drainage while diffusion and revascularization are occurring. Its greatest disadvantage is that sutures usually cannot be used; therefore, skin cannot be stretched as much as it can when other techniques are utilized. More skin is required to graft a wound by open technique than when the graft is stretched and molded into the shape of the wound by an occlusive dressing. If the wound is convex in shape, such as a wound of the lateral chest wall, sutures can be used and the graft stretched over the surface. Stretching the graft over a convex surface will not elevate it from the wound surface as when it is stretched over a concave wound crater. If sutures are used and the graft is placed under tension over wounds which are other than convex in contour, the graft will not fit into recesses or crevices as closely as desirable. Pockets of pus or serum beneath the graft will then cause spotty or no take. It is important to take more skin than necessary when grafting a wound by open technique because grafts undergo some immediate shrinkage when removed from their dermal frame. Moreover, open grafts need to be tucked or fitted into every crevice of the wound; this takes more skin than a casual estimate of the dimensions of the wound surface indicates. A fibrin seal will occur rapidly in most wounds, and the graft should be stuck to the surface within a few minutes after it is applied. No dressing is used, but a protective frame should be constructed over the graft to keep bed linen or other materials from mechanically disturbing it.

Within six to eight hours after grafting of an infected wound, small bubbles of pus and gas may be seen under the surface. The graft

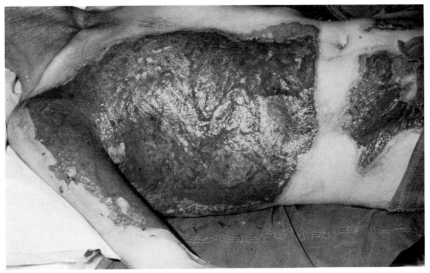

Figure 7–67. Properly prepared granulation tissue for open grafting of a third degree burn wound of anterior chest and axilla.

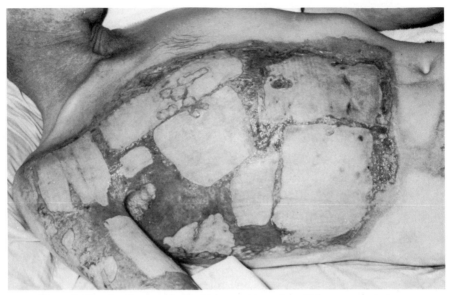

Figure 7–68. Application of split-thickness skin grafts utilizing open technique.

will be lifted away from the wound surface in that area and, if the graft was covered, these bubbles would soon coalesce into a massive unilocular abscess. The object of open grafting is to prevent abscess formation by making it possible to spot focal points where deep infection is producing surface drainage. These are the points where external drainage must be provided. Accurate external drainage is accomplished by making small holes in the graft over the center of the bubbles. Usually it is a good idea on the following day to place warm compresses over the graft to insure drainage by capillary attraction. If compresses are applied carefully, the fibrin seal beneath the graft will prevent it from moving and the wet compresses will provide, in addition to capillary drainage, external pressure to keep the graft close to the wound surface. In a badly infected wound, considerable difficulty may be encountered in trying to keep up with subsurface exudate. Portions of the graft may be lost by the open method. Some portions of the graft invariably will take, however; in only mild infections, all of the skin may survive if accurate spot drainage is provided as soon as need for it is recognized. Excellent grafts covering difficult surfaces can be obtained by the open technique. Its only real disadvantage is that skin does not go as far as when it is sutured under mild tension.

Another application of the open technique is for surfaces which cannot be completely immobilized. Extremities seldom are grafted by the open technique except when it is necessary to cover chronically infected wounds. Extremity wounds usually can be made surgically clean and immobilized satisfactorily during wound healing. Wounds of the chest, abdomen, buttocks, and perineum, however, not only are more difficult to render surgically clean, but also present difficult problems of adequate postoperative immobilization. In considering this problem, it should be remembered that, in all layers of the wound and its dressing, the least surface tension exists between the undersurface of a new graft and the surface of the wound. This means that motion in the dressing sufficient to move it in relation to the body wall, or motion of the body wall beneath the dressing, will result in shearing stress between the graft and the wound. Hence, huge circular casts are not good fixative devices for grafted wounds. A splint on one side of an extremity provides just as good joint stability without adding the weight or pendulum effect of a full circular cast. Compact fabric dressings, reinforced occasionally by small plaster splints, can immobilize an extremity as satisfactorily as a cast. They are lighter and more accurate than a cast; thus the pendulum effect is negligible. When the wound surface cannot be kept from moving (because of respiration, peristalsis, and so forth), a dressing that holds the graft in one position will inhibit take by accentuating the shearing force between the movable wound and the stable graft. Open grafting will eliminate this problem, as the graft and the bed can move together if there is no external fixation producing inertia in the graft. Open grafting should be used, therefore, in most areas where motion cannot be controlled.

Another adjunct to open grafting is the use of small postage stamp

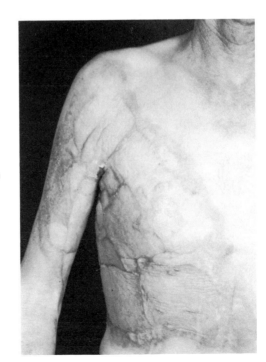

Figure 7–69. Same patient shown in Figure 7–68 following healing.

grafts (sometimes called Thiersch grafts). When motion is considerable or drainage is profuse, a group of small grafts with open spaces between them will permit better drainage than small holes placed in a single graft. To keep such grafts from becoming rolled upon themselves, many surgeons have found it useful to take a large drum of skin with a Reese dermatome and then to cut the tape and graft into small pieces, leaving the relatively rigid rubber backing on the graft. This maneuver makes it easier to spot a large number of small grafts than if each had to be spread out and teased into position individually. The rubber backing separates with desquamation of epithelium several days after revascularization has occurred. When rubber backing is maintained on the grafts in curved areas or in areas where motion is unavoidable, it is important to separate the grafts slightly so there will be room for individual graft motion in relation to the overall bed and to other grafts. A single large sheet of skin covered by stiff rubber backing is splinted by the rubber, and may not move adequately with the wound. An important factor to remember, however, is that the use of multiple grafts, whether they be pinch grafts or postage stamp grafts, converts the wound into a number of small wounds, each of which will heal by contraction and epithelization. The epithelized areas will not contain dermis as the grafted areas do; the total area and effect of a group of little wounds undergoing contraction and epithelization will be essentially the same as if a single wound of similar size had healed without dermis. Recent acclamation for a mechanical device to overcome this fundamental biological principle has resulted in marketing of several dermatomes advertised to make skin go further by dicing it. Of course a larger area can be sprinkled with tiny fragments of skin than can be covered with a sheet of skin, or a sheet can be stretched to cover a larger area if it contains a large number of small perforations. But the perforations will still create open wounds, and healing can occur in these wounds only by epithelization and contraction. Perhaps a better way to think of perforating a graft or sprinkling a wound with small fragments of skin is that the procedure divides the wound into a number of little wounds — not that it makes more skin by mechanically dividing or stretching it.

Some surgeons claim an advantage to dividing a wound into numerous small ones. The surgeon who dices or stretches skin by placing holes in it under the impression that he can provide skin where there was not enough before will be disappointed if wound contraction or healing by epithelization are complications he was attempting to avoid by transplanting skin from another area.

A monumental step in the care of burn wounds was made when Blair, Brown, Davis, Pagett, and others perfected instruments and techniques which have made it possible for most surgeons to transfer large sheets of skin. Before these men made their monumental contributions, burns were treated by applying small grafts in the form of pinch

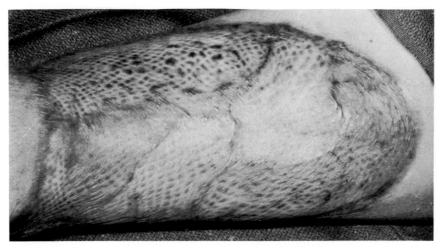

Figure 7–70. Typical appearance of wound grafted with open mesh graft. Note that holes created by expansion of mesh are really only third degree wounds which are healing by epithelization and wound contraction.

or Thiersch grafts. Although wounds could be made to heal by these techniques, functional and cosmetic results were atrocious by modern standards. This was particularly true for the lowly pinch graft which, in addition to being so small that little was accomplished by successful transplant, is of such variable thickness that a single graft is practically full-thickness in the center and a very thin, split-thickness graft on the edges. The donor site produced by taking pinch grafts is a negative deformity; the overall effect, therefore, is a positive cobblestone surface in the recipient area and a negative cobblestone surface in the donor site. Wound contraction is usually severe, and the cosmetic and functional results of pinch grafting are often hideous. The only reason to revert to the use of tiny small grafts of any type in preference to large sheets of skin is the possibility that life can be salvaged only by doing so. Of course, under these circumstances, cosmetic and functional aspects of the healed surface are unimportant. The proponents of using punctured grafts and scattering wound surfaces with tiny fragments of skin justify their recommendations on the basis that such maneuvers may be the only way to obtain a closed wound when skin is in short supply. As long as enthusiasm for such technical manipulations is not based upon unsound biological principles, no damage will be done. The notion that life may have been saved which could not have been saved with conventional sheets of skin is still to be evaluated. Unfortunately, however, in the understandably human search for still another technical miracle, we may have taken a backward step by asking too much of the process of dicing skin. There are no miracles on the wound healing horizon at this time. To repeat: realization that skin is a complex organ without regenerative capacity and acquisition of sound biological knowledge about the basic phenomena by which wounds heal are the most dependable and useful tools the restorative surgeon can acquire.

Important technical adjuvants in the transfer of partial-thickness skin include the various types of available dermatomes. Of course the simplest method of removing a portion of the thickness of skin is with a sharp knife. Although freehand excision of split-thickness skin with a large sharp knife can produce a graft of unlimited size, it is not a popular method except among people who use it frequently; the freehand technique requires more manual skill than any other method of taking skin. So the surgeon who performs occasional skin grafts prefers to rely almost entirely on some type of mechanical dermatome. For him, development of various dermatomes has been of inestimable value in reconstructive surgery. It has made possible split-thickness skin grafts from almost any available donor site. Moreover, grafts removed with a dermatome are uniform in thickness—a very desirable quality for skin destined to be transplanted to the face or hands. Perfect uniformity in thickness is almost impossible to achieve by the freehand technique. The major disadvantage to using a dermatome is that the width of grafts is restricted to the width of the dermatome surface. Dermatomes which depend upon having skin adhere to the frame are also limited in the length of grafts they can take. Oscillating dermatomes will take a continuous graft, although the width of these grafts is limited by the relatively narrow width of the oscillating blade. Except in burned patients, who often need large sheets of split-thickness skin, a single drum of skin from a mechanically operated dermatome usually suffices. Mastery of the use of a dermatome is an essential part of any modern surgical education.

The question of how thick a split-thickness graft should be or whether a full-thickness graft should be used is one which usually can be decided on a biological basis. The key to such reasoning is that, with the exception of providing a watertight seal, most of the qualities desirable in skin are qualities of dermis. Such concerns as texture, elasticity, color, sensation and reception, and lubrication arise or develop within dermis. When we think of restoring these qualities to a denuded or scarred area, therefore, we are thinking in terms of transferring dermis. The age-old principle of not getting something for nothing holds true in restorative surgery of skin. What we take from a donor site in the way of dermal qualities, the donor site will permanently lack. The basic process which occurs following abrasion of skin is reepithelization, and reepithelization occurs without regeneration of complex dermis. If any restoration of thickness of skin below scarred epithelium occurs, it is the result of fibrous protein synthesis; the almost plaque-like scar which occasionally occurs following healing in some split-thickness donor site wound (even to the point of frank keloid formation) should never be mistaken for highly specialized dermis.

The following facts are basic in the selection of a graft of proper thickness for restorative procedures. First and foremost, compound tissues do not regenerate; thus a finite amount of skin exists in any site. When one removes a portion of skin or bowel or nerve, he leaves a deficit in the donor area; the old adage of robbing Peter to pay Paul was never more applicable than for skin. Even in the case of bone, where regeneration of a sort occurs in some defects, the length of time required and the type of bone that regenerates usually is such that, for practical purposes, the same reasoning holds. The decision is really no more complicated than the answer to the question: How severely is one willing to mutilate one area of the body to restore another? In the case of skin, the decision often is easy. All that must be remembered is that when the surgeon transfers certain properties of skin by split-thickness grafting, he takes away similar properties from the donor area. If all of the properties of skin are needed in a wound where all of the properties have been lost, nothing short of a full-thickness skin graft will suffice. All of the qualities of skin are found only in all of the dermis. Such a procedure, however, "transfers" the wound as well as skin, because the defect in the donor area becomes a full-thickness deficit similar to the recipient wound before grafting was performed. If the original wound is small, in an area where there is no extra skin, and if the donor site can be placed in an area where there is extra skin, the solution is obvious. It makes sense to pay Paul out of Peter's bank when Peter's bank contains adequate resources. If the donor site cannot be closed as a primary wound, split-thickness skin from still another donor site must be obtained. Thus, qualities of dermis can be split between two donor sites (where all the qualities of dermis are not needed in either) to provide one full-thickness graft containing all of the qualities of normal skin.

Examples of two extremes which illustrate application of skin and wound healing biology to the selection of a graft of proper thickness are as follows: As one example, consider a 2 cm. diameter circular defect in the cheek of an adolescent girl. No extra skin is available in this area, and stretching the remaining skin with sutures or by wound contraction would result in distortion of the lower eyelid or elevation of the corner of the mouth. Replacement of skin obviously will produce a patch surrounded by a circular scar. How noticeable the patch will be, however, depends to some extent on how well the patch matches surrounding skin. A circular scar will be inevitable in any case, but characteristics of the patch, such as hue, texture, and thickness, are controllable by proper selection of a donor site and thickness of the graft. A split-thickness graft never becomes as thick as a full-thickness graft. It tends to have more melanin than surrounding skin, and it often has a shiny, brittle appearance presumably because of absence of glands, among other things, located in the deeper layers of dermis. The thicker the graft, the less pronounced these deficits appear; a full-thickness graft is usually completely normal in appearance after six to nine months in its new location. It is important, however, to match full-thickness skin grafts with surrounding skin at the site of the wound. Thickness, hair-bearing potential, and vascularity (color) are transplanted intact, and these important characteristics are not altered by surrounding skin in the recipient area. In the case of the small defect in the youngster's cheek, only a full-thickness graft will suffice to replace the characteristics of the recipient area. The donor site is no problem, as the graft needed is small enough to be removed from many places, such as behind the ear, the supraclavicular region, groin, or inframammary area. These potential donor sites all contain enough redundant skin so that a wound no more than a centimeter or two in diameter can be closed with sutures. There are usually too many red tones in skin of the ear in males, and the supraclavicular region should not be used in females. Scarring frequently is excessive in the supraclavicular region in young people, and any type of scar in this area in females is only slightly less objectionable than a scar on the face. The groin is an excellent donor site if hair-bearing skin is carefully avoided in taking grafts destined for transplantation to non-hair-bearing areas.

Because the cheek wound is small and does not involve vital structures such as nerve or tendon it can be completely excised or debrided as necessary; and, because the wound is aseptic and does not contain granulation tissue or scar tissue, it will be ideal for both diffusion and revascularization. The thickest possible graft can be used because the best of circumstances prevails. Thus, there is no question that a full-thickness graft (from the standpoint of both the donor and recipient area) is the procedure of choice.

An example of how consideration of the biological principles involved in both take of the graft and healing of the donor site can lead to the selection of a very thin split-thickness graft can be found in a typical severely burned patient. The recipient area in the burned patient is likely to be far from ideal. Even if granulation tissue is present, the wound is not as suitable for diffusion and vascularization as an excised one. Healthy granulation tissue is superior to many surfaces, but it is not as satisfactory for graft survival as many nongranulating surfaces; the biological basis for this assertion already has been discussed. In summary, however, a wound which is covered with granulation tissue is old enough to have many other processes going on in it, such as contraction, fibrous protein synthesis, and epithelization. Moreover, edema and inflammation also are likely to be present. As every surgeon knows, free skin grafts will take superbly on most granulation tissue; in some wounds a granulating surface is the best that can be achieved. Nevertheless, very thick grafts often will not take, and full-thickness grafts usually will not take if placed on a granulating surface.

In the case of the burned patient, donor site restrictions are even more critical in selection of thickness of a graft than factors imposed by the conditions in the recipient area. If the burn is extensive, survival may depend upon quick healing of donor sites, so that it will be possible to remove two or three crops of skin from the same area. Actually, what is required is that dermis be split into four layers. Three layers will be transferred elsewhere, and the fourth allowed to remain. The quicker a new epithelial covering can be regenerated for each layer so that the next lower layer of dermis with its new epithelial surface can be removed, the better the patient will have been managed. An unintentional deep cut through dermis, or development of a complication (such as infection which inhibits reepithelization or causes a partial-thickness injury to become a full-thickness injury) is disastrous. Thus, biological principles in donor site healing argue strongly for taking very thin grafts in the burned patient.

Between these two extreme examples, many different types of wounds and potential donor site considerations may create more complex problems which do not have solutions as obvious as those just cited. The basic biological considerations remain the same, however, and the first decision always is a judgment in which the donor site cost is weighed against predicted gains in the recipient area. Desirable objectives in the recipient area often must be compromised, however, because the risk of not achieving diffusion or revascularization under less than optimal circumstances cannot be overcome. With all these variables, closure of a wound by transfer of skin can be even more intellectually challenging and rewarding than closure of a laceration. Failure to achieve satisfactory results in recipient area or donor site may be the result of looking only at conditions in one area or selecting a particular graft out of habit.

Dressing Grafts

A frequently overlooked use for split-thickness skin grafts is in dressing difficult wounds in all areas of the body. Reluctance of many surgeons to use split-thickness skin as a dressing material usually stems from the feeling that placing skin over a wound closes it in the same manner as suturing wound edges together. But when thin split-thickness skin grafts are utilized to cover a wound, it is not closed any more tightly and therefore more dangerously than if only a layer of gauze or some other dressing had been utilized. An example of a type of wound in which a dressing graft can be used to great advantage is a gunshot wound of the thigh or leg with extensive soft tissue damage over an undefinable area. After all obviously devitalized skin, fascia, and muscle have been excised, a gaping wound remains which often still contains an unknown amount of foreign material such as pellets and clothing, and may also contain partially damaged tissue. Edema and hemorrhage may cause the muscle and fat to bulge out of the wound, and loss of skin may add to the futility of trying to coapt skin edges under these circumstances. Even if skin is not missing and soft tissue swelling is minimal, many surgeons would not choose to bring skin edges together because of fear that unrecognized devitalized muscle and contaminated material remained. The usual practice in these circumstances is to insert a medicated gauze dressing and attempt to close the wound by a skin graft or coaptation of the edges at some future date. In many cases, the five or six days the surgeon planned to leave the wound open stretches to five or six weeks as wound complications such as infection and continuing necrosis occur. An alternate form of management, based on the biology of graft take, is to dress the wound with a thin split-thickness skin graft. If one is skilled with the use of a freehand knife, such a graft can be obtained in most operating rooms almost as quickly as dressing material; use of a dermatome takes only slightly longer. Only a few strategically located sutures are necessary to prevent the graft from shifting while an occlusive dressing is applied. A wound dressed in this manner is not closed any more tightly or dangerously than a wound closed with Vaseline gauze. The part of the graft which is in contact with an adequately debrided surface will take; even if only 5 per cent of the graft follows this course, the wound will be that much nearer healed because skin was used instead of an artificial fabric. Usually all of the graft will take because, in most instances, the wound is more adequately debrided than the surgeon realizes. Biological scavenger activity may be able to take care of areas which are not completely debrided surgically. Even when a wound has not been debrided completely (particularly if contamination is not severe) take of a graft can produce a closed wound even though internal absorption and replacement of necrotic tissue by deep scar must still occur. Secondary infection in these cases is actually prevented by closure of the wound. If, on the other hand, gross contamination and inadequate debridement are severe and infection and more necrosis occur, only a few square centimeters of epithelium and less than a millimeter thickness of dermis from the donor area will have been lost. Certainly nothing is endangered in the recipient wound, for pus, bacteria, and various enzymes will take care of the flimsy split-thickness covering with ease. In patients in whom serious infection is encountered after a wound has been dressed with split-thickness skin, not even a trace of the graft may be recognizable.

Thus, a dressing graft offers the possibility of closing all or some portion of a difficult wound; if deep complications which prevent wound closure from being completely successful arise, all or part of the graft will disappear and nothing of importance will have been lost. Grafts of this type applied in this manner do not impede drainage or otherwise interfere with open wound healing.

Allografts and Xenografts

A form of dressing graft which is more popular than isografts described in the preceding paragraphs is the use of an allograft or a xenograft. Porcine skin, usually obtained from a commercial distributor, is an example of a xenograft which is readily available. The use of allografts and xenografts in the treatment of massive burns may be lifesaving, particularly when infection of eschar has occurred. Allografts are not needed as often now that topical agents to prevent bacterial invasion of eschar are available. A properly cared for sterile eschar is just as effective in sealing a burn wound for many months as an allograft or a xenograft. If eschar has not been properly cared for and must be removed before donor sites can provide sufficient isografts, an allograft or a xenograft can be lifesaving and should be used. The authors' preference is for allografts. Although specific antigens have not been found in skin which could account for acute rejection of organs (hyperimmune condition), the cause of immediate hyperimmune rejections has not been elucidated. It seems reasonable, therefore, to protect patients from, rather than expose them to, antigens crossing major histocompatibility lines until more is known about the hyperimmune state.

Allografts and xenografts, including amniotic membrane, also

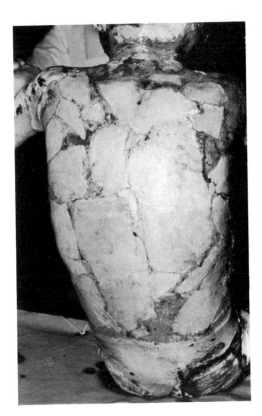

Figure 7–71. Extensive burn wound of the back covered temporarily with allografts. Allografts provide a superb biological dressing for temporary closure of the wound while autograft donor sites are healing and nutrition is restored.

have been used with increasing frequency as a biological dressing for second degree injuries of skin. The idea is that epithelization proceeds more rapidly and with fewer complications under such surfaces than beneath a scab or artificial dressing. It is important to remember when using amniotic membranes that the shiny side (epithelial side) should be facing the surgeon and the dull side should be against the wound. Data to support the claim that healing is enhanced by the use of allografts are not convincing at this time. Again, critical analysis takes into consideration all of the other benefits which accrue to a wound treated by an allograft as compared to one that is allowed to epithelize or contract naturally. Certainly skin is as good as other materials; the authors prefer an allograft rather than a xenograft even if one is willing to overlook expense, as the surgeon often is; availability of porcine grafts, however, has made them generally more attractive than allografts. Although considerable debate has raged over whether xenografts actually become vascularized before being rejected, the argument is largely academic. Most surgeons agree that dressing xenografts applied to surfaces undergoing epithelization should be removed and reapplied before take occurs.

Pedicle Flap Grafts

When more than full thickness of skin is missing, the use of a free graft, except in limited situations where composite tissue grafts will survive or microvascular anastomosis of free composite grafts is possible, is not practical. Diffusion and revascularization are possible through all layers of skin only if nothing is interposed between skin and the wound surface. Fat, muscle, and fascia present a mechanical obstacle to diffusion and revascularization. Thus, skin grafts which carry these tissues also must carry their own blood supply. The principle of the pedicle flap is to excise partially composite tissue grafts so they can be moved out of their original site and into a new area without ever being separated entirely from original blood supply. Such flaps usually are in the shape of a trapdoor—detached on three sides but remaining attached on the fourth side. They are moved to new areas by rotating the flap to the wound, or by bringing the wound to the flap as when an extremity is moved beneath an elevated abdominal pedicle flap. Successful transfer of composite tissues by the flap technique requires unfailing judgment in determining how much of the flap can be elevated and detached without compromising the circulation to a point beyond which cell survival is possible. The more narrow the base of the pedicle, the more freedom the flap has for movement to another area. The wider the base of the flap, the safer the blood suppy within it will be. The essence of perfection in narrowing the base so that 360 degrees' freedom of rotation is possible, without compromising dangerously the blood

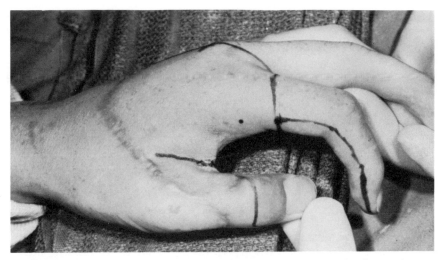

Figure 7–72.   Outline of incisions to convert index finger into a rotation skin flap to release an adduction contracture of web between thumb and index finger.

supply and distal cells, is the production of an island pedicle flap. In an island pedicle flap, the tissue to be transferred is completely excised from the donor area except for a single artery, vein, and sometimes a nerve. Thus, connection with the general circulation is a point rather than a broad base; flaps developed in this manner can be rotated 180 degrees without embarrassing their circulation. Free transplantation of

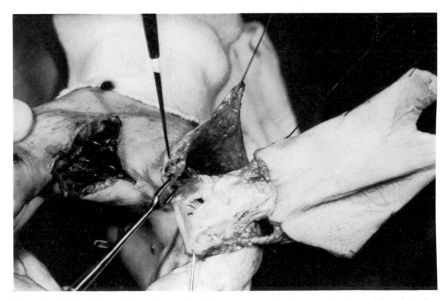

Figure 7–73.   Excision of scar tissue in web to release adduction contracture of thumb. Index finger has been converted into a local island pedicle flap.

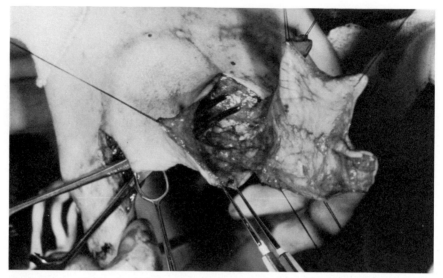

Figure 7–74. Clamp introduced beneath skin of web to pull skin flap from index finger into defect on radial side of thumb.

a composite tissue graft to a new site, followed by microvascular anastomosis of at least one artery and one vein, is a further technical refinement or exploitation of this principle.

Only in certain areas, such as the hand or scalp, can composite tissue grafts or free transplants and revascularization be designed so that

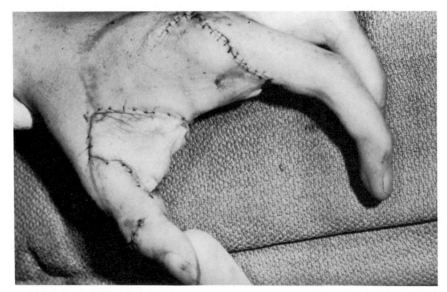

Figure 7–75. Skin flap from index finger restoring abduction by replacing scar tissue in damaged web.

they are supplied by one artery and vein arising from a single point. Most flaps are rotation flaps nourished by a number of small blood vessels in a broad base. The ratio between width of the base and length of the flap varies between different areas of the body. A flap in the face or scalp can be several times longer than it is wide, while a flap on the back may not be safe if it has more than a 1:1 ratio of width to length. Experienced surgeons usually are able to estimate fairly accurately what the size and shape of a skin flap will have to be to achieve successful transplantation, but a satisfactory test or measurement of circulatory efficiency is badly needed. A number of tests have been proposed and evaluated, including circulation of agents which produce local effects on skin such as histamine or epinephrine, clearance of radioactive labeled substances, and simple tests of capillary filling and emptying following digital pressure. The important parameter, however — cell oxygenation — at present can only be measured directly with an oxygen electrode. Although instruments which measure tissue oxygen are available, they have not been perfected to a point where they are suitable for clinical use. The outline and construction of flaps presently is based largely on judgment and experience, not on any sound biological test.

A technical maneuver which improves safety during transfer of a relatively long pedicle on a narrow base has been to delay transfer of the flap by reducing its blood supply in stages. The biological basis for the delaying technique is not clear, but there is no question that a long flap with a narrow base in a relatively avascular area of the body can be rotated successfully only if the blood supply is reduced gradually. This is accomplished by making an incision along one or two sides only of a proposed flap and suturing the incision immediately. After a period of ten days to two weeks, the remaining outline of the flap is incised and another eight to ten days is allowed to elapse. Finally, the entire outline of the flap is incised and undermining is started. Each step cuts across more blood vessels so that, by the time the flap can be incised on three sides and undermined completely, the only remaining blood vessels are in the one intact side or base. Whereas these blood vessels would not have been adequate to nourish the flap had all of the other blood vessels been cut in a single incision, they will be adequate after other blood vessels have been cut in several stages. Many flaps can be elevated and rotated after only one delay; others require several delays. That the principle of delay is effective is certain, but how it works is not clear. There is often considerable difference of opinion about how much can be done safely in one stage, how long one should wait between stages, and how the stages should be designed for maximal speed and safety. As usual, when data obtained from direct measurements are not available, there is ample room for speculation, deductive reasoning, and authoritative declarations.

At the time the principle of delay was discovered, it was thought

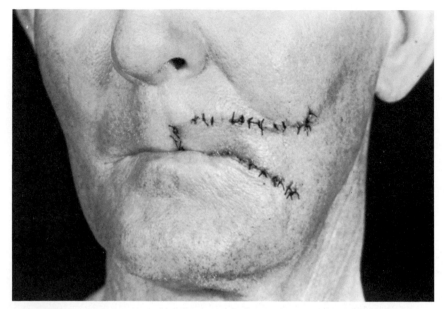

Figure 7–76.   Simple advancement flap from redundant tissue in cheek to reconstruct left side of the lip.

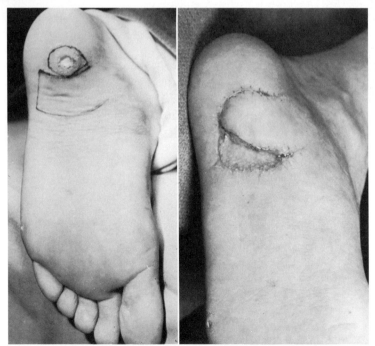

Fig. 7–77   **Fig. 7–78**

Figure 7–77.   Simple rotation flap from non-weight-bearing surface of foot to resurface deep radiation ulcer on weight-bearing surface of heel.
Figure 7–78.   Same foot shown in Figure 7–77. Note that split-thickness graft over donor site is on non-weight-bearing surface while full-thickness pedicle has been rotated to weight-bearing area.

that the basic biological alteration produced was to teach the cells in the flap to get along with less oxygen so they could survive when circulation was embarrassed. Modern knowledge of cell biology strongly suggests that such an explanation is unfounded. Moreover, a few observations made recently in laboratory animals indicate that blood supply through the intact base is measurably increased by staged interruption of other vascular channels. A clinical observation supporting the assumptions of these measurements is the occasional appearance of dilated vessels which literally become racemose just beneath epithelium in the base of the pedicle while delaying procedures are being performed. Whether these dilated vessels represent *de novo* development of new vessels or whether they are the result of changes in preexisting vessels which carried little or no blood before circulation was partially interrupted is not known. There may be nothing more to the principle of delay than production of a sterile inflammatory reaction. Recent work by Myers and others strongly suggests that an epinephrine effect producing necrosis, inflammation, and angiotaxis may be the fundamental process involved in improvement of blood supply by a surgical procedure. Edema and dependency have been shown by these investigators not to be factors of major significance in the delay phenomenon. The liberation of various amines in a sterile inflammatory reaction could result in closing of precapillary shunts or opening of capillary networks so that preexisting vessels become functional on a sustained basis. The main reason this appears to be an oversimplified explanation, however, is that the effect of delay lasts too long to be the result of visible inflammatory reaction. Once delayed, flaps can be safely elevated many months after all the visible effects of reactive inflammation have subsided. Of course, once dilated by the inflammatory reaction, vessels might stay competent without outside influence. To say that they do so because they are needed, however, is to apply to the problem a teleological twist which is hard to justify in an objective analysis. Tissue subjected to partial interference of blood supply becomes acidotic, and the effect of excess accumulation of metabolites also could conceivably exert an effect on intact vessels or development of new ones.

Examination of the base of a pedicle flap during and after delays has shown that an increased number and size of subdermal vessels occurs. How and why these vessels became enlarged and more numerous, however, is unknown; this is a pity, as the problem is suitable for research by modern biological techniques. A great deal of expense, time, and uncertainty during management of tissue transfer problems could be prevented if present techniques of numerous delays could be based accurately on some reliable measurement. The practical implications of being able to control the rate and intensity of vascular proliferation are obvious. Control of the procss will be dependent, however, upon understanding of basic physiology involved. Clinically, about all that can be done now is to recognize that blood supply can be increased

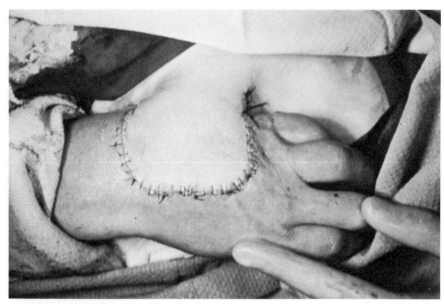

Figure 7–79. Abdominal pedicle flap to resurface dorsum of hand.

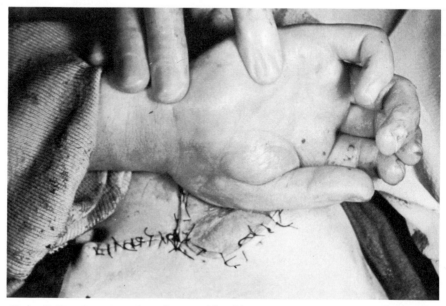

Figure 7–80. Scar tissue from dorsum of hand has been reflected onto abdominal wall to provide temporary closure.

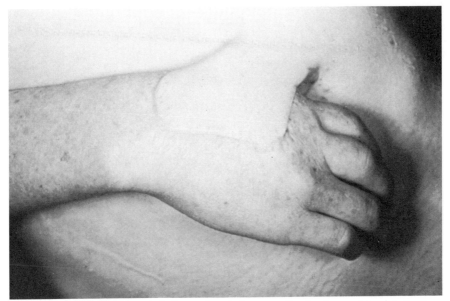

Figure 7–81. Abdominal pedicle flap on hand after wound healing is complete and all sutures have been removed. Because abdominal donor site also was resurfaced, no dressing is required and ambulation is permitted. (From E. E. Peacock, Jr., in *Principles of Surgery*, edited by S. I. Schwartz. Copyright 1969, McGraw-Hill Book Company. Used with permission of McGraw-Hill Book Company.)

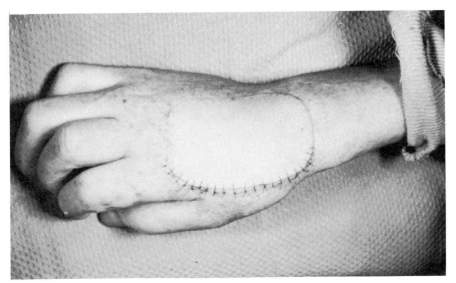

Figure 7–82. Abdominal pedicle flap immediately after detachment from abdomen. Note restoration of contour by utilizing full-thickness skin and subcutaneous tissue from abdominal wall.

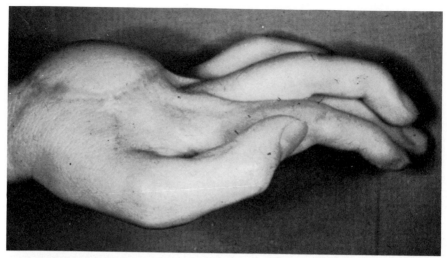

Figure 7–83. Typical appearance of abdominal pedicle flap of inadequate proportions placed on a healing wound. Note that wound contracture was not stopped and that grafted tissue is now converted into a small mound surrounded by a circular scar. Note checkreining of fingers in hyperextension by attachment of extensor tendons to deep scar. (From E. E. Peacock, Jr., in *Reconstructive Plastic Surgery,* vol. IV, edited by J. M. Converse, Philadelphia, W. B. Saunders Co., 1964.)

in the base of a flap by interrupting other blood vessels deliberately in stages. Time between stages usually is governed by allowing inflammatory reaction, such as edema and erythema, to subside and by waiting for all objective signs of grossly deficient circulation (cyanosis) to disappear before another stage is undertaken. Failure of delays to prepare an area of skin for transfer by the pedicle method usually is the result of improper design of the stages, haste in proceeding to a subsequent stage before results of the previous delay have become stable, or development of an infection or some other wound complication. Because the biological principles of delaying procedures are so vague, there is no point in going into the various gimmicks or techniques which many surgeons believe are important in preventing these complications from occurring. Such factors have been dignified sufficiently in the many technique books on restorative surgery.

The most frequent cause of failure during transfer of composite tissue flaps is development of venous insufficiency. Flaps seldom fail for lack of arterial perfusion; they frequently are in serious trouble from congestion caused by inadequate venous or lymphatic drainage. As described under management of cutaneous wounds, a sharp line of color demarcation in a flap is a serious sign of venous insufficiency. If something is not done rapidly when this sign develops, thrombosis and necrosis are inevitable. If a flap is only dusky in appearance and there is no sharp line of color differentiation between normal and dusky skin, an occlusive dressing removed often for inspection of the flap and reapplied to keep mild pressure on the flap may be all that is needed to overcome congestion. Occasionally flaps can be improved by light digital stroking in the direction of the base. If this is done every 10 to 15 minutes for a few hours after transfer, venous drainage may become sufficient — presumably because of relief of smooth muscle spasm. If a sharp line of demarcation develops, however, much more aggressive measures should be resorted to. These include removal of as many sutures as necessary to restore proper color and transfer of the flap back to its original bed. A sharp line of demarcation must be gotten rid of, regardless of what is involved. Once the flap has been elevated and rotated, one might ask what good can be accomplished by simply returning it to its original site — blood vessels which have already been divided will not be reestablished. Presumably the flap would never have been elevated in the first place, however, and certainly it would not have been rotated to the recipient area if circulation had not appeared adequate after it had been incised and undermined. It is this state that one is trying to retreat to when the flap becomes congested in its new area; the slight gain achieved by correcting torsion at the base, plus relieving tension by removing sutures, can mean the difference between survival and necrosis.

Dextran was thought to show promise of aiding sluggish circulation by reducing the viscosity of blood. Theoretically, heparin also would be indicated during a period when venous drainage was sluggish. Heparin, hyperbaric oxygen, and local amines have all shown some beneficial effect on the survival of congested flaps in laboratory animals. Adequate control observations to support these data often are lacking, however, and results in human beings suggest that the problem at the moment should be considered as more mechanical than biological. Therefore, mechanical alterations which increase venous drainage are more reliable than physiological or pharmacological measures.

Failure of a portion or all of a flap to survive will produce an eschar which should be treated exactly as an eschar in any other type of wound. Usually immediate excision and replacement with another type of graft is the treatment of choice. Depending upon the size and area of the necrotic wound, however, other treatment may be indicated. Rarely, for instance, a portion of the full thickness of the skin may be lost, yet a deep layer of dermis or subcutaneous tissue may remain viable so that a free graft is possible where it could not be done before the pedicle was transferred. The experienced reconstructive surgeon usually is able to plan flaps so that sufficient length or width can be developed by further advancement or rotation should a small portion of the original flap not make the grade.

An alternate method of closing the wound should be a part of planning for any pedicle transfer. Planning an entire restoration on the end of a narrow-based flap which cannot be extended or rotated any further, so that even one centimeter of distal necrosis will expose a critical portion of the wound (such as that covering an exposed tendon, bone or fistula), is a mistake that usually is avoidable. Sometimes this type of planning is inevitable, but getting into such situations usually can be avoided by not planning complex transfers without large safety margins, including alternate routes of approach. In this regard (also as far as color match, time, expense, and so forth are concerned), local flaps nearly always are superior to distant ones. Although full-thickness skin and fat can be moved literally from one end of the body to the other by use of an extremity as a carrier or by multiple jumping or walking techniques, every transfer sets up another complex biological abnormality which must be considered. Flaps may survive transfer over a long distance, but months of impaired circulation, edema, and surgical insult often take a toll which, although not measured in loss of tissue, is measured by change in characteristics of the tissue, including fibrosis and loss of important skin appendages. Tissue so affected may arrive at a distant recipient area resembling typical scleroderma and without some of the characteristics which were important in the selection of the donor site. This should not be interpreted to mean that skilled restorative surgeons frequently are not able to move tissue over great distances and, in spite of potential hazards, still have it arrive at its final destination in near perfect condition. However, such feats of technical skill and judgment are not the essence of the best and safest restorative surgery. In most cases, an element of biological safety can be built into the restorative plan so that everything is not dependent on perfect mechanical execution and judgment. As in most surgical problems, optimal conditions exist when sound biological planning is combined with superb technical performance. Although outstanding ability to do one can sometimes make up for minor deficiencies in the other, the object of good restorative surgery is not to crowd luck to one side or the other and see what one can get by with. It is to plan and carry out a procedure with margins of safety so extensive that, even if something unexpectedly goes awry, built-in safety factors will insure ultimate success.

Although no adequate biological tests are available to determine when new blood supply from peripheral vessels in the recipient area can nourish a flap sufficiently so that the last remaining connections with the donor site can be divided, most flaps have picked up adequate nourishment from the recipient bed by 14 to 18 days. If as much as 90 per cent of the flap was applied to the wound at the initial transfer, final detachment from the donor site can be performed in one stage. If only 50 per cent of the flap was set in at the first stage, a delay in cutting across the base may be indicated. This is accomplished by cutting halfway across the base at the first stage and waiting approximately ten days to divide the remainder of the pedicle. In a simple rotation flap, the entire base usually does not ever have to be divided; only a dog-ear or unacceptable wrinkle where rotation occurred will require

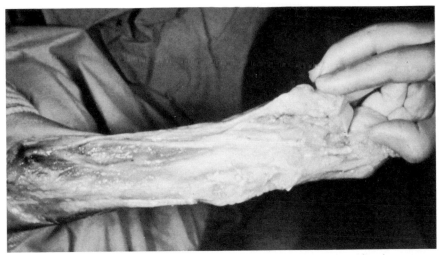

Figure 7–84.   Severe avulsion injury of soft tissue of forearm and hand.

revision. Flaps resurfacing wounds caused by short-wave radiation should never be detached from their donor blood supply. The important biological difference in these wounds is vasculitis, which prevents adequate circulation. A flap that is nourished adequately as long as the base is intact may become an island of necrotic tissue if the base is divided. Actually, the main reason for performing a flap in radiation

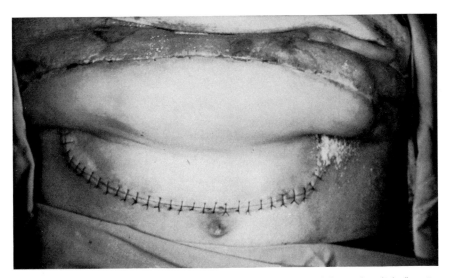

Figure 7–85.   Immediate coverage of forearm and hand with an abdominal pedicle flap. Because only 50 per cent of the flap could be set in at the initial procedure, there was a delay before the flap was detached from the abdominal wall. When as much as 90 per cent of the flap can be set in at the first stage, as shown in Figures 7–79 to 7–83, delay procedures are not necessary.

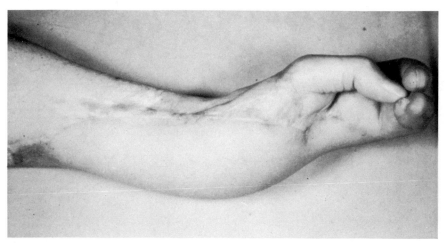

Figure 7–86.   Same hand shown in Figure 7–84. Note contour reconstruction with abdominal pedicle flap.

wounds is to bring blood vessels into the area. The skin may not be so badly damaged that it cannot heal itself, yet a flap is still indicated to improve the circulation in the entire area. These flaps should be regarded as permanent blood-carrying flaps and should be transferred by the island pedicle method or by a rotation which is planned so that it is never necessary to divide the base. It is amazing how the texture and physical characteristics of surrounding tissue often will be improved by

Text continued on page 356

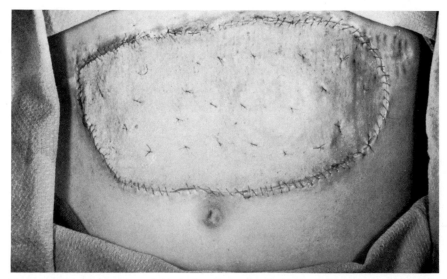

Figure 7–87.   Donor site on abdominal wall resurfaced with a split-thickness skin graft at the time abdominal flap was detached.

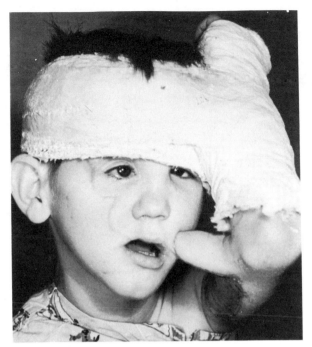

Figure 7–88. An arm flap lined with a split-thickness skin graft has been passed through an old wound of the cheek to reconstruct the hard and soft palate following a mutilating injury of the central third of the face. Same patient as shown in Figures 11–8 to 11–10. (Reproduced by permission from E. E. Peacock, Jr., Amer. Surg., *24*:639, 1958.)

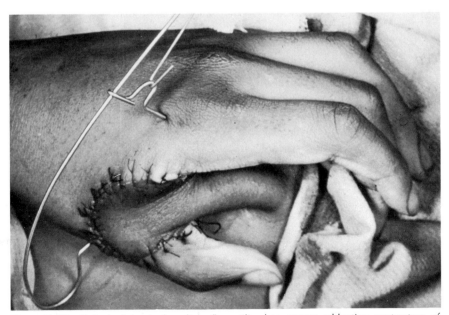

Figure 7–89. Tubed abdominal pedicle flap utilized to correct adduction contracture of thumb. (From E. E. Peacock, Jr., in *Reconstructive Plastic Surgery*, vol. IV, edited by J. M. Converse, Philadelphia, W. B. Saunders Co., 1964.)

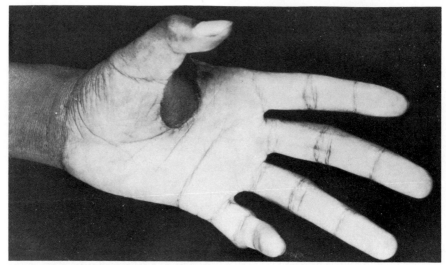

Figure 7–90. Release of adduction contracture of the thumb by bringing tubed pedicle flap shown in Figure 7–89 into palm. (From E. E. Peacock, Jr., in *Reconstructive Plastic Surgery,* vol. IV, edited by J. M. Converse, Philadelphia, W. B. Saunders Co., 1964.)

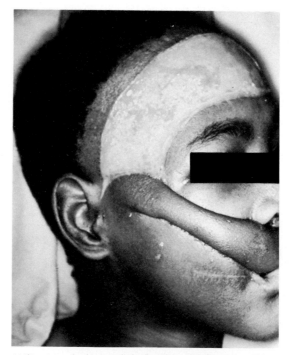

Figure 7–91. Utilization of tubed pedicle flap from forehead to reconstruct upper lip.

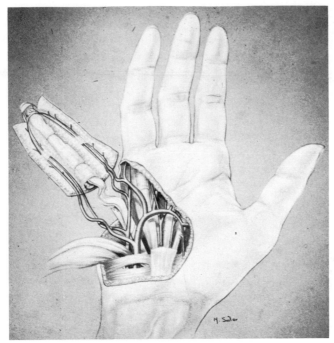

Figure 7–92. Artist's concept of exploded digit to show dual radially oriented neurovascular bundles. Soft tissue from any digit can be moved anywhere in the hand or wrist as a composite island pedicle graft. (Reproduced by permission from E. E. Peacock, Jr., Plast. Reconstr. Surg., 25:298, 1960. Copyright 1960, The Williams & Wilkins Co., Baltimore, Md. 21202, U.S.A.)

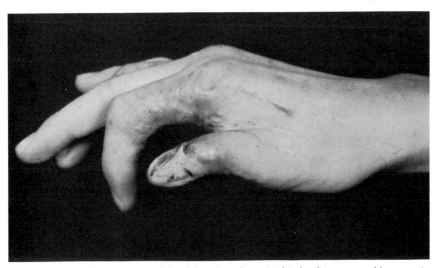

Figure 7–93. Mutilating injury of distal thumb and proximal index finger caused by a moving belt. (From E. E. Peacock, Jr., in *Surgery: Principles and Practice*, 4th edition, edited by C. A. Moyer, J. E. Rhoads, H. N. Harkins, and J. G. Allen, Philadelphia, J. B. Lippincott Co., 1970.)

the effect of blood vessels in the flap. Treatment of a radiation effect in skin which leads to an ulcer that does not heal should be viewed primarily as transfer of intact functioning blood vessels. In addition to increasing the badly needed oxygenated blood supply the transplant also brings into the radiated area stem cells with capacity to divide and produce fibroblasts, myofibroblasts, and other stem cells which seem to have lain along blood vessels and to have been permanently lost from that area when destroyed by ionizing radiation. Finally, of course, a permanent blood-carrying pedicle brings coverage in the form of skin with its own nutrition when it is needed. One cannot expect such important skin coverage to heal or survive if the primary requisites of blood supply and stem cells are not provided on a permanent basis by the transfer.

After composite tissue grafts have been transplanted by the pedicle technique, the biology of transplanted skin is different for many months from that of undisturbed full-thickness skin. Many of these differences should be remembered during care of the flap for the first few months after transfer. From a practical standpoint, sensitivity to change in temperature is the most important such biological alteration. Flaps are extremely sensitive to heat. Deep second and third degree burns can be caused by temperatures (particularly wet heat) which would not even be uncomfortable to normal skin. Because flaps can be destroyed completely by relatively small increases in temperatures, the problem is not one of simple inability to appreciate temperature because of anesthesia. It is more likely that the circulation in a new flap is barely adequate during the first few months after transfer, and an island of full-thickness skin without normal circulation probably does not have the dynamic flexibility of normally vascularized and innervated tissue. It cannot, therefore, participate in skin temperature control by undergoing dilatation or constriction of surface blood vessels to maintain homeostasis during changing environmental conditions. Thus a newly transferred flap is, in a sense, similar to the skin of cold-blooded animals. The vascular flexibility needed to maintain a constant temperature is not present. This explanation for sensitivity of flaps to temperature change is sheer hypothesis. No direct measurements are available which can tell us precisely why recently transferred flaps will develop a second or third degree burn after exposure to temperatures which would produce no more than transient erythema in normal skin. The whole subject of fragility of denervated skin is one which needs study now that sophisticated qualitative and quantitative methods are available for measuring collagen synthesis and lysis. In the meantime, the practical point that recently transplanted skin is extremely heat-sensitive must be recognized and protective measures must be taken if loss of extensive coverage is to be avoided during the immediate postoperative period. Recently transplanted composite tissue flaps are excellent models, of course, for studying denervated skin.

Another unexplained phenomenon in flaps is how they eventually regain sensation to some degree. Numerous direct measurements have revealed that distant flaps, completely separated from their previous donor sites, ultimately regain protective sensation. Data on the amount and type of sensory reception which develops are not conclusive. Our impression is that the type and amount of sensation that returns can better be correlated with the type of skin that was transplanted than with the site to which it is transplanted. For example, abdominal flaps transplanted to the hand seem to regain sensation much more like that of abdominal skin than skin of the hand. Cross-finger flaps regain modalities and a degree of sensibility more like hand skin than distant flaps. If true, such impressions suggest strongly that the type of sensation regained is dependent upon the number and type of receptors which are available. This is a problem of tremendous importance, because reinnervation of other anesthetic areas such as following division of a major peripheral nerve does not occur to the same extent as reinnervation of free grafts and flaps.

Skin recently transplanted by the pedicle method is also more susceptible to short-wave radiation than nontransplanted skin. It will

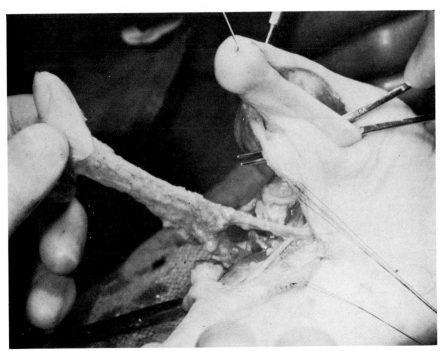

Figure 7–94.   Utilization of island pedicle principle depicted in Figure 7–92 to transplant distal end of index finger to amputation stump of thumb. (From E. E. Peacock, Jr., in *Surgery: Principles and Practice,* 4th edition, edited by C. A. Moyer, J. E. Rhoads, H. N. Harkins, and J. G. Allen, Philadelphia, J. B. Lippincott Co., 1970.)

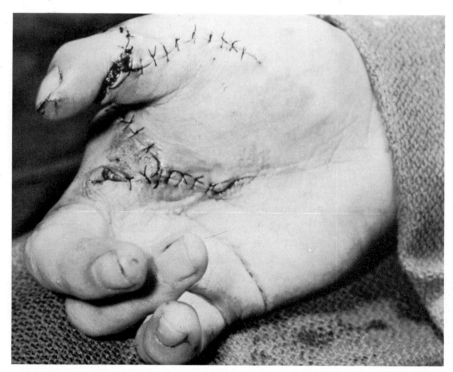

Figure 7–95.   Index finger tip shown in Figure 7–94 transplanted to distal end of thumb.

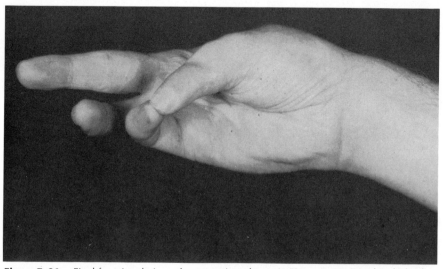

Figure 7–96.   Final functional view of same patient shown in Figure 7–93. Distal end of index finger has been transplanted as an island pedicle flap to end of thumb amputation stump. (From E. E. Peacock, Jr., in *Surgery: Principles and Practice,* 4th edition, edited by C. A. Moyer, J. E. Rhoads, H. N. Harkins, and J. G. Allen, Philadelphia, J. B. Lippincott Co., 1970.)

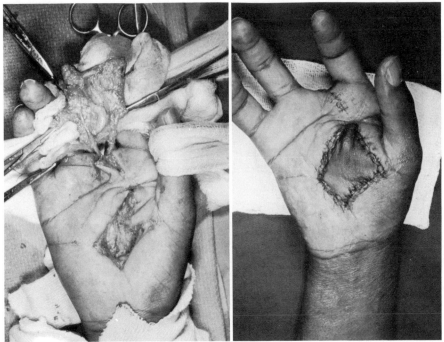

Fig. 7-97   **Fig. 7-98**

Figure 7-97. Island pedicle flap nourished by two neurovascular bundles from the long finger. Flap will be passed through the palm to resurface a proximal wound caused by excision of scar tissue to release an adduction contracture of thumb. (From E. E. Peacock, Jr., in *Principles of Surgery,* edited by S. I. Schwartz. Copyright 1969, McGraw-Hill Book Company. Used with permission of McGraw-Hill Book Company.)

Figure 7-98. Island pedicle flap from long finger resurfacing defect of the palm. Dark skin was on dorsum of finger; light skin was on volar surface. (Reproduced by permission from E. E. Peacock, Jr., Plast. Reconstr. Surg., *25:*298, 1960. Copyright 1960, The Williams & Wilkins Co., Baltimore, Md. 21202, U.S.A.)

respond to solar radiation by developing deeper pigment than surrounding tissue. Flaps on exposed areas of the body should be protected from solar radiation for at least one year if a dark appearance is to be avoided. Very acute exposure will result in deep second degree burns, just as exposure to longer-wave radiation is more dangerous in transplanted skin. Exposure to sun that produces no more than mild erythema in normal skin may produce a deep second degree burn in an adjacent flap. A permanent loss of pigment-producing cells may occur following such an injury.

The propensity for subcutaneous fat to accumulate is transferred with abdominal skin even if abdominal subcutaneous fat was not included with the graft. As long as 20 years after transfer of abdominal pedicle flaps which contain no subcutaneous fat at the time of transfer, an unsightly mound will develop on the hand if the patient begins to add subcutaneous tissue in the abdominal region. The biological basis for this observation apparently is at least partially under the control of

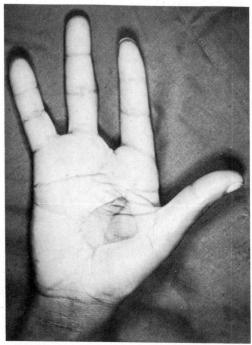

Figure 7–99. Same hand shown in Figure 7–97 following release of adduction contracture with an island pedicle flap from long finger.

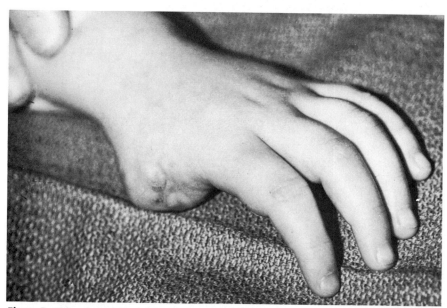

Figure 7–100. Amputation of thumb through base of first metacarpal. (Reproduced by permission from E. E. Peacock, Jr., in *Hand Surgery,* edited by J. E. Flynn. Copyright 1966, The Williams & Wilkins Co., Baltimore, Md. 21202, U.S.A.)

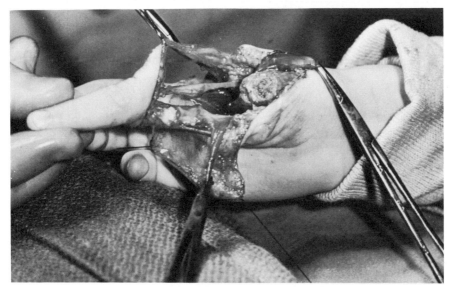

Figure 7–101. Utilization of island pedicle principles to transplant the entire index finger as a composite tissue graft to the base of first metacarpal. Note that finger is nourished by two neurovascular bundles. (Reproduced by permission from E. E. Peacock, Jr., in *Hand Surgery*, edited by J. E. Flynn. Copyright 1966, The Williams & Wilkins Co., Baltimore, Md. 21202, U.S.A.)

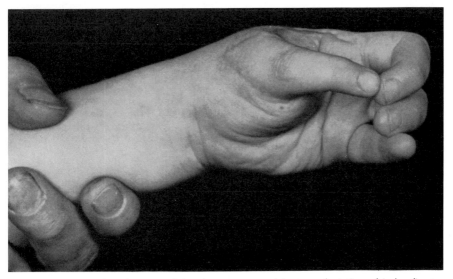

Figure 7–102. Prehensile view of thumb reconstructed by transplantation of index finger.

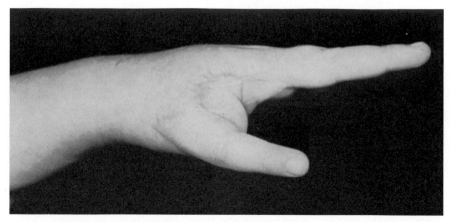

Figure 7–103. Same hand shown in Figure 7–100 following reconstruction of thumb by transplantation of index finger as a composite tissue graft.

dermis. Whatever the controlling mechanisms may be they are implanted intact with a pedicle flap to some other area of the body. Another example suggesting that subcutaneous tissue composition and properties may be at least partially induced by overlying dermis is the occasional patient with severe Dupuytren's contracture who repeatedly re-forms dense fibrous tissue beneath palmar skin. Excision of overlying skin is now the only known method of stopping subcutaneous proliferation of fibrous tissue in these unfortunate individuals. Similar observations have been made for plantar fibromatosis.

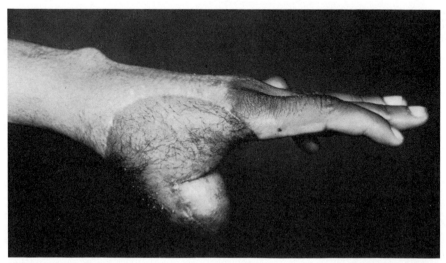

Figure 7–104. Reconstruction of thumb by means of large abdominal pedicle flap stabilized by a bone graft. Although occasionally indicated, this type of thumb reconstruction is not as satisfactory as transplantation of an index finger. (Reproduced by permission from E. E. Peacock, Jr., in *Hand Surgery,* edited by J. E. Flynn. Copyright 1966, The Williams & Wilkins Co., Baltimore, Md. 21202, U.S.A.)

WOUNDS CAUSED BY DEHISCENCE OF LARGE SKIN FLAPS

A distressing complication of a radical neck dissection, breast excision, or groin dissection may be complete dehiscence of skin flaps and exposure of deep structures such as the carotid or femoral vessels. These wounds are worthy of special consideration because ill timed or injudicious intervention can turn a relatively innocuous complication into a nightmare of restorative complications with dangerous implications. The initial approach is often one characterized by feeling that something radical must be done quickly to protect the structures which are exposed. Because dehiscence may be the result of closure under too much tension, and always will result in additional tissue loss, simple replacement of skin flaps by suturing them together is almost never advisable. Flaps which are left hanging from the wound rapidly develop a sort of bursal lining caused by continued motion of the flap against the underlying base. This appearance is caused by coagulation of serum and lining of the flap with connective tissue elements so that a shiny smooth appearance is produced. When two such surfaces are opposed to each other, friction is minimal and motion is constant; healing either does not occur at all or is greatly prolonged.

The first guide to successful management of acute dehiscences is to realize that loss of skin coverage does not produce a serious hazard to deep structures if adequate wound care is provided. The vasa vasorum of large vessels will nourish the vessel adequately whether it is covered by skin or not. Unless the vasa vasorum has been damaged or obliterated by an irradiation- or infection-induced vasculitis, a "blow out" of an exposed vessel is not a serious possibility provided good wound care is available. It is not necessary, therefore, to try to mobilize further inflamed and already deficient tissue or to begin transferring complicated distant flaps to cover blood vessels as quickly as possible. Unless the vessel is abnormal, granulation tissue will develop and cover the adventitia along with the rest of the wound. Major vessels have been exposed for several months in noninfected, nonirradiated wounds without apparent damage. Infection in a wound with an expanded exposed major vessel is a potential hazard. Adequate drainage, antibacterial therapy, proper dressing, and so forth should be utilized as skillfully as possible. Dehiscence in an irradiated wound also is reason for concern but the important point in these problems is that both infection and irradiated wounds respond quickly and more satisfactorily to conservative wound therapy than to heroic surgical maneuvers. Expressed simply, emergency surgery during active infection and upon deficient amounts of tissue, or irradiated tissue, is certain to worsen the problem of wound coverage. Healing can be obtained much faster by promoting wound contraction and epithelization than by bringing distant skin into the area by pedicle transfer. If an irradiated artery is exposed, precaution should be taken to achieve rapid ligation if further destruction of the wall occurs. A heroic emergency surgical procedure to get local tissue over the wound not only has a high incidence of failure but also probably delays wound contraction and formation of valuable granulation tissue.

Conservative management of a dehisced wound consists of expert application of dressings until flaps become attached to underlying tissue and wound contraction occurs. After contraction has occurred, the remaining uncovered wound surface can be covered by small split-thickness skin grafts with the open grafting technique. The dressing is designed to prevent organization of connective tissue and fibrin to form a smooth pseudolining. Once such a lining develops, motion is virtually assured between flap and wound bed; adherence between the two will not occur under these conditions. An oversimplification of the principle used to prevent organization of a pseudolining on dehisced skin flaps is to provide a mild irritant surface for the entire wound surface to heal against. This can be accomplished with a plain fine mesh gauze, as a preventive measure, or by impregnating the gauze with a mild irritant such as iodine (iodoform gauze) or balsam of Peru, if the membrane already has formed. Balsam of Peru is especially useful as it stimulates a neutrophil response.

The technique of applying the dressing is important. Copious irrigation with weak hydrogen peroxide solution is performed at each dressing, to be sure that drainage throughout the recesses of the wound is adequate. The gauze is then carefully laid in the wound so that it is in contact with the entire wound surface (roof as well as floor). The wound is *not packed.* Packing a wound interferes with drainage, prevents obliteration of the cavity by the healing process, and ultimately promotes formation of organized ·connective tissue on all surfaces. This is particularly true after two or three dressings when fine strands of fibrin begin to bridge the wound cavity, heralding the obliteration of the cavity by scar formation between flap and bed. As the cavity begins to be obliterated by fibrin and fibrous tissue synthesis, the gauze is even more cautiously inserted—only enough to insure drainage and keep unagglutinated surfaces apart. Once adherence begins, the entire flap will become attached in 24 to 48 hours if dressings are applied carefully. Until adherence begins, dressings may have to be changed three or four times a day to keep transudate and exudate from accumulating beneath the flaps. If the necessary care is used during this period, a rather sudden cessation of transudation occurs, and an adhesive stage begins.

The surgeon may become concerned as adherence begins because of what appears to be a reduction in size of the flaps. The flaps appear to be retracting in a peripheral circumferential manner, leaving a relatively large area of the base uncovered. This phenomenon is the beginning of the wound contraction stage, and because the flap is the most movable tissue involved, contraction is first represented by retraction of skin edges in a circumferential manner. Any attempt to lessen the retraction of skin flaps will interfere with the more important process which is also going on—adherence of the flaps to the base of the wound. As contracture continues, the entire circumference of the wound will move in a centripetal fashion so that the exposed area in the base of the wound will be reduced; what was lost in the way of early peripheral contracture will be made up before contraction ends. The result will be a relatively small wound, surrounded by skin flaps which are attached to the base, and an exposed base which has healthy granulation. The fundamental biological consideration being relied upon is that contraction is the desired activity and contraction will not occur as long as the lateral margins of the wound are not attached to the base. As attachment begins by adherence of the flaps to the base in the lateral recesses of the cavity, the more easily movable central skin is retracted peripherally. As the central margins of skin become attached, however, the contraction phenomenon also occurs at the point of attachment of the flap to the base. The overall result is a wound of surprisingly small dimensions which can be easily grafted by the open technique. In areas such as the chest wall or neck the open technique is mandatory as motion cannot be prevented in these structures. Also, subclinical infection undoubtedly prevails and a dressing only promotes collection of pus beneath the graft.

The main objection to this plan of treatment in dehiscence following neck dissection is that contraction and synthesis of scar produce an annoying constricting sensation which sometimes causes considerable fear. Swallowing may be difficult for a short period of time. Patients can be reassured, however, that secondary remodeling of scar will do much to alleviate the tight feeling. Rarely a secondary procedure, such as a revision of external scar or addition of more skin, may be needed.

In summary, refraining from embarking on complicated transfers of tissue, calm and patient conservative care of the wound, relying on and aiming for wound contraction as the main biological phenomenon desired, and finishing the job with a small free graft after contraction is over will invariably correct the most terrifying-appearing dehiscence faster than any other method. Satisfactory management of such a case can be one of the most gratifying experiences in which application of fundamental biology to practical aspects of wound repair is possible.

SUGGESTED READING

Artz, C. P., and Gaston, B. H. A Reappraisal of the Exposure Method in the Treatment of Burns, Donor Sites and Skin Grafts. Ann. Surg. *151*:939, 1960.

Artz, C. P., Rittenbury, M. S., and Yarbrough, D. R. Appraisal of Allografts and Xenografts as Biologic Dressings for Wounds and Burns. Ann. Surg. *175*:939, 1972.

Artz, C. P., and Thompson, N. J., Jr. Early Excision of Large Areas in Burns. Surgery *63*:868, 1968.

Baxter, C. R. Topical Use of 1.0% Silver Sulfadiazine. In: *Contemporary Burn Management.* Edited by H. C. Polk, Jr. and H. H. Stone. Boston, Little, Brown & Co., 1971, p. 217.

Blocker, T. G., Jr., Lewis, S. R., Grant, D. A., Blocker, V., and Bennett, J. E. Experiences in the Management of the Burn Wounds. Plast. Reconstr. Surg. 26:579, 1960.

Brown, J. B., and McDowell, F. Massive Repairs of Burns with Thick Split-Skin Grafts. Ann. Surg. *115*:658, 1942.

Brown, J. B., McDowell, F., and Fryer, M. P. Radiation Burns, Including Vocational and Atomic Exposures. Treatment, and Surgical Prevention of Chronic Lesions. Ann. Surg. *130*:593, 1949.

Caldwell, F. T., Jr., Casali, R. E., and Boswer, B. On the Failure of Heat Production in the Immediate Post-Burn Period. J. Trauma *11*:936, 1971.

Cortese, T. A., Jr., Sams, W. M., and Sulzberger, M. B. Studies on Blisters Produced by Friction. II. The Blister Fluid. J. Invest. Derm. *50*:47, 1968.

Cramer, L., McCormick, R., and Carroll, D. B. Progressive Partial Excision and Early Grafting in Lethal Burns. Plast. Reconstr. Surg. *30*:595, 1962.

Giacometti, L., and Montagna, W. The Healing of Skin Wounds in Primates. II. The Proliferation of Epidermal Cell Melanocytes. J. Invest. Derm. *50*:273, 1968.

Gibbons, J. R. Migration of Stratified Squamous Epithelium in Vivo. Amer. J. Path. *53*:929, 1968.

Grillo, H. C., Watts, G. T., and Gross, J. Studies in Wound Healing: I. Contraction and the Wound Contents. Ann. Surg. *148*:145, 1958.

Higton, D. I. R., and James, D. W. The Force of Contraction of Full-Thickness Wounds of Rabbit Skin. Brit. J. Surg. *51*:462, 1964.

Jackson, D., Topley, E., Carson, J. S., and Lowbury, E. J. L. Primary Excision and Grafting of Large Burns. Ann. Surg. *152*:167, 1960.

Jelenko, C., III, and Ginsburg, J. M. Water-Holding Lipid and Water Transmission Through Homeothermic and Poikilothermic Skins. Proc. Soc. Exp. Biol. Med. *136*:1059, 1971.

Jelenko, C., III, Mendelson, J. A., and Buxton, R. W. The Marfanil Mystery. Surg. Gynec. Obstet. *122*:121, 1966.

Lowney, E. D., Baublis, J. V., Kreye, G. M., Harrell, E. R., and McKenzie, A. R. The Scalded Skin Syndrome in Small Children. Arch. Derm. *95*:359, 1967.

Luccioli, C., Kahn, D. S., and Robertson, H. R. Histologic Study of Wound Contraction in the Rabbit. Ann. Surg. *160*:1030, 1964.

Madden, J. W., Morton, D., Jr., and Peacock, E. E., Jr. Contraction of Experimental Wounds. I. Inhibiting Wound Contraction by Using a Topical Smooth Muscle Antagonist. Surgery *76*:8, 1974.

Montagna, W. The Skin. Sci. Amer. *212*:56, 1965.

Moyer, C. A., Brentano, L., Gravens, D. S., Margraf, H. W., and Monafo, W. W., Jr. The Treatment of Large Human Burns with 0.5 Per Cent Silver Nitrate Solution. Arch. Surg. *90*:812, 1965.

Myers, M. B., and Cherry, G. Design of Skin Flaps to Study Vascular Insufficiency. J. Surg. Res. *7*:399, 1967.

Myers, M. B., and Rightor, M. Augmentation of Wound Strength by Pretreatment with Epinephrine. Plast. Reconstr. Surg. *54*:201, 1974.

Odland, G., and Ross, R. Human Wound Repair. I. Epidermal Regeneration. J. Cell Biol. *39*:135, 1968.

Ramirez, A. T., Soroff, H. S., Schwartz, M. S., Mooty, J., Pearson, E., and Raben, M. S. Experimental Wound Healing in Man. Surg. Gynec. Obstet. *128*:283, 1969.

Robb, H. J. Dynamics of the Microcirculation during a Burn. Arch. Surg. *94*:776, 1967.

Ross, R., and Odland, G. Human Wound Repair. II. Inflammatory Cells, Epithelial-Mesenchymal Interrelations, and Fibrogenesis. J. Cell Biol. *39*:152, 1968.

Stone, H. H. Wound Care with Topical Gentamicin. In: *Contemporary Burn Management.* Edited by H. C. Polk, Jr., and H. H. Stone. Boston, Little, Brown & Co., 1971, p. 203.

Stone, P. A., and Madden, J. W. Biological Factors Affecting Wound Contraction. Surg. Forum *26*:547, 1975.

Vaughn, R. B., and Trinkaus, J. P. Movement of Epithelial Cell Sheets *in Vitro.* J. Cell Sci. *1*:407, 1966.

Watts, G. T., Grillo, H. C., and Gross, J. Studies in Wound Healing: II. The Role of Granulation Tissue in Contraction. Ann. Surg. *148*:153, 1958.

Whitson, T. C. The Development of Topical Chemotherapy in the Management of Burns. Amer. J. Surg. *116*:69, 1968.

Zahir, M. Contraction of Wounds. Brit. J. Surg. *51*:456, 1964.

Zahir, M. Formation of Scabs on Skin Wounds. Brit. J. Surg. *52*:376, 1965.

Zawacki, B. E., Spitzer, K. W., and Mason, A. D., Jr. Does Increased Evaporative Water Loss Cause Hypermetabolism in Burned Patients? Ann. Surg. *171*:236, 1970.

Chapter 8

REPAIR OF TENDONS AND RESTORATION OF GLIDING FUNCTION

The healing of injured tendons is one of the most interesting yet perplexing problems in the biology of tissue repair; diametrically opposite objectives seem to be required in the same wound. The objective of healing in some collagenous tissues, such as fascia or bone, is simply to gain tensile strength as rapidly and effectively as possible; "overhealing" is neither a serious consideration nor an undesirable end result. Following repair of other collagenous structures, such as serosa of bowel, physical strength is not needed as much as development of a watertight seal without adherence to other organs. Successful restoration of injured tendons, however, requires the best of both processes. For a single scar to provide strength in one area, yet not restrict motion in another, an extremely complex series of events must occur. Because so much of what must occur is only barely understood, the history of surgeons' attempts to improve tendon healing is not particularly exciting. No other chapter in the history of surgery, however, brings out so vividly the necessity for understanding fundamental biological processes before designing and altering surgical manipulations.

Frustrated by inability to understand or control complex phenomena during healing of tendons, surgeons understandably have relied almost entirely upon empirical manipulations. Although the effect of empiricism in this field is difficult to assess, a few general principles and specific technical maneuvers have emerged which appear to be significant in assuring both a strong anastomosis and an adequate gliding function. Almost simultaneously with the development of empirical technical maneuvers and a few broad principles, a greater understanding of fundamental connective tissue biology has emerged. This body of knowledge has given us some insight into the reason some technical manipulations have improved results of tendon repairs and others actually may have been harmful. More important, however, future approaches to biological and technical control of the healing process in tendons will be based on sound biochemical and biophysical knowledge of the changes which must take place for a scar to produce great tensile strength yet permit movement through a relatively long amplitude.

Future surgeons probably will be less dependent upon exacting surgical technique than we are at present, but right now success in restoring function in tendons with long amplitudes of motion is best assured by mastering meticulous surgical techniques based on a sound understanding of connective tissue metabolism. Moreover, as important as the surgeon's skill during repair of divided tendons is the postoperative care he provides. Fundamental collagen biology is just as applicable to this part of patient therapy as it is to operative technique. Although such information is not yet complete enough to provide us with the answers to all postoperative problems, it does provide some insight into what is happening during remodeling of scar tissue in and around a repaired tendon, so that harmful or ineffective measures are not instituted.

FUNDAMENTAL PRINCIPLES IN TENDON HEALING

An important general principle in the biology of tendon healing is the "one wound-one scar" concept. This phrase encompasses a great deal of our knowledge about the fluid stage of healing when even fibrous protein is held in a viscous suspension able to permeate every recess of the wound. A tendon should be considered part of a compound wound which can be compared to a saucer or crater containing the cut ends of a number of tissues. In addition to divided tendon ends, the cavity also contains injured fat, blood vessels, dermis, and possibly even bone or cartilage. The scar which ultimately amalgamates all of these structures is, at one time, a single viscous medium which permeates the entire wound. Thus each structure in the wound is connected with all the others during one phase of scar evolution.

Although the term "one wound-one scar" and the principle it defines sound simple enough, many of the unsuccessful operations which have occupied surgeons' time and thought during the last 20 years have been based on the assumption or hope that at least two

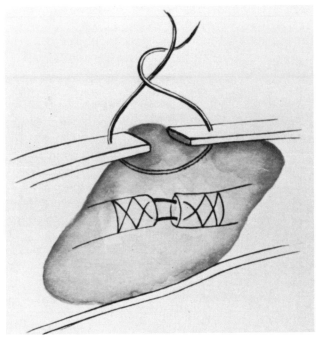

Figure 8–1.   Diagram of one-wound concept of tendon healing. Wounds of skin, subcutaneous tissue, tendon, and deep structures are continuous and can be thought of as a single container which ultimately will be filled with all the products of the healing process.

wounds and two scars existed or could be produced. There is no question that if the wound between two tendon ends could be managed independently of the wound of overlying skin or underlying bone, the problem of tendon repair could be vastly simplified. Treatment directed toward a single objective, such as development of tensile strength between two tendon ends, would be no more complicated than repair of a hernia or fractured bone. Similarly, if the wound surrounding the tendon also could be managed independently, the objectives of preventing excessive fibrous protein synthesis and development of significant physical strength could be controlled by pharmacological or surgical methods. The inescapable fact, however, is that only one wound exists and that every attempt so far to separate a wound containing divided tendons into compartments, either in the mind of the surgeon or by some physical manipulation, has resulted in faulty analysis of the problem or in worsening of the clinical result. All available knowledge, whether clinical, basic, or theoretical, strongly suggests that the one wound-one scar concept is fundamental and that anything surgeons devise to improve the results of tendon repair must take it into consideration.

The biological basis for the one-scar concept is found in a number of laboratory experiments and clinical observations which suggest strongly that mature tendons do not contain cells capable of synthesizing fibrous protein. The majority of cells in a mature tendon are spindle-shaped cells, which probably are relatively inactive fibrocytes. Although there is an increase in number of many types of cells soon after injury to a tendon, it seems likely that these cells are mostly inflammatory cells delivered by the intrinsic blood supply, or multipotent cells which have migrated into the region of repair from outside the tendon. Fibrocytes found in uninjured mature tendon apparently are end cells, which have little capacity to divide or synthesize fibrous protein in amounts necessary to develop strong union between tendon ends. Actually, the appearance of lacerated tendon ends completely isolated from the surrounding wound is characterized by atrophy and resorption. There is no evidence of regeneration or synthesis of new protein. Grossly, the cut end of a tendon becomes rounded, as collagenolytic activity apparently causes resorption of stringy bundles of fibers; it becomes shorter and smaller in diameter during the first few weeks after injury. Microscopically, there is disappearance of connective tissue cells in the area of injury. The entire process seems to support the hypothesis that most tissues are naturally endowed with cells which have the capacity to synthesize new connective tissue and heal by formation of a scar.

The blood supply to tendons is more adequate than is generally appreciated. If blood-borne cells have potential for synthesizing scar

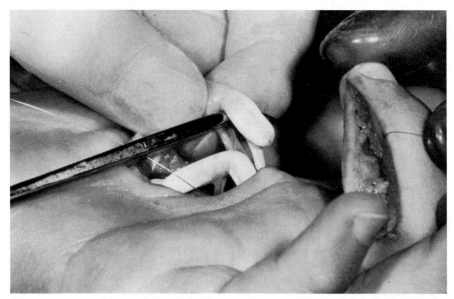

Figure 8–2. Atrophic rounded end of a flexor tendon cut within the digital sheath. Note absence of any proliferation of tissue from cut end of tendon.

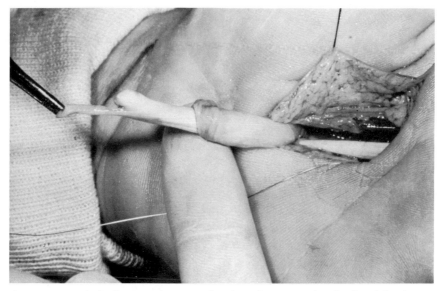

Figure 8–3. End of a flexor tendon cut within the palm, proximal to the digital sheath. Note rounded, atrophic end of the tendon; longitudinally oriented scar tissue has been misinterpreted as proliferation of tendon but actually is a condensation of dense, newly synthesized connective tissue around the tendon.

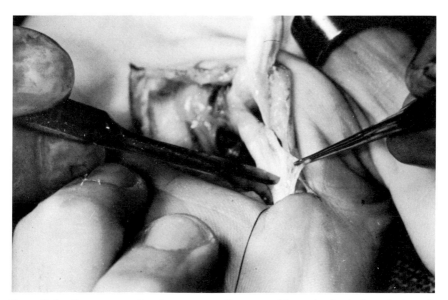

Figure 8–4. Dense connective tissue surrounding severed flexor tendon in the palm is easily distinguished from mature tendon. It can be dissected cleanly from tendons.

tissue, it seems likely that a scar could be produced at the end of a tendon even though the tendon was isolated from surrounding tissues. When the ends of a tendon are isolated from surrounding loose connective tissue, however, restoration of tendon continuity does not occur; thus we assume that repair of a tendon by formation of a dense connective tissue scar is dependent upon migration of cells from other areas which have the ability to synthesize fibrous protein, mucopolysaccharides, and so forth. Interestingly, cells with such reparative potential apparently are not located in the digital sheath of long flexor tendons. This conclusion is based on the clinical observation that tendons which break within an intact sheath or retract into an uninjured portion of sheath also undergo atrophic changes without evidence of regeneration. This finding has important clinical implications in the repair of digital flexor tendons.

When the end of a severed tendon retracts or is left in loose connective tissue, an interesting development occurs which has led many observers to the erroneous conclusion that severed tendon ends have regenerative potential similar to that of the severed end of a peripheral nerve. Over a period of six to eight weeks, the loose connective tissue (presumably all newly synthesized in the wound crater) becomes remodeled in opposite directions. The effect may be so perfect that casual observation leads to the conclusion that the tendon has sprouted new collagenous bundles which have grown out and become attached to a fixed structure. What has actually happened, however, is that the tendon stump has become atrophic and rounded, as is the case when the injury occurs within a digital sheath or an artificial barrier. In an area where cells have the ability to synthesize new connective tissue, the wound then becomes filled at first with gelatinous, and then with dense fibrous scar. Following synthesis of such a scar, an uncanny remodeling may occur which sometimes results in a portion of the previously nonpolarized scar becoming longitudinally oriented while another area of the same scar becomes oriented in a transverse direction. Thus, an early invisible, and later grossly discernible, plane develops, with the result that a new tendinous structure appears to lie in a new fibrous sheath. Close examination of both the longitudinally and transversely oriented areas of the remodeled scar reveals, however, that neither structure is identical with normal tendon or normal tendon sheath. The color of the newly synthesized tissue is a paler white than tendon or sheath, and the cellular components are both qualitatively and quantitatively different from that found in normal tendon or sheath. Moreover, careful gross dissection and microscopic examination of the juncture between severed tendon and new regenerate reveals that there is no continuity between the end of the tendon and new connective tissue. The new tissue is superbly woven *around* the tendon, but one can dissect it easily from the injured tendon without cutting across a major collagen bundle. The entire effect has been produced by an unbelieva-

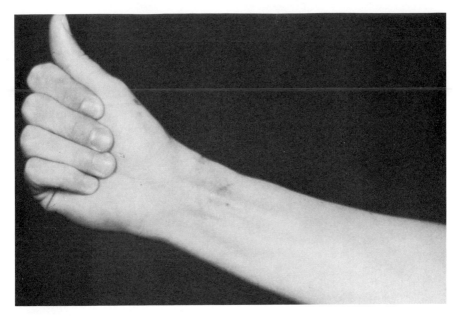

Figure 8–5.   Forced flexion view of wrist to show apparent reconstitution of the flexor carpi radialis longus after laceration. The flexor carpi radialis tendon in this patient was *not* repaired.

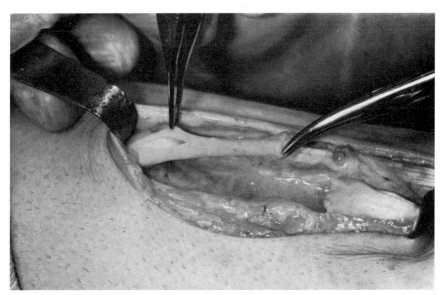

Figure 8–6.   Operative view of same wrist shown in Figure 8–5. Note that newly synthesized dense connective tissue connecting ends of flexor carpi radialis longus is clearly discernible and easily dissected from mature tendon. Between tendon ends it is longitudinally polarized, while around the tendon it is transversely oriented to provide a gliding surface. Thus two areas in the same scar have become remodeled in opposite directions to provide continuity between tendon ends and a nonadherent gliding surface. (From E. E. Peacock, Jr., Surg. Clin. N. Amer. 45:461, 1965.)

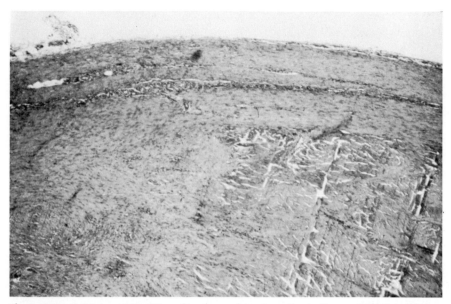

Figure 8–7. Microscopic junction of tendon and newly synthesized connective tissue shown in Figures 8–5 and 8–6. Note that newly synthesized connective tissue surrounds the old tendon but does not appear to be a proliferation of tissue from within it.

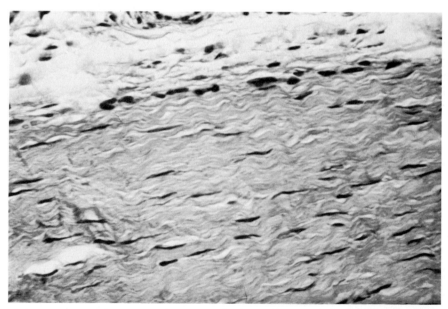

Figure 8–8. Microscopic view of interface between newly synthesized longitudinal scar and gliding surface shown in Figures 8–5 and 8–6. Note longitudinally oriented dense connective tissue surrounded by transversely oriented vascular and loosely arranged tissue. At one time both tissues were part of a single homogeneous scar.

bly efficient secondary remodeling process which has caused collagen fibrils that are not longitudinally oriented to disappear while longitudinally oriented fibrils accrue more monomeric particles in that portion of the scar. Simultaneously, the reverse is occurring in another area of the scar with the result that transverse polarity is developed. The final product is a remarkably efficient yet abortive attempt to reform—not regenerate—a tendon with gliding potential. Although the appearance of such a reaction may suggest that gliding function could occur, the authors have seldom seen a tendon formed in this manner actually develop gliding function over a substantial amplitude. In other words, the effect of regeneration looks better than it works, although in some areas, such as the volar surface of the wrist and forearm, a reformed flexor carpi radialis, which normally has a relatively small amplitude of motion, may contribute some power to gross function such as flexion of the wrist.

The process just described, which often results in what appears to be a regenerating tendon, occurs predictably when tendons have been lacerated in loose connective tissue such as in the wrist or midpalm of the hand. Almost as predictably, tendons lacerated within a digital sheath are found with rounded atrophic ends and with no evidence of regeneration. These findings suggest that tendon and tendon sheath usually do not contain cells with the potential to synthesize new

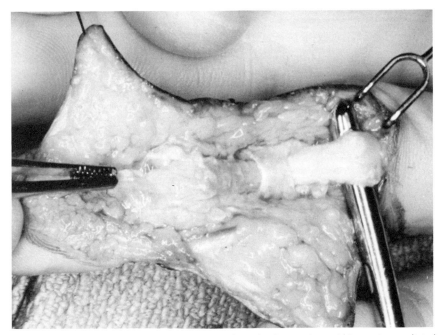

Figure 8–9. Apparent regeneration of ruptured profundus tendon within an intact digital sheath. No gliding function was detectable. In the author's experience, this condition is found only when rupture occurs in a distal portion of the tendon.

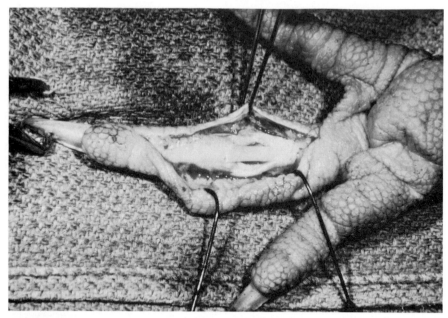

Figure 8–10. Operative view of flexor profundus and flexor sublimis tendons in the long digit of a chicken's foot. Passage of the profundus tendon through the sublimis within an annular sheath is very similar to that of the flexor tendons and sheath in a human finger. (Reproduced by permission from J. W. Madden and E. E. Peacock, Jr., Surgery, 63:288, 1968.)

collagen and that regenerate is the product of externally derived cells. When the digital sheath has been lacerated and the lacerated tendon end remains in the sheath wound and does not retract into an uninjured portion of the sheath, scar tissue remodeled to resemble tendon regenerate may be found at the end of the divided tendon similar to that encountered at the end of divided tendons outside the sheath. Such observations do not weaken the hypothesis that mature tendon cannot synthesize new dense connective tissue; practically every ruptured tendon within an intact sheath is found with rounded atrophic ends. Once in the author's (E.E.P.) experience a ruptured flexor profundus tendon within an intact sheath was found to be connected to beautifully remodeled, newly synthesized dense connective tissue strongly resembling regenerated tendon connecting the distally avulsed profundus tendon with the distal phalanx. No gliding function was present, however. Others have reported an occasional case of what appeared to be regeneration of tendon within an intact sheath. In the author's case, regeneration was relatively distal and it may be that the wound of the periosteum where Sharpey's fibers were broken was the wound that produced cells with synthetic capability. Other cases, if observed accurately, may have similar explanations or may simply be the exception which accompanies every biological rule.

DEVELOPMENT OF GLIDING FUNCTION

Although remodeling of a large scar to resemble a whole new tendon and bed is seldom functional, the potential for selective morphological change, as shown in Figure 8-3, is probably fundamental to development of gliding function following repair of all injured tendons. Restoration of an entire section of a tendon and sheath is simply more than the secondary remodeling process can accomplish, but secondary remodeling of a relatively small scar between two accurately coapted tendon ends and the tissue which surrounds the junction is well within the realm of biological possibility. The end result of the process has been fairly accurately defined; the exact mechanisms by which it produces gliding function and the measures which a physician might take to assure success are still vague.

The sequence of events which leads to gliding function can be hypothesized by speculating as to what might bridge the gap between what has been observed in animal experiments and what has been found during dissection of human tendons which functioned or failed to function following surgical repair. Although most surgeons are thoroughly familiar with the gross and microscopic findings in various tissues involved in the healing of a tendon repair or graft that did not function, there has been little opportunity to study the same tissues in human tendon restorations that did function satisfactorily. The intricate and biologically specific anatomical arrangement of flexor tendons found in human digits does not exist in any other species, with the possible exception of some primates. Therefore, although some valuable general principles about how scar is synthesized and repair occurs in injured tendons have been gained from animal experimentation, some of the most important details upon which gliding function in human tendons depends simply cannot be studied in animal extremities.

The experimental animal which has been found so far to be best for study of gliding function in long tendons is the chicken. The flexor profundus tendon to the long central digit in a chicken has many of the anatomical configurations which characterize the flexor mechanism in human fingers. The most important difference in the chicken flexor mechanism, compared to that found in human digits, is that the central long digit in chickens has more than one sublimis tendon.

MECHANISM OF HEALING

The complex anatomical arrangement of mesentery-nourished flexor tendons passing through each other and coursing along an elaborate system of pulleys so that direction is changed at appropriate levels also is found in the hands of some primates, but the small size of the structures and the lack of cooperation during postoperative training and study have discouraged most investigators from working with them. From data that have been obtained from animal experiments and from observations surgeons have made during operations on human fingers, the following sequence of events can be assumed to occur following surgical coaption of a divided long tendon: Fibroblasts from surrounding loose connective tissue migrate into the wound which includes the space between tendon ends. That some tissues through which tendons may be injured are more highly endowed with these specialized cells than others is a likely assumption with important clinical implications. Fibroblasts synthesize and discharge monomeric collagen and various mucopolysaccharides needed for synthesis of mature scar into the intercellular milieu. Rapid polymerization of monomeric subunits converts the initial fine reticular network immersed in a viscous ground substance into discernible fibrils and finally into a dense connective tissue scar. At this early stage, the scar is uniform in consistency, physical properties, and distribution throughout the wound. In long tendons which are destined to regain useful amplitudes of motion, however, the uniformity of the process is interrupted as selective differentiation of various parts of the scar begins to occur.

It is easy to understand why, before the importance of secondary remodeling of scar tissue was recognized, so many efforts were directed toward attempting to influence the synthetic phase of scar development. Almost every conceivable substance was evaluated as a potential artificial barrier between healing tendon and the rest of the wound. Blood vessels, amniotic membrane, and foreign body-produced scar tissue are but a few examples of biological membranes which were mechanically interposed between repaired tendons and the wound in which they lay. After World War II, practically every new synthetic substance with intriguing physical properties also was evaluated. All of these experiments confirmed what was surmised from studies performed in 1929: namely, that healing between tendon ends is dependent upon migration of cells from outside the tendon into the defect between tendon ends. Successful isolation of a tendon anastomosis from tissues which naturally contain these cells invariably results in failure of healing other than formation of a serum and fibrin clot. More sophisticated studies on the blood supply of tendons later revealed that although tendon is surprisingly well endowed with longitudinally oriented intrinsic blood vessels, the vessels are not capable of nourishing more than one-fourth of the tendon without collateral connections from larger external vessels. To add insult to injury, successful isolation of a tendon over any significant distance not only prevents healing, by denying cells with synthetic potential access to the wound, but also produces necrosis of a critical portion of the tendon because of impairment of revascularization. The last brief flare of excitement over the possibility of isolating tendon from surrounding scar was provoked by

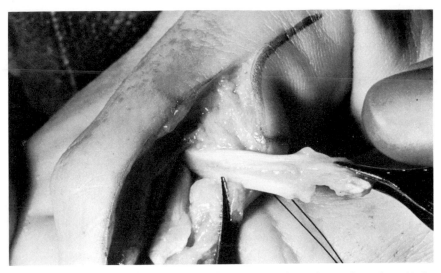

Figure 8–11.   Mesentery containing specialized coiled blood vessels on volar surface of index flexor profundus tendon.

development of Millipore membrane. The proponents of a Millipore sheath or barrier to separate a tendon wound into separate sections hypothesized that Millipore interstices would permit diffusion of gases and nutrients to the tendon but not passage of large cells and collagen

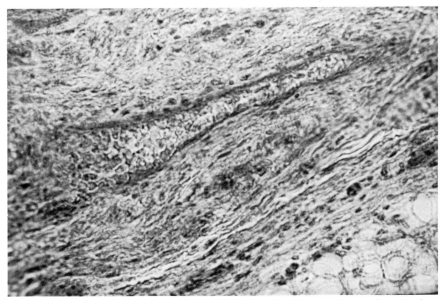

Figure 8–12.   Longitudinally oriented intrinsic blood supply of a mature human flexor tendon. (Reproduced by permission from E. E. Peacock, Jr., Ann. Surg., *149*:415, 1959.)

subunits. Failure of Millipore membranes to isolate adequately an area of tendon repair put to rest for a while the intriguing, but biologically unsound, notion that surgical isolation of an area of repaired tendon was feasible. Accumulation of data on the mechanism and importance of secondary remodeling of deep scar tissue has channeled the thoughts of most investigators along more biologically oriented lines during the last decade.

Dissection of scar tissue surrounding flexor tendon grafts which have developed an amplitude of motion sufficient to provide finger flexion reveals a different type of tissue from that encountered around grafts or anastomoses which do not glide. Thus, failure to glide seems to be related to physical characteristics of scar tissue surrounding the graft and not to the absence, deficiency, elasticity, or breaking of scar tissue. It is important to note that, within certain limits, the amount of scar tissue surrounding a tendon does not seem to be as critical as the physical characteristics of scar tissue. Of course, abnormally large deposits of scar which are seen occasionally, particularly after a complication such as hematoma or infection, markedly restrict motion, and it seems reasonable to predict that remodeling has a better chance to lessen the restrictive qualities of scar if the scar is a small one. Within the limits of usual or normal amount of scar, however, gliding or restriction of gliding can be produced by relatively large or small

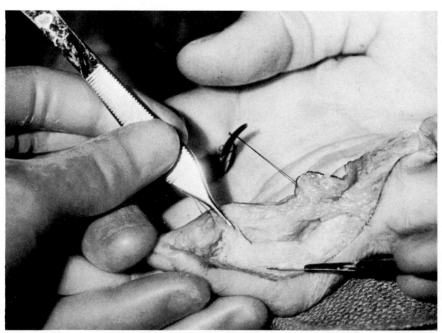

Figure 8–13. Postoperative adhesions restricting motion in a repaired flexor tendon. (From E. E. Peacock, Jr., Surg. Clin. N. Amer. *45*:461, 1965.)

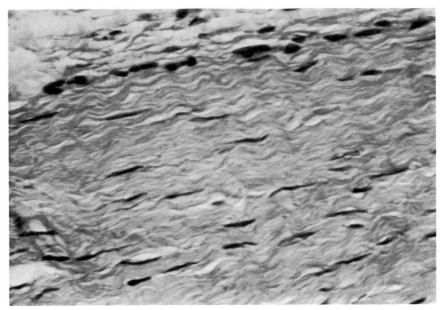

Figure 8–14. Microscopic appearance of adhesions in Figure 8–13. Note compact longitudinally oriented collagen fibers and cells. Secondary remodeling of tissue in these adhesions resembles normal tendon and resists longitudinal deformation necessary for movement of the graft. (From E. E. Peacock, Jr., Surg. Clin. N. Amer. *45*:461, 1965.)

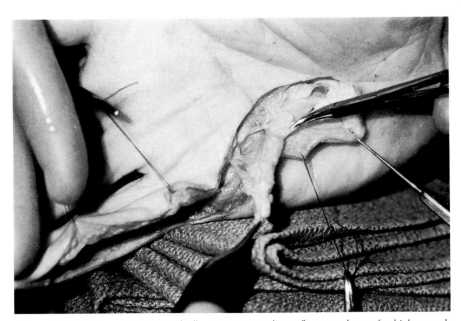

Figure 8–15. Gross appearance of adhesions surrounding a flexor tendon graft which moved adequately for normal flexion. Note the length and flimsy nature of adhesions. (From E. E. Peacock, Jr., Surg. Clin. N. Amer. *45*:461, 1965.)

amounts of fibrous tissue. Adhesions are not absent or even noticeably diminished around functioning grafts. Moreover, they are not elastic and do not differ in any other perceptible way from restricting adhesions except in their length. Gross examination in the evolution of nonrestrictive scar tissue suggests that, at some time, reduction in lateral cross-linking or friction between subunits permitted longitudinal slipping so that elongation of the entire adhesion occurred. The inescapable conclusion would seem to be that repaired tendons either glide or fail to glide because circumferential adhesions elongate or fail to elongate. This is an important consideration, for, if true, it changes many prevailing concepts concerning postoperative activation of repaired tendons. Currently popular techniques of occupational and physical therapy are based almost entirely on the concept of breaking or stretching adhesions, just as many equally popular surgical maneuvers are based on the concept of preventing adhesions. In all probability neither concept is accurate. Considerable evidence is available to show that adhesions are part of normal wound healing and that blood vessels intermingled with fibrous elements are needed for nourishment of the tendon. The very nature of the progress patients undergo while reactivating repaired tendon indicates that, usually, there is no sudden breaking of restricting forces. An almost imperceptible gradual gain in motion strongly suggests that slowly developing changes in the physical properties of dense connective tissue are responsible for increased motion. The end result leads us to the idea that the remodeling process primarily develops length in bundles of collagenous fibers.

If this hypothesis is correct, the mechanism by which length is gained becomes crucial in a biological approach to restoration of gliding function. Microscopic examination of adhesions which restrict motion reveals that the type of fibril organization in them is very different from that in adhesions which are not restrictive. Both types of adhesions are vascular, but the more vascular appearance of nonrestricting adhesions suggests either that blood vessels are more plentiful or that they are more coiled so that the same vessel is seen several times. The most striking microscopic features in restricting adhesions are regular organization, compact arrangement, and longitudinal polarity of collagen fibers. Although the physical arrangement of various fibrils is so different that one might wonder if one structure is actually not elastic and the other rigid, such gross physical differences are not discernible. It does not take much imagination to suppose, however, that application of longitudinal force would be more effective in causing elongation for one than it would for the other. To pursue this question further, one needs to know whether longitudinal slippage occurs at a molecular, fibril, fiber, or fiber-bundle level. Although the question is definitely open to research with modern techniques of measuring cross-linking and by three-dimensional scanning electron microscopy to visualize the effect of stress and strain on fibrous material, we simply do not have

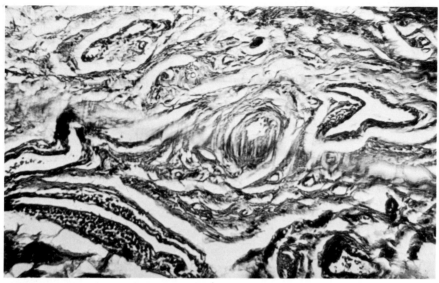

Figure 8–16.   Microscopic appearance of adhesions shown in Figure 8–15. Note vascularity and disorganized arrangement of collagen fibers. (From E. E. Peacock, Jr., Surg. Clin. N. Amer. 45:461, 1965.)

data at this time which permit anything more than speculation as to the exact plane where lengthening occurs in human adhesions. Because chemical bonding is relatively strong and the distances which can be spanned are so small, it seems more likely that alteration occurs in the physical weave of relatively large subunits rather than in chemical cross-links. Certainly the different appearance of restricting and nonrestricting adhesions in the light microscope points to the fiber and fibril level as the plane where secondary alterations providing increased length occur. The distances between units of this magnitude are in the range of several micra, or roughly 2000 times too great to be influenced by chemical bonds. In laboratory preparations, however, artificial insertion of amide or methyl cross-links so dramatically alters physical properties of connective tissue that manipulation and alteration of cross-links must not be eliminated from investigation at this time.

The only evidence that chemical cross-links may be involved in alteration of physical properties of newly synthesized adhesions is that similar tissue in the scar of a healing incised and sutured wound of dermis can be influenced significantly by adding cross-links no more than a few angstroms in length. The significance of this finding is not clear, however; at present most investigators subscribe to longitudinal slippage or friction-induced instability of fibers and fibrils as the most probable method by which additional length is obtained. Why some bundles are woven together in extremely efficient longitudinally oriented units while others respond to longitudinal force by undergoing fibril slippage and becoming elongated is not clear. The answer probably lies in the effect of selective collagen aggregation and collagenolytic activity. The final appearance of restricting adhesions suggests that longitudinally oriented fibrils accrue more monomeric particles, while transverse or nonoriented fibrils are gradually removed by selective collagenolytic activity. This hypothesis could be tested by present methods of measuring collagen synthesis and lysis, provided an appropriate experimental model could be developed.

Microscopic examination of adhesions which restrict motion of tendons reveals that the alignment of cells and fibers is very similar to that in normal tendon. Examination of nonrestrictive adhesions reveals a striking similarity to the architecture of loose areolar tissue commonly found around tendons with long amplitudes of motion outside a fibrous sheath. This material is often referred to as paratenon; it is vascular and randomly arranged and does not contain large fiber bundles. In contrast, the scar between two surgically coapted tendon ends remodels to look almost exactly like normal tendon. The new connective tissue is packed densely, oriented longitudinally, and arranged in large bundles. One can literally predict what the architectural arrangement of remodeled scar tissue will be by noting the effect the scar has on tendon function. The important question, of course, is what causes secondary remodeling to follow one course in some patients and another course in others. Even more perplexing, why does one portion of the scar remodel to produce great physical strength while another portion of the same scar remodels in a way to permit elongation in response to longitudinal force? A possible answer to these questions, which also would support the clinical impression that care in handling and suturing tendons influences the amount of motion they regain, follows.

From a morphological standpoint, it appears that newly synthesized scar tissue remodels according to the architecture of tissue with which it is in juxtaposition. This statement seems particularly true with newly synthesized tissue which remodels in close proximity to injured tissue. Almost invariably, new connective tissue synthesized between two tendon ends, and therefore in contact with the cut surface of tendon, will remodel to look almost exactly like the tendons it joins. Similarly, if a tendon is damaged along its longitudinal surface by rough handling or a partial laceration so that the interior of the tendon is exposed, scar tissue in that area often will exert a severe restricting influence and be found to resemble normal tendon. These two facts are fairly certain, as many observations on adherent immovable tendons have been made in animal and human extremities. Because we have so few histological observations on functioning human flexor tendons, however, the next supposition, that nonrestricting adhesions have remodeled to resemble paratenon, is not nearly so certain. The few observations we have on functioning human grafts, plus the general notion most surgeons support that careful handling of a tendon reduces the restrictive nature of postoperative adhesions, suggest that if a thin film of paratenon is maintained around a tendon, scar tissue which forms around it will remodel so that it has the same characteristics as normal paratenon. If this hypothesis is true, it would seem that mature connective tissues exert a sort of induction influence on newly synthesized connective tissue and that secondary remodeling can be influenced by assuring that newly synthesized fibrous tissue comes in contact only with the type of tissue one would like the scar to resemble ultimately. Although the hypothesis that an inductor influence controls secondary remodeling is pure speculation at this time, it is mentioned now because it provides a biological basis for some of the technical maneuvers which seem to have influenced favorably the results of surgical repair of flexor tendons. Even if other factors, such as chemical, electrical, or mechanical influences, ultimately are shown to influence secondary remodeling of tendon adhesions, the present working hypothesis that remodeling is influenced, to some extent, by the amount of trauma and subsequent tissue damage probably will still be useful in surgical repair of these structures. Having covered the known facts and advanced several theses by which these facts can be related and explained, we will now consider how technical maneuvers can be analyzed and how decisions in clinical situations can be reached on a biological basis.

TECHNICAL ASPECTS OF TENDON REPAIR

A consideration of the technical aspects of tendon repair should be divided with respect to wounds involving extensor tendons and wounds involving flexor tendons. Extensor tendons have such relatively short amplitudes of motion (5 mm.) that mild restriction of motion does not significantly retard active extension of a digit. The main objective usually cited in repairing an extensor tendon is to obtain structural continuity without changing the overall length of the musculotendinous unit. The objectives are very different in repair of a flexor tendon, which may have to pass through a 5 to 7 cm. range of motion to flex the long finger completely.

Principles of Extensor Tendon Repair

The most serious complication following repair of an extensor tendon is adherence over a long distance while the metacarpophalangeal joint is immobilized in extension. The checkrein effect of an adherent extensor tendon is much more serious when the metacarpophalangeal joint is in extension than when it is in mid- or complete flexion. A moderate checkrein effect on the long extensor tendon is usually reflected more in proximal interphalangeal function than metacarpophalangeal joint function. Most movements of the hand are embarrassed more by limitation of motion in the interphalangeal than metacarpophalangeal joints. A patient with adherence of an extensor to osseous callus surrounding a fractured metacarpal shaft usually can flex the metacarpophalangeal joint by completely extending the distal and proximal interphalangeal joints. The proximal interphalangeal joint and the distal interphalangeal joints can be flexed (and then only partially), however, only when the metacarpophalangeal joint is maintained in extension. Active extension of all joints usually will be possible even though complete flexion of the joints simultaneously is impossible. The important principle is that a greater amplitude of motion of the extensor hood is required for simultaneous flexion of all three finger joints than is required for simultaneous extension. The intrinsic muscles extend the interphalangeal joints, even if proximal adhesions permit only enough movement of the long extensor to extend the metacarpophalangeal joint. Simultaneous flexion of all finger joints requires rather extensive mobilization of the extensor mechanism, and thus even slight restriction of movement of this structure will be more disabling during flexion than extension.

Divided extensor tendons can be repaired in any wound in which skin can be closed primarily. They usually should be repaired, unless an immovable structure such as a metacarpal also is injured at exactly the same level. In addition to obvious displaced fractures, other injuries such as partial saw cuts into a metacarpal or severe abrasions denuding a large area of bone should be considered unfavorable wounds in which to repair tendons. To repair an extensor tendon in the wound with an immovable structure which also is going to be healing means that, although active extension may be restored, full passive flexion of distal joints will not be possible, and a second operation will be needed. In wounds where a segment of extensor tendon has been lost by injury or debridement, it is even more important not to replace the lost tendon with a graft when bone is also damaged. Invariably, the metacarpophalangeal joint will become tenodesed in extension. During the three weeks required for tendon healing and the four to six weeks which elapse before the patient and his physician realize that mobilization of the joint is impossible, collateral ligament and joint capsule become permanently shortened so that capsulotomy and collateral ligament excision may be needed to regain passive flexion. This complication can be avoided by delaying extensor tendon restoration until after the fracture has healed and soft tissue planes are reestablished.

A maneuver which can be used to restore extension of the central two digits (ring and long) during primary repair of a dorsal metacarpal injury is to bypass the proximal wound and insert extensor power in the form of circumferential or lateral tendon transfers which are inserted into the extensor mechanism distal to the injury. The long and ring fingers frequently are injured selectively by penetrating wounds in the center of the hand, and occasionally a dorsal cut or blunt injury also will involve only these tendons. When central tendons alone are damaged, the primary wound in the center of the hand can be debrided, fractures reduced and stabilized, and soft tissue closed. As a sort of finale to the main operation, the surgeon can then make tiny (5 mm.) transverse incisions over the neck of all four finger metacarpals. Through these incisions the common extensor tendon to the index finger can be detached and displaced ulnarward for insertion into the extensor mechanism of the long finger. The common extensor tendon of the small finger can be detached and shifted radialward to empower the extensor mechanism of the ring finger. These small transfers add only a few minutes of operating time, do not change significantly the mechanism of hand function, and restore central digit extension primarily without introducing the hazard of adherence of long extensor tendons at the site of a healing fracture. It is very important while performing these procedures (or during preparation of any dorsal wound where extensor tendon fragments and bone are exposed) to debride the distal tendon fragments thoroughly so that they do not cause a distal tenodesis by adhering to an immovable structure.

Most surgeons do not attempt to repair extensor tendons in a wound in which bone is exposed; yet the incidence of metacarpophalangeal joint damage is still high because even an unrepaired distal tendon fragment can become incarcerated in dorsal scar. No matter what secondary procedure is planned, divided distal tendons should be excised as far distal in the wound as necessary to leave them in movable uninjured tissue. If adequate soft tissue is not present between the wound and the metacarpophalangeal joints, distal tendon fragments should be removed distal to the metacarpophalangeal joint so that the joint cannot possibly be held in extension. Whether a free graft or an appropriate transfer ultimately is selected to provide active extension, the procedure will not be complicated by the necessity to construct the proximal tendon unit long enough to insert into the extensor hood distal to the metacarpophalangeal joint.

The mechanical aspects of extension are designed to produce rapidity of motion rather than power or precise control. The extensor tendons exert their force on the fingers close to the axis of rotation of the metacarpophalangeal joints; they are not mechanically efficient to move a long lever arm. The length of the motor unit which provides extension, therefore, is much more critical than in other tendons which have a different mechanical advantage. It follows that adjustment of tension during repair by tendon graft or transfer is more important than in repair of some other tendons. Although adherence of an extensor tendon to an immovable object may tenodese a finger in extension, a transfer or graft which is slightly too short will not prevent distal flexion, provided it is movable. Excursion of the tendon is so small, and the mechanical advantage so poor, that almost any amount of motion in the tendon will permit useful flexion. The reverse condition is not true, however. A tendon transfer or graft which is even slightly too long produces a very significant deformity, and in most cases complete extension is not possible even with the wrist in midflexion.

Because a motor unit which is too short is seldom disabling (provided it is movable) and a motor unit which is even slightly too long is very disabling, many hand surgeons have adopted the principle that an extensor restoration cannot be made too tight provided it is movable. Certainly the wrist and metacarpophalangeal joints should be in extension while tension is adjusted. The familiar practice of placing all of the finger and wrist joints in extreme hyperextension for three weeks during tendon healing should not be continued. Proximal and distal interphalangeal joints simply cannot be immobilized safely in an extreme position for that length of time without a high risk of permanent stiffness.

EXTENSOR TENDON GRAFTS.   The technique of performing a distal anastomosis in an extensor tendon graft should be considered in some detail. Although it has not been apparent in human tendon anastomoses (largely because there seldom has been an opportunity to examine a human tendon junction during the first few weeks following repair), the gap which invariably develops between tendon ends during the second and third week of healing is a striking feature of tendon healing in experimental animals. The gap in a chicken flexor profundus tendon repaired by a buried figure-of-eight wire may be as long as 4 mm. It is probably caused by a loss of transverse stability between collagen bundles as the secondary remodeling stage begins. Even a slight loss of transverse stability permits sutures to pull through the tendon just enough to create a small gap between tendon ends. The gap occurs at a time when the ends are held together by only a relatively weak gel and when collagenolytic activity also is increased. The scar produced at this time may be 3 or 4 mm. in length and will elongate the entire motor unit by that amount. Although a few millimeters' elongation in a flexor tendon unit is unimportant, the efficiency of an extensor unit operating within a small range of motion at the base of a long lever arm often is significantly impaired.

The best technique to prevent gap formation and elongation of a restored extensor unit is to suture the graft to the distal extensor mechanism in an overlay fashion. Because adhesions at the site of insertion are not of any functional significance, it is not necessary to perform a perfect end-to-end approximation of tendon ends. The distal end of a graft or transfer should be scarified on the underside and placed on top of a similarly scarified strip of central tendon of the extensor mechanism. At least three permanent mattress-type sutures are used to attach the graft to the central slip. Although some elongation may occur after an anastomosis of this type, the danger of clinically significant elongation is usually eliminated by having a broad area of contact between tendons and by using multiple strong permanent sutures to maintain the scarified tendon surfaces in close approximation. The proximal anastomosis in an extensor tendon graft causes a greater problem, because a bulky anastomosis cannot be put in the retinacular area. Even though the dorsal retinacular ligament is broad, and considerable portions of it can be excised without producing a bowstring effect, extensor tendons are very superficial in the wrist and dorsal metacarpal areas, and a large subcutaneous mass is unsightly and subjectively annoying. The best solution to the problem is to place these anastomoses in the most proximal position possible. An anastomosis placed high in the forearm just distal to the musculotendinous junction is both more functional and less visible than one placed in the wrist or metacarpal area. Short extensor tendon grafts seldom are as functional as long grafts which can be atraumatically threaded through the retinacular space so that a bowstring effect is not produced. One should not try to remove the proximal end of a damaged tendon, for the many lateral connections and dense fibrous adhesions which develop after injury often make it impossible to withdraw the tendon through a single proximal incision. It is usually necessary to open the entire extensor space to take out an extensor tendon, and this should not be

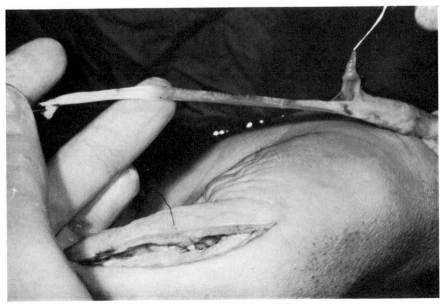

Figure 8–17.   Appearance of an end-weave anastomosis of flexor tendons three weeks after repair. Area of anastomosis is approximately 2.5 times the size of the tendon and is surrounded by adherent soft tissue.

done during a secondary reconstructive procedure. The damaged tendon should simply be bypassed with as little trauma as possible.

SIMPLE REPAIR OF EXTENSOR TENDONS.   Repair of a severed extensor tendon where loss of tendon has not occurred is relatively simple as far as restoring complete extension is concerned. It should be remembered, however, that restoration of extension following damage to an extensor tendon is not the only objective. Another important objective, which is frequently overlooked, involves avoiding loss of simultaneous full flexion of all finger joints. This complication is usually thought to be due to joint stiffness, or it is assumed that it will improve spontaneously with passage of time, and if active extension is present after repair of the tendon, the result is usually classified as successful. In our experience, however, a substantial number of such patients, even though they are able to extend the fingers superbly, are unable to flex the proximal and distal interphalangeal joints completely without extending the metacarpophalangeal joint to nearly 180 degrees. Because this is not a serious disability for most people and because it is thought to be only temporary by some observers, this complication of extensor tendon repair usually is not mentioned. Perfection following repair of an extensor tendon injury is difficult to obtain, however, and imperfections usually can be measured in terms of loss of passive flexion arc, not in failure to restore active extension.

Perfection in extensor tendon restoration requires special attention to a number of technical details. To begin with, it is important to be certain that repair of a tendon is not done unnecessarily. Sometimes extensor tendons are repaired simply because they are lacerated, not because active extension of a digit has been lost. Particularly in the central two digits, there is such a complex network of tendon ramifications that a proximal division of a common tendon may not impair active extension. In addition, some patients have more than one communis tendon to all of the digits, and many patients have two or more common extensor tendons to the long and ring fingers. Extensor tendons do not retract after they have been divided; they are usually visible in the soft tissue wound if the surgeon can locate the correct plane. If finger extension is normal after division of a single tendon in the proximal metacarpal or wrist area, both ends of the divided tendon should be pulled out of the wound as far as possible and cut so they will retract into undamaged soft tissue where adherence to central scar will not occur. To repair such a tendon not only would not improve hand function, but would provide an opportunity for subsequent adherence of the tendon which might limit passive finger flexion.

A second reason for not repairing some tendons primarily is that they would have to be anastomosed in an unsatisfactory wound. A wound in which injured bone is exposed, for instance, is clearly not a satisfactory wound for primary repair of tendons. Other conditions, such as extensive undermining of soft tissue, introduction of large

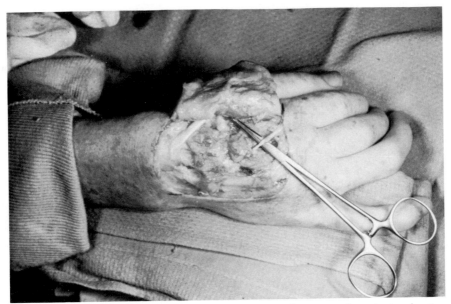

Figure 8–18. Adherence of a divided extensor tendon to callus surrounding a fractured metacarpal. Distal ends of lacerated extensor tendons should never be left in such a wound as they invariably will adhere to the fracture site and restrict flexion of the metacarpophalangeal joint.

amounts of foreign material, and damage to tendon over a relatively long distance, also militate against primary repair in patients in whom perfect flexion is needed in addition to active extension. The distal bypass principle described previously is applicable to these wounds and is a good solution to complicated wounds involving central digits. When a distal transfer is not a feasible procedure, debridement of injured tendons back into normal tissue is preferable to repairing a damaged tendon in a bad bed. An old principle of tendon surgery which has been helpful in making these decisions is that a good tendon can be passed through a bad bed or a bad tendon can be passed through a good bed, but good results cannot be expected when a bad tendon is placed in a bad bed. This rule was developed almost entirely for guidance in restoring flexor tendons, where an injury within the sheath mechanism, almost by definition, means a bad bed. If perfection is sought, however, the rule has important connotations in extensor tendon repair also.

There are differences in degrees of bad and good for both the tendon and the bed; these differences must be recognized when the above rule is applied to an extensor mechanism injury. Whereas any anastomosis in a flexor tendon restoration must be considered a bad tendon at that point, a carefully repaired extensor tendon is not necessarily a bad tendon, and a neatly repaired extensor tendon can function in a good or a bad bed if other conditions are favorable. An extensor tendon which has been abraded or frayed a considerable distance may be a bad tendon, regardless of how well it was repaired. If a damaged tendon remains in a bad bed, incarceration with limitation of distal finger flexion usually will occur. An abraded or partially avulsed extensor tendon in a relatively uninjured soft tissue bed where immovable structures are not exposed and surrounding soft tissue can heal with minimal chance of complication usually will function adequately. Tendons which are in continuity, even though severely damaged, should not be debrided or removed, regardless of how badly frayed or abraded they are. In wounds where damaged tendons are still in continuity, the surgeon's effort should be directed primarily toward improving the bed. The bed for a damaged tendon can be improved surgically by debridement and shifting of uninjured tissue to lie against the damaged tendon. A distant flap may occasionally be needed to provide a satisfactory cover, but this usually should be resorted to only when skin is missing and tendons are intact.

Anastomoses should be simple yet strong. An end-to-end anastomosis is adequate if special precautions are taken to avoid gap formation. Such precautions include using the largest practical suture which can be buried completely within the tendon, crossing the suture within each end of the tendon at least three times, making the passage through the tendon more horizontal than longitudinal, and tying the suture under enough tension that the tendon becomes ruffled in an accordion-like manner. Invariably, the suture will slip through the tendon during the healing process; if one merely coapts the ends of the tendon without "drawing up" or "pleating" a little bit that portion of the tendon through which the suture passes, gap formation may be a problem. Of course, simply bringing tendon ends together with a single loop stitch may be sufficient to restore active extension. A more accurate approximation of tendon ends is advisable, however, if complete restoration of passive flexion also is to be achieved.

In the case of an extensor tendon graft, there is ample tendon for a more complex anastomosis. An end-weave technique, in which the tendon graft is woven at right angles to the proximal tendon, will provide a large surface contact between tendons, thus decreasing the danger of gap formation. Strong permanent sutures passed through both tendons assure immediate strength in an anastomosis of this type. The cut or raw end of the proximal tendon can be buried by wrapping the graft around it, a technique developed by Brand and shown in Figure 8–43. This is probably the most elegant tendon anastomosis now in use, but it cannot be used in tight spaces such as in a finger or on the dorsum of the hand or wrist because it is a bulky anastomosis. It is also not suitable for repairing a simple laceration, because considerable tendon substance is used in performing the proximal weave and shrouding the distal end of the proximal stump.

Extensor tendon restorations should remain immobilized for three weeks, but the proximal and distal interphalangeal joints of involved fingers should not be immobilized during this period. With the wrist and metacarpophalangeal joints in full extension, the interphalangeal joint can be put through a complete range of active and passive motion without significantly altering tension on the healing anastomosis. As soon as the restraining splint or dressing has been removed—at the end of three weeks—the first objective should be to develop flexion of the metacarpophalangeal joints and, later, the wrist joint. If adequate wrist and metacarpophalangeal joint flexion can be obtained, active extension usually will follow. Active motion at the metacarpophalangeal joints can sometimes be improved by having the patient hold both interphalangeal joints in complete flexion while the metacarpophalangeal joints are flexed and extended rapidly. Flexion of the interphalangeal joints lessens the effect of the intrinsic muscles, and thus makes it possible for the patient to concentrate almost entirely on pure metacarpophalangeal joint extension produced by the long extensors. Active extension usually will be recovered almost simultaneously with attainment of passive flexion. If active extension does not return after passive flexion of the finger joints is possible, elongation of the extensor unit by dehiscence or gap formation should be suspected. As long as flexion is not complete, an adhesive process may account for inability to extend the digit. Because so much more long tendon excursion is needed to flex all of the finger joints simultaneously than is needed to obtain only metacarpophalangeal joint extension, disruption or elongation of a restored motor unit must be suspected if complete flexion is possible and active metacarpophalangeal joint extension is absent.

Failure of a restored extensor mechanism to extend actively the metacarpophalangeal joints because of elongation and dehiscence can be corrected only by reoperating upon the extensor mechanism. Failure to develop complete flexion of the interphalangeal joints, however, cannot be solved so simply. A period of physical therapy may result in a gradual release of the extensor mechanism. Splinting often is of little value; it is very difficult to design a splint which will exert effective force on all of the interphalangeal joints at the end of their flexion arcs. A trial of nonoperative measures designed to produce longitudinal tension on the extensor mechanism is justifiable, however, on the basis that the restricting scar tissue undoubtedly undergoes secondary remodeling which might be favorably influenced by application of mechanical stress. From a biological standpoint, the weakness of this hypothesis is that there are so few data available about the effect of mechanical stress on scar tissue that we are not certain what the effect of mechanical stress on scar tissue is, much less when is the best time to apply such force. An excellent case can be made for suggesting that no physical force should be applied to a remodeling scar because application of unidirectional tension might enhance internal stabilization of the scar to resist external force.

The remodeling of bone appears to be mechanically directed, and the end result in that tissue is exactly the opposite of what is desired in tendon adhesions. One might also ask, if any appreciable effect of mechanical stress is reflected in secondary remodeling of fibrous tissue: Would not connective tissue between tendon ends be similarly affected? Of course, the only answer to this question is that, with our present understanding, we have to start almost with the supposition that remodeling in tendon scars must be radically different in various areas or no possibility of success exists. The fact that we do not understand *how* different types of remodeling can occur in separate areas of the scar does not keep us from developing a logical approach to activation of incarcerated tendons based on the fundamental premise that various types of remodeling do occur.

Considerable data are available to suggest that mechanical force could produce the exact opposite effect of what is sought in remodeling tendon scar, but there are also data to support the hypothesis that collagenous tissue reacts differently in some places than it does in others. Although mechanical force seems to influence the synthetic phase of collagen metabolism, secondary remodeling is not necessarily affected after periods of maximal collagen synthesis are over. For instance, skin wounds in areas where physical tension is great, such as around the shoulders or breasts in women, often are characterized by hypertrophic scars which may even approach keloid dimensions. That tension causes excess collagen production (or possibly decreased collagen degradation) is strongly supported by the fact that the most certain way to correct a hypertrophic scar is to relieve tension on skin by inserting more tissue or changing the direction of the scar. Both skin wounds and unwounded skin in laboratory animals contain significantly more extractable and total collagen when the wound or skin is under tension. That there is any difference in the internal organization of scars or normal skin, or that their overall reaction to external deformation is altered by mechanical force, has not been proved directly. There is evidence, however, that the collagenous structure around normal and some abnormal joints can be altered by continued mechanical stress. The contortions of a dancer or circus acrobat are familiar examples of the increased range of motion which can be developed by applying mechanical stress to restraining ligaments and membranes around movable joints. After the period of rapid collagen synthesis is complete in a healing skin wound, tension across the scar often produces a wide atrophic scar. Thus there is considerable evidence to support either hypothesis; the important thing to recognize now is that we simply do not have data needed to recommend with any degree of biological certainty that physical stress in a remodeling scar is either beneficial or detrimental.

The fact that pulling on a recalcitrant fibrous tissue scar has been followed in some instances by release of a contracture or development of motion where none existed before has been the basis for the faith many physicians have in physical manipulations. The extent of such faith is often more than present biological data can support, however. Time is an extremely important factor in the change of fibrous tissue scars. It is so easy for a group championing some discipline or approach to a problem to arrive on the scene at a time when naturally maturing or remodeling fibrous tissue processes are occurring, and thus assume that a cause-and-effect relation exists between observed changes and the treatment they administered. It is important to remember that no one has ever really challenged many time-honored principles of physical medicine, such as application of physical tension and change in temperature of tissues. For instance, no one has ever been willing to keep a tendon graft immobilized for six months to see if lack of mechanical tension on circumferential adhesions would cause them to become reduced in strength and internally deranged so that they could not resist longitudinal force. Of course, small joints would have to be put through a passive range of motion to prevent joint stiffness during such an extended period, but this could be accomplished without great difficulty.

TENOLYSIS.   An extensor tendon restoration which has become incarcerated in dorsal scar and does not respond to nonoperative treatment should be operated on if restriction of finger flexion is disabling. The results of surgical release of tendons are variable according to the area of the tendon involved. The most satisfactory results from tenol-

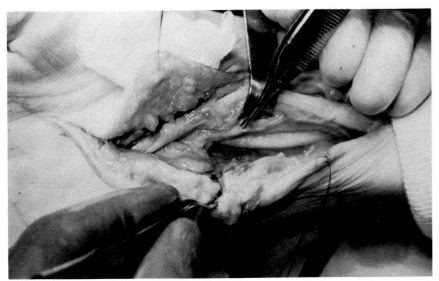

Figure 8–19. Appearance of an anastomosed tendon at the wrist three months after repair. Note flimsy quality of surrounding soft tissue. Although all of the tendons are connected by this tissue and move together, attachments to immovable structures have disappeared.

ysis in the hand can be achieved in the extensor mechanism if the scar is a small one producing adherence of the tendon in only one area. An example of a favorable situation is a sharply localized adherence of a finger extensor to a small callus surrounding a healed metacarpal or phalangeal fracture. Surgical therapy of this condition involves release of tendons, restoration of a soft tissue plane between the movable and immovable scar, wound healing without complications, early postoperative mobilization and flexion, and active and passive motion as soon as soft tissue healing permits. The only difficulty which might be encountered in this procedure is restoration of a soft tissue barrier between fixed and movable portions of the scar. When possible, a local flap of subcutaneous fat or superficial fascia or both can provide a satisfactory bed for the scarred tendon. Such an approach is dependent, however, upon being able to find adequate subcutaneous tissue in the immediate vicinity of the adherent tendon. In young children there is usually an abundant layer of fat beneath skin which can be split to form a separate layer to pass beneath a liberated tendon. Older children and adults lose excess subcutaneous tissue on the dorsum of the hand; in these patients, or in those in whom subcutaneous scar has replaced soft tissue, a free graft may be needed. A number of synthetic substances have been advocated for interposition between scarred tendons and immovable structures. At present a very thin sheet of Silastic membrane seems most satisfactory. As will be discussed later, Silastic polymer causes a distinctive type of foreign body reaction in the hand which seems to be more conducive to establishment of gliding function than other synthetic materials. The authors have always preferred a biological material, although use of such material is more empirically than biologically defensible.

PARATENON TRANSPLANTS. Tendons which are not encased in a thick fibrous tissue sheath, such as the digital theca around long flexor tendons, characteristically are surrounded by a distinctive type of loose areolar tissue commonly referred to as paratenon. Although paratenon is definitely areolar connective tissue as far as its gross microscopic classification is concerned, it has special characteristics not found in loose connective tissue elsewhere in the body. For instance, the blood vessels in paratenon are highly specialized coiled elastic vessels which nourish it without restricting amplitude of motion. More striking, however, is the slippery feel and appearance of paratenon. Although the biochemical composition of this interesting tissue has not been studied in depth, we do know that it has a high glycoprotein content as evidenced by increased sialic acid. The tissue has almost a mucoid character, which makes it nearly ideal for providing a low-resistance covering for unsheathed tendon. Paratenon is difficult to handle surgically, as it sticks to itself tenaciously and becomes rolled into a mucoid ball when handled like other tissues. A careful surgeon can take a graft of paratenon, however, by using traction sutures to outline the graft and then handling it only by the sutures. The volar surface of the flexor carpi ulnaris is a convenient donor site. Sutures are passed through the paratenon at the four corners of the proposed graft and an incision is then made outside the sutures. The free graft is lifted from the surface of the muscle by the sutures and passed immediately beneath the liberated tendon. The same traction sutures are then utilized to maintain the graft in its new position. Although there is no question that such a paratenon graft appears to influence favorably the outcome of a small tenolysis procedure, the more important question of why this is true is not so easy to answer. Transplantation of a copious amount of paratenon with a free tendon graft has not been nearly so effective in assuring adequate range of motion as it has in providing spot separation of movable and immovable scar from motor units with small amplitude of motion.

Paratenon is esthetically appealing, and a decade ago surgeons almost routinely advocated opening the forearm and leg along the entire course of a proposed tendon graft so that a graft could be lifted out of its bed with a generous supply of paratenon. Now, most surgeons not only do not advocate taking a free graft in this manner but actually take precautions to dissect redundant paratenon from a graft before it is placed in a new location. The reason for this change is that grafts surrounded by copious amounts of paratenon seem to become surrounded by a greater amount of scar tissue than grafts surrounded by only a thin membrane. Although more will be said about preparation of tendons for free grafts, it should be emphasized now that there is some reason to suggest that paratenon is highly endowed with cells capable of synthesizing fibrous tissue. Transplanting large quantities of paratenon to insure gliding in many situations, therefore, is suspect. The experience of the authors has been that in establishing a small localized barrier between an adherent extensor tendon and a metacarpal or phalangeal callus, a thin free paratenon graft from the volar surface of the flexor carpi ulnaris is of definite benefit.

FIBROSIS OF EXTENSOR MECHANISM.   Adherence of an extensor restoration is not always a localized problem, and the surgical approach to more generalized adherence may be disappointing. One of the most difficult problems in restorative hand surgery is involvement of the entire dorsum of the hand by a sort of sclerosing fibrosis which changes the consistency and other physical characteristics of many of the soft tissues. The initial injury leading to such a complication may be only a small laceration, although more characteristically it is caused by blunt trauma followed by massive edema. The biological pathway by which sclerosing fibrosis develops is not known precisely, but the end results are familiar. Surgical exploration of a hand several months after a severe dorsal injury that was followed by significant edema reveals that the entire extensor mechanism to single or multiple digits is adherent to surrounding tissues. Perhaps even more important than the fact that the tendons are adherent is the change in characteristics of the usual movable tissue to which the tendons have become adherent. These tissues are no longer movable, and the pathological process which has occurred is a general one which can be so extensive that subcutaneous fat, loose areolar tissue, and sometimes intrinsic muscles are affected.

In some patients, even though a direct injury to a tendon did not occur, the entire surface of the tendon may be attached to surrounding tissue. Surrounding tissues are not typical paratenon or subcutaneous fat, but are almost granular in appearance and consistency. Subcutaneous fat is lighter in color and much less elastic than normal. Although quantitative and qualitative measurements have not been made on these tissues, there seems little doubt that fibrous tissue elements have undergone proliferation and factors which contribute to elasticity and plasticity have been diminished.

The surgical approach to extensor fibrosis of the dorsum of the hand frequently produces less than optimal results. It is usually necessary to open the hand extensively to release an extensive incarceration of the extensor mechanism; this always involves more surgery than was originally planned. It is usually worthwhile to try to liberate the extensor mechanism, however, even though the extremity may have to be dissected from distal forearm to metacarpophalangeal joints. After the tendons have been released, it should be possible to place all of the finger joints in complete flexion simultaneously. On the mechanical premise that more amplitude of motion is needed to make a tight fist than to extend the metacarpophalangeal joints actively, the fingers should be put into flexion and maintained there during the healing period. Since a tendon anastomosis has not been performed, there is no reason to wait longer than the time required for the hand to become relatively painless before beginning passive, and active, exercises. Unfortunately, the dorsum of the hand is rather sensitive after extensive superficial dissection; it may be seven to ten days before patients will permit extensive physical manipulations. During this time it is important to keep all joints in tight flexion so that recurrent adherence of the extensor mechanism will occur with the entire mechanism in the most distal position. Return of active extension of the metacarpophalangeal joints may be a little tardy if patients are slow to perform active and passive motion, but it usually will return in six to eight weeks.

TENDON SUBSTITUTES.   Only a word need be said about substitutes for extensor tendons, as almost any fibrous structure seems to suffice. Some patients are able to extend their fingers adequately by a combination of flexion of the wrist and tightening of scarred dorsal skin, without the use of any extensor tendons. This is most often seen in a burned hand. The phenomenon demonstrates how little amplitude of motion is required to extend the metacarpophalangeal joints and why either a superficial or a deep scar can serve as a tenodesis when normal wrist flexion is possible. When soft tissue is more pliable, particularly

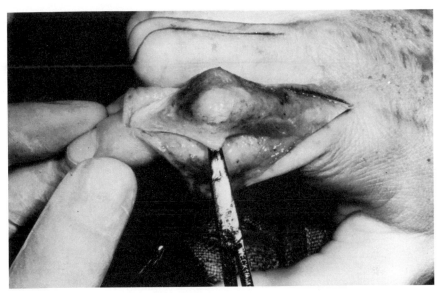

Figure 8–20. Typical lateral displacement of the extensor mechanism in a boutonniere deformity. There was no direct injury of the extensor mechanism over the proximal phalanx of the index finger but a long period of immobilization following a burn resulted in attenuation of transverse fibers and subluxation of lateral bands below the axis of the joint.

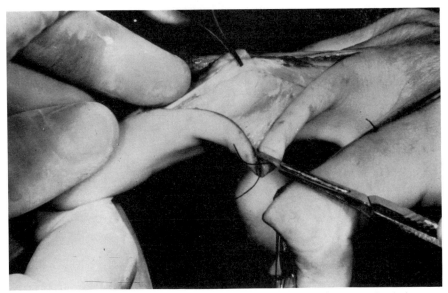

Figure 8–21. Elevation of lateral bands above the axis of rotation during repair of a boutonniere deformity.

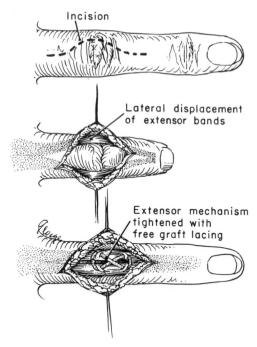

Figure 8–22. Diagrammatic representation of boutonniere repair using a free tendon graft to lace the extensor mechanism in the dorsal midline. (From E. E. Peacock, Jr., in *Reconstructive Plastic Surgery,* vol. IV, edited by J. M. Converse, Philadelphia, W. B. Saunders Co., 1964.)

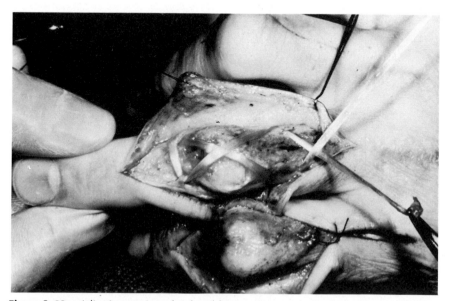

Figure 8–23. Adjusting tension of a dorsal boutonniere repair. Correct tension is extremely important or flexion of the proximal interphalangeal joint will not be possible. Many patients with boutonniere deformity can be treated conservatively by proper splinting.

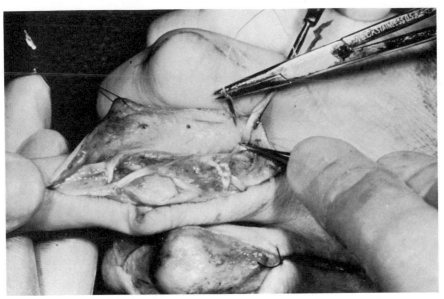

Figure 8–24.   Onlay method of anastomosing extensor tendon graft to prevent change in tension by production of gaps after end-to-end anastomosis.

after resurfacing of the dorsum with an abdominal pedicle flap, missing extensor tendons must be replaced. A plantaris tendon will provide two grafts, and a palmaris longus tendon will provide one, if the defect is not too long. Toe extensors are the correct size and shape, although technical difficulties attendant to taking these grafts have discouraged most surgeons from using them except when multiple long grafts are required. The long extensors to the toes are often a common tendon over a third or more of their course through the foot and ankle. This means that a "many-tail graft" can be obtained by taking the graft through the area of the ankle and dorsal foot. Such a graft is usually reserved for cases in which a central mass of proximal scarred tendon in the forearm is all that can be utilized for a motor unit. When a single motor unit is attached to all of the fingers by means of a single proximal anastomosed "many-tail graft," it is important to set the fingers under different tension by careful separate adjustment of distal anastomoses. The index finger should be under the most tension, the long finger under more than the ring, and so on. The fingers ideally should be elevated in order, starting from the radial side. If the order of extension is reversed or even eliminated by placing ulnar grafts under more tension than radial grafts, patients will not be able to grasp large objects easily. The natural tendency for the fifth metacarpal head to drop as the movable transverse arch of the hand deepens contributes to the subtle but efficient mechanism for preparing the fingers for strong grasp.

Strips of fascia lata and synthetic substances also have been used to replace extensor tendons. From the variety of materials which have been reported as successful and from our knowledge that some extension is possible by a tenodesis effect of movable scar, it is likely that some synthetic substances may merely create a foreign body reaction which crosses two joints. In this regard, it should be emphasized (as pointed out in the discussion in Chapter 7 on skin replacement) that an intact tendon should not be debrided before a pedicle flap is applied. This important principle in extensor tendon repair is more mechanical than biological. Proper length, position, and movability of the extensor mechanism is of more importance than other biological considerations. Having a set of extensor tendons the right length and in the right position, regardless of how badly burned or frayed and abraded they may be, is a real asset. They should be covered without regard for viability, for length and position are more important than variations in healing on the extensor surface. If the fingers are kept in a flexed position so that the only motion that will be needed is to extend the metacarpophalangeal joints, adequate function usually will be obtained. If adherence does occur with the extensor mechanism in a proximal position, secondary release is a better procedure than replacement of multiple extensor tendons by free grafts. Even heat-denatured collagen can serve as a biological scaffold of exactly the right dimensions into which new cells can migrate, and an organized scar or new tendon can be developed.

TENDON TRANSFER.   When an extensor motor unit has been destroyed at the musculotendinous junction, so that neither primary nor secondary repair is physically possible, transfer of an appropriate motor unit should be considered. Many texts on reconstructive surgery of the extremities have reviewed the advantages and disadvantages of various muscle transfers. From the standpoint of the wound through which these transfers are performed, however, it should be remembered that the same mechanical principles apply to tendon transfers as to muscle transfers, namely, the need for more tension on the index finger than the small, and the realization that complete flexion of all joints and all digits requires more in the way of technical perfection than does active extension. A tenodesis effect (primarily providing finger extension as the wrist drops into flexion) can be obtained by almost any type of transfer performed in almost any manner so long as a strong scar crossing two joints is produced. An actively functioning transfer which will extend the metacarpophalangeal joints with the wrist also in extension and which will also permit complete finger flexion requires exacting technique. It is important to provide a large window in the ulnar fascia which separates the flexor and extensor muscle compartments on that side of the forearm. The muscle belly of the flexor carpi ulnaris, often utilized to empower the finger extensors, should be passed through the window so that the tendon has a direct approach to the finger extensors. A right-angle passage of a distal tendon through a small hole in the fascia usually results in a tenodesis effect and failure of the fingers to flex completely. Excision of fixed structures, such as an adequate segment of the dorsal retinaculum in the area where the transfer joins the extensor tendons, also is important.

It is tempting to use one of the radial wrist extensors for a motor transfer to paralyzed or irreparably damaged finger extensors. Although it can be done, wrist extensor transfers to finger extensors should be avoided if other units are available. Wrist extension, particularly radial wrist extension, is a force that is indispensable for power grip. It is a little wasteful to use so much power needed for the valuable function of power grip to do no more than provide a positioning maneuver for the fingers.

Repair of Flexor Tendons

Flexor tendons are quite different from extensors in that they have long amplitudes of motion, change direction several times, and are arranged to provide power and accuracy during finger and wrist movement. The relatively long amplitude of motion required for a flexor profundus tendon to flex the distal tip of a finger completely makes restorative surgery a technically difficult and biologically complex problem. The degree of difficulty and complexity varies with the level of the injury and is directly proportional to the amplitude of motion of the tendon at that level. For example, the amplitude of motion of a flexor motor unit is zero at the origin of the muscles and insertion of the tendon. Repair at either level is a relatively simple problem. In the center of the unit (midpalm in a flexor profundus tendon) the amplitude of motion may be as much as 5 cm., and both technical and biological considerations significantly affect the end result. Flexor tendons in the wrist or midfinger (distal to insertion of sublimis) have an amplitude of motion and potential for successful restoration of gliding function intermediate between the two extremes just described.

WHEN TO REPAIR. One of the first problems encountered in repair of a wound of a flexor tendon is whether to perform a primary or secondary repair. At the wrist, the answer is simple because flexor tendons at that level do not have restraining structures such as the lumbrical muscle or vincula. As a result, severance of a long flexor tendon at the wrist results in retraction of the proximal end of the tendon into the forearm muscle compartment. If the proximal tendon is not recovered and restrained in a forward position as a primary procedure, that motor unit will be lost permanently. Intramuscular fibrosis and shortening of the entire unit makes secondary anastomosis of tendons at the proximal wrist level virtually impossible. A good general rule for treatment of severed tendons distal to the wrist, however, is that, if there is any doubt whether a primary repair should be done, only skin should be closed. If a digital nerve has been divided also, it can be repaired during primary wound closure. The important principle in this rule is that, although some flexor tendon injuries can be repaired satisfactorily as a primary procedure, most tendon injuries can be handled just as satisfactorily (and in some instances, even more so) in a secondary procedure. Because some of the complications of primary tendon repair can be ruinous to development of gliding function, the recommendation to repair tendons as a secondary procedure if there is any doubt about the feasibility of a primary repair is sound.

As already stated, divided tendons in wrist wounds must be repaired at the time the rest of the soft tissue is closed. An extensive laceration of the volar surface of the wrist is second only to amputation in destructive potential, and quite often neither the patient nor the surgeon realizes the extraordinary functional loss which has been produced by division of all the structures which pass into the hand. To try to repair these structures (two blood vessels, two nerves, 11 tendons, and skin) requires four or five hours of tedious and exacting surgery. It is too much to do at one time under most circumstances, and thus proper staging of restorative procedures is important. The possibility of a good result from an initial restoration is enhanced if only a minimal number of structures are repaired in the least amount of time. Four flexor profundus tendons and the flexor pollicis longus are the minimal number of tendons which can be repaired without leaving a serious functional deficit. The three wrist flexors are not important enough to justify the hour of additional operative time required to anastomose them accurately. Moreover, an important problem in the volar wrist compartment is that there must be adequate space for the large number of structures which must pass through it. Three large tendon anastomoses and the foreign suture material which must be introduced to repair them securely take up space needed for other tendons and nerves. Few people require powerful wrist flexion; thus repair of wrist flexors is not mandatory so long as finger flexors function adequately.

There is some difference of opinion concerning the advisability of repairing the flexor sublimis and the flexor profundus tendon at the same level. In the judgment of the author, only the profundus should be repaired in most patients for the following reasons: There is a considerable difference in amplitude of motion between flexor sublimis and flexor profundus tendons. When cross-union occurs between these two tendons, both tendons will move only with the amplitude of motion of the one with the shorter range. Remembering the dispersion stage of the healing process and the one wound-one scar concept of tendon healing, it seems likely that repair of sublimis and profundus tendons at the same level inevitably will be followed by cross-union in a common scar. Although it is conceivable that an intricate secondary

Figure 8–25. The hand and wrist are divided into five zones for consideration of repair of tendons and nerves. *Zone I* injuries are best treated by advancement of profundus, tenodesis, fusion of the distal interphalangeal joint, or insertion of a free graft through the intact sublimis. In *Zone II*, primary repair of a single tendon within the sheath can be done by experienced surgeons, but secondary flexor tendon grafting is the more reliable procedure. In *Zone III*, repair of profundus tendons should be accomplished by primary suture; sublimis tendons usually should not be repaired. In *Zone IV*, interposition grafts probably should be used if multiple tendons are injured. The restricted passage of tendons through a fibrous canal duplicates many of the problems of repair of flexor tendons in Zone II. In *Zone V*, primary repair of the flexor profundus tendons takes precedence over repair of any other tissue. Secondary repair usually is not possible in Zone V as there are no restraining influences on the proximal ends of tendons severed here. Sublimis tendons and wrist flexors usually should not be repaired.

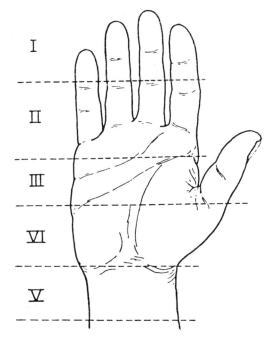

remodeling process could separate the scars of the two tendons (as well as separate the scar of both tendons from nonmovable structures), in actual practice such separation does not occur with predictable regularity. A few scattered reports claiming independent sublimis and profundus function following repair of both tendons at the same level have appeared; such occurrences are relatively rare, however, and cannot be counted upon following repair of tendons at the wrist. A profundus unit with no more amplitude of motion than its sublimis counterpart is less than optimal, even if the repaired sublimis regains a full range of motion. It is unlikely, therefore, that combined profundus and sublimis repairs produce any better functional result than a sublimis repair alone, and usually the result is not as good as that of repair of a profundus alone. Because successful repair of a profundus tendon will provide distal as well as proximal finger joint flexion, requires less time to perform than repair of both tendons, and leaves considerably more space in the carpal canal than when sublimis and profundus tendons are repaired, most surgeons agree that only the profundus tendon to the fingers and the flexor pollicis longus tendon to the thumb should be repaired. The only flaw in this reasoning is that the sublimis muscle is the better motor unit of the two; it provides independent digital flexion and is more powerful than other finger flexors. Most surgeons agree, however, that loss of power and independent function is permissible in most patients in order to gain the added certainty of long flexor activity which a shorter operation involving repair of only the profundus tendon usually provides. A compromise is to repair one or, at most, two sublimis tendons such as the ring and long finger tendons. One reason for doing this is so that later one or both tendons can be dissected out of scar tissue and utilized as a motor unit for an intrinsic transfer if median and ulnar nerve repairs are not entirely successful.

Throughout the rest of the palm and fingers, the problem is really not so much one of whether primary or secondary repair should be performed but whether a primary repair or secondary replacement of the tendon will provide better gliding function. The real core of the problem is expressed again in the rule previously stated, that a good tendon can be put through a bad bed or a bad tendon through a good bed, and so on. For a tendon which must move through a 5 to 6 cm. range, most of the distal palm and all of the fingers must be considered a bad bed. Specifically, the area between proximal wrist and midpalm and between distal palmar crease and midproximal phalanx are areas where flexor tendons change direction abruptly, pass through constricted nonmovable fibrous tunnels, and pass through each other at one site. A single scar involving tendon and nonmovable, tightly fitting structures in these areas may not undergo secondary remodeling sufficient to restore more than a fraction of the needed range of active motion. A few technical maneuvers such as excision of some of the surrounding theca in the area of the anastomosis or interposition of local viable tissues may help; but, generally speaking, the one wound-one scar principle in these areas results in scar tissue being formed which permanently restricts full finger flexion. Thus the midpalm and distal phalangeal areas of the fingers are the only sites other than the proximal wrist where primary repair is feasible for the average surgeon. A helpful approach to the problem of lacerated tendons in sheath areas (often referred to as "no man's land") has been to accept the fact that the bed at the site of injury will always be a bad bed and that an anastomosis of a flexor tendon will always be a bad tendon at that site. Following the rule, therefore, the anastomosis and the original sheath injury must not be in the same wound. To avoid this, the wound is first allowed to heal; after soft tissue scar reaction has subsided, a new wound is made in another plane and a new tendon is inserted. The tendon graft spans the old wound site with new tendon and paratenon, and the anastomotic areas (bad tendon) can be put where conditions are more favorable. This usually means that the proximal anastomosis is placed in the wrist or midpalm, and the distal anastomosis is an attachment of tendon to bone at the distal phalanx. The distal attachment is of no consequence as far as gliding is concerned; a rigid scar is all that is desired, for the relative amplitude of motion of tendon to movable structures at that point is zero. The proximal anastomosis in the palm or wrist can be placed so that it is surrounded by movable muscle or fat. Moreover, the possibility of favorable secondary remodeling, plus the potentially movable character of the bed, provides a combination of conditions which can lead to 5 to 6 cm. of active motion. Biologically speaking, the wrist is probably a more ideal place for a proximal anastomosis of a tendon graft than is the midpalm. Most of the tendons in the wrist move together to some extent because of specialized paratenon connection. Also, the amplitude of motion of all of the tendons in the wrist is less than in the palm. Proximal anastomoses of free tendon grafts in the wrist have not been popular, however; the reasons probably are that most surgeons still prefer a sublimis or palmaris tendon graft and believe that there is some virtue in retaining the lumbrical muscle. Neither a palmaris nor a sublimis graft (distal sublimis following laceration of both tendons) is long enough to reach from fingertip to proximal wrist except in the small finger. Although there are some reasons to suspect that it may even be desirable to eliminate the lumbrical in a grafted digit, the natural reluctance of restorative surgeons to sacrifice a normal structure is understandable.

The first factor in considering whether to attempt primary repair of a tendon in the wrist or digital sheath area is that data upon which a definite answer could be based are not available. This statement may evoke disbelief in the beginning student in view of the enormous number of tendon repairs which have been performed and the prominence the subject has enjoyed since World War II. Many observations have been made and recorded, but, for the most part, observations are all that we have; most of the data cannot be analyzed or correlated because of a lack of adequate control information.

To begin with, there still has not been any universal acceptance of the best way to evaluate results of a flexor tendon repair. Commonly used methods such as measuring the distance from fingertip to palm are of little value; the amplitudes of motion of flexor tendons required to flex the fingertip to palmar skin are variable among fingers and individuals. Moreover, some individuals are able to develop abnormal motion in their metacarpophalangeal joints while striving to achieve active flexion in proximal and distal interphalangeal joints. We have seen a few patients develop enough motion in the metacarpophalangeal joint to bring the tip of the finger to within less than an inch of palmar skin without a single degree of proximal or distal interphalangeal joint motion.

A second important factor in assessing any flexor tendon restoration is ability of the patient to extend the digit. A permanent flexion contracture of some degree is not unusual following replacement of the entire flexor mechanism, and this condition can vary in severity from a 15 to 20 degree contracture of only the distal interphalangeal joint to midflexion fixation of both proximal and distal joints. Such unfortunate individuals may be able to flex their fingers until the tip touches palmar skin by using only the metacarpophalangeal joints. The fact that they are not able to develop a single degree of active or passive interphalangeal joint motion is not incorporated in the distance measurement as it is commonly reported. Another factor which causes tip-to-palm measurements to be misleading is failure to specify position of the metacarpophalangeal joint while measurements are being made. If the metacarpophalangeal joint is maintained in extension while the interphalangeal joints are flexed, more flexion of the distal joints is possible than if the metacarpophalangeal joint is also allowed to flex. This is true for several reasons, which will be analyzed in detail when considering reactivation of flexor tendon grafts.

Finally, the factor of strength in a restored flexor unit is also of importance for some individuals. It is possible, following restoration of the distal flexor mechanism, to move the tip actively through a measurable flexion arc without that range of motion being useful because of inadequate power. Several factors contribute to this condition; they will be considered in detail in subsequent sections. It is sufficient to point out now that the many variables encountered in evaluating postoperative results of flexor tendon repairs have made comparison studies almost impossible at this time. A review of the published reports of flexor tendon repair reveals such a wide range of results that one can only conclude that all are not counting the same thing in the same way.

The decision between primary repair and secondary graft in the critical zones probably can be approached best on a biological basis. To begin with, it must be acknowledged that primary repair of long flexor tendons within the digital sheath can be done by experienced surgeons and that excellent function can be restored. (The term excellent function as used in the rest of this chapter includes extension to 180 degrees and flexion of the fingertip to touch the palm.) Excellent function can also be obtained by merely closing skin primarily and performing a full-length flexor tendon graft as a secondary procedure. The consensus has been, however, that excellent results following primary repair are not as predictable as those following secondary grafts and that considerably more technical skill and judgment are needed to repair tendons primarily than to graft them secondarily. Although reliable data are not available to prove or disprove this hypothesis, the biology of tendon healing and reestablishment of gliding function strongly suggests its truth. Even the strongest proponents of primary repairs concede that patients must be selected carefully and that conditions must be ideal. Ideal circumstances include a clean laceration, definitive surgical care within a few hours after injury, a low order of contamination, superb facilities, and a surgeon with considerable experience in tendon repair. Such criteria eliminate many candidates, which indicates that a greater margin of safety exists when performing a secondary graft. The reason for this probably lies in the degree of secondary remodeling which must occur in the different procedures.

Continued interest and improvement of surgeons in flexor tendon repair and continued improvement in education of patients and referring physicians have resulted in more primary repairs being performed successfully than was thought possible in the past. The chances of a patient with cut flexor tendons in a digital sheath reaching a surgeon with technical and biological expertise within a reasonable period after injury have improved to the extent that apparently about as many primary repairs are being performed successfully now as secondary grafts. Results of both procedures seem to continue improving although no major breakthrough in the form of a new technique or procedure has evolved.

The greatest advantage of a secondary graft is that the surgeon controls the site of the wound. Thus optimal conditions in surrounding tissue are predictable. In a primary repair, the surgeon begins by having to concede the location of the anastomosis as the one the injury selected. This is an important factor when one realizes that if the wound also involves an immovable structure, the only hope for even a flicker of active tendon motion depends upon a biological process about which we understand very little and over which we have pathetically little control at present. If the surgeon controls the site of the wound, he can be sure that it will be possible for the entire scar to move to some extent even though selective remodeling does not occur, and thus he controls more factors which influence gliding motion. Because the synthetic phase of collagen metabolism in a developing scar is influenced considerably by the technical proficiency of the surgeon, the demands on technical performance are greater during primary repair. Where selective collagenolysis is important in releasing tendons from attachment to a movable object, the total amount of scar tissue to be degraded may be important.

In summary, although it is recognized that experienced surgeons operating under ideal conditions are able to restore excellent function by primary repair of lacerated tendons within the digital sheath, a greater allowance for error in judgment and technique exists with a secondary graft. Present knowledge concerning collagen synthesis and degradation following tendon repair suggests that the surgeon has more control over the final outcome of a secondary graft than he has following primary repair, where gliding function is totally dependent upon selective remodeling of scar tissue. Such statements should not prevent well trained and experienced surgeons from performing primary repairs when conditions are favorable. Secondary grafting still provides an excellent "fall-back position" and provides even the uninitiated with justification for doing nothing but closing a soft tissue wound when there is any question about what the best course is.

TECHNIQUE OF PRIMARY REPAIR.   When primary repair is chosen, the surgeon should remove fibrous sheath in the immediate vicinity of the tendon anastomosis. Because of introduction of a foreign body to hold tendon ends together and the unavoidable trauma associated with introduction of the suture, the greatest inflammatory reaction in the wound will be at the site of anastomosis. On the basis that a dense scar will be produced at the site of maximal tissue inflammation, it seems advisable to place the tendon anastomosis in tissues which are movable to some extent. Also, an anastomosed tendon more than doubles in diameter during the healing period; if nonyielding sheath is left around that portion of the tendon, sheath and tendon may fuse because of lack of space for the tendon anastomosis to enlarge. Removal of the sheath on both sides of the anastomosis is biologically as well as mechanically sound and probably should be done over as extensive an area as possible without producing bowstring deformity. Excision of sheath primarily was also believed to be advantageous when a secondary graft was to be performed, but recent knowledge of the healing process and the function of the sheath has changed thinking about removing normal theca. The disadvantages of having sheath in the wound of a primary repair, however, are so severe that sheath should be excised over a sizable distance if the best opportunity for gliding function is to be provided.

A minimal amount of suture material is desirable when performing a primary repair. Most surgeons use only a few small permanent sutures to provide fine adjustment of the cut surfaces of the tendon; other fixative devices are utilized to provide physical strength for the anastomosis. The ends of the tendon often are kept from separating by an ingenious procedure, designed by Verdan, which involves driving straight needles across the sheath and tendon on both sides of, and at some distance from, the anastomosis. Such transverse fixation of the tendon to the immovable sheath will immobilize the anastomotic site so that only one or two fine sutures at most will be needed to adjust the surfaces of the juncture accurately. Although there is a hypothetical danger of transfixing a tendon to immovable sheath so that a permanent fusion develops, this has not been observed.

The question is often posed: Why not perform a primary graft instead of a direct anastomosis in a bad bed? Actually, primary grafts have been performed in carefully selected patients. Excellent functional results can be obtained, but primary grafting is the most dangerous of all of the procedures discussed so far. The entire flexor tendon-sheath mechanism has to be dissected or exposed for a graft, and most surgeons do not want to open a hand to this extent through a traumatically induced wound. An infection following simple closure of skin is a nuisance, and an infection following a primary tendon repair is locally disastrous, but a postoperative infection following a flexor tendon graft is a catastrophe for the entire hand. Occasionally, however, a sharp incision made by a clean instrument, in a clean hand, when it occurs near a good hospital and an experienced surgeon, may be treated by a primary graft rather than a primary anastomosis because of the experience or preference of the surgeon.

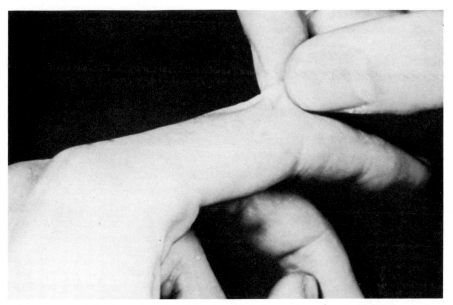

Figure 8–26.   A simple test based on skin edema to indicate when a hand is ready for secondary reconstructive tendon or nerve surgery.

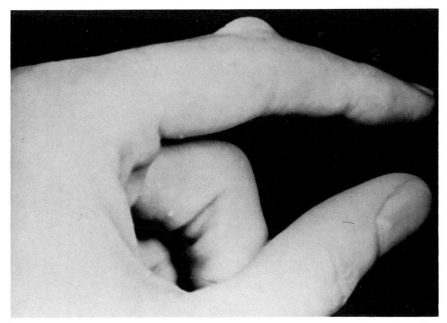

Figure 8–27.   Skin without significant edema will remain elevated for several seconds. Failure of skin to remain elevated suggests that edema is present and that secondary surgery should be delayed.

TECHNIQUE OF SECONDARY REPAIR.   Another procedure which has been considered is secondary suture of divided tendons. The basis for recommending a secondary repair of tendons by direct anastomosis is that immediate closure of only soft tissue can serve as a test for sterility of the healing wound. Proponents of this approach reason that if several days after closure of overlying soft tissue there is no evidence of inordinate soft tissue reaction, the danger of infection from the original wound can be considered to be over. The repair of tendons can be done then with more assurance than at the time of original wound closure. The question also might be raised whether a three to five day old wound does not have some advantages from a biological standpoint. Reports on a group of patients with secondary tendon repairs suggest that such an approach to repair of flexor tendons can produce some good functional results. From a hypothetical standpoint, however, a three to four day old wound would seem to be, biologically, a poor substrate for definitive repair. If nothing else, the secondary wounding phenomenon would be coming into play at this time, and most people who have worked with this biological process would predict that attempts to repair tendon at that time would be followed by increased synthesis of fibrous tissue and production of a wound with scar which possessed more than usual tensile strength. If secondary repair is to be accomplished, however, it must be done within several days; after a

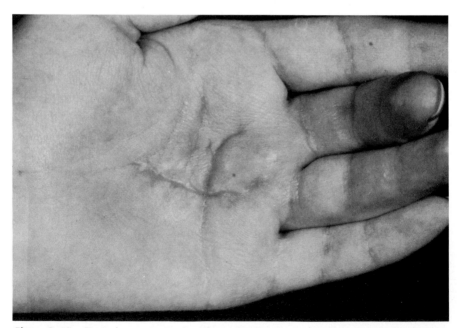

Figure 8–28.   Typical appearance of a palmar wound in the active period of wound contraction and secondary remodeling of scar tissue. Secondary surgery should be avoided during this stage as the secondary healing effect will be prominent.

longer period of time, the proximal ends of the divided flexor tendon cannot be advanced to the distal tendon end without putting the finger under too much volar surface tension. Secondary anastomosis of tendons is mentioned in this chapter for completeness, but all that can be said about it at this time is that a few cases apparently have been successfully managed in this way. The biological basis for such an approach is not clear; from a theoretical standpoint, primary repair in highly selected cases or secondary grafting in the remainder of cases appears more sound.

TECHNIQUE OF SECONDARY GRAFTING.   The technique for repairing a wound of flexor tendons by secondary grafting can be planned to take advantage of recent knowledge concerning the healing process of soft tissues in general and the specific phenomena in the healing of tendons. The best time for performing a secondary tendon graft is usually between 6 and 12 weeks after the original injury. The actual time is not so important, however, as the condition of skin, scar tissue, joints, and proximal motor unit, which must be accurately assessed. Most of these tissues will be in good condition for secondary grafting by eight weeks, but in some patients more time will be needed. On the basis that inflamed tissues react to additional injury by synthesizing more collagen and that persistent inflammation often signals that bacteria remain in scar tissue, grafting should not be done in a wound created by incising red or tender scar tissue. Edema should have subsided in the entire hand and the soft tissue scar should be movable before definitive tendon repair is attempted. Surface scar tissue which shows no sign of secondary remodeling in the direction of removing excess collagen and developing movability probably does not cover scar tissue which can be expected to release an incarcerated tendon graft during the maturation phase of tendon healing. From a biological standpoint, the maturation of the primary soft tissue scar is not so much a signal of the time when secondary grafting can be performed as it is a sign that healing and scar maturation in that patient can be of a type through which gliding function can be expected to occur. We do not have data to prove the point conclusively, but deductive reasoning based on considerable clinical experience strongly suggests that many of the bad results from tendon repairs were inevitable because of biological variations in the healing process in that individual. Expressed more simply, even a skilled surgeon experienced in tendon repair cannot predict the outcome of flexor tendon restoration with nearly the certainty he can for other procedures. Flexor tendon repair, even under the best of circumstances, has to be classified as a somewhat unpredictable procedure because not all individuals with similar injuries react the same way to operative repair of tendons. Until we know precisely why some individuals react differently, we can only take cognizance of the fact that everything that affects maturation of scar tissue is neither understood nor controllable at this time. The best we can do under these circumstances is to use all of the signs we have to predict which patients will react favorably during the maturation phase. Experience has shown that patients who develop hard, red scar tissue which does not become movable in a reasonable period of time are not good candidates for reconstructive surgery designed to provide gliding function. The reaction to soft tissue repair cannot be used alone, however. For instance, in elderly people soft tissue wounds usually heal without excess production of collagen. Moreover, secondary remodeling in these individuals is often rapid and effective in producing a movable hairline scar. Yet, elderly people are generally not good candidates for tendon grafts because of their propensity to develop stiff joints. Rapid development of a movable, mature, soft tissue scar, therefore, does not in itself guarantee that a properly performed tendon graft will provide excellent function. Patients who do not show any evidence of this type of differentiation of soft tissue scar, however, probably will not develop gliding function and, in most instances, should not be subjected to an extensive flexor tendon restoration.

The question of how long one should wait before performing a secondary restoration also should be considered. The time which can be permitted to elapse before performing a tendon graft is limited by changes in extensibility of the proximal muscle belly. A sublimis tendon divided completely in the proximal finger area will retract several centimeters because of the normal tone of the muscle fibers. If left in a shortened position for several months, it usually cannot be extended again to a distance sufficient to provide a normal range of motion. Although profundus tendons lacerated at the same level do not retract quite as severely as a sublimis tendon because of the limiting effect of the lumbrical, the muscle belly does shorten following division of a profundus tendon, and a measurable reduction in amplitude of motion may become permanent. Our impression is that if such a reduction in amplitude of motion exists for more than three months, it should be considered permanent. Profundus motor units examined at this time usually have such a short range of motion that it has not seemed wise to use them to empower a new graft.

Occasionally vincula, or tendon mesentery, keep a proximal tendon from retracting significantly. When this occurs, the length of time between injury and grafting is not critical; distally attached tendons have been grafted successfully several years after injury. The most unfavorable tendon injury in a finger, as far as the effect of time is concerned, is avulsion of a profundus tendon during violent activity. Although some congenital or acquired mechanism such as cystic degeneration of the tendon may be involved, sudden violent extension of the distal interphalangeal joint while the profundus muscle is undergoing maximal contraction can suddenly avulse the profundus tendon completely out of the finger. Sharpey's fibers entering the distal phalanx, both vincula, and the mesotendon all may be ruptured. When this happens, the tendon will be found coiled in the midpalmar space. If the diagnosis is made immediately, repair by rethreading the tendon through the digital sheath and intact sublimis and attaching it to the distal phalanx may be possible. More often, however, the diagnosis is not made for a week or ten days, and after this period of time, the tendon usually cannot be advanced to the distal phalanx. In these cases, a graft should be performed through an intact sublimis tendon. Because there is no surface scar to contend with, secondary grafting of avulsion injuries can be done through an optimal bed as soon as the diagnosis is made; some of the best results in flexor tendon restorations can be expected following technically proficient repair of these injuries.

When a freshly avulsed tendon can be reattached to the distal phalanx without putting the finger in a nonextensible flexion contracture, the digital theca should be opened in one area to guide the tendon over the undulating volar surface. The best place to open the theca is at the level of the proximal interphalangeal joint, where the sheath is thin and no volar restraint is needed to prevent bowstringing. An incision at this point is adequate to withdraw and expose the opening in the sublimis tendon for passage of the profundus. For reasons which will be discussed in more detail when considering technique of flexor tendon grafting, it is advisable to save as much of the sheath as possible. A free graft, or an avulsed profundus tendon, can be threaded through the proximal half of the digital theca, passed through the

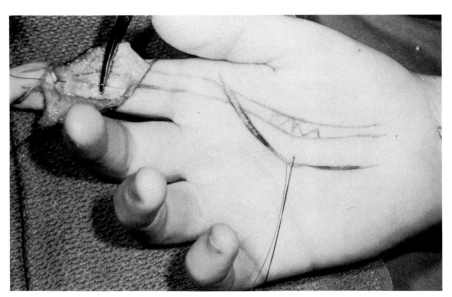

Figure 8–29.   Placement of a wire through an intact flexor tendon digital sheath in preparation for inserting a free tendon graft. The sheath has been opened only over the proximal interphalangeal joint; the rest of the digital sheath is carefully preserved as it presents an ideal surface for subsequent gliding function.

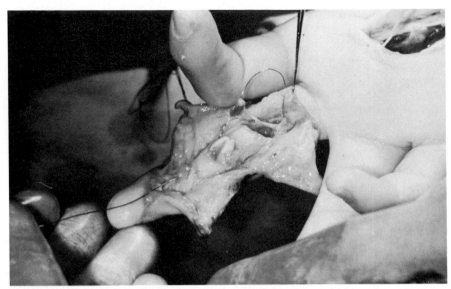

Figure 8–30.   Preservation of the insertion of the sublimis tendon over the proximal inter-phalangeal joint. Decussation of the sublimis tendon in this area provides an ideal gliding surface for a tendon graft and should be carefully preserved. Careless injury to or removal of the insertion of the sublimis tendon over the volar plate frequently results in uncorrectable flexion contractures or a serious recurvatum deformity of the proximal interphalangeal joint.

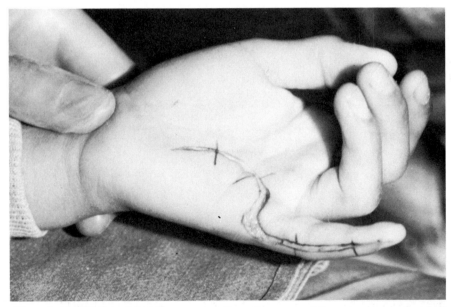

Figure 8–31.   Midlateral incision to expose the entire course of flexor tendons in the small finger. The resulting scar does not change dimensions regardless of the position of the finger, and will not limit subsequent flexion or extension.

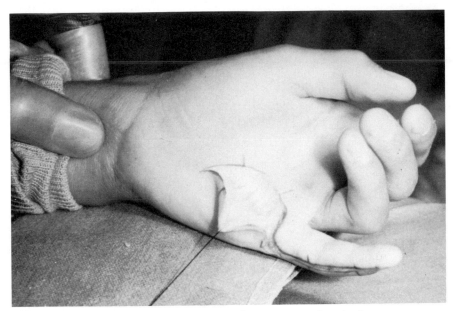

Figure 8–32.   Reflection of skin flap to expose palmar fascia.

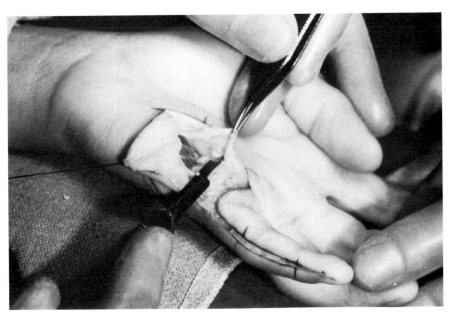

Figure 8–33.   Excision of palmar fascia as in treatment of Dupuytren's contracture. Because palmar fascia is fixed in three planes, it should be removed so that the subsequent scar involving all tissues in the palm will not be attached to an immovable structure.

opening in the sublimis tendon, and directed distally through undamaged sheath by making a single incision in the sheath over the proximal interphalangeal joint. At the conclusion of this maneuver, the sheath edges usually will fall together if the finger is placed in slight flexion. Because a minimum of collagen synthesis is desirable, sutures should not be used to close the incision in the digital sheath.

Unless the sublimis has been damaged at the point where the profundus normally passes through it, an opening usually can be located. Tendons do not contain cells capable of synthesizing collagen, and unless the opening is actually involved in the healing process of the original wound, fibrous obliteration of the sublimis opening does not occur. Use of a blunt probe is the best way to locate the opening, particularly when the tendon is being stretched by being pulled into a small wound in the sheath. The opening frequently is filled with fibrin and loose connective tissues, but exploration of the area with a smooth blunt probe will reveal the normal passage for the profundus tendon. Usually when the surgeon cannot locate the opening it is because he does not realize how far proximal the profundus tendon passes through the sublimis.

If the normal opening in the center of the sublimis tendon is closed, a free tendon graft can be passed along the side of the sublimis. It is important to remember, however, that the flexor profundus tendon does not pass through an opening between two insertion slips of the sublimis tendon. The sublimis is literally perforated by the profundus at a site proximal to the division of the sublimis into its terminal slips for insertion into the middle phalanx. The normal split of the sublimis tendon occasionally has been recommended as a site for passing a profundus tendon, but there are several reasons why this may not be a good idea. Distal division of the sublimis into its terminal insertion slip occurs over the proximal interphalangeal joint. This means that a profundus tendon which became superficial by passing between the sublimis slips would have an abnormal course between the sublimis and the attachment of the volar plate to the proximal phalanx. As will be discussed in more detail later, the attachment of the volar capsule and plate to the proximal phalanx is an area of critical importance for normal interphalangeal joint function. Moreover, abnormal passage of a tendon beneath the sublimis at this point interferes with the blood supply and the fibrous tissue attachments which are important to sublimis function. The chance of developing nonyielding adherence of the sublimis to the volar plate is enhanced by blunt dissection in this zone.

If the normal passage in the sublimis cannot be reopened, lateral free passage of a tendon graft is preferable to creating a false passage through the sublimis or to utilizing the split between the terminal insertion slips. Lateral passage causes the profundus, which is beneath the sublimis as it enters the digital sheath, to form a 180 degree spiral around the sublimis so that it emerges on top of it in the midfinger. A

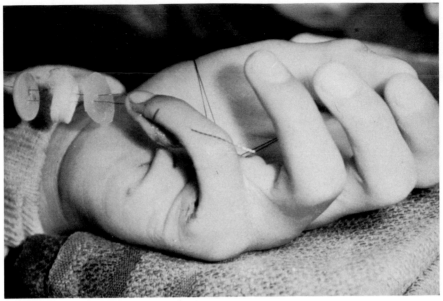

Figure 8–34. Protection of distal pulp of small finger with a pull-out wire tied over a button.

plantaris or palmaris graft is thin and flat; it conforms perfectly to the sublimis during its intrathecal course, and the shape of the sublimis tendon as it passes over the volar capsule forces the graft around the sublimis to a superficial position.

Distal attachment is usually accomplished by a pull-out wire. As far as gliding function is concerned, the distal attachment is not important; a complication of tendon grafting, however, is detachment of the graft from the distal phalanx during the first few weeks of active motion. Relative frequency of dehiscence at the point of terminal attachment suggests that this area is vulnerable and that some attention should be given to technique of joining tendons to bone. Fragility of a tendon-bone junction can be due to necrosis of the graft or interposition of other soft tissue. Necrosis usually is the result of threading a crossing permanent suture through 7 or 8 mm. of distal tendon, drawing the suture through the bone too tightly, and securing it to an immovable object such as fingernail or button. Necrosis is seldom observed when the pull-out wire is threaded through a piece of cotton dental roll before it is passed through the button. Use of a section of cotton dental roll between the button and skin makes it more difficult to keep the area clean for four weeks than when the simpler method of placing a button over the fingernail is used, but if wires emerge through skin some padding should be placed between the button and skin to prevent ischemia and possible necrosis of skin.

The author has found it helpful to ream out a small crater on the volar cortex of the proximal phalanx to receive the distal tendon. This is accomplished by making a few turns with a very small drill point until the cortex is broken. A large needle can then be used to go through the rest of the bone and fingernail. This provides a crater in the phalanx into which most of the tendon which contains suture material can be buried. Periosteal healing is, therefore, at a site slightly proximal to the suture; if distal necrosis does occur in the sutured portion of the tendon, the periosteal-tendon junction may still be strong. Of course, no matter what method of attaching tendon to bone is used, careful attention must be given to keeping redundant fat from the distal pad, and fragments of old tendon or fascia from becoming interposed between tendon and periosteum.

Immediately following avulsion of a tendon from its point of insertion or division of a profundus tendon within 1 cm. of the insertion, an opportunity exists for advancement of the proximal stump to the distal tip. The limiting factor in this procedure is the length of remaining tendon. Approximately 1 cm. of tendon can be lost without putting the finger under too much volar tension. The only sure test for being able to advance the proximal tendon is to see if extension is possible after the tendon has been sutured in its new position. If it is not possible to obtain nearly normal extension, a full-length graft should be used. Proximal manipulations of the muscle belly and lengthening of the muscle-tendon unit in more proximal areas are unsatisfactory when performed in conjunction with a tendon advancement procedure. An important consideration in the biology of tendons and their function is that tendons are not static bowstrings or "leaders." Tendons are more comparable to bowel in their relation to the cavity in which they lie. From musculotendinous origin to Sharpey's fibers, tendons are attached to surrounding tissue by specialized loose connective tissue. Only rarely does proximal manipulation such as cutting partway through a muscle belly or performing a sliding advancement in the proximal tendon produce significant release of tension at the distal end. Of course, such maneuvers can influence distal tension if connections along the course of the tendon are divided, as when "stripping a tendon." Once this has been accomplished, however, the tendon is a free graft from a biological standpoint; there are several reasons why a free graft from a distant site may be preferable to advancing a proximal tendon by dividing lateral connections in this manner. Certainly no better results occur from using the original tendon after it has been stripped from its surroundings, and the usual excellent results expected following advancement of a tendon to the distal phalanx often are compromised if it is necessary to convert the tendon to a free graft by a stripping procedure.

Selection and removal of a tendon graft is a step in restoration of finger flexion which also can be based on sound biological knowledge. When selecting a graft, the surgeon should be influenced by knowledge that free grafts become enlarged several times normal size during the second week following transplantation. An inflammatory reaction in surrounding wound tissue and death and necrosis of cells within the graft contribute to post-transplantation swelling. Grafts should not be so large in diameter, therefore, that they cannot be accommodated by immovable structures surrounding them. A graft which can barely be compressed into a fibrous sheath usually will remain firmly adherent to the sheath after it has been pressed tightly against it during the edematous stage. A second important fact is that autogenous tendon grafts ultimately require vascularization to maintain their original architecture and develop gliding function. For both revascularization and diffusion to be most effective, a graft of small diameter is desirable. These considerations are most applicable when the possibility of using a sublimis tendon as a graft for the profundus exists. Sublimis tendon grafts, although popular at one time, are not used often now because necrosis and replacement by disorganized scar has been observed. Actually, sublimis tendons make excellent free flexor tendon grafts, provided the fundamental biology of graft nourishment and healing is considered. Application of these principles usually leads one to the conclusion that sublimis tendons from some index fingers and most small fingers make excellent free tendon grafts. The sublimis tendon from the long or ring finger may make a satisfactory graft for a child, but the relatively enormous size of these tendons in adults renders them unsuitable for free transfer.

The main advantage in using a sublimis graft is that it is more nearly normal in size and shape for flexor tendons than distant grafts are. A sublimis tendon of correct size is usually the proper diameter for perfect end-to-end anastomosis with the proximal profundus tendon. The proximal sublimis tendon from the index and small fingers will usually be just the right length for grafting a profundus tendon between the origin of the lumbrical and the attachment to the distal phalanx. Removal of a normal sublimis tendon from an uninjured finger to graft a profundus tendon in an injured finger is not recommended. The sublimis motor unit is valuable from an active and passive standpoint. Not only are valuable power and independent control lost when a sublimis is removed, but development of a deformity called sublimis minus imbalance will occur in about one of 15 patients who lose sublimis tendons. This distressing deformity is most likely to occur in patients who have abnormal joint mobility (popularly called "being double jointed"). Scientifically speaking, the condition is caused by proximal interphalangeal joints which have an unusual range of motion because of redundant volar capsules. In these patients, normal tone of the sublimis motor unit is all that prevents hyperextension of the proximal interphalangeal joint, which then produces a flexion deformity of the distal interphalangeal joint. The two deformities together are sometimes referred to as a swan-neck deformity.

Choice between palmaris longus and plantaris tendon grafts usually should be made on the basis of how long the graft should be. Both tendons may be absent; but when both are available, length of the graft usually is the deciding factor in selecting one over the other. A palmaris longus may be too short to provide very much choice in a section for a graft for the long finger unless muscle from the proximal end of the graft is removed, particularly if the graft has to be extended into the wrist. When two grafts are required, a plantaris tendon should be selected, for it is long enough to supply both grafts and provides some choice in size and condition of paratenon. Both plantaris and palmaris are thin flat tendons which fit easily into the digital sheath of most digits.

Although the most undesirable tendon for a flexor graft is a toe extensor, if a number of tendons are required, or if neither palmaris nor plantaris tendons can be found, a toe extensor can and probably should be used. Toe extensors cannot be stripped out of the foot and ankle by cutting loose fibrous connective tissue in the same way that the palmaris longus and plantaris tendons can be removed. The long toe extensors are arranged much the same as the long finger extensors; they are interconnected with tough tendon-like bands. The entire course of the tendon from midankle to proximal phalanx of the toe must be exposed to find a satisfactory segment for a graft. Even then, intratendinous connections will have to be divided, and this produces a cut surface along the longitudinal surface of the tendon. In addition, the inadequacies of toe extensors as tendon grafts are reflected in damage to the donor site. Particularly in patients over 35 years of age, extensive dissection of the dorsum of the foot and ankle often causes prolonged edema and discomfort. All factors considered, toe extensors should be used only as a last resort.

Synthetic tendons have been evaluated exhaustively in animals and, to a lesser extent, in human beings. The search for a substance so inert that substitution for a flexor tendon seems practical has often been rewarded by finding that such a material cannot be attached reliably to muscle or bone. The relatively enormous strain placed on flexor tendons over a lifetime probably requires more in the way of physical stability than most synthetic substances can provide. A self-renewing mechanism is almost mandatory for structures which are called upon to transmit mechanical force over a course of changing direction, and relatively long amplitude, for 60 to 75 years.

It has already been stated that removal of flexor tendon grafts so that large amounts of loose areolar tissue are transferred with the tendon is not desirable. Although esthetically appealing, tissue surrounding palmaris and plantaris tendons is apparently very reactive when damaged. Excessive collagen seems to be produced by this tissue following the trauma of transplantation. Moreover, adequate space in relatively restricted areas is needed during the healing phase; a minimal amount of surrounding connective tissue assures adequate passage of the graft, even when edematous, through the restricted thecal space. The question of just how much paratenon should be left on free tendon grafts is probably best approached for the present by assuming that the previously expressed hypothesis concerning induction of secondary remodeling of scar tissue by other tissues is true. Tendon grafts surrounded by a very thin membrane of loose aerolar tissue have appeared to most observers to glide better than those with an excessive amount of areolar tissue. The objective would seem to be, therefore, to transplant a tendon with no more surrounding areolar tissue than is necessary to assure that longitudinally oriented and compact bundles of dense connective tissue within the tendon are not exposed to surrounding wound tissues. Actually, a limiting membrane, capsule, or outer sheath is not present on long tendons. A sort of imaginary plane must be conceived, therefore, and a pseudomembrane developed by dissecting away the connective tissue around a tendon graft just short of exposing the longitudinally oriented bundles. Successful execution of this concept will produce a free tendon graft around which secondary remodeling scar usually will resemble loose areolar tissue. Inadvertent exposure of longitudinally oriented dense connective tissue by careless handling of the graft or by being forced to use a toe extensor can cause remodeling scar tissue to take on the characteristics of mature tendon. Although this is precisely what is desired between tendon ends, it can be disastrous when it occurs along the longitudinal surface of the ten-

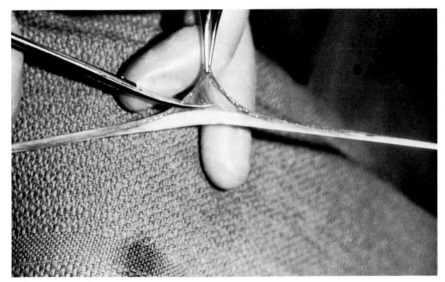

Figure 8–35. Cautious dissection of loose areolar tissue surrounding plantaris tendon. Note that only a tiny film of loose areolar tissue remains. (From E. E. Peacock, Jr., Surg. Clin. N. Amer. 45:461, 1965.)

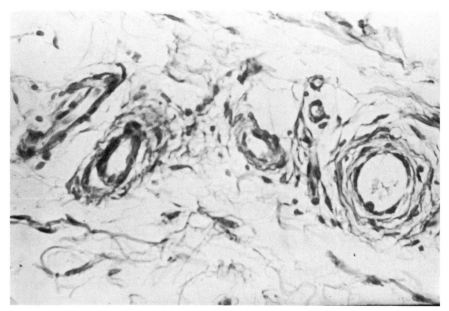

Figure 8–36. Microscopic appearance of film of loose areolar tissue surrounding plantaris tendon. It is hypothesized that this tissue will act as an inductor for secondary remodeling of newly synthesized scar tissue.

don. Removal of excess paratenon without exposing dense connective tissue is best accomplished by stripping the tendon from its bed through a small incision. The graft can then be suspended under optimal conditions, while paratenon is dissected carefully with fine instruments.

Once excess paratenon has been removed, the graft is in a precarious condition; the thin film of loose connective tissue which remains around the graft becomes the most important concern at this point. Delicate areolar tissue must not be allowed to dry, cells must not be subjected to unphysiological concentrations of salt or water, and mechanical abrasion of any type must be avoided. Obviously, the best place for such tissue is the recipient tissue bed. The more quickly it can be transplanted to that site, the better the chances are that collagen synthesis will be minimal and that secondary remodeling will produce tissue of desirable physical characteristics. Wrapping a graft in a sponge or placing it in a bowl of water or saline while further preparation of the bed is carried out is not biologically sound.

A great deal of attention has been focused on methods of performing a proximal anastomosis. Because the proximal anastomosis often is in an area where the tendon must have maximal amplitude of motion in relation to fixed structures, and because the anastomotic site will become the area of largest diameter, strict attention to certain technical details is essential. The importance some surgeons attach to technical details, however, suggests that they believe adhesions around the anastomotic site are the main cause of failure of tendon grafts to develop gliding motion. Although the restricting effect of adhesions in the area of the proximal anastomosis undoubtedly contributes significantly to failure of a tendon graft to glide, the author has never explored a nonfunctioning graft and found adhesions around the anastomosis which, when excised, released the graft. The entire length of a nonmovable graft usually is involved, and it is only rarely that a technical error at the junction is responsible for localized adhesions preventing movement of the tendon. Because there is more opportunity to have the cut surface of tendon exposed at the anastomotic area, however, the biologically oriented surgeon will concentrate upon coapting the ends in a way designed to reduce as much as possible exposure of the interior of either tendon.

The advantage of performing an end-to-end anastomosis is that the ultimate diameter of the anastomosis is smaller than that which follows any other type of juncture. The disadvantages of an end-to-end anastomosis are that technical perfection is difficult to achieve, and a perfect union of cut surfaces is impossible if there is significant discrepancy in the diameter of tendons. End-to-end anastomosis probably should be reserved for experienced surgeons anastomosing tendons of near equal diameter. When a graft is utilized to restore continuity of the flexor mechanism, end-to-end anastomosis should usually be used

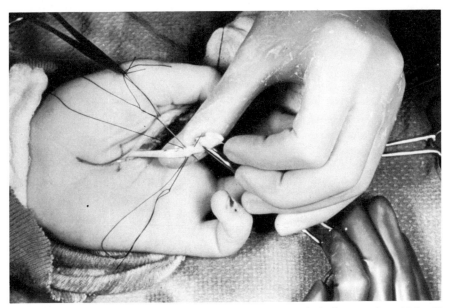

Figure 8–37. The crossing suture is inserted in the proximal end of a flexor tendon which will be anastomosed by end-to-end technique. Note that both needles are placed simultaneously to prevent fragmentation of the suture by a needle.

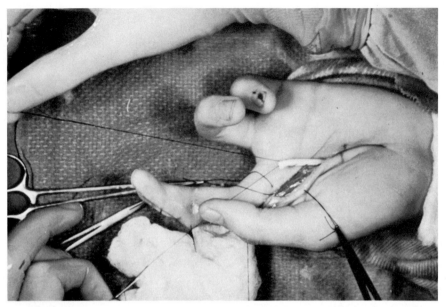

Figure 8–38.   The suture is pulled into the center of the tendon so that there is no exposed silk on the external surface.

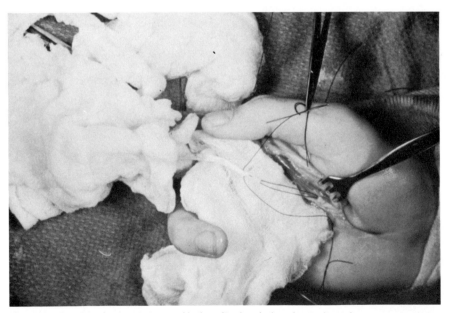

Figure 8–39.   Distal suture is inserted before distal end of tendon is slipped over suture to meet proximal surface.

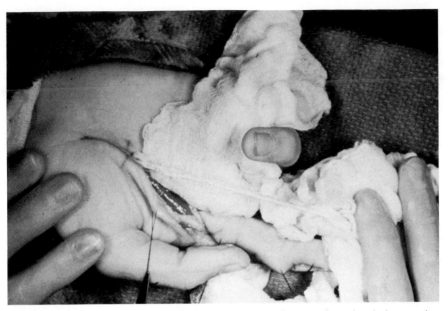

Figure 8–40. Completed end-to-end anastomosis. Note that suture can barely be seen beneath surface of tendon.

only when a proximal sublimis tendon is selected for a graft. When tendons of different diameters must be joined, some type of end-weave or splice is preferable. An end-weave is stronger than an end-to-end junction, but it also has disadvantages which must be taken into consideration. More length is required for an end-weave anastomosis; thus it is not a suitable junction for lacerated tendons when a graft is not used. The diameter of the anastomosis is nearly twice that of an end-to-end anastomosis; thus it should not be performed in tight places such as the digital or carpal retinaculum. Raw tendon ends will be exposed unless some measure is taken to bury them. This can be accomplished by wrapping the tendon graft around the proximal tendon stump so that the cut end of the stump will not be exposed to newly synthesized scar tissue.

The type of suture material used is not important so long as it is strong, permanent, and relatively nonreactive. Synthetic monofilaments are not recommended because so many knots are required to keep them from untying. An end-to-end anastomosis is probably enhanced by use of a suture with high frictional resistance such as braided wire or silk. Internal slippage of the suture through the tendon so that a gap develops is less likely when sutures with a high coefficient of friction are used than when monofilament sutures are used. Sutures have been designed with barbs to prevent the suture from slipping through the tendon but there is no evidence that such specialized sutures have significantly influenced the results of tendon repairs.

Text continued on page 433

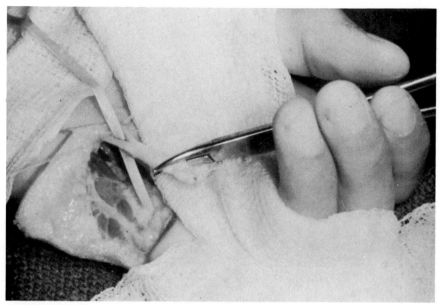

Figure 8–41.   First step in an end-weave anastomosis. Distal graft (small tendon) has just been passed through an incision in larger proximal tendon.

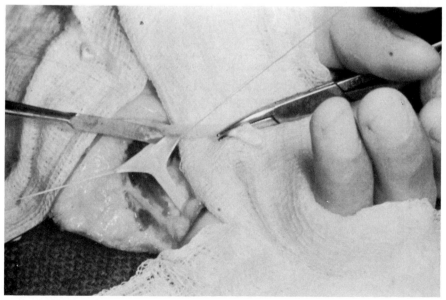

Figure 8–42.   Lateral attenuation of tendon graft to receive distal end of proximal tendon.

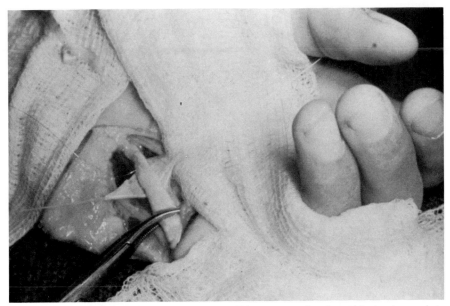

Figure 8–43.   Distal end of proximal tendon will be amputated to lie within the sleeve of attenuated plantaris tendon graft which will be wrapped around it according to the method of Brand.

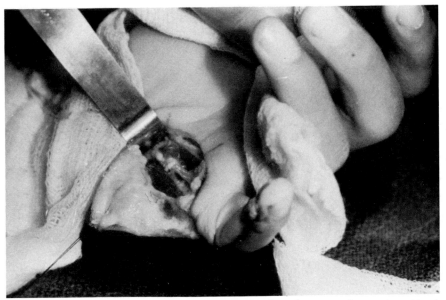

Figure 8–44.   Completed proximal anastomosis within hypothenar muscles on ulnar side of the hand. Note that no immovable tissue is in contact with anastomosis.

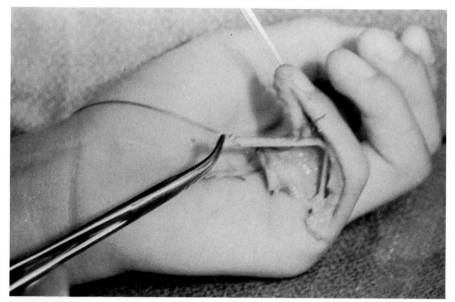

Figure 8–45.   Adjusting tension of a tendon graft so that grafted finger assumes a natural position in relation to other digits.

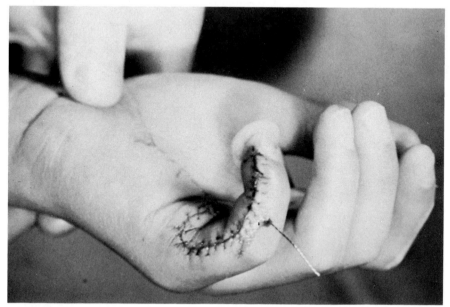

Figure 8–46.   Correct position of finger after tension on tendon graft has been adjusted and skin closed.

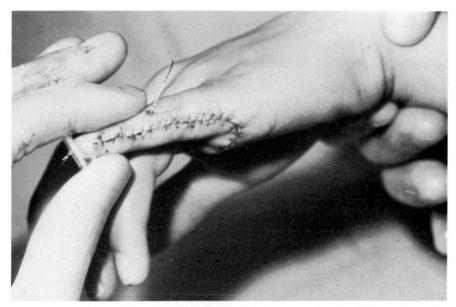

Figure 8–47. At completion of a tendon graft procedure, extension should be possible with the wrist in slight flexion.

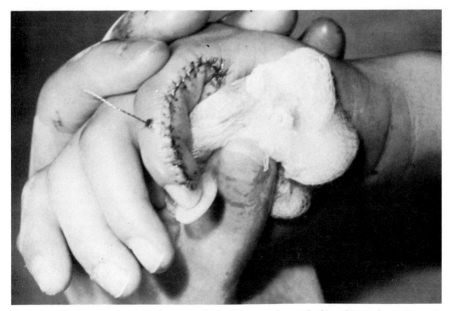

Figure 8–48. Spot pressure on the wound of a flexor tendon graft after release of tourniquet. It is best to close the wound with the tourniquet inflated, but approximately five minutes should be allowed to elapse before the final dressing is applied to be sure that a hematoma does not develop.

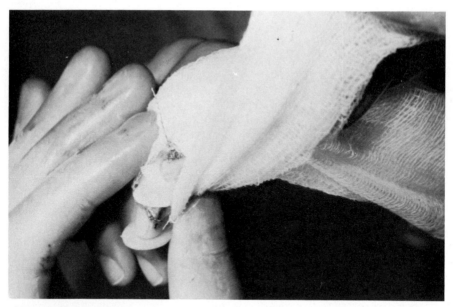

Figure 8–49. Use of damp gauze to mold a grafted finger in proper position. Note that most flexion is in the proximal interphalangeal joint with only 5 to 10 degrees' flexion in the distal interphalangeal joint.

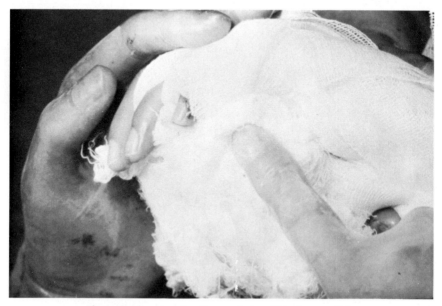

Figure 8–50. Use of cotton waste to add bulk accurately.

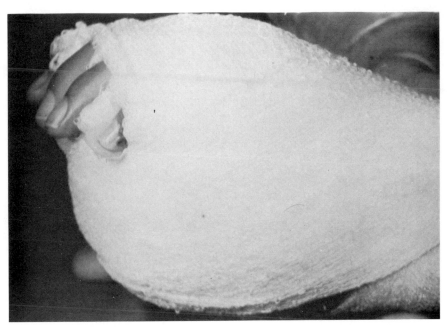

Figure 8–51. Completion of the dressing shown in Figures 8–48 to 8–50 with gauze rolls. A small plaster exterior can be used to maintain the position of sponges, cotton waste, and gauze.

The proper adjustment of tension for the motor unit is an important step in restoring flexion by tendon grafting. Grafts which are too long will not function through a full flexion arc; grafts which are too short may produce a permanent flexion contracture. A helpful guide to adjusting the length of a new tendon graft is to perform the proximal anastomosis first and then put in the distal suture so that the grafted fingertip will be pulled into slightly more flexion than surrounding digits. Passive extension of the finger should then be attempted. With the wrist in a neutral position, the grafted finger should be extendible. If the proximal muscle is not elastic enough to permit almost full extension after tendon length has been adjusted, a compromise between full flexion and full extension may have to be reached. It is usually better to have the flexion arc shortened at both ends than to have only a flexion contracture or only weakness of flexion. This type of decision usually is necessary only when muscles have become shortened from remaining in a relaxed state for a long period of time.

As soon as the graft is attached at both ends, the tourniquet should be released and pressure applied to the wound. Unless a major digital or palmar arch artery has been divided, ligatures should not be placed in a wound containing a tendon repair. Elevation and pressure will stop hemorrhage other than from a major artery. The proximal tendon anastomosis can often be wrapped with the lumbrical muscle by using a few small sutures to direct the muscle around the tendon. The skin should be closed without subcuticular or subcutaneous sutures. The subdermal and palmar fascial planes in most hands are very reactive to foreign substances. Deep sutures in this area usually become surrounded by hard nodules of scar tissue, and a hand which contains such sutures may resemble one in the nodular phase of Dupuytren's contracture. The wound should not be drained, although a layer of moist gauze is frequently placed against the surface to assist capillary drainage.

It has been recommended previously that the wrist be placed in midflexion following repair of a flexor tendon. Although longitudinal tension on the suture line unquestionably is relieved by flexing the wrist, the disadvantages of keeping the wrist in a flexed position for three weeks are so outstanding that most surgeons do not recommend it. When the wrist is flexed, inordinate tension is placed on the extensor mechanism, which may be at least partially responsible for improper use of the extensor muscles after removal of the cast. The danger of producing shortened collateral ligaments in the metacarpophalangeal joints of older people also is increased by placing the wrist in flexion.

RECONSTRUCTION OF TENDON SHEATH. Another approach to a badly scarred bed and destroyed sheath has been to insert a Silastic rod in the tendon bed and close the finger without doing anything else. Approximately eight weeks later, the rod can be removed through small proximal and distal incisions, and a conventional flexor tendon graft passed through the tunnel which the rod pro-

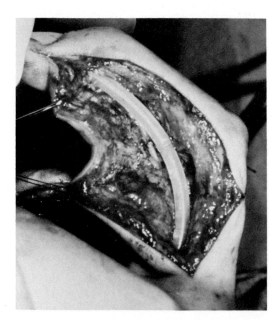

Figure 8–52. Silastic rod in digital bed where sheath was too badly damaged to be utilized.

duced. The biological principle underlying this approach is old. As early as 1920, glass rods and other foreign bodies were placed in scarred tendon beds to induce a foreign body reaction in the shape of a tunnel. The first stage in these restorations was successful in that a circular wall of fibrous tissue was induced around the implant and removal of the implant left a hollow tunnel lined with compressed fibrous tissue through which a tendon graft could be passed. In spite of encouraging early function, grafts placed in fibrous tissue tunnels produced by foreign bodies inexorably became part of the fibrous tissue reaction and blended with the dense connective tissue through which they passed. It is possible also that grafts in these tunnels could not acquire an adequate blood supply; necrosis may have contributed to their final demise. There is no doubt, however, that a fibrous tissue sheath induced by a Silastic implant is a different structure, from a biological standpoint, from the sheath which developed around other implants. A number of clinical investigations in recent years have shown that excellent sustained gliding function can be obtained by placing grafts through Silastic rod-induced tunnels. Unfortunately, there have not been any well controlled studies to compare clinical features of these grafts with more conventional preparations, but the number of good results reported indicates that a different order of fibrosis is being induced than was observed with other implants.

The most important difference we have observed in patients who have had flexor tendon grafts passed through a Silastic-induced sheath is that the range of motion possible immediately after removal of the splint and the relatively rapid progress which the patients make during the first week of mobilization are superior to those following conventional techniques. After the first week, the course of a patient with a Silastic-induced sheath does not seem significantly different from that of other patients. At one time during a period of study of Silastic rod implants, we encountered an inordinate number of avulsions of the distal anastomosis during the first postimmobilization week. Although we surmised first that rupture of the tendon-bone junction was due to impaired blood supply, other factors such as forceful manipulation and technical errors in performing the anastomosis could not be ruled out. Immediate exploration of the graft site afforded an opportunity to study the relationship of the sheath and tendon.

The first interesting finding in these patients was that in tendons within a Silastic rod-induced sheath there were definite vascular and fibrous adhesions between the sheath and the longitudinal surface of the tendon. Adhesions in the fingers we examined were more typical of loose areolar than dense connective tissue. The most striking feature, however, was not the adhesions, but the sheath around the tendon. The sheath in all of the cases examined was remarkably movable in a longitudinal direction. Even though grafts within the sheath were adherent, some flexion had occurred because of movability of a condensate of fibrous tissue which is surprisingly thin and semitrans-parent. The new sheath does not appear to be a physically strong structure, although its fate following long use as a restraint for flexor tendons has not been studied. Our cases showed considerable bow-string deformation, which suggests that Silastic foreign body reaction may not be strong enough to withstand the pull of a flexor motor unit at a point where it is changing direction within the finger.

Foreign body reaction to a Silastic implant is not great. The newly synthesized connective tissue appears to cling to the rod rather than spread out to involve other structures. A real three-sided tunnel, with the periosteum and volar plate of the finger as the floor, is not produced. The tunnel is a floating conduit which is only loosely, if at all, attached to the skeleton or any other tissue in the finger. It is a sort of artificial paratenon which is stronger than loose areolar tissue nor-mally found around a tendon, but unable to restrain a tendon and cause it to change direction. A Silastic-induced tendon sheath is more comparable to a flexible synovial membrane than to a rigid fibrous pulley. As such, it is probably most effective when induced within at least one fibrous pulley. A Silastic rod passed beneath a preexisting fibrous tissue pulley can induce a synovial membrane which improves the chances of early longitudinal motion without bowstring deformity. If such a pulley can be salvaged, one might raise the question of whether rapid early return of active flexion is worth the cost of a sec-ond operation and two month delay before inserting the graft. The an-swer to this question is that in some patients it is unquestionably better to stage the reconstruction in this manner. The reason is that the sheath in the pulley area, although present, may be inseparably fused with old tendon or so badly damaged by infection or trauma that a gliding surface on the inside cannot be restored. To force a tendon graft through such a pulley results in fixation of the graft at that point.

The same biological principles involving the secondary remodeling of collagen on the damaged surface of a tendon apply to the internal surface of the sheath. Sheath with a wound (healed or just created) is a bad sheath, and a good tendon must pass through it for any possibility of gliding function. A pulley created by reaming a core of old tendon and scar from the center of a block of dense connective tissue is more than a bad bed—it is a terrible bed; even with a good tendon passing through it, incarceration usually will occur. Thus a movable membrane type of foreign body reaction which Silastic can induce may serve as a cushion within a segment of biologically destroyed sheath. As such, it may turn out to be a valuable, although limited, contribution to our restorative armamentarium.

At present, Silastic preparation of a tendon bed is utilized for sev-eral types of restoration: when normal sheath and pulleys exist, when the sheath has been destroyed completely and cannot be salvaged as a pulley in any area, and when there is damaged but salvageable sheath in the pulley area. When there is a usable sheath, it has not seemed to us that results were worth the cost and delay of a second operation. When the sheath is completely destroyed so that Silastic rods have to be "floated free" in the finger, the bowstring effect following insertion of the tendon has made this method of restoring flexion less desirable than complete restoration of the sheath and tendon with a composite tissue allograft (see later). The best indication for a two-stage reconstruction, in which the bed is prepared first by Silastic induction of a synovial membrane, seems to be to salvage a badly damaged sheath which otherwise would have to be debrided.

COMPOSITE TISSUE ALLOGRAFTS.   An alternative to induction of an artificial sheath by the use of a foreign substance is to insert a graft of the entire flexor mechanism, including sheath, blood vessels, and tendons. The graft consists of an intact flexor tendon sheath surrounding two flexor tendons and the specialized blood vessels and vincula which connect the sheath and tendon. The hypothetical basis for clinical use of such a graft is that the healing process will occur primarily between the scarred tendon bed and the exterior of the intact tendon sheath. The highly specialized internal gliding surfaces between tendon and sheath should not be involved as long as the sheath remains intact. Nourishment of tendons within the sheath is through normal vascular connections in the mesotendon and vincula. Such a composite tissue graft of the flexor mechanism must be an allograft, however, as the rather unique relation of tendon, sheath, and mesentery occurs only in the digits of human beings and some primates.

A composite tissue allograft of flexor tendons and digital sheath is essentially a homostatic graft. All of the donor cells disappear within ten days, leaving primarily a nonliving collagenous structure. Host cells migrate into the graft over a 21 day period after donor cells have

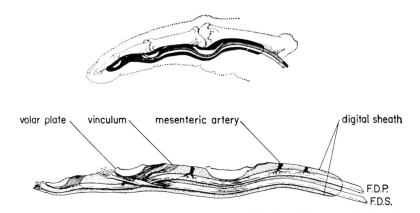

Figure 8–53. Diagram of composite tissue allograft of the digital flexor mechanism. (Reproduced by permission from E. E. Peacock, Jr., and J. W. Madden, Ann. Surg., *166*:624, 1967.)

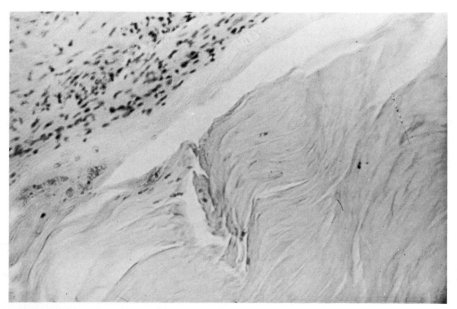

Figure 8–54. Microscopic view of composite tissue allograft of digital flexor mechanism. Note host cells outside the sheath and absence of cells within the sheath and flexor tendons.

disappeared. During this period there may be enlargement of regional lymph nodes, such as the epitrochlear node, when the ring or small finger has been grafted.

Destruction of cells eight days after transplantation and enlargement of regional lymph nodes suggests that an immune reaction is involved. The number of cells contributing antigen is relatively small, however. The dose of antigen does not appear to be great enough to induce a second-set rejection, as measured by challenging a tendon recipient with a skin graft from the tendon donor. Examination of host serum by complement-fixation techniques in which reconstituted collagen from the tendon donor is used as an antigen has not revealed a significant titer of collagen antibodies. Although there is some evidence suggesting that soluble collagen may be species-specific and able therefore to induce antibody production in susceptible animals, most data support the notion that insoluble mature collagen is not antigenic. It is virtually impossible to separate collagen completely from physically entrapped noncollagenous components of connective tissue such as various mucopolysaccharides. Some of these entrapped substances contain glycoproteins and other proteins which contribute to the antigenicity of the connective tissue. It is possible that such substances are responsible for the minimal antigenicity of soluble collagens reported by a few investigators. However, recent studies indicate that collagen, *per se,* may be antigenic and that the antigenic site may reside in the amino-terminal portion of the $\alpha 2$ chain. Clinically, however, collagen can be considered as an extracellular, partially crystalline, aggregate which is freely transplantable across major histocompatibility lines.

There seems to be little doubt that transplanted collagen (and probably all other collagen for that matter) is replaced and remodeled constantly. Some histological observations suggest that remodeling occurs at an increased rate in a large tendon allograft as compared to an autograft or normal tendon. The rate of remodeling or replacement of collagen is not clinically significant, however, as far as transmission of power in a longitudinal direction is concerned. A change in the physical properties of tendons in a composite tissue allograft which is clinically significant is the decrease in transverse stability. The physical weave of major collagen bundles in tendons primarily confers longitudinal stability. What transverse stability there is in a tendon is probably the result mainly of ground substance with a high content of glycoproteins and chondroitin sulfate. Although quantitative histochemical data are not available to substantiate the belief that ground substance disappears following transplantation of a tendon allograft, histochemical staining techniques indicate that this is so. Clinically, there is no question that allografts lose significant transverse stability between the tenth and twenty-first post-transplantation days. They do not regain anything resembling normal transverse stability until host cells have migrated into the interstices of major collagen bundles. Reappearance of ground substance after cells have invaded the tendon suggests that transverse stability is due to extrafibrillar substances, presumably elaborated by cells within the tendons. The clinical significance of these observations is that tendon allografts must not be subjected to physical stress for 28 days.

As more studies on the rate of collagen synthesis during healing of tendon are performed, it is increasingly clear that the suture material and technique of inserting sutures in tendons is more important than was realized in the past. Transferring data obtained from studying healing in dermis of rats and guinea pigs has been somewhat misleading, in that in these animals wounds of the skin heal rapidly and effectively with a very short phase of collagen synthesis. The collagen synthesis phase of healing between tendon ends is much more prolonged and really becomes maximal only a full week after removal of splints and activation of the muscle in most patients. The suture, therefore, is responsible for a considerable portion of the strength of the anastomosis during the first few weeks following removal of the cast. Effectiveness of tendon sutures is determined, to a considerable extent, by transverse stability of the tendon. Sutures pull easily through longitudinally oriented collagen bundles which are not held together transversely by some sort of cementing substance. (As might have been predicted, the first composite tissue allograft became dehisced at the proximal anastomosis when motion started at the end of a conventional

21 day immobilization period.) Immobilizing composite tissue allografts for 28 days and waiting an additonal week before applying significant force to flex or extend the finger has prevented dehiscence in subsequent grafts.

The clearest indications for using a composite tissue allograft to reconstruct the flexor mechanism are failure of a conventional autograft to provide flexion and destruction of the digital sheath by a complication, such as tenosynovitis, so that utilization of any portion of it for a pulley would not be practical. Because tendon allografts are homeostatic grafts (survival of cells does not occur), the length of time between death of the patient and removal of the graft is not important. Patients with infections obviously should not be selected as donors, and for medicolegal reasons patients with neoplasms probably should not be used. The age of potential donors does not seem to be important, but the size of the digit should be taken into consideration. A graft does not necessarily have to go into the same finger in the recipient's hand that it came out of in the donor hand but the length of the fingers should be approximately the same. The small finger of a mature woman may provide a graft exactly the right size for the index finger of a child, and so forth. The left hand should be used as the donor because the right hand is frequently exposed when the body is on display. Grafts should be removed in the operating room under the same conditions used for insertion of flexor tendon grafts in human patients, i.e., with concern for sterility, assistants, instruments, and surgical skill. One of the real disadvantages to the use of composite tissue allografts on a large scale is that the time and skill required to obtain a graft are considerable. Dissection is tedious and frequently requires about 45 minutes, or half as long as it takes to insert a conventional autograft.

To remove a composite tissue allograft, the finger, palm, and wrist are opened through a single longitudinal incision extending down the center of the volar surface. It is important to remember that the flexor mechanism is projected in a volar direction by the cartilaginous plates over the interphalangeal joints. At the level of the interphalangeal joints almost no subcutaneous tissue exists between skin and filmy tendon sheath. It is easy to open the sheath inadvertently over the proximal interphalangeal joint as the skin incision is being made. Once the entire course of the flexor mechanism from proximal muscle to distal interphalangeal insertion has been exposed, removal of the graft can be started. The graft is outlined by incisions made in the periosteum of all three phalanges in a midlateral line. A subperiosteal dissection is started at the tip of the finger so that the entire theca is elevated without exposing tendon in any area. The dorsal layer of the tendon sheath blends with the volar periosteum and fibrocartilaginous volar plates. They are elevated with and retained with the graft. Special care is required in the area of insertion of profundus and sublimis tendons.

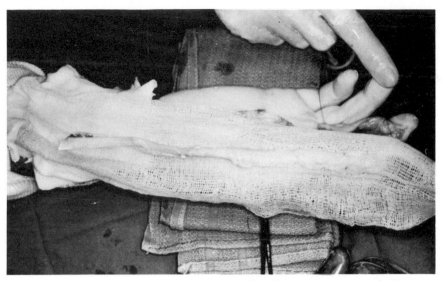

Figure 8–55. Composite tissue allograft with intact digital sheath removed from the finger of a recently deceased cadaver.

The knife has a tendency to follow Sharpey's fibers in these areas, with the result that the sheath inadvertently is entered. By keeping the blade directed into the bone in an exaggerated manner, the intact sheath and attached volar plate can be dissected from the digital skeleton and delivered out of the finger. In the palm and wrist, proximal to the beginning of the digital sheath, both tendons should be elevated, together with a minimal, but definite, envelope of paratenon. Vessels should be clamped and tied; seepage of embalming fluid is a problem for undertakers.

The graft should be gently wrapped in a gauze sponge saturated with saline to which penicillin and streptomycin have been added. The sponge is then rolled loosely and placed in a bottle, which is sealed sufficiently to prevent evaporation. Refrigeration at 37° F. is all that is required to preserve the graft. Although we have transplanted most grafts in human beings the day after death of the patient, grafts have been transplanted successfully to animals after six months' storage at 37° F. In all probability, protection against contamination and growth of mold is all that is required for indefinite preservation.

It also has been shown that composite tissue tendon grafts can be lyophilized and stored indefinitely. Lyophilized grafts have been stored for a period up to six months and then transplanted to the hands of primates and human beings. In the limited investigations performed so far, gliding function of lyophilized grafts appears as good as fresh allografts. Such studies suggest that a tissue bank could provide lyophilized composite tissue allografts of the flexor tendon mechanism from human beings on a commercial basis. If so, the greatest impediment to the use of composite tissue allografts—availability—would be eliminated. An allografted intact flexor tendon sheath is superior to a Silastic-induced tendon sheath in at least three ways: elimination of an operative procedure, protection against bowstring effect, and elimination of digital adhesions.

The recipient hand should be opened as in preparation for a conventional autograft. The only difference is that no attempt is made to preserve digital sheath in any area. The volar plates are left on the interphalangeal joint, and special precautions are taken to avoid damaging the volar capsule. Small tags of periosteum are preserved in the center of the distal phalanx and on each side of the middle and proximal phalanges. These tags will be used to anchor the allograft in its new location. The tourniquet should not be removed until the digital wound has been closed. There is just enough soft tissue to close the finger after an allograft has been inserted; if the hand is allowed to become engorged and the tissues edematous before closure is attempted, difficulty will be encountered. The reader has probably already surmised that there will be two volar plates in the reconstructed finger; one volar plate remains with the graft and the other is left attached to the joint of the recipient finger. Skin over the interphalangeal area is normally tight during extension of the digits; a second volar plate in the area is about all that one can add and still close soft tissue safely.

The allograft is draped over the volar surface of the digital skeleton so that insertions of profundus and sublimis tendons are in proper

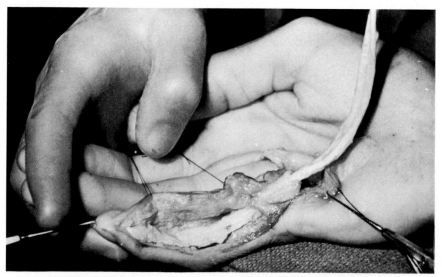

Figure 8–56. Composite tissue allograft being placed in small finger.

position. The graft is sutured to the periosteal tags with fine wire sutures. No direct tendon-to-bone junctions are attempted. After the fine wire sutures have been inserted, proximal pull on sublimis and profundus tendons should produce independent flexion at the proximal interphalangeal joint. Soft tissue of the finger then can be closed and the tourniquet released.

Although almost any combination of proximal anastomoses can be used, anastomosis of the sublimis in the palm and profundus at the wrist usually is the best choice. One of the advantages of composite tissue allografts is that both sublimis and profundus function can be restored. If either the wrist or the palm is not ideal for a tendon anastomosis, only one tendon should be repaired. The same problems of anastomosing tendons with different amplitudes of motion exist in inserting an allograft as in performing a primary repair in the palm or wrist. Preservation of normal lumbrical function could be considered as a reason for making the profundus junction in the palm, but because the amplitude of motion of the profundus is the greater of the two tendons, we have thought it preferable to suture the profundus in the wrist. The absence of a proximal attachment for the lumbrical muscle has not made a discernible difference in digital function.

The tendon ends are usually exactly the same size. A buried-wire, end-to-end anastomosis has been a satisfactory method for anastomosing these ends. Length of the motor units is adjusted so that the finger will be in slightly more flexion than it is after a conventional autograft. For some reason, allografts seem to elongate (perhaps some gap formation occurs in the proximal suture line) more than autografts in which an end-weave proximal anastomosis often is utilized.

Postoperative care following insertion of a composite tissue allograft is no different from that following insertion of an autograft except in the length of time before active motion is permitted. The danger of loss of passive motion in interphalangeal joints is greater than following an autograft because of the more extensive dissection and time of immobilization. Because allografts usually are selected for fingers in which there have been devastating complications or which failed to respond to conventional procedures, the interphalangeal joints may be in a rather precarious condition. Often the finger will have some degree of flexion contracture which cannot be overcome by physical measures. One of the unexpected rewards of an allograft, however, is that such a contracture frequently can be corrected in preparation of the finger to receive the graft. The extensive excision of all fibrous tissue on the volar surface of the digit usually makes it possible to extend the digit completely. Such radical preparation of a finger means that radical healing will follow, however, and this is probably why a finger with an allograft requires just as much, if not more, attention to prevent interphalangeal joint stiffness during the postoperative period. Fortunately this is easy to achieve by removing the dressing at regular intervals and putting the interphalangeal joints through a complete range of motion. Recovery of active motion in an allografted tendon follows almost exactly the same course as in an autografted one. Progress is rapid during the first week; about 30 per cent of normal range of motion usually can be achieved during that time. The remainder comes slowly and only with persistent exercise and attention to details as outlined in this chapter.

Allografted fingers appear more swollen in the early postoperative stages than autografted ones. The extra volar plate does not make any perceptible difference, however, after a few weeks have elapsed. Regional lymphadenopathy also disappears by six weeks. Analysis of ten-year results of allografting at the time this chapter was prepared revealed that 70 per cent of patients who receive allografts recover complete extension and active flexion sufficient to touch the midpalm with the fingertip. This represents a 70 per cent salvage rate of fingers which were 100 per cent failures following a more conventional approach. Exploration of fingers which failed to flex actively after receiving an allograft revealed that the transplanted sheath remained intact and that adhesions had not formed between the internal surface of the sheath and the enclosed tendons. Failure to achieve flexion in all patients was due to incarceration of the proximal exposed tendon in dense nonyielding cicatrix. Although the composite graft apparently has solved the problem in the digital theca area, biological variations of healing and remodeling in the remainder of the hand still plague some patients and probably will continue to do so until more precise biochemical and biophysical data explaining these variations can be obtained.

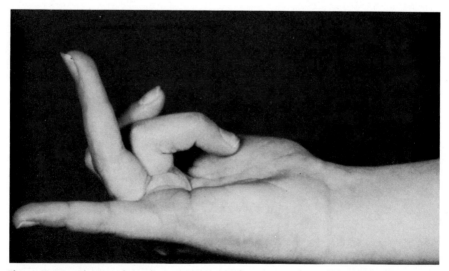

Figure 8–57. Flexion of ring finger in patient with composite tissue homograft. Note relative independence of motion when suture lines are staggered in the palm and in the wrist.

POSTOPERATIVE CARE OF REPAIRED TENDONS

If a technically good anastomosis has been performed, dehiscence will not occur with the wrist in a neutral position (thumb on a straight line with radius). Tension can be relieved by flexing the metacarpophalangeal and proximal interphalangeal joints. The distal interphalangeal joints should remain almost completely extended (180 degrees). The biological basis for immobilization is not to prevent tension on the anastomosis from causing dehiscence; it is to allow revascularization to occur. The dressing should remain undisturbed for three weeks in young patients. In patients over 35, the dressing should be removed in seven to ten days so that joints can be put through a passive range of motion. Of primary concern at this stage is the prevention of proximal interphalangeal joint stiffness. When dressings are changed, the wrist should be flexed while the proximal interphalangeal joints are moved passively through a full range.

Although there are conflicting clinical impressions and recommendations regarding early active motion, everything we know about fundamental processes of tendon healing suggests that active motion should not be attempted before three weeks. The concept that a bursal type of lining for the graft can be created by moving the tendon continually is without biological basis. The evidence is particularly striking following tenolysis procedures. To be certain that a tendon released from old scar tissue by a tenolysis procedure kept moving during the entire healing period, one of the authors once attached a long No. 34 wire to the musculotendinous junction of the liberated flexor profundus unit. The tendon had been incarcerated in scar at the wrist and, after scar tissue had been excised, it was possible to put the finger through a complete flexion arc by pulling on the proximal muscle mass. The wire at the musculotendinous junction was passed through the center of the forearm and brought out on the posterior surface of the elbow. By pulling the wire, one could move the flexor profundus unit through a full range of motion. Twice daily, beginning on the day after tenolysis, the profundus tendon was pulled by the wire through a range sufficient to produce full flexion and extension of the digit. After the fifth day, the force required to flex the finger by pulling on the wire became noticeably greater; by the ninth day it was almost impossible to flex the finger. An attempt to do so on the tenth day resulted in the wire cutting through the tendon, and no further increase in range of motion of the motor unit could be accomplished. Collagen synthesis and remodeling around the tendon in the midwrist area had become so effective that continued motion was impossible. Blood supply was not a factor during the ten days, as the tendon at wrist level is so large that it did not break before the wire pulled through it.

A different sequence of events occurs if early motion is forced upon a relatively small tendon graft in the digital area. Usually, active motion is possible within the limits imposed by pain and postoperative swelling. As time goes by, however, less motion is possible; by six weeks, active motion may no longer be possible. Moreover, the finger frequently is restrained in a flexion contracture. Exploration of a finger which has lost active motion following early activation of a small graft reveals that the graft has been replaced by dense fibrous tissue; the graft may not even be recognizable. A logical explanation for this series of events is that early motion prevented revascularization of the graft; loss of architecture and gliding function is inevitable when this occurs. Some surgeons have reported success with limited active motion during the early part of the healing process. Success under these circumstances probably was due to the fact that motion was not extensive enough to prevent the graft from developing a new blood supply. The old concept that tendons should be immobilized for three weeks because the anastomosis requires that long to become strong is fallacious. Tendon grafts are immobilized three weeks primarily to allow them to develop a new blood supply.

Studies on healing of long tendons indicate that increased collagen synthesis occurs for a longer time than in skin or muscle. Increased collagen synthesis has been measured for as long as 35 days following a tendon anastomosis; there is nothing critical about 21 days as far as tensile strength is concerned. Although a sensible amount of active power can be generated to mobilize a tendon graft after three weeks' immobilization, forceful muscle contraction, particularly against forced resistance, can break a tendon graft or cause dehiscence of an anastomosis five weeks after surgery. The distal attachment is usually the weakest point. The pull-out wire invariably produces some necrosis in the end of a tendon, and many weeks may be required before collagen synthesis and remodeling produces a scar which will replace tendon in that area. Attempting to flex a finger against forced resistance usually is the exercise that causes dehiscence of a tendon-bone junction. It should be remembered, however, that normal tendons can be avulsed by powerful flexion against forced resistance. Moreover, hard contraction of the profundus muscle against forced resistance probably exerts a net force of near zero on restricting adhesions. Probably the only benefit occurring from isometric contraction of a grafted profundus unit is increased strength of the muscle belly. There is no evidence that changes in collagen leading to gliding function of an incarcerated tendon occur faster or more effectively in response to great mechanical stress. Most individuals who place reliance on brute force to activate incarcerated tendons are still thinking in terms of rupturing adhesions, rather than applying stimuli to encourage secondary remodeling of scar tissue.

Because we are not certain of the various physical stimuli which affect the remodeling process, we are not able at present to outline with confidence a program to restore gliding function after three weeks of immobilization. Although a few manipulations and exercises, when performed correctly, appear to influence favorably the return of active motion, it must be remembered that controlled studies have not been performed on this phase of tendon repair. We do not have direct evidence that anything of a physical nature has a cause-and-effect relation on secondary remodeling of newly synthesized scar. The following program has been associated with return of active motion in a relatively short period of time, however. It is recommended until more data are available.

The first objective is to recover full range of passive motion in interphalangeal joints if it has not been maintained throughout the healing period. It is not necessary in youngsters, who regain active motion so quickly, to put interphalangeal joints through a passive range of motion during the three-week healing period. In people over 35, however, the splint should be removed and the interphalangeal joints put through a passive range of motion as often as necessary. During the first week after the cast has been removed (fourth postoperative week), only passive flexion should be performed. Passive extension is dangerous during this time because it may result in dehiscence of the distal anastomosis. Again, however, the key to management of a flexion contracture is not to let it occur. Loss of the final 10 to 15 degrees of distal interphalangeal joint extension is a common complication of flexor tendon reconstruction which can be prevented more easily than it can be corrected. One method of preventing flexion contracture of the distal interphalangeal joint is to keep the tip of the finger extended during the immobilization period. With the wrist and metacarpophalangeal joints flexed, the proximal and distal interphalangeal joints can be extended safely.

The pull-out wire used in the distal anastomosis should be left in place during the first week of exercise. If the tip is involved in a flexion contracture, the pull-out wire should be left in during the second week of exercise also, while passive extension and splinting are continued.

At the same time passive flexion is started (first week after removal of splint), active flexion can be started cautiously. Active flexion at this time usually is dependent upon movement of the whole scar and one cannot, therefore, expect more than a flicker of flexion. It is important for the patient to see a flicker of motion at this time, however, as it provides needed encouragement for the remainder of a long slow course. When a graft has been properly transplanted, a flicker of motion at the end of three weeks usually is possible, and a surgeon should take whatever time is needed to demonstrate to the patient that a tendon capable of flexing the tip is in place and is working to some extent. Sustained forceful contraction at this stage is inadvisable. Forceful contraction of the profundus muscle will not be of any real value at this time and may set the stage for improper use of the extensor mechanism during subsequent weeks. Any active motion which is

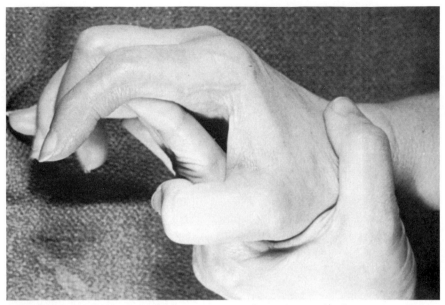

Figure 8–58. First exercise in mobilizing a flexor tendon graft. Note that the metacarpophalangeal joint only is blocked in extension. Motion should be gained in the proximal interphalangeal joint before significant distal interphalangeal joint motion is attempted.

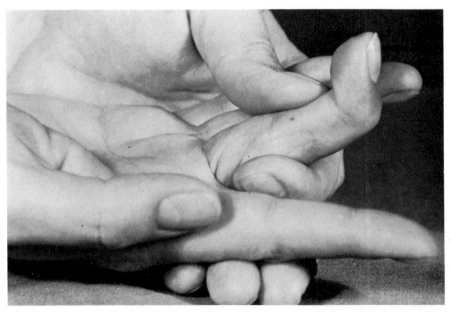

Figure 8–59. Incorrect method of beginning motion following placement of a flexor tendon graft or repair of a flexor tendon. Hyperextension of the proximal interphalangeal joint while distal interphalangeal joint flexion is attempted may result in recurvatum deformity of the proximal interphalangeal joint and a flexion contracture of the distal interphalangeal joint. (Reproduced by permission from E. E. Peacock, Jr., Surgery 45:415, 1959.)

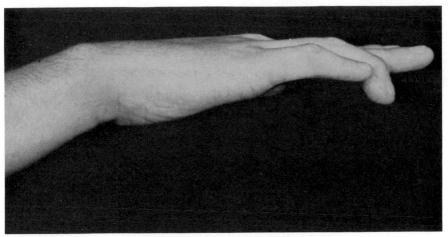

Figure 8–60. Typical appearance of a finger in which distal interphalangeal joint motion was obtained too early by incorrect methods.

possible during the first training session should be performed with minimal effort. Difficulty in obtaining a flicker of flexion at the first training session is usually due to fear, discomfort, or confusion. Demonstration of a small amount of motion can almost always be obtained, however, if the surgeon takes time to overcome these problems by instruction and reassurance.

The patient should attempt active flexion first by blocking the metacarpophalangeal joint in full extension with the pad of the thumb of the other hand pressed against the volar surface of the proximal phalanx. This maneuver tightens the flexor tendon by molding it against the concave surface of the proximal phalanx, thus placing the entire flexor mechanism under maximal tension and insuring that any additional tension generated by the proximal muscle will be transmitted to the proximal interphalangeal joint. Careless performance of this exercise can be harmful, particularly if the proximal interphalangeal joint also is blocked so that motion is gained first in the distal interphalangeal joint.

There is always a danger that fingers with only a single tendon will develop a sublimis minus deformity. Pressure against the middle phalanx which forces the proximal interphalangeal joint into hyperextension can produce such a deformity because it adds tension to the flexor surface of the distal interphalangeal joint. Part of the protection against the sublimis minus deformity is the tenodesis effect of operative scar and mild contracture of the volar capsule. This tissue is subject to mechanical deformation during the first week following removal of the splint, just as it is hoped that connective tissue along the tendon is influenced. It is extremely important, therefore, that flexion be developed first and extension be achieved last in the proximal interphalangeal joint. When flexion inadvertently appears in the distal interphalangeal joint while the proximal interphalangeal joint remains extended, a cylindrical cast should be placed on the distal joint so that all flexion must occur in the proximal area. If even the slightest tendency to develop a recurvatum deformity is noted in the proximal interphalangeal joint, a protective splint or cast should be used to hold the joint in mild flexion while remodeling of tissue on the volar surface occurs. In summary, during the first week of remobilization, the objective is to obtain a full range of passive flexion in all joints, and to develop a limited range or active flexion in the proximal interphalangeal joint.

During the second week of remobilization (following removal of the splint), passive extension of the proximal interphalangeal joint should be started and more vigorous and sustained active flexion encouraged. The pull-out wire can be removed at the end of the first week (fourth postoperative week), but flexion against forced resistance or extremely forceful passive extension should not be performed yet. Active flexion should be continued, with the opposite thumb restricting the metacarpophalangeal joint in extension, until approximately 90 degrees of active flexion of the proximal interphalangeal joint has been achieved. Only then should the proximal interphalangeal joint be blocked in extension while the patient works specifically on distal interphalangeal joint flexion. By the end of the second immobilization week (fifth postoperative week), the volar checkrein effect of new scar tissue and capsule remodeling will be stable enough to permit pressure on the middle phalanx.

A frequent and often severe complication sometimes appears during this time, and should be diagnosed early and treated vigorously. The condition is best described as improper use of the extensor mechanism during attempts to flex a digit. Biologically, it is difficult to be any more specific than to point out that protective reflexes, in which the extensor mechanism overpowers the potentially more powerful flexor motor units, occur very rapidly after an injury, particularly if the injury involves the volar surface of a digit. Almost instantly the extensor mechanism will contract as if it were attempting to remove the involved finger from the rest of the hand. (One of the authors was watching his own index finger once at the time a tip laceration occurred. It was amazing to note that the long extensor and intrinsic components of the extensor mechanism produced full extensor rigidity before pain of any type was appreciated.) During the week after soft tissue healing has occurred and scar tissue remains sensitive, improper use of the extensor muscles may become reflex. The result is that the involved finger becomes "physiologically amputated" by being held in maximal extension while the rest of the hand is in a semiflexed or prehensile position. Although the mechanism for inciting and developing this reflex may be entirely central at first, the role of the lumbrical also may be a contributing factor when the profundus has been cut distal to the origin of that muscle. The profundus is really a tendon with both volar (flexor) and dorsal (extensor) insertion by virtue of its attachments to the extensor hood through the lumbrical. Following division of the profundus distal to the origin of the lumbrical, the only attachment the profundus has to bone is through the lumbrical muscle. Understandably, contraction of the proximal muscle mass, whether intentional or unintentional, places strain on the extensor mechanism and upsets the entire flexor-extensor balance in the involved digit. Whether or not this triggers or increases the tendency to contract the long extensors inappropriately is unknown, but that patients unknowingly splint their fingers in extension by contracting the extensor muscle units at a time they think they are contracting only the flexor muscles is undeniable. A simple test which should be performed during the second week or whenever the patient begins serious active exercises is to have the patient flex the digit as powerfully as possible and hold it at the end of the flexion arc. The examiner should then attempt to continue flexing the digit passively by pushing the finger tip into the palm. If the extensors are checkreining the finger at this point in the flexion arc, resistance will be encountered and further passive flexion at the end of the active flexion arc will not be possible. After the patient has been told to relax, flexor and extensor muscles usually will relax simultaneously; the finger tips can then be pushed easily through the full flexion arc. The patient usually is amazed to see that passive flexion is not possible while he is attempting active flexion. Most patients can be shown that, while they are attempting to flex, the extensor mechanism on the dorsum of the hand is standing out because it is under such tension. Some patients need only to be shown that improper use of the extensor muscle is contributing to their inability to flex; they seem to know instinctively how to break the habit. Other patients require hours of instruction and utilization of a number of tricks to break the habit of using extensor muscles when flexion is desired. If improper use of the extensor muscles continues during attempts to flex, however, there is no point in proceeding any further until the problem has been solved. When fully developed, it is an extremely effective physiological block to restoration of finger flexion.

After approximately 90 degrees of proximal interphalangeal joint flexion has been obtained with the metacarpophalangeal joint restrained in extension, exercises should be performed without blocking the joint. It is usually at this point that the first real evidence of improper use of the extensors occurs. Progress in flexion of all joints simultaneously is best assisted and recorded by having a patient exercise against a ruler placed in the center of the palm. The fingernail serves as an indicator to measure the distance that flexion of the tip has to cover before grasp is complete. By working against a ruler, progress

sion, during the second week; and active flexion directed by a ruler in the palm after 90 per cent flexion of the proximal interphalangeal joints with the metacarpophalangeal joint extended is possible. Development of distal interphalangeal joint flexion before proximal interphalangeal joint flexion, appearance of a recurvatum deformity (sublimis minus) in the proximal interphalangeal joint, improper use of extensors, and development of abnormal mobility of the metacarpophalangeal joint are complications which must be diagnosed early and corrected before progress can continue. The most serious complication—dehiscence of the distal anastomosis—usually is caused by flexing the tip of the finger against forced resistance or an error in technique of attaching tendon to bone.

Most tendon grafts or restorations will continue to develop an increased range of motion for 10 to 12 weeks after the cast has been removed. The small finger usually develops active flexion most rapidly and successfully; the index finger requires more time and is least successful. The flexion arc in the little finger is the smallest, and this probably accounts for the high rate of success in reconstructing its flexor mechanism. Not only does the index finger require a longer range of motion to flex and extend the tip, but the tendency to physiologically amputate this digit, if it is not in perfect condition, is more pronounced than for any other finger. It is instinctive to "throw an abnormal index finger out of the hand" and use the radial side of the long finger as an opposable surface. As a result, real concentration is required to use a damaged index finger. This, of course, is not true for the small finger, which forms the vital fulcrum or trailing edge of the hand during many types of power grasping function. Finally, most of the work performed by the index finger is done in tandem with the thumb. Only about 45 degrees' flexion of the proximal interphalangeal joint and no distal interphalangeal joint flexion is needed to oppose the index finger to the thumb. Thus, as soon as this amount of flexion is recovered, many patients lose stimulus to continue exercising and develop no more active motion.

Treatment of Complications

If, after three to four months have elapsed, satisfactory flexion has not been regained, the question of whether a second operation should be performed arises. The first consideration at such a time is the status of small joints. If a satisfactory range of passive motion in the interphalangeal joints has been achieved and active motion has not returned, the possibility of regaining function by a second procedure is much better than if passive motion also has been lost. If a complication has caused the tendon to become replaced by dense volar scar or incarcerated by a nonyielding proximal adhesion, interphalangeal joints will be tenodesed in flexion, and operative intervention is recommended as soon as possible. Joints tenodesed in this manner can be released by excising the volar scar early. If volar scar is not excised relatively soon, secondary changes in the joints may occur which are not amenable to further therapy.

The next consideration involves the possibility of correcting a mistake or complication which occurred during the first operation. If the original procedure was performed under ideal conditions and no known technical irregularity or postoperative complication occurred, the case for a repeat performance of the original procedure is not good. If, however, a primary repair was performed originally, it is possible that a secondary graft would have a better chance of producing flexion. If inadequate postoperative care is suspected and better care can be assured the next time, the case for another attempt to restore flexion by surgery is sound. The essence of the question is whether failure to glide is due to factors which the surgeon can control, such as selection of a proper procedure, technical perfection, postoperative management, and so forth, or whether adherence of the tendon can be attributed to noncontrollable factors and must therefore be assigned to biological variations in the healing process. One, of course, is amenable to correction by a second operation; the other is not, until other methods for controlling the physical characteristics of scar tissue are available.

If a second operative attempt to provide flexion is decided upon, the timing of the procedure may be important. When dehiscence of a primary repair or a secondary graft has occurred, it is best to open the hand as soon as possible. One usually cannot be certain about the level of separation, and the possibility that the proximal motor unit is completely relaxed because of a dehisced distal attachment must be considered. If dehiscence occurred at the junction of tendon and bone, it may be possible to advance the tendon without having to perform another graft—provided it is done within 48 hours. If failure to glide is the complication for which the second procedure is designed, however, not only is early operation *not* desirable; it may even be detrimental.

When the repaired tendon is judged to be intact, the danger of proximal muscle fibrosis and shortening is insignificant; the condition of the interphalangeal joint and maturity of soft tissue scar are the most important considerations. Particularly when small joints already have been immobilized for a long time and have not regained normal motion, it is important to do what can be done to remobilize them before performing a second operation with its attendant period of immobilization. Even if several months are required to regain passive motion, reduce swelling, and eliminate pain, it is worthwhile to wait several months to prevent further inevitable damage caused by a second operation, further immobilization, and vigorous remobilization. On the other hand, if a bowstring effect, caused by an adherent flexor tendon, is preventing extension of interphalangeal joints, excision of scar tissue or the entire graft may be needed early to protect the joint from intrinsic damage and permanent fixation.

The maturity of the scar and subsidence of soft tissue reaction also must be considered when a second operation appears advisable. A definitive secondary procedure, such as a tendon graft, should not be performed through immature scar. It also should not be done in a digit or hand which is inflamed or edematous from previous injury, surgery, or physical manipulations. For such a hand, when there is evidence that a primarily repaired tendon is unremittingly checkreining the finger in a flexed position, two operations definitely are better than one. The first operation should consist of opening the finger distal to the metacarpophalangeal joint and removing the flexor mechanism only where it is causing restriction of interphalangeal extension. In most fingers, particularly in digits which have received a free graft of the profundus tendon, the effect of the graft will not be that of tenodesis. Checkrein effect for scar tenodesis usually can be diagnosed preoperatively by simply determining if change in position of the proximal joint, such as the wrist or metacarpophalangeal joint, releases the flexion contracture in the proximal or distal interphalangeal joints. In most cases, change in position of a proximal joint does not affect contracture of distal joints; when these fingers are opened, the graft either has been replaced by a solid diffuse band of scar or is attached to everything along its entire course. If the entire graft has been replaced by scar tissue, the sheath also is usually unrecognizable. Most of the sheath may have been removed at the first operation, and the one or two small pulleys which were preserved usually become inseparably amalgamated with scar tissue. If recognizable pulleys can be found and the tendon passing through the pulleys is not fused to them, this portion of the previous restoration should be preserved for future use. Under these circumstances, only the tendon and scar tissue between the pulley should be removed; tendon within an intact pulley should be preserved to maintain a space through which a subsequent graft can be passed. Removing all of the sheath lessens enormously the possibility of a successful secondary restoration and means that a pulley reconstruction of some type will be necessary if bowstringing is to be avoided. Intact pulleys with movable tendons within them should be preserved in the center of the proximal phalanx (and middle phalanx, also, if possible). Scar tissue binding the proximal tendon to the base of the proximal phalanx also should be preserved to prevent release and retraction of the motor unit. The rest of the scar tissue and old tendon should be excised over a large enough area on the volar surface of the proximal and distal interphalangeal joints to permit passive extension of these joints. The volar plate should not be excised, as interphalangeal joint function is seldom retained after this important structure has been removed. Failure to achieve immediate interphalangeal joint extension during the operation should not be regarded as a sign that extension cannot be achieved. After volar scar tissue has been removed surgically, the contracted volar capsule, which may often limit joint extension, may respond to splinting and physical therapy over a moderate period of time. Following excision of an old graft or volar scar tissue or both, three or four months may be required for recovery of interphalangeal joint motion, subsidence of edema, and disappearance of traumatic arthritis. Only then should a new tendon graft be inserted.

A finger in which a flexor tendon graft has been inserted under optimal circumstances and in which no known postoperative complication developed which might be avoided during a second attempt to restore flexion may recover complete extension and passive flexion without recovering any significant active flexion. This condition strongly suggests that a biological variation of the healing and remodeling process was responsible for permanent incarceration of the tendon. In these patients, a repeat of the same procedure would result only in similar failure to restore gliding function. A trick that sometimes works in such fingers is to wait until soft tissue reaction has subsided and then to insert a subcutaneous tendon graft without disturbing the old one. This can be done through a small distal incision in the tip of the finger and a larger proximal incision in the palm. A small tendon graft can be passed through the finger on top of the old one in a complex subcu-

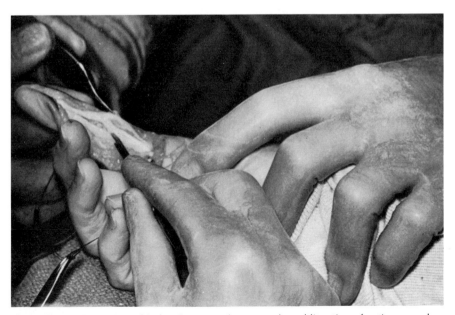

Figure 8–64. Dissection of index finger to show complete obliteration of entire space between digital sheath and damaged flexor tendons. This is usually the result of an unskilled attempt to repair flexor tendons in an initial procedure or a complication such as tenosynovitis.

taneous plane. The old proximal anastomosis is exposed, and the motor unit is transferred to the new graft. Palmar fascia and old scar in the vicinity of the new anastomosis should be removed. A subcutaneous graft inserted in this manner usually will function well, but a real compromise in overall finger activity results because of pronounced bowstringing effect. Function can be improved after soft tissue healing by having the patient wear a ring which acts as an external pulley. It is possible to reconstruct a fibrous tissue pulley in a finger with a subcutaneous graft after bowstring type of flexion has been achieved. Insertion of a pulley as a secondary procedure is always hazardous, however. The danger of losing amplitude of motion in the graft is responsible for the justifiable hesitancy of most surgeons to correct the bowstring effect.

Reconstruction of a pulley around a functioning flexor tendon graft should not be undertaken unless the bowstring effect of an unrestrained graft is objectionable and wearing a ring on the involved finger is not satisfactory. The most important technical part of reconstructing a pulley is to find a soft tissue plane which will not endanger longitudinal motion of the graft. The pulley should be superficial so that substantial subcutaneous tissue will remain between it and the tendon. A pulley usually is inserted on the dorsal side of the finger and threaded blindly around the volar surface. The tendon passer should be just beneath skin while the finger is held in a flexed position. If the

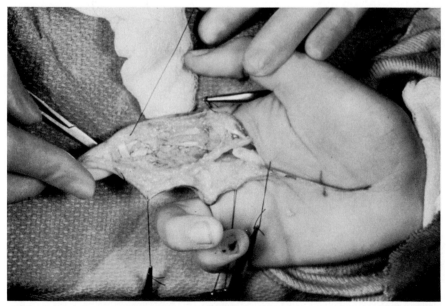

Figure 8–65. Reconstruction of distal pulley by use of a free graft of plantaris tendon. Note that anastomosis is pulled to dorsal side of finger with a suture.

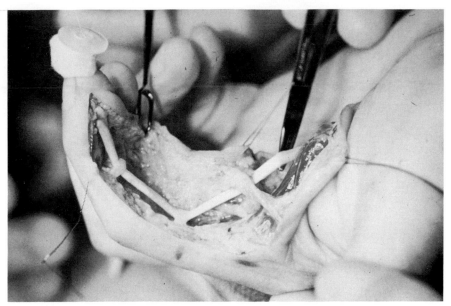

Figure 8–66. Simultaneous replacement of proximal and distal pulleys and insertion of a flexor tendon graft. It is usually preferable to place the graft first and insert the pulleys as a secondary procedure to relieve a bowstring effect. Placement of graft and pulleys at the same time often results in restricted motion of the flexor tendon graft. (From E. E. Peacock, Jr., in *Surgery: Principles and Practice,* 4th edition, edited by C. A. Moyer, J. E. Rhoads, H. N. Harkins, and J. G. Allen, Philadelphia, J. B. Lippincott Co., 1970.)

finger is held in extension while a passage for the pulley is being made, skin and tendon will be in close approximation, and damage to the tendon will be inevitable. A palmaris longus or plantaris graft split longitudinally makes an ideal graft for a pulley reconstruction. The pulley should not suspend a tendon as the mesotendon or vincula do, however. It should be nonmovable and should draw the tendon close to the volar surface of the proximal phalanx. This can be accomplished by duplicating the decussating fibers of a natural pulley. Examination of the arrangement of fibers in a digital sheath reveals that, in the pulley area (between the interphalangeal joints), the sheath is thick because of a figure-of-eight weave of large fiber bundles. A similar arrangement can be constructed in an artificial pulley by passing the graft in a figure-of-eight configuration so that a pendulum type of motion is impossible and minimal contact between graft and pulley is established. The dorsal anastomosis of the graft to itself is usually made on the lateral side of the phalanx. The graft usually is passed beneath the extensor mechanism, although it also works satisfactorily dorsal to the extensor mechanism.

A four week immobilization period is advisable before active flexion is started. At first, the thumb of the opposite hand should be used to reinforce the pulley, as in the first exercises following a flexor tendon graft. If active motion cannot be regained after an adequate period of exercise, it should be assumed that the tendon is attached to the pulley and the pulley should be removed.

Tenolysis

Tenolysis following suture of a digital tendon or insertion of a flexor tendon graft has not been a reliable procedure in our experience. Others have reported some success with tenolysis, but the general consensus seems to be that it is not reliable unless adhesions have developed in an area where there was no external wound. Examples of this type of condition are a superficial burn, severe contusion, closed fracture, and soft tissue infection. Following healing of these wounds in some patients, active flexion may not be equivalent to passive range of motion in spite of arduous physical therapy. Regardless of the fact that the original wound did not involve directly a single flexor tendon, all of the digits may be involved. Exploration of the flexor mechanism may reveal a few sharply localized fibrous condensates between flexor tendons or between a flexor tendon and the sheath. An adhesion adjoining the two flexor tendons can be very effective in limiting active motion, for the range of motion of the sublimis tendon is only about

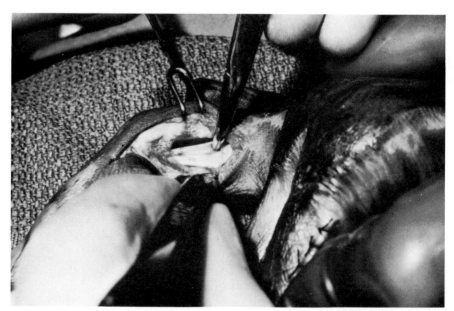

Figure 8–67. Adherence of sublimis and profundus tendons following a closed superficial burn of the hand. Amalgamation of these structures is secondary to immobilization of an edematous extremity. The pathway by which edema fluid and fibrin become replaced by collagen is not understood at this time.

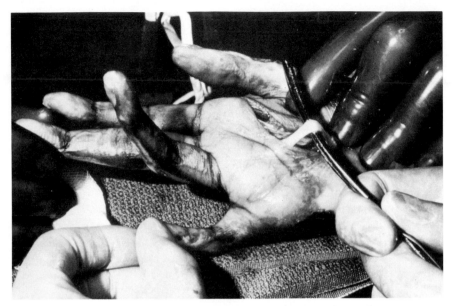

Figure 8–68.   Retraction of sublimis tendon in the palm following release of the scar between tendons in the distal finger still does not result in flexion of the distal finger. The tendons are attached along their entire course. In this instance, excision of the sublimis tendon was necessary before active flexion of the profundus could be developed.

two-thirds that required to flex the tip of the digit. If excessive callus formation during healing of a fracture involves a flexor tendon directly, it is easy to see how longitudinal motion in the tendon can be restricted. If no wound of the tendon sheath or bed occurred, however, one is left with the conclusion that a pathway must exist to convert loose connective tissue into densely organized collagen. The exact pathway by which this occurs is unknown, but the end result leaves little doubt that immobilization of an edematous hand is dangerous from the standpoint of increasing the collagen content between movable planes. On the dorsum of the hand, subcutaneous tissues and intrinsics may be involved, as described previously, while in small joints the capsule and collateral ligaments are remodeled. Within a digital sheath flexor tendons can become adherent to each other; if infection occurs within the sheath, the entire sheath-tendon relationship often is destroyed and no hope for restoring motion by tenolysis exists. If the sheath is intact or if bacteria did not actually penetrate the theca, adhesions may be sharply localized and can be excised with good results.

Motion should be started following tenolysis as soon as soft tissue healing permits. If the process is more diffuse and adhesions bind the tendons to each other more than to the sheath, the sublimis tendon should be removed. This provides more room for the profundus within the digital compartment and removes completely the site of attachment of the profundus. If the adhesive process involves the digital sheath as well as the tendons, the sheath should be removed except for two strategically located pulleys over the proximal and middle phalanges. Results are encouraging and may even be dramatic if the original injury did not involve tendons directly.

None of the above-described procedures has been effective for us following direct repair of a digital flexor tendon or insertion of a flexor tendon graft. Tenolysis is of some value in the wrist or palm, but in the digital area it has been very disappointing. A flexor tendon graft can be stripped completely of restricting adhesions, but the same processes which produced adhesions during healing of the original wound seem to recur. Sometimes it seems that the secondary healing phenomenon may actually produce stronger adhesions more rapidly than in the first wound. The biological basis for different response to tenolysis following healing of open and closed wounds is speculative. Of course, the degree of involvement in closed wounds often is less than in open ones; there may be nothing more involved. It is possible, however, that collagen fibrils developing along fibrin-oriented matrix in structurally intact but injured tissues are different in some way from collagen produced in an open healing wound. In addition, the secondary healing phenomenon may be accountable, although this phenomenon has not been studied in deep scar tissue as extensively as it has in skin wounds.

Biological Control of Scar Tissue

The statement that biological variations of healing and remodeling in the remainder of the hand will continue to be responsible for unpredictable results introduces a wide range of speculation which will be summarized at this time by saying that one intriguing approach to many of the problems discussed in this chapter is the biological control of physical properties of scar tissue. Although a number of possibilities (many still unappreciated) exist for controlling synthesis, assembly, and remodeling of collagen, the lathyrogenic phenomenon at present seems to be nature's revelation that specific alteration of the collagen system is within the scope of manipulation at this time. The hope that general protein synthesis inhibitors such as actinomycin and puromycin might be of value in solving problems of tendon adhesions was never a realistic one; these agents are too nonspecific to be useful in manipulating scar tissue in healing wounds. Even such alterations as producing ascorbic acid deficiency or interfering with specific enzyme systems such as proline hydroxylase (by chelating or removing valuable metal. co-factors) have been too nonspecific, although they are more specific for the collagen system. Lathyrogenic agents, such as β-aminopropionitrile, which interfere selectively with intermolecular and intramolecular cross-linking of collagen, have produced spectacular results, however, in alteration of physical properties of adhesions around animal tendons. Even if β-aminopropionitrile does not turn out to be the actual substance which ultimately is used to produce similar effects in human beings, the principle by which it exerts its effect suggests that biological control of processes which surgical manipulation now, at best, can only partially control, is possible. The greatest handicap, of course, is need for a suitable experimental model.

In the search for pharmacological control of tendon adhesions, the results of experiments evaluating proline analogs such as cis-hydroxy-1-proline, 3,4-dehydroproline, or azetidine-2-carboxylic acid for inhibiting net collagen synthesis and deposition are disappointing. Proline analogs are effective in tissue culture preparations in reducing collagen synthesis; several reports suggesting a beneficial effect in animals appeared several years ago. More recent investigations in the author's (E. E. P.) laboratories, however, have indicated that the toxicity of proline analogs in doses sufficient to inhibit significantly collagen synthesis was too great to proceed to Phase III or clinical testing in human beings. Other analogs will be tested and, if any are found sufficiently nontoxic to be used in human beings, it seems likely that this approach will be most useful in postoperative care of patients undergoing tenolysis procedures.

Whereas dangerous drugs with known generalized toxicity can be administered experimentally to patients with incurable diseases, administration of such agents to patients whose only infirmity is a severed flexor tendon cannot be tolerated except under the most exacting controls. Development of the chicken foot preparation as an animal model and the increasing interest of biologically oriented surgeons in gaining as much information as possible from human tissues, which previously have been disregarded, are making differences in our present outlook. The new information coming out of such studies will be applicable to other organ systems, such as the cardiovascular or hepatobiliary system, where scar tissue of undesirable quality and quantity offers an even more serious threat to health.

SUGGESTED READING

Brockis, J. G. The Blood Supply of the Flexor and Extensor Tendons of the Fingers in Man. J. Bone Joint Surg. *35B*:131, 1953.

Cameron, R. R. Freeze-Dried Composite Tendon Allografts: An Experimental Study. Plast. Reconstr. Surg. *47*:39, 1971.

Chacha, P. Free Autologous Composite Tendon Grafts for Division of Both Flexor Tendons Within the Digital Theca of the Hand. J. Bone Joint Surg. *56A*:960, 1974.

Craver, J. M., Madden, J. W., and Peacock, E. E., Jr. Biological Control of Physical Properties of Tendon Adhesions: Effect of Beta-aminopropionitrile in Chickens. Ann. Surg. *167*:697, 1968.

Graham, W. C. Delayed Tendon Repairs. Amer. J. Surg. *80*:776, 1950.

Green, W. L., and Niebauer, J. J. Results of Primary and Secondary Flexor-Tendon Repairs in No Man's Land. J. Bone Joint Surg. *56A*:1216, 1974.

Greenlee, T. K., Beckman, C., and Pike, D. A Fine Structural Study of the Development of the Chick Flexor Digital Tendon: A Model for Synovial Sheathed Tendon Healing. Amer. J. Anat. *143*:303, 1975.

Hueston, J. T., Hubble, B., and Rigg, B. R. Homografts of the Digital Flexor Tendon System. Aust. N. Zeal. J. Surg. *36*,269, 1967.

Hunter, J. M., et al. Flexor Tendon Reconstruction in Severely Damaged Hands. A Two-Stage Procedure Using a Silicone-Dacron Reinforced Gliding Prosthesis Prior to Tendon Grafting. J. Bone Joint Surg. *53*:829, 1971.

Jaffe, S., and Weckesser, E. Profundus Tendon Grafting with the Sublimis Intact. An End-Result Study of Thirty Patients. J. Bone Joint Surg. *49A*:1298, 1967.

Kleinert, H. E., Kutz, J. E., Atasoy, E., and Stormo, A. Primary Repair of Flexor Tendons. Orthop. Clin. N. Amer. *4*:865, 1973.

Lindsay, W. K. The Fibroblasts in Flexor Tendon Healing. Plast. Reconstr. Surg. *34*:223, 1964.

McFarlane, R. M., Lamon, R., and Jarvis, G. Flexor Tendon Injuries within the Finger. A Study of the Results of Tendon Suture and Tendon Graft. J. Trauma *8*:987, 1968.

Peacock, E. E., Jr. A Study of Circulation in Normal Tendons and Healing Grafts. Ann. Surg. *149*:415, 1959.

Peacock, E. E., Jr. Biological Principles in the Healing of Long Tendons. Surg. Clin. N. Amer. *45*:461, 1965.

Peacock, E. E., Jr. Fundamental Aspects of Wound Healing Relating to the Restoration of Gliding Function after Tendon Repair. Surg. Gynec. Obstet. *119*:241, 1964.

Peacock, E. E., Jr. Some Technical Aspects and Results of Flexor Tendon Repair. Surgery *58*:330, 1965.

Peacock, E. E., Jr., and Hartrampf, C. R. Collective Review. The Repair of Flexor Tendons in the Hand. Int. Abstr. Surg. *113*:1, 1961.

Peacock, E. E., Jr., and Madden, J. W. Human Composite Flexor Tendon Allografts. Ann. Surg. *166*:624, 1967.

Peacock, E. E., Jr., and Madden, J. W. Some Studies on the Effects of Beta-aminopropionitrile in Patients with Injured Flexor Tendons. Surgery *66*:215, 1969.

Peacock, E. E., Jr., and Madden, J. W. Some Studies on the Effect of Beta-aminopropionitrile on Collagen in Healing Wounds. Surgery *60*:7, 1966.

Potenza, A. D. Critical Evaluation of Flexor-Tendon Healing and Adhesion Formation within Artificial Digital Sheaths. An Experimental Study. J. Bone Joint Surg. *45-A*:1217, 1963.

Potenza, A. D. Effect of Associated Trauma on Healing of Divided Tendons. J. Trauma *2*: 175, 1962.

Potenza, A. D. Prevention of Adhesions to Healing Digital Flexor Tendons. J.A.M.A. *187*: 99, 1964.

Urbaniak, J. R., Bright, D. S., Gil, L. H., and Goldner, J. L.: Vascularization and the Gliding Mechanism of Free Flexor-Tendon Grafts Inserted by the Silicone-Rod Method. J. Bone Joint Surg. *56A*:473, 1974.

van der Meulen, J. C. Silastic Spacers in Tendon Grafting. Brit. J. Plast. Surg. *24*:166, 1971.

Chapter 9

FASCIA AND MUSCLE

FASCIA

Fascia is important during care of wounds when it becomes infected or when there is not enough to provide structural support. Although fascia is usually classified as a tissue (dense connective tissue), like tendons and skin, it is best considered as a compound organ by surgeons confronted with an inadequate amount during repair of a wound. Although fascia heals superbly by fibrous protein synthesis and remodeling of collagen fibers, its regenerative powers are limited. Thus a wound in which fascia needed for structural stability has been destroyed is going to require transplantation of new fascia from either local or distant sources. Structural stability is rarely regained by regeneration of fascia, particularly when other soft tissue protrudes through a major fascial defect. Although the abdominal wall, diaphragm, and pelvis are areas where inadequate fascia most frequently causes clinical disability, small defects in fascia of the lower extremities occasionally cause symptoms because of herniation of underlying muscle. Such defects are usually slit-like tears in the tough lateral fascia of the thigh or upper leg and usually can be repaired without difficulty by excising a small amount of muscle and suturing fascial edges together. Defects which cannot be repaired in this way usually can be made asymptomatic by enlarging the window.

Abdominal Wall Defects

Defects in the anterior abdominal wall are the most frequently encountered wounds in fascia which have clinical significance. Acute conditions include disruption following abdominal surgery or omphalocele in newborn infants; chronic wounds are hernias and may be the result of either operative, congenital, or metabolic factors. In this chapter, indirect inguinal hernias, spigelian hernias, and umbilical hernias will be considered as congenital wounds of fascia, incisional hernias as chronic surgical wounds, and direct inguinal hernias as biological variations of collagen metabolism in the inguinal area. Other hernias such as diaphragmatic hernias do not fall clearly into this classification and may be the result of abnormal stress secondary to physiological abnormalities of longitudinally oriented esophageal muscle and other defects. Although inguinal hernias usually are not thought of as wounds in the conventional sense, biological considerations of the cause of inguinal hernias which are important in selecting and performing successful restorations are so closely allied to the biology of healing of fibrous tissue that classification in this manner may be useful to the surgeon.

Wound Dehiscence

Dehiscence of an abdominal wound is a major surgical complication which carries a mortality rate of between 15 and 20 per cent if evisceration also occurs. Because the cause of death following dehiscence usually is septic peritonitis, there is some basis for optimism that the mortality is being reduced by better antibiotic therapy. Abdominal wounds have been observed to disrupt as late as 25 days after surgery but the highest incidence of disruption is between the fifth and eighth postoperative days. Warning of dehiscence usually is given in the form of a brown serosanguineous discharge from the wound 24 hours before gross dehiscence occurs. Dehiscence is not an infrequent complication; it occurs approximately once in every 250 abdominal operations. Although attempts to correlate disruption of abdominal wounds with various systemic diseases and conditions have not been generally successful, malignancy, old age, vitamin depletion, azotemia, anemia, hormone deficiencies or excesses, and other factors have been suspected but seldom positively identified as certain causes of failure of fascia to heal. The effect of neoplasms, anemia, azotemia, and hormone imbalances has been examined in animals under controlled laboratory conditions. Perhaps the most interesting of these studies involves the study of healing in animals with large neoplasms.

Surgeons have believed for a long time that patients with advanced neoplasms were more susceptible to wound dehiscence than other patients. Although experimental evidence for some systemic inhibiting effect by neoplasms on the healing process is available, the degree of measurable inhibition is not of an order likely to result in complete abdominal dehiscence. Moreover, analysis of data on dehiscence of human patients does not reveal a significant correlation between disruption in human beings and the presence of a neoplasm. In an attempt to see if there was a reduction in rate of gain in tensile strength in rats with large neoplasms, tensile strength studies have been carried out, under controlled conditions, on healing incised and sutured abdominal wounds in rats with neoplasms. A statistically significant decrease in tensile strength gain was measured in rats with neoplasms, but the order of inhibition was not sufficient to be clinically significant in human beings under most conditions. Tumor-bearing rats also had mild protein depletion and anemia. Correction of protein depletion by dietary supplements and treatment of anemia by transfusion did not alter the decreased rate of gain in tensile strength in the wound. An alcoholic extract of tumor was selected because alcoholic extracts of neoplasms have been shown to interfere with other vital metabolic functions. Data from such work are not complete and this undoubtedly is a fertile field for further investigation.

Because urea has been shown to break hydrogen bonds, and thus denature collagen, some surgeons have suggested that azotemia might be responsible for failure to heal by interfering with collagen assembly. This also has been studied under controlled laboratory conditions and the result of the studies is that markedly azotemic rats show a decrease in rate of gain in tensile strength of wounds. The decrease cannot be corrected by correcting dehydration which often is observed during urea loading experiments in rats. Apparently there is no correlation between the amount of inhibition of wound healing and the serum urea level. Also, inhibition of tensile strength gain in rats is in a range which would be unlikely to cause complete abdominal disruption. These results are not surprising because it would require a blood urea level of 24,000 mg. per 100 cc. to denature collagen; a level one-hundredth of that would presage a fatal outcome.

Anemia and protein depletion also can produce a mathematically significant decrease in rate of gain in tensile strength in laboratory animals. The degree of protein depletion and anemia needed to inhibit healing in animals, however, is more severe than that encountered in human patients. Moreover, the effect is never more than measurable retardation—not almost complete failure of collagen synthesis as occurs in ascorbic acid depletion. It almost seems as if a healing wound has first call on vital substances and, even when they are in relatively short supply, the healing process is seldom embarrassed. It should be pointed out, however, that the length of time a patient has severe protein deficiency may make a difference. The effect of long-term depletion states on blood volume and viscosity may be more important to wound healing than reduction in building blocks for repair.

Addition of hormones such as corticosteroids inhibits collagen synthesis but does not prevent it completely. Clinical experience has shown that patients may be operated upon safely while being treated with relatively enormous amounts of corticosteroids and that, although the gain in tensile strength of the wound may be delayed, healing eventually will occur and abdominal disruption is not a serious hazard.

In spite of the fact that many general conditions have been shown mathematically to interfere with gain in tensile strength of abdominal wounds in laboratory animals and undoubtedly these same conditions exert a similar statistical effect in human wounds, the causes of complete dehiscence in surgical patients almost always are local in the wound and are seldom the result of systemic abnormalities. Local causes include infection, hematoma, and mechanical problems such as bringing out colostomies in the incision and breaking or cutting tissues with sutures. The direction of incisions has been thought by surgeons to be important but the few studies which are available do not substantiate this clinical impression. Some studies do, however, substantiate the clinical impression that upper abdominal incisions dehisce more often than lower ones.

There is not much that can be said about prevention of infection or hematoma that is not obvious to any well trained surgeon. The mechanical aspects of abdominal closure still are controversial, however, and the few facts we have are worthy of additional emphasis. No matter what type of closure the surgeon has selected, pulmonary complications and abdominal distention can cause dehiscence. These two conditions have been shown repeatedly to influence the rate of dehiscence and it does not seem likely at this time that the type of closure has very much to do with the outcome when these complications are severe. Surgeons have believed for many years that external support from devices such as a scultetus binder or internal support from through-and-through retention sutures affords additional protection for patients with abdominal distention, pulmonary complications, or systemic conditions such as neoplasms. Again, data are not conclusive but analysis of existing reports suggests that, although through-and-through retention sutures are effective in preventing evisceration after wound dehiscence, actual rate of dehiscence is not significantly affected. This is not an insignificant contribution because sepsis is the major cause of death when dehiscence occurs. As far as selection of a suture material or a tissue plane in which to use the sutures is concerned, however, the way the suture is used is more important in preventing dehiscence. If the simplest fundamentals of tying secure knots without necrosing tissue and accurately approximating fibrous tissue layers are followed, the type of suture material used does not seem to make a difference in the incidence of wound separation.

The factor of mechanical tension has been studied experimentally from the standpoint of effect on gain in strength of abdominal wounds. These studies can be summarized by stating that the effect of tension is actually beneficial to fascial strength in the abdominal wall, up to a point where it produces necrosis or causes a suture to cut through a layer of fascia. Experiments which were cited in the discussion of repair of skin under tension suggest that collagen synthesis may be increased when dermis is placed under increased tension.

Another possibility is that orientation of new collagen fibers by tensile forces may result in a more compact arrangement which makes them more resistant to collagenolysis. Creation of moderate tension in the fascia of an abdominal wound results in a significant increase in rate of gain in tensile strength of the entire wound. Of course, tension created by a shortage of fascia is clearly different from increased abdominal tension created by severe distention of an abdominal viscus or excessive diaphragmatic excursion. As stated before, these conditions markedly increase the incidence of wound dehiscence, but a moderate shortage of fascia which permits approximation of the fascial edge under slight tension not only does not interfere with fascial healing but may actually increase the rate of gain in strength of the entire wound.

Bringing a drain out through an abdominal incision does not increase the hazard of a dehiscence. Although it is believed that this practice does increase the incidence of a postoperative incisional hernia, there is no evidence that the incidence of acute dehiscence is increased. This is not true for the practice of bringing out a colostomy through the end of an abdominal incision, however. In one study, abdominal wounds containing end colostomies dehisced six times more frequently than similar wounds when the colostomy was brought out through a separate opening.

In summary, the prevention of abdominal wound dehiscence is the prevention of pulmonary complications, abdominal distention, and local sepsis. Systemic disease, suture materials, technique of closure, drains, and moderate tension seem to make little, if any, difference. An end colostomy in an abdominal wound significantly increases the rate of dehiscence, however, and upper abdominal wounds appear to have a higher incidence of dehiscence than lower ones. The question which surgeons often discuss and are frequently very opinionated about—whether a longitudinal abdominal wound is more likely to undergo dehiscence than a transverse one—has not been studied under accurately controlled conditions. Available data strongly suggest that there is no significant difference in dehiscence of a transverse and a longitudinally oriented wound, but the question is definitely open to research and undoubtedly will be answered more definitively in the future.

Hernia

Although an abdominal wall hernia is not classically considered a wound, a few paragraphs in a text on wound healing should be directed to consideration of hernia because of the technical and biological differences which such considerations can make. Actually, no apology is needed for inclusion of hernia in a treatise on wound healing as there is considerable value in viewing a hernia as a chronic wound of the fascia even though only a few such wounds actually are traumatic in origin. Many biological principles of fundamental importance in the care of other wounds can be applied to the problem of hernia repair and some recently gained information in the field of collagen metabolism in healing wounds is essential to modern understanding of the pathophysiology of some abdominal hernias.

DIRECT INGUINAL HERNIAS. One example of the importance of the impact which modern collagen biochemistry has made on both understanding and treatment of abdominal hernia is the special case of direct inguinal hernia. Classically, we have been taught that elderly men develop a chronic weakness of, or, because of excessive strain, develop an acute wound of, the transversalis fascia in the floor of the inguinal canal. This is not, however, exactly what the surgeon finds when he explores the inguinal region. The transversalis fascia actually appears to be missing or to have become replaced by fat. If this is indeed what has happened, the pathophysiology of direct inguinal hernia belongs more understandably with metabolic disorders than with traumatic disorders of collagen.

Information gained from study of the disease lathyrism probably sheds some light on the type of metabolic defect which could result in a direct hernia. Rats fed lathyrogenic agents develop large hernias of the anterior abdominal wall which pathologically resemble in many respects the lesion in the transversalis fascia of human beings with large direct inguinal hernias. Whereas the lesion in indirect or incisional hernias is usually a sharply delineated aperture surrounded by normal fas-

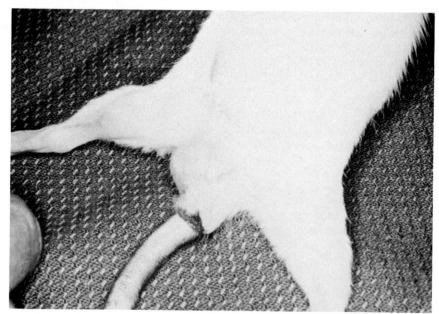

Figure 9–1. Direct inguinal hernia in rat with lathyrism produced by feeding sweet pea seeds.

cia, the defect in a large direct hernia is more diffuse and really consists of an attenuation of fascia over a poorly defined area. The end result strongly suggests that the normal equilibrium of collagen metabolism has been upset in favor of collagen lysis over collagen synthesis. Of course, the same end result could be produced if there was only a diminution in collagen synthesis or assembly of fibrils so that normal lytic activity was relatively unopposed. Such an imbalance could be infinitesimally small (far too small to be detected by present methods of measuring collagen synthesis or degradation), yet over many years the inexorable result would be thinning, attenuation, and gradual weakening of an already vulnerable section of the anterior wall. Why the groin is selectively affected and why the condition occurs more often in elderly men than in other individuals is not clear.

The hypothesis that direct inguinal hernia is a localized metabolic disorder of collagen is supported by some data. Studies performed several years ago by Read and Waugh suggested that the basic defect in collagen metabolism in patients with direct inguinal hernia was a decrease in net collagen synthesis and deposition. The data were obtained by measuring total collagen and rate of collagen synthesis and deposition in anterior wall fascia of patients with direct hernia. Controls were individuals undergoing elective replacement of the abdominal aorta because of aneurysm. We have several objections to these data. The first objection is that the kinetics of collagen synthesis in the anterior abdominal wall do not necessarily reflect the kinetics of collagen synthesis in the groin. Secondly, patients with abdominal aneurysms are not necessarily good controls; aneurysm may be an indication of a serious connective tissue abnormality to which inhibition of collagen synthesis may be critical. Finally, measurements of collagen synthesis provide only half of the equation needed to assess accurately the metabolic turnover of dense connective tissue; the kinetics of collagenolysis also must be measured before conclusions can be made about the state of collagen turnover.

To support some of the objections to the measurements just cited, the authors have measured net collagen synthesis and deposition in fascia surrounding defects in the transversalis fascia of patients with and without direct inguinal hernia. Controls were specimens of fascia from the identical location in the transversalis fascia from the contralateral groin of the same patient. Thus each patient served as his own control. These studies revealed that collagen synthesis during early development of fascial defects, before complete hernia was recognizable, is markedly increased over control values in the majority, although not all, of patients. Increased synthesis of collagen in an area where defects in collagenous structure can be identified can be explained only by hypothesizing that collagenolysis also is increased or that, for some reason, newly synthesized collagen in the area of the defect is not being incorporated into the collagenous structures. Qualitative determinations of collagenolytic enzyme activity at neutral pH have revealed that tissue collagenases are active in the groin of patients with inguinal hernias; badly needed quantitative determinations are not available now. In summary, all that can be stated at this time is that there are definite structural abnormalities in the transversalis fascia of patients with recurrent groin hernia. These abnormalities appear to be the result of an imbalance between collagen synthesis and deposition, and collagenolysis. Such studies strongly suggest that, until the exact abnormality is defined and corrected, continued attempts to repair structural defects will only result in more recurrences of the hernia.

The most important therapeutic principle which consideration of direct hernias and collagen disorders dictates is that there may be no clear line of demarcation between normal and abnormal fascia. It also raises the uncomfortable possibility that the conditions which affected equilibrium of collagen synthesis and degradation are indigenous to the area and are not inherent within that particular collagenous tissue. Whichever the case may be, one must conclude that bringing new, uninvolved fascia into the area is a sound principle if early repetition of the entire process is to be prevented. Considered in this light, success or failure of direct inguinal hernia repair will be determined in large measure by whether or not reconstruction of the inguinal floor is performed with uninvolved tissues—not whether the technique of performing the repair is perfect, as is often necessary during repair of an indirect or incisional hernia. In most patients a successful result implies that the defect was not widespread; the relatively high rate of recurrence of direct inguinal hernia, however, also suggests that involved tissues are used to reconstruct the inguinal floor more often than is commonly appreciated. That recurrence of a direct inguinal hernia is usually due to a defect in surgical technique, or to selection of a suture material, as commonly ascribed, is not as plausible to a biologically oriented surgeon as the possibility that a defective building material might have been used in the repair.

Two technical recommendations which seem to have improved the results of inguinal hernia repair during recent years, and which may be based on the principle of a metabolic defect being the cause of the hernia, are the utilization of Cooper's ligament and the preperitoneal approach. It is possible that the apparent success of both technical maneuvers may be due to the fact that they assure a better chance of utilizing tissue which is not involved in a local collagen metabolic disorder. Certainly one is impressed with the replacement of fascia by fat more in superficial layers of the inguinal region than in deep layers. Thus utilization of deep structures such as Cooper's ligament and the iliopubic band (which can be defined accurately only through a preperitoneal approach) may offer the best possibility of replacing deficient local tissues with tissues that are sufficiently stable metabolically so that prolapse of abdominal contents in the medial inguinal region is not possible. Another process which has been helpful in some cases has been advancement of fascia into a deficient area by means of a local pedicle. This is accomplished by a bipedicle flap when relaxing incisions are made in tissue superior to the defect. It is also accomplished by means of a rotation pedicle when a flap of anterior rectus abdominis fascia is rotated into the inguinal wound. Biologically speaking, the result of both is to transplant uninvolved fascia to an area where fascia has apparently undergone severe metabolic derangement.

The free fascial graft probably is as good as any other procedure for restoring fascial continuity with normal collagen. Although it is not nearly so popular as other complicated techniques of advancing local fascia into the wound, it has a sound biological basis and effectively replaces deficient fascia with normal fibrous tissue. It has the marked advantage of guaranteeing that the material from which the new inguinal floor will be constructed is not involved in a localized metabolic disorder. The graft is easily obtained from fascia lata and can be inserted either as a strip which is used to reinforce a conventional local tissue repair or as a sheet or patch of fascia which is used to resurface an entire area. Strip replacement is most often used as a fascial suture which literally laces the local tissue together. Although this is a distinct improvement over using an artificial fiber such as catgut or silk to lace local tissues, it is not as biologically sound as reinforcement of an entire area by placing a sheet of fascia as a free graft over the defect and sur-

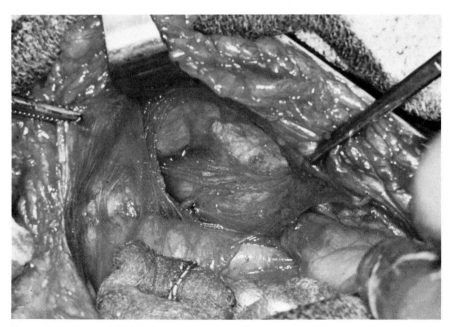

Figure 9–2. Large defect in transversalis fascia in a patient with recurrent groin hernia. Exposure is through a preperitoneal approach.

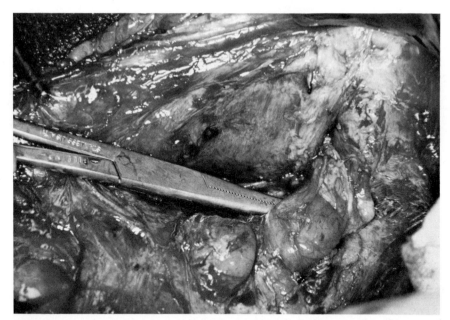

Figure 9–3. Large defect in transversalis fascia exposed by preperitoneal approach. Sutures from previous repair through a groin incision can be seen superficial to new disease. Bilobed sac (saddle hernia) is being retracted by hemostat. Preperitoneal approach reveals that previous repair is intact; present recurrence appears to be the result of continuing disease deep to old wound and sutures.

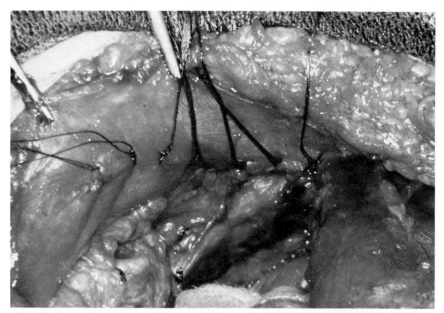

Figure 9–4. Defect in transversalis fascia closed by silk sutures through a preperitoneal approach.

rounding tissues alike. Just as utilization of Cooper's ligament during an anterior approach and utilization of the iliopubic ligament through a preperitoneal approach have significantly decreased the recurrence rate following repair of direct hernias, so is there further reason to presume that consideration of direct hernia as a metabolic defect will result in more use of free fascial grafts with a corresponding improvement in the recurrence rate. Certainly this sort of reasoning is more appealing than sacrificing a testicle because the inguinal canal seemingly cannot be made strong as long as a structure passes through it.

During the last five years, one of the authors (E.E.P.) has operated upon 25 patients with recurrent groin hernias by the preperitoneal approach. In addition to repairing the defect in the transversalis fascia as classically described by Nyhus and others, the author has resurfaced the entire pelvic floor with a massive free graft of fascia lata. The concept requires that virtually all of the fascia lata from one thigh be utilized for the graft. The graft extends from one lateral pelvic wall to the other, similar to an airplane wing passing uninterrupted through the body of an airplane. The single graft insures that no medial recurrences are possible. Inferiorly the graft is attached to both pubic rami; superiorly it is attached to the anterior abdominal wall at the level of the transverse abdominal preperitoneal incision. Laterally the graft is draped over the femoral vessels and attached to the lateral pelvic walls. Medially it is draped over the rectum and bladder and is attached to

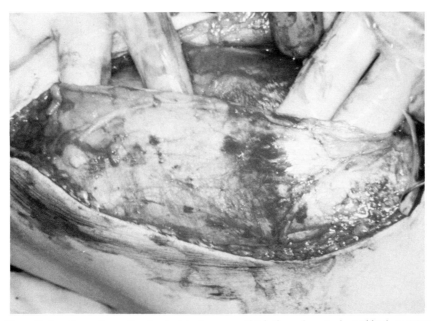

Figure 9–5. Removing entire fascia lata from one thigh through a single midthigh incision.

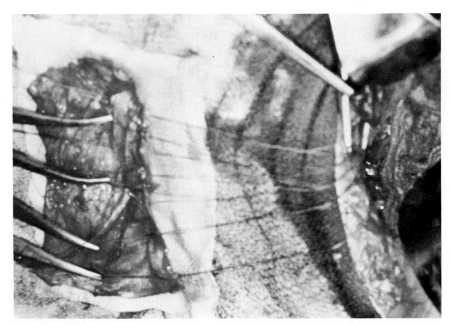

Figure 9–6. Threading fascial graft down preplaced sutures in pelvic rami.

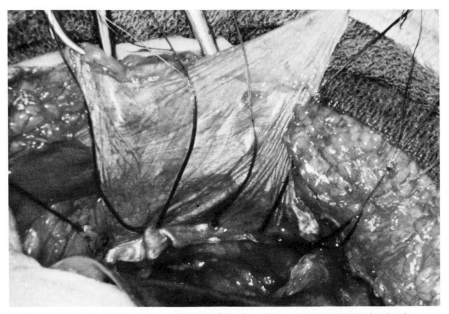

Figure 9–7. Graft being "snugged" into place by tying sutures in ramus of pubic bone.

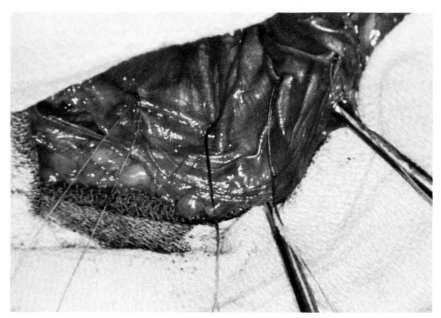

Figure 9–8. Graft in place overlying entire endopelvic fascia and extending to inferior edge of transverse abdominal incision.

the deep side of the symphysis pubis. The effect is a complete restoration or resurfacing of endopelvic fascia in a preperitoneal plane by a massive onlay graft.

Two grafts have been visualized as long as two years following transplantation. Metabolic studies in these grafts reveal that, in addition to being structurally intact, they were synthesizing and depositing collagen at almost ten times the rate measured at the time of transplantation. Total collagen in the grafts was reduced by approximately 10 per cent, suggesting that collagenolysis also was increased over normal. Subsequent studies on the ability of transplanted fascia to induce collagen synthesis and deposition in unwounded fascia have been interpreted as revealing that induction of unwounded tissue does not occur. Transplantation of fascia, or simply wounding fascia *in situ* by making an incision, causes a tenfold increase in net collagen synthesis and deposition which persists for as long as we have measured it. Although transplantation of fascia may contribute biological as well as structural benefits, data to support such a hypothesis have not appeared yet.

Three of the twenty-five patients with multiple recurrences treated by fascial graft of the entire endopelvic fascia have developed recurrences during the one to five year period they have been followed. One patient had a typical medial recurrence of a direct hernia which was the result of a unilateral graft rolling laterally and permitting peritoneum to enter the old defect. This cause of recurrence apparently has been eliminated by utilizing a single graft extending from one pelvic side wall to the other. Two patients had indirect recurrences following repair of direct hernias. In one case, the hernia recurred so soon after placement of the graft (six weeks) that the question has been raised whether an internal ring protective mechanism was disturbed or paralyzed by extensive dissection of the pelvic floor required for placement of the graft. Subsequently the internal ring has been reinforced with a few sutures and the direction of the cord has been changed by suturing it directly, or with a small fascial sling, to the pelvic floor. It is possible that an indirect sac was missed in both patients but this does not seem likely in view of the superb exposure which a preperitoneal approach provides. Repair of the two indirect recurrences of direct hernias was very easy through an external groin approach. The excellent, almost redundant, transplanted fascia made a repair to Cooper's ligament very easy. These patients have provoked interesting speculation about such basic questions as the protective or sphincteric action of the internal ring, the persistence in adult life of congenital peritoneal sacs, and the differences, if any, between a direct and an indirect inguinal hernia other than the side of a relatively unimportant blood vessel on which a basic biological phenomenon happens to appear.

Diagnosis is the key to the biological approach to direct hernia repair—just as in most superficial wounds or defects. The question

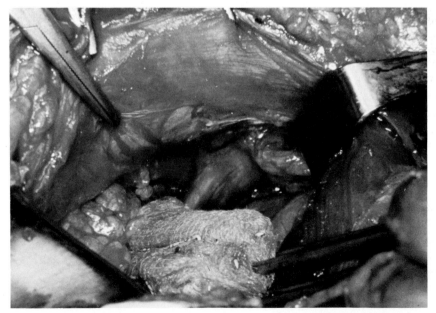

Figure 9–9. Transversalis fascial defect in recurrent hernia exposed through a preperitoneal approach. Clamp points to defect.

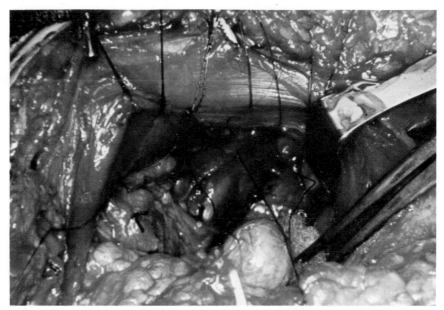

Figure 9–10. Closure of same recurrent direct hernia shown in Figure 9–9 through a pre-peritoneal approach. Note that peritoneum has been retracted out of pelvis so that a sac will not be missed.

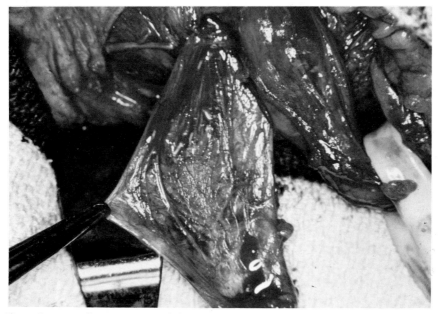

Figure 9–11. Indirect sac exposed through a groin incision six weeks following procedure shown in Figures 9–9 and 9–10.

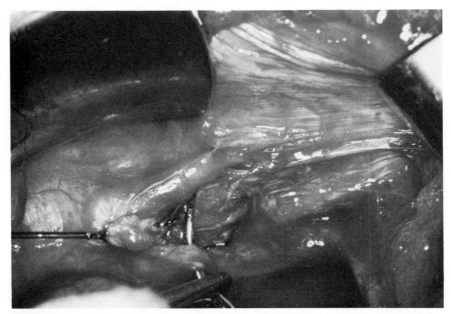

Figure 9–12. Repair of indirect hernia following removal of sac shown in Figure 9–11. Graft placed through preperitoneal approach six weeks previously is easy to locate and suture to Cooper's ligament without tension.

must be asked: What is missing? If the answer can be given accurately, it usually makes quite clear what steps must be taken to restore normal relationships. Just as some of the effects of wound healing (contraction and epithelization, and so forth) may have to be removed or, as is frequently stated, the defect has to be re-created before restoration begins, normal relations in the inguinal region such as direction of the cord and location of the internal ring may have to be reconstituted before the actual restorative procedure is begun. If the decision is clear that a wound characterized by absence of fascia is responsible for the protrusion of abdominal contents, the surgeon should be prepared to bring new fascia into the wounded area. If local tissues are normal, they should be used; if local tissues are not clearly free of metabolic derangement, there should be no hesitation in bringing distant tissue in as a free graft.

INDIRECT INGUINAL HERNIAS. Indirect inguinal hernias are caused by peritoneum persisting in an area where obliteration of the peritoneal cavity normally occurs. Thus an abnormal passage for peritoneal contents is preserved. Correction of this abnormality consists primarily of obliterating the abnormal peritoneal extension; reconstruction of fascial layers is necessary only when the peritoneal extension is large and has been present for a long time. A large peritoneal sac can so distort the internal and external inguinal rings that reconstruction of normal anatomical relations between cord, muscles, and fascia may be necessary after the peritoneal sac has been removed. Because the problem in these patients is primarily one of long-term stretching and dilatation of an aperture, there usually is an adequate amount of normal fascia in the local area to restore proper relationships without the necessity of transplanting fascia from a distant site. Local fascia usually is perfectly adequate except in elderly patients in whom metabolic changes in inguinal fascia have become apparent. In these patients, a combination of removal of the peritoneal sac and excision of defective collagenous tissue may be required; in some patients a local flap or a free graft of fascia lata may be required.

INCISIONAL HERNIA.   An incisional hernia is a clear example of a traumatic wound of fascia; the problem is a deficiency in fascia in most cases. Although some treatises on repair of incisional hernia have stated that it is not necessary to open the peritoneal sac while repairing an incisional hernia, the authors have found that opening the sac can be very helpful in diagnosing the true condition of fascia surrounding the wound. The major difference between an incisional hernia and other abdominal hernias characterized by deficiency of collagenous tissue is that wound healing has occurred in the incisional hernia site. This means that contraction may or may not have occurred and that fibrous protein synthesis has altered tissues. The result is that the actual size of the fascial defect may be obscure and that a considerable proportion of what appears to be fascia is not normal fascia but only deep fibrous scar tissue. As explained in Chapter 6, on repair of integument, surface scar tissues are subject to remodeling deformation many months after they appear to be structurally stable. Just as a surface scar (unsupported by subcuticular sutures in uninjured, naturally woven fibrous protein layers) inexorably widens with passage of time, so will a deep scar undergo similar physical changes. Apparently the physical weave of young scar tissue simply is not efficient enough to resist physical stress, although the relatively high turnover of remodeling collagen in a young scar is reason enough to account for change in overall dimensions with passage of time and application of deforming forces.

A critical factor in the repair of incisional hernia is the ability to recognize accurately the products and results of wound healing. The first step in restoration of the abdominal wall is to re-create the defect by excising products of wound healing so that they will not be used inadvertently in the reconstitution of the abdominal wall. It is not difficult to distinguish normal fascia from recently synthesized scar tissue *provided* both are visible so that the comparison can be made. It may be extremely difficult to recognize scar tissue which has become remodeled in a horizontal plane so that it resembles a sheet of fascia if it is the only tissue visible in the wound. It is important therefore to cut through various planes of scar tissue in a vertical direction until by sight and feel one can appreciate that one type of tissue has been left behind and another entered. The safest maneuver for making this distinction is to open the peritoneal sac at an appropriate site under direct vision, and then enlarge the opening so that bowel can be separated safely from the undersurface of the abdominal wall. Then it will be possible to hold the abdominal wall between the thumb and fingers of the noncutting hand. All layers of the abdominal wall should be incised until there is a clear delineation of normal fascia, muscle, and peritoneum. An important distinguishing sign between scar and fascia can be readily appreciated at this point because anterior rectus fascia does not blend inseparably with peritoneum as the posterior layer does in some areas or as scar tissue always does. Thus an area where the various fascial and muscle layers can be identified in the wound serves as a locus to begin circumcising the entire wound so that all products of previous wound healing can be removed and only undamaged tissue remains.

After the defect has been re-created, an assessment of remaining tissue must be made before one can decide how the defect will be reconstructed. A small defect often can be closed by merely approximating various layers of the abdominal wall as in closure of any incision. No special measures such as extra strong sutures, overlapping fascia, or free grafts will be needed if excision of the wound was complete. Moderate tension is not undesirable as long as fascia is not torn and a large enough suture is selected.

In most patients the deficiency of fascia is such that closure by

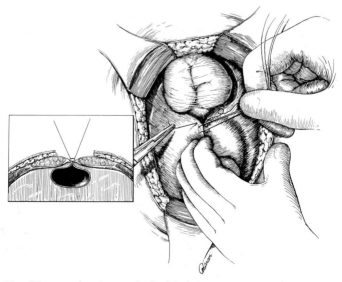

Figure 9–13. Diagram showing method of imbricating incisional hernia in anterior abdominal wall by inverting sac, scar tissue, and preperitoneal fat. Sutures are not under tension. (Reproduced by permission from J. B. Lippincott Co. E. E. Peacock, Jr., Ann. Surg. *181*:722, 1975.)

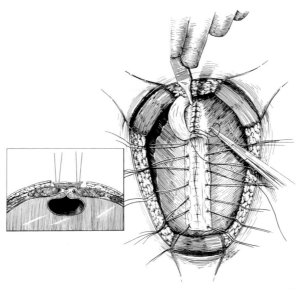

Figure 9–14. Diagram showing placement of lateral sutures maintaining free fascial graft over imbricated sac. (Reproduced by permission from J. B. Lippincott Co. E. E. Peacock, Jr., Ann. Surg. *181:*722, 1975.)

simple approximation of the edges of the new wound is impossible. In these patients, need for a fascial transplant by flap or free graft is clear. Wide lateral incisions allowing medial shift of local fascia are adequate for defects of moderate size; free grafts from a distant site nearly always are needed for large openings. One layer is sufficient if the fascia is from an area such as the lateral thigh. Adding several layers of fascia is destructive to the donor site and unnecessary to reconstruct the abdominal wall. As in other free grafts, during periods of revascularization diffusion of gases and nutrients may be important in maintenance of cell viability. As was learned by experience with composite tissue tendon grafts, structural stability is affected by cell survival — probably because of the effect on mucopolysaccharides elaborated by living cells. When all of the fibers in a graft are parallel in longitudinal array as in a tendon, transverse stability produced by collagen-mucopolysaccharide interactions may not be so important in determining physical characteristics. Nevertheless, all of the elements which make a naturally woven fascial structure such as fascia lata structurally dependable should be preserved when fascia is transplanted to provide strength in a weak area. Successful transplantation of cells definitely is enhanced by transplanting only single sheets of fascia rather than piling layer on top of layer to increase the bulk or thickness of the abdominal wall at that point.

If the fascial defect in an incisional hernia is small and approximation of fascial edges is easy without applying force, a simple repair

more proximal such an injury occurs, the less retraction of the muscle belly will occur. When no distinct internal or external fibrous band can be located, the authors have had some success with weaving a figure-of-eight silk or wire suture through the distal tendon several times until a secure purchase on the tendon has been obtained. The suture is then passed longitudinally through the center of the muscle parallel to the muscle fibers. The entire muscle mass is traversed by the suture which is then brought out external to the muscle proximal to its origin where it is tied over a button or some other bolster. A pull-out wire on the tendon side makes it possible to remove the entire suture after reattachment of muscle fibers to tendon has occurred. As much contact as possible between muscle and tendon is desirable in this type of repair. The distal joints traversed by the tendon should be flexed or extended so that as much length of tendon as possible passes through the muscle belly. The procedure is followed by immobilization for three to five weeks, depending upon the extremeness of joint position, age of the patient, and so forth.

Tears of complex structures such as the rotator cup of the shoulder joint or quadriceps tendon require special judgment and mastery of important technical details if adequate function is to be restored. More simple repair of the biceps muscle or division of the musculotendinous junction in a forearm or lower leg muscle can be managed by using the general principles just outlined. When repairing shoulder or knee wounds of muscles and tendons, however, the surgeon should be thoroughly familiar with various technical maneuvers and substitution patterns which orthopedists have devised for repairing injuries in these areas.

Volkmann's Ischemic Contracture

Classically, Volkmann's ischemic contracture of muscle is described as an acute and chronic wound of muscle secondary to vascular complications following a supracondylar fracture of the humerus. The condition has been taught so expertly and publicized so widely that the incidence of classic Volkmann's ischemic contracture following a supracondylar fracture is remarkably low. Serious restriction of range of motion of digits of the upper extremity secondary to fibrous replacement of the healing process in forearm muscles is not rare, however. It is the result of healing following a wide variety of muscle injuries which are more frequent than commonly appreciated. Such injuries as burns, large hematomas, infection, direct pressure or crushing injuries of the forearm and, in recent years, inadvertent instillation of narcotics into the forearm compartment have produced a typical syndrome of limitation of finger flexion, varying degrees of median and ulnar nerve palsy, and a small distal forearm with a firm, contracted proximal group of muscles. Although the cause of such a contracture may not be ischemia

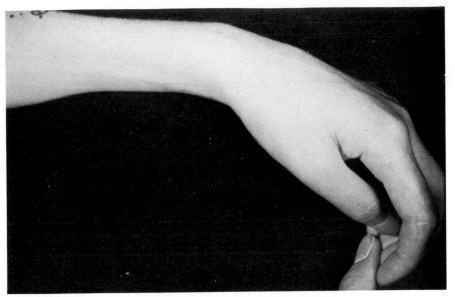

Figure 9–19. Typical appearance of Volkmann's ischemic contracture of forearm muscles. Note intrinsic palsy and flexion contracture of wrist and fingers.

secondary to major arterial damage, the end result, as far as appearance and function of the forearm and hand are concerned, may be identical with that which follows a supracondylar fracture. Moreover, it is not certain that production of a forearm flexion contracture following a supracondylar fracture is due to simple ischemia from major vessel damage. Until more is known about the production of this devastating complication, it is probably best considered as a direct wound of muscle which heals by fibrous protein synthesis. In all probability, muscle can react in only one way to serious injury and the end result is the same whether the initial injury is ischemia, congestion, direct trauma, or infection. The pathological change secondary to all such injuries is replacement of contractile and extensor motor units with nonextensible fibrous tissue. Considered as such, the condition is a major complication of wound healing which deserves special study.

Actually, the condition has been surprisingly well studied from both a biological and a surgical standpoint. The most significant information to come out of such studies has been that development of a typical Volkmann's contracture apparently is not the result of a pure arterial or pure venous obstruction. Simple ligation of the brachial artery may or may not produce gangrene in the distal extremity, depending upon the competence of collateral vessels around the elbow. If arterial insufficiency is created by a specific arterial lesion, however, the characteristic pathological condition is gangrene. Moreover, gangrene is more severe in distal tissues beginning with the fingertips; skin is affected more severely than muscle. Pure venous obstruction caused by individual ligation of major veins produces much the same result except that the initial reaction is characterized by engorgement and cyanosis.

In a typical Volkmann's contracture following a supracondylar fracture of the humerus there usually is an element of arterial obstruction, venous obstruction, and lymphatic obstruction. It is probably significant, however, that complete obstruction of any of the three does not exist. The rather peculiar end result (most pronounced in the deep flexor group—flexor digitorum sublimis and profundus and flexor pollicis longus) in the proximal forearm must be, therefore, the result of partial obstruction of all three systems. Thus the biological disorder is a complex one and treatment directed toward the arterial, venous, or lymphatic system alone is likely to be ineffective.

The best management appears now to be preventive, with the objective being maintenance of competency in the three vascular systems, and therapeutic, in changing the potentially dangerous anatomical relationships of the major nerves in the forearm. Expressed differently, everything that can be done to prevent fibrosis of muscle should be attempted by means of manipulation of the circulatory system. Failing this, however, it is important not to lose the opportunity, before irreversible intrinsic paralysis occurs, to prevent the median and ulnar nerves from becoming involved in a severe muscle cicatrix. This can be accomplished by transplanting the major nerves into a subcutaneous position so that they will not become incarcerated during the collagen-synthesizing and contracting phase of muscle healing.

The inexperienced surgeon is understandably more familiar with and therefore more concerned about the severe wrist flexion and forearm pronation contractures following elbow injuries than with other aspects of Volkmann's contracture. Actually, the flexion and pronation contractures are not nearly so devastating as the effect muscle fibrosis may exert on the median and ulnar nerves. Because these structures have an amazingly competent internal longitudinal blood supply and because embarrassment of nerve conduction may not appear for several days (occasionally several weeks) after the initial injury, it seems likely that loss of nerve conduction is truly the result of axonotmesis caused by external compression of the nerve rather than immediate vascular insufficiency elsewhere in the arm. This is an important hypothesis because, if true, it means that special attention to the nerve during the first 48 to 72 hours could result in preservation of nerve function even though remaining structures in the forearm compartment became irreversibly fibrosed because of inability to restore normal circulatory dynamics soon enough. The authors would like to emphasize this point, as most other treatises on the subject have dealt primarily with early restoration of vascular competency or late relief of major nerve entrapment. Our experience with a small number of cases, coupled with the biological reasoning already summarized, leads us to recommend strongly that early surgery for impending Volkmann's ischemic contracture include not only an aggressive approach to restoration of vascular dynamics but also an anatomical rearrangement of the two major nerves to insure that they will not become entrapped within deep muscle cicatrix. The reason for making such a special point of this aspect of preventive surgery is that, although sensation can be restored as long as one year after entrapment of a major nerve in a forearm cicatrix, recovery of intrinsic motor function characteristically does not occur after late secondary release of an entrapped nerve. Prevention of intrinsic paralysis is possible by preventive surgery, however, as shown by the following case.

The patient was an eight year old boy with a typical supracondylar fracture of the humerus. The fracture was reduced without difficulty and the arm was placed in a flexed position by a well trained surgeon. Within several hours the hand became pale in color and swollen, and lost considerable amplitude of radial pulsation. All dressings and plaster were removed and the elbow was extended. Although some return in radial pulse amplitude was thought to have occurred, the condition of the hand worsened and small blebs appeared on the skin of the upper forearm and elbow. A sympathetic block was performed and an extensive fasciotomy including excision of the lacertus fibrosus and exposure of the brachial artery was done. No discrete arterial lesion was found and the radial pulse was greatly improved. Two days later the patient began to lose sensation in the median and ulnar nerve distributions, however, and he was transferred to a larger hospital. An immediate operation revealed the most extensive involvement of the muscles in the forearm which the authors have ever encountered. As was discovered later, the muscle degeneration and beginning contraction involved not only all of the usual muscles but also the extensor compartment, although to a lesser extent than the flexor area. The muscle was neither engorged nor ischemic. It had the typical gray, flaky appearance which is not characteristic of either venous or arterial insufficiency alone. The muscle was completely nonreactive but there was no evidence of venous or arterial thrombosis and some arterial and venous flow could be demonstrated throughout the forearm. The flow was very sluggish, however, and it was clear that the entire vascular system was embarrassed. The obviously involved superficial muscles and some of the deep muscles were excised. The median and ulnar nerves were then carefully dissected out of their normal passages between muscle groups and were transplanted into a subcutaneous position on the volar surface of the forearm. The ulnar nerve was transplanted from behind the medial epicondyle to the volar surface of the elbow. The hand was so badly swollen at the time of operation that adequate sensory and intrinsic motor examination could not be performed. As edema subsided over the ensuing ten days, however, sensation improved and intrinsic motor function returned rapidly. Although some sensation definitely was lost prior to surgery (this was the reason for emergency referral of the patient), it is likely that intrinsic motor function was never completely lost. A typical wrist flexion contracture and a mild finger contracture did, of course, develop but the hand was never completely anesthetic and an intrinsic claw deformity was never present. As will be discussed later, correction of a wrist and finger contraction is often not a serious problem and it is never comparable to the problem of correcting an anesthetic hand and an intrinsic claw deformity. Although it is possible for sensation to be restored as long as several years after injury, in this case it seems

elongated position or because the flexor mass has been advanced in the forearm, complete flexion will not be possible because the reduced amplitude of motion will be expended in the first portion of flexion arc. Failure to splint the fingers or wrist will result in a range of motion that is confined almost entirely to the terminal flexion arc; flexion will be powerful and complete but extension will be sharply limited. In summary, once preventive surgery is over, the amplitude of motion is probably fixed and the object of postoperative care becomes that of placing the amplitude of motion which will be possible by a compromised muscle in a position where it will be most useful both in positioning the fingers (extension) and in grasping various sizes of objects (flexion). The most important factor in this objective is preserving a wide range of active and psssive motion of the wrist. Normal wrist motion is the key to adequate hand function in a severe Volkmann's contracture as partially damaged muscle will have to remain in order for active flexion to occur and yet the amplitude of motion possible is not enough to flex and extend the fingers through a full arc. Thus splinting and physiotherapy during the healing period following the initial injury should be directed toward maintaining full passive motion of the wrist joint and active flexion of the fingers.

Secondary restoration of typical forearm contracture usually is directed toward restoration of median nerve sensation, replacement of paralyzed intrinsic muscles, and adjustment of long flexor power to the most useful portion of the finger flexion arc. Sensation often can be

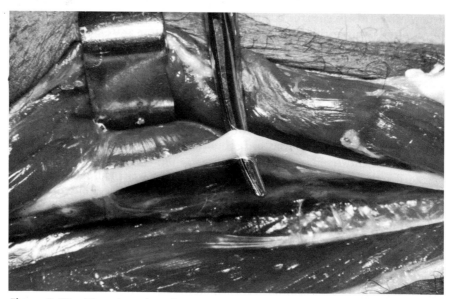

Figure 9–23. Dissection of median nerve in forearm showing fascial compartment on under surface of sublimis muscle. Note that retraction of sublimis muscle does not liberate median nerve from connective tissue compartment.

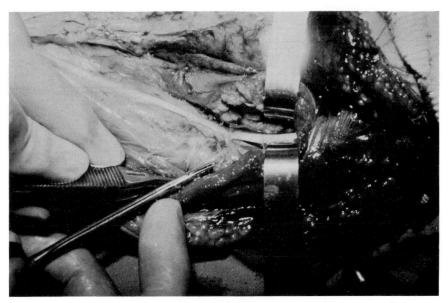

Figure 9–24. Small motor branches of median nerve in antecubital space which occasionally must be sacrificed to transplant median nerve into a subcutaneous position.

regained as late as two years after incarceration of the median nerve and possibly even later. The nerve should be approached with the objective of releasing it from external entrapment by fibrosed muscle. This usually involves exposure of the nerve from upper arm to lower forearm and excision of the entire sublimis muscle and superficial portion of the pronator if they are involved in the fibrosis. The nerve should then be examined carefully to determine whether direct trauma occurred at the time of the original injury. Partial lacerations with or without neuromas or in-continuity intraneural neuromas may be detected by palpating and observing the nerve carefully. Obvious lesions, particularly a neuroma found proximal to the point of injury, usually should be excised and a primary anastomosis of the nerve ends should be performed. The problem of partial or irreparable nerve injury is discussed in the next chapter and will not be discussed here other than to say that extensive decompression by excision of all involved fibrosed muscles superficial to the nerve may be all that is required to restore sensation. This is particularly true for a hand that has become progressively anesthetic over a period of several days during the healing phase of a lower arm or upper forearm injury. If simple decompression fails to restore sensation, a more extensive plan will have to be developed as there is generally no point in proceeding further with motor restorations if some sensation cannot be regained. Restoration of sensation following irreparable damage to the major nerves of the upper extremity is covered in detail elsewhere.

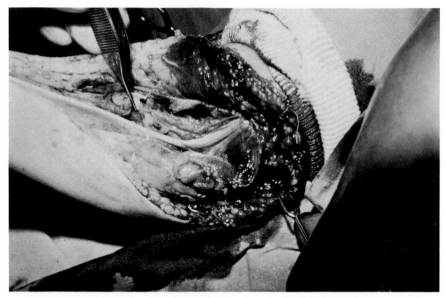

Figure 9–25. Subcutaneous position of ulnar nerve following transplantation from posterior surface of medial epicondyle. (Reproduced by permission from E. E. Peacock, Jr., J. W. Madden, and W. C. Trier, Ann. Surg. *169*:748, 1969.)

After sensation returns, attention can be directed to restoration of function. Long finger flexor units and wrist flexors and extensors should be approached before replacement of intrinsic muscles is considered. The first objective should be to obtain normal wrist motion. In many patients the only possibility of obtaining anything near normal finger action is by changing position of the wrist joint (semitenodesis effect of shortened finger flexors). Restriction of wrist excursion is most often the result of fibrosis in major wrist flexors, although unsuspected fibrosis of the extensor carpi radialis longus and brevis may be even more detrimental to finger function. Severe involvement of forearm muscles includes the radial wrist extensors more often than is usually appreciated. This should always be suspected when difficulty is encountered in restoring a full range of passive wrist flexion.

A not uncommon finding in Volkmann's contracture is inability to flex the wrist following a three to five week course of finger and wrist splinting with the wrist in dorsal extension. After removal of the splint, inability to flex the wrist may be attributed to a tight dorsal capsule so that extensive physiotherapy is prescribed. Failure to gain substantial wrist flexion following intensive physiotherapy is a sure sign that wrist extensors have become fibrosed and shortened so that the radial carpal joint is maintained by extensor tenodesis. Exploration of the extensor compartment usually reveals that one wrist extensor is more completely involved than the others. The brevis is the more valuable of the two radial carpal extensors and should be preserved as a wrist extensor if a choice exists. The better of the two muscles should be maintained as a wrist extensor, however, while the other is detached and threaded to the volar surface to act as a wrist flexor if all of the wrist flexors have been sacrificed; this can be either a primary or a secondary procedure. If it is necessary to lengthen the remaining radial wrist extensors to provide full wrist flexion, this should be done by a Z-plasty or interposition graft. Valuable power will be lost if a partially fibrosed and shortened wrist extensor is lengthened, but wrist flexion is so important when extensive damage has occurred to the finger flexors that whatever adjustment is needed to obtain adequate wrist flexion will result in overall improvement of hand function. A combination of sacrifice of the most fibrosed and shortened extensor; transfer of the unit, if there is any activity left in the proximal muscle and the wrist flexors are gone; and lengthening of the remaining radial extensor tendon to whatever degree is necessary, so that active and passive wrist flexion will be possible, may be all that is needed to provide adequate finger extension. Such patients will be able to extend their fingers by flexing the wrist, and by using wrist extensors to provide 25 to 30 degrees of finger flexion they will be able to bring the hand into a position from which the remaining amplitude of long finger flexion can complete the flexion arc.

Muscle advancement performed at the origin of long muscles in the forearm is mentioned only to be condemned. Such procedures are difficult, are often dangerous because additional muscle fibers may be lost, and — most important — transfer whatever range of muscle remains to the intermediate or first portion of the flexion arc rather than the terminal portion where power is needed for grasp of small objects. Such transfer of power is too great a price to pay for being able to position the fingers in a more natural attitude. Wrist flexion, although perhaps not a pretty way of obtaining finger extension, is by far the simplest and most mechanically sound approach to obtaining adequate position of the fingers before the flexion arc begins. If long flexor activity is not sufficient to close the fingers in useful grasp after the wrist is extended, a flexor transfer should be added. The brachioradialis is the best muscle to transfer into the long flexor units. It is innervated by the radial nerve, is usually spared in the ischemic process, and is about the only muscle innervated by the radial nerve with an amplitude of motion sufficient to restore even 50 per cent of finger flexion. Most experienced surgeons combine a brachioradialis transfer with a tenodesis of the profundus tendons when little or no function remains. Actually, the profundus group usually is already fixed to some extent by fibrosis but if the wrist and fingers were splinted in extension, the tenodesis may require shortening to allow wrist extensors to make their contribution at a point where power is needed. Again, extensive wrist motion, including powerful extension, is a prerequisite to success of volar transfers and profundus tenodesis.

Intrinsic transfers should be considered only after long tendon and proximal joint function has provided maximal coarse grasping efficiency. Intrinsic transfers should be used primarily to strengthen thumb adduction and to provide active metacarpophalangeal joint finger flexion. The severe shortage of motor units eliminates the possibility of using the usual finger and wrist flexors so that only the most important objectives such as thumb adduction and metacarpophalangeal flexion should be sought. To use one of the few remaining motor units that has been spared on the dorsum of the hand to restore abduction of the thumb is a serious mistake. Opposition, of course, is only a position movement and an abductor may be useless if there is not a powerful adductor to bring the thumb to the fingers or palm after a position of abduction has been obtained. The relatively refined thumb motion required for pulp-to-pulp pinch usually will not be possible after severe mutilation of the forearm and paralysis of all intrinsic muscles. Useful key pinch utilizing the intact extensor pollicis longus to position the thumb and transfer of a powerful tendon such as an extensor carpi radialis longus prolonged with a free graft to adduct the thumb against the side of the index finger is a realistic objective which can make a useful addition to hand function. Simultaneous fusion of the first metacarpophalangeal joint will add stability to the thumb and increase the usefulness of the transfer. A small amount of intrinsic muscle fibrosis, or normally tight collateral ligaments and volar capsule of the finger metacarpophalangeal joints, may make an intrinsic transfer to the fingers unnecessary. Only when abnormal extensibility of these joints occurs so that they go into hyperextension during attempts at distal finger extension should an intrinsic transfer be considered. Details of the technique and selection of intrinsic transfers have been given in preceding chapters.

SUGGESTED READING

Alexander, H. C., and Prudden, J. F. The Causes of Abdominal Wound Disruption. Surg. Gynec. Obstet. *122*:1223, 1966.

Betz, E. H., Firket, H., and Reznik, M. Some Aspects of Muscle Regeneration. Int. Rev. Cytol. *19*:203, 1966.

Bitterman, W., Gemer, M., and Lutwak, E. M. Wound Dehiscence. Increased Intra-abdominal Pressure after Repair of Diaphragmatic Hernia. Arch. Surg. *94*:178, 1967.

Brooks, B. Experimental Study of Volkmann's Paralysis. Arch. Surg. *5*:188, 1922.

Brooks, B., Johnson, G. S., and Kirtley, J. A. Simultaneous Vein Ligation. Surg. Gynec. Obstet. *59*:496, 1934.

Church, J. C. T., Noronha, R. F. X., and Allbrook, D. B. Satellite Cells and Skeletal Muscle Regeneration. Brit. J. Surg. *53*:638, 1966.

Conner, W. T., and Peacock, E. E., Jr. Some Studies on the Etiology of Inguinal Hernia. Amer. J. Surg. *126*:732, 1973.

Gilbert, R. K., and Hazard, J. B. Regeneration in Human Skeletal Muscle. J. Path. Bact. *89*: 503, 1965.

Godman, G. C. On the Regeneration and Redifferentiation of Mammalian Striated Muscle. J. Morph. *100*:27, 1957.

Guiney, E. J., Morris, P. J., and Donaldson, G. A. Wound Dehiscence. A Continuing Problem in Abdominal Surgery. Arch. Surg. *92*:47, 1966.

Higgins, G. A., Jr., Antkowiak, J. G., and Esterkyn, S. H. A Clinical and Laboratory Study of Abdominal Wound Closure and Dehiscence. Arch. Surg. *98*:421, 1969.

Lavine, D. M. Personal communication of unpublished data.

Lehman, J. A., Jr., Cross, F. S., and Partington, P. F. Prevention of Abdominal Wound Disruption. Surg. Gynec. Obstet. *126*:1235, 1968.

Levene, A. The Response to Injury of Rat Synovial Membrane. J. Path. Bact. *73*:87, 1957.

Mendoza, C. B., Jr., Watne, A. L., Grace, J. E., and Moore, G. E. Wire versus Silk: Choice of Surgical Wound Closure in Patients with Cancer. Amer. J. Surg. *112*:839, 1966.

Peacock, E. E., Jr. Subcutaneous Extraperitoneal Repair of Ventral Hernias: A Biological Basis for Fascial Transplantation. Ann. Surg. *181*:722, 1975.

Peacock, E. E., and Madden, J. W. Studies on the Biology and Treatment of Recurrent Inguinal Hernias. II. Morphological Changes. Ann. Surg. *179*:567, 1974.

Peacock, E. E., Jr., Madden, J. W., and Trier, W. C. Transfer of Median and Ulnar Nerves during Early Treatment of Forearm Ischemia. Ann. Surg. *169*:748, 1969.

Robertson, H. T. Preperitoneal Approach in the Repair of Inguinal Hernias. Amer. J. Surg. *112*:627, 1966.

Thompson, N. Autogenous Free Grafts of Skeletal Muscle. A Preliminary Experimental and Clinical Study. Plast. Reconstr. Surg. *48*:11, 1971.

Thompson, N. Investigation of Autogenous Skeletal Muscle Free Grafts in the Dog with a Report of a Successful Free Graft of Skeletal Muscle in Man. Transplantation *12*:353, 1971.

Thorngate, S., and Ferguson, D. J. Effect of Tension on Healing of Aponeurotic Wounds. Surgery *44*:619, 1958.

Wagh, P. V., Lererich, A. P., Sun, C. N., White, H. J., and Read, R. C. Direct Inguinal Herniation in Men: A Disease of Collagen. J. Surg. Res. *17*:425, 1974.

Webb, P. The Effect of Innervation, Denervation, and Muscle Type on the Reunion of Skeletal Muscle. Brit. J. Surg. *60*:180, 1973.

Wirtschafter, Z. T., and Bentley, J. P. Hernias as a Collagen Maturation Defect. Ann. Surg. *160*:852, 1964.

possible to define accurately the proximal extent of the injury so that anastomoses are not made distal to free-flowing axoplasm.

Allowing normal healing processes to occur at the end of the proximal segment also permits undesirable changes to occur which may make secondary suture more difficult and thus less successful. Not the least of these is the wild distribution of regenerating axons which double back, loop in every direction, and seemingly explode the distal end of the proximal segment by forming a typical neuroma. Proliferation of longitudinal and circularly oriented connective tissue causes compression of axons and loss of extensibility of the proximal segment.

Another serious drawback to primary suture is the loss of time that invariably occurs if judgment turns out to have been faulty. Once primary repair has been undertaken, three to nine months may elapse before the result of the procedure is known. An even more serious problem is that a partial return of function following primary suture raises the question of whether a second repair is indicated. Whether to sacrifice what function has been gained by excising the neuroma at the site of a previous anastomosis and performing a secondary repair is an agonizing decision for the surgeon; if he decides to do so he forces the patient to make an enormous expenditure of time on what amounts to a gamble. Secondary suture performed relatively early, before any function returns, prevents this problem from arising. Unless a known preventable complication occurs, there usually is no reason to suspect that repetition of the anastomosis will provide any better return of function when a delayed anastomosis was performed the first time.

Clinical experience strongly suggests that, within the limitations produced by complications (known and unknown), primary repair of a nerve is desirable when possible. The word possible in this statement refers primarily to the condition of surrounding tissue, the suitability of the wound for primary closure (which includes implantation of foreign suture material), and the ability to judge the longitudinal extent of injury in both segments of nerve. In certain types of wounds such as a blast injury, caused by a high-velocity missile, or a crushing or contusing injury inflicted by a blunt object, the surgeon probably should not even attempt to assess the longitudinal extent of damage to the nerve but should plan a secondary anastomosis on the basis of the history alone. Several weeks after the primary wound has healed and scar tissue has become mature, diagnosis of the extent of neural injury can be more accurate. Even though definitive preparation is not done, it is advisable, when possible, to coapt the two nerve ends with a single suture so that excessive length will not be lost during healing and maturation of deep scar tissue. One might ask why a technically complete anastomosis should not be done in all patients at the time of wound closure, reasoning that if assessment of damage in either end has been inadequate, nothing has been lost; a secondary reanastomosis should be just as effective regardless of whether primary suturing was done. In our opinion, there are at least two reasons. First, some slight return of function almost always occurs if the nerve ends are joined. Return of even a tiny amount of function provides a measure of false hope that a second operation will not be required, and the decision to perform a secondary anastomosis is unnecessarily delayed. Even worse, however, the patient or the physician may decide to accept a mere fraction of the function that could have been restored had no alternative to a second procedure been introduced. Second, and perhaps more important, some neural tissue is lost after every unsuccessful repair. Moreover, fibrosis around and within the nerve is significantly increased by manipulation and insertion of sutures. This costly loss of neural tissue and even a small increase in fibrous tissue should be avoided when possible.

Most experienced surgeons feel that a primary repair should be performed when a clean soft tissue laceration has resulted in relatively atraumatic division of a nerve and there are no contraindications to closure of the wound. This is particularly true if the nerve laceration is sharply localized and there is no history or evidence of damage except at the point of laceration.

When the limits of damage to the nerve are indefinite or surrounding tissue is traumatized excessively, a single suture can be used to coapt the nerve ends so that secondary scar formation around and within the nerve will immobilize it in a position of maximal length and extensibility. Such a suture invariably will cause a 180 degree rotation of the most movable segment if any tension exists. The result is that the inferior margin of one end will touch the superior margin of the other and none of the remaining circumference or diameter of the ends will be in contact. It seems impossible that a single proximal axon could find a channel in the distal segment under such circumstances, yet it is almost certain that some distal function will occur if adequate time is allowed. On secondary exploration the nerve ends will be found perfectly polarized. Rotation of one or both nerves around the axis of a single suture apparently brings the cross-sectional surfaces of both into proper alignment. The exact mechanism by which this phenomenon occurs is unknown. One can speculate, however, that axons and Schwann cells extend from the distal end of the proximal segment while connective tissue extends from the proximal end of the distal segment to become amalgamated into a single scar. Secondary remodeling occurs, and an effective rotation of the entire junction into proper alignment results. In our experience, return of function has sometimes been so effective following temporary coaptation of nerves in this manner that a secondary repair was not justified even though the nerve ends were so diffusely damaged at the original injury that a definitive repair was impossible. It should be pointed out that most of these cases have been in children, whose regenerative potential is quite high. It does raise the question, however, of whether a single point of fixation which permits rotation during regeneration might not be preferable to the usual method of fixation with multiple sutures so that rotation is not possible. Once the second suture is tied, rotation of the nerve becomes impossible, regardless of biological factors that might have been effective in matching axons with distal tubes if a mechanical impediment had not been present. This subject will be treated more fully in the discussion of techniques for repairing nerves, but we should point out here that the excellent return of function occasionally observed following coaptation of badly damaged nerve ends with a single suture suggests that minimal foreign body reaction and the ability to rotate and remodel intervening scar (in response to currently undefined biological stimuli) may be more important than perfect fixation of minimally traumatized ends by multiple sutures so that rotation during regeneration is not possible. Such a hypothesis is pure speculation at this time, but it is speculation based on observations made during secondary exploration of forearms (for tendon transfers) following nerve repairs by only a single suture to maintain length until a definitive anastomosis could be achieved. The question raised by remarkable return of function and direct visual evidence that nonpolarized segments became polarized when the potential for rotation was not eliminated could be fundamental in revising our techniques for restoration of continuity of divided nerves.

Partial return of function following inaccurate approximation of badly damaged nerves raises the problem of speculating whether a better result could be obtained with a definitive preparation of the ends and reanastomosis. The longer one waits to answer this question, the more unlikely it becomes that there will be an opportunity to know. It is extremely difficult for patients and physicians to agree to sacrifice regained function even though there is a possibility of regaining considerably more function. It would seem, therefore, that if, in the judgment of the surgeon, the nerve ends cannot be properly prepared because of serious damage or indefinite extension of injury, a secondary repair should be scheduled as soon as overlying soft tissue scar is mature and before any return of function occurs. We will discuss in more detail later whether or not the secondary repair, after excision of external and internal scar, should be performed with a single point of fixation as suggested by the preceding discussion or by more conventional techniques. Just as primary repair, when possible, appears to have several advantages over secondary repair, early secondary repair has significant advantages over late secondary repair.

Not the least of the several advantages of primary repair over secondary repair or early secondary repair over late secondary repair is the factor of return of motor function. Time is of the essence when motor return is expected and early repair is particularly important in nerves in which a significant number of motor fibers are present. In the upper extremity, for example, early repair of the radial nerve at the elbow is much more important than early repair of the median nerve at the wrist. The median nerve at the wrist, primarily a sensory nerve except for one motor funiculus supplying an easily replaced muscle group in the thenar eminence, can be repaired with excellent return of sensory function as long as two years after injury. Degeneration of motor end plates and subsequent changes following denervation of striated muscle make return of motor function in the forearm unlikely after six months and virtually impossible thereafter. Recent demonstrations that sensory end organs such as pacinian corpuscles degenerate within a few weeks or months after proximal nerve section cannot be correlated with clinical return of sensory function. Apparently end organs regenerate when axoplasm reaches terminal nerve filaments; on the basis of histological changes in sensory end organs, there does not seem to be any time when protective sensation cannot be retained.

TECHNIQUE OF NERVE REPAIR

The general principle underlying most techniques for repair of peripheral nerves is coaptation of segments as accurately as possible so that axoplasm may flow uninhibited into a distal neurolemmal tube. As suggested previously, however, it is possible that, within reasonable limits, physical position of opposing channels may not be nearly as important as biological guidance, which could be the result of chemical, electrical, or even undefined energy. Suffice it to say, however, that we do know that seemingly improbable physical gaps can be overcome with amazing return of function, and that approximation that is grossly nearly perfect sometimes is followed by enormous neuroma formation and negligible return of function. Such observations make it imperative to keep an open mind about factors which may influence axonal regeneration and to be willing to look at measures for improvement of regeneration other than those aimed primarily at reducing the size of the gap. Certainly, early concern with reduction of the size of the gap and with increasing the immediate physical strength of the union by introducing as many sutures as possible increases significantly the amount of fibrous proliferation within and around the anastomosis. Although the method may not be practical to apply in many patients, present data strongly suggest that the smaller the number of sutures utilized, the less likely it is that interference of axon regrowth by interneural and intraneural connective tissue will occur. Ideally in a nerve repair no foreign material should pass through the highly reactive epineurium or perineurium. Practically, however, the nerve ends must be maintained in reasonable proximity in some way; at the present time, fine sutures are the best way to accomplish this. Enthusiastic supporters of funicular suture, who apparently are willing to insert all manner and number of sutures to try to improve matching of funiculi, seem to have lost sight of the fact that every suture creates fibrous tissue reaction.

An important difference between healing in nerves and healing in tendons that has both theoretical and practical implications is that during healing of tendons no significant scar is generated within the tendon and restoration of strength by scar tissue is dependent entirely upon ingrowth of highly specialized connective tissue. Thus, successful isolation of a tendon suture line from surrounding soft tissue invariably defeats the objective of repair—to develop a connective tissue scar between the ends. Exactly the opposite is true during repair of a peripheral nerve. Any external or internal tissue proliferation other than restoration of the delicate neurolemmal tubes will interfere with distal flow of axoplasm. There is some evidence that the connective tissue of peripheral nerves, unlike that of tendons, is highly specialized tissue with unusual regenerative capacity and possibly is able to influence axoplasm flow as well as to restore physical integrity to the anastomosis. Therefore it is both theoretically and practically desirable to isolate a repaired nerve from surrounding healing connective tissue.

An excellent example is the superb regeneration of a severed facial nerve within the facial canal of the temporal bone. Such regeneration actually is better when the two nerve ends are not sutured; a gap of several millimeters between nerve ends is permissible within the bony canal. Regeneration under these conditions often is better than if the laceration occurred distal to the bony canal and the nerve ends were sutured fastidiously but left in a bed of healing connective tissue.

It is easy to see, therefore, why quite an exhaustive search has been made for methods to isolate a nerve anastomosis from surrounding tissues. Present data suggest that improvement in regeneration can be obtained by artificial isolation of a nerve anastomosis, but practical considerations in obtaining such isolation have been formidable. So far, definitive laboratory experiments have not been possible.

Some of the most difficult problems have centered around implementation of an isolation technique without creating ischemia, restriction of lymph flow, or, worst of all, restriction of distal axoplasmic flow. Proximal enlargement of a nerve after an attempt to isolate an anastomosis is evidence that distal flow of axoplasm has been restricted. If an artificial barrier does not produce complete isolation, it is virtually useless; if a barrier is applied tightly enough to assure complete isolation from surrounding connective tissue at the time the nerve is repaired, subsequent edema within the nerve may compromise internal circulation. All types of biological membranes and tubular structures—blood vessels, amnion, skin, and so forth—have been tried, as have a variety of inorganic and organic substances. Long-chain polymers placed around the nerve in liquid state and then polymerized by addition of an activator have produced a fairly effective barrier in laboratory animals. Siloxane seems to be one of the most effective agents in creating a sleeve or custom-fitted tube to isolate a nerve anastomosis. Satisfactory evaluation of peripheral function is difficult, however. At best, such technical adjuvants can only be described now as biologically sound but extremely difficult to apply and evaluate.

The most impressive clinical observations supported by laboratory studies in primates strongly suggest that tension must be prevented if a nerve anastomosis is to have the best opportunity for axonal regeneration. Literally, tension must be eliminated even if a graft is required. Millesi has taken this principle further than necessary, in our judgment. It is not necessary to put in free nerve grafts for virtually every nerve laceration as Millesi seems to advocate. Electrical conductivity studies performed by Terzis confirm that a primary nerve anastomosis performed without tension is the best operation a surgeon can perform today. Although a graft requiring two anastomoses definitely is superior to a single anastomosis made under tension, grafts do not conduct evoked potentials as well as a single anastomosis performed without tension. Millesi's clinical reports do not contain control observations; electrical conductivity data performed in primates constitute the soundest base for deciding whether to graft a nerve or perform a simple anastomosis. Present data support a primary single anastomosis when possible without tension and performing an interposition free graft when tension cannot be overcome by flexing joints or rerouting a nerve.

Selection of the best suture to coapt nerve endings has provoked considerable thought and disagreement among surgeons. There are three major choices—natural fibers, metallic sutures, and synthetic fibers.

Very fine (No. 40) steel or tantalum sutures were introduced by neurosurgeons and became popular during World War II for three reasons. Such sutures have minimal coefficients of friction and thus can be passed through the delicate epineurium of small nerves with relatively little trauma. They produced less tissue reaction than any other suture available at that time. They can be visualized by x-rays and thus serve as a marker during the months of convalescence to show whether the suture line has dehisced. There are three objections to metal sutures. They are more difficult than fibers to handle because of their tendency to kink and break during placement of the suture and setting of the knot. They emit radiant energy which can cause damage to the nerve if an unsuspecting physiotherapist uses radiant energy in treatment of the extremity (this happened in many cases). Although they are clinically inert, metal sutures are mechanically irritating and will stimulate soft tissue reaction in the area where small joints are being put through a wide range of motion. This, of course, is the most important objection and it applies particularly to the hand and fingers. A nerve anastomosis in the midfemur or midforearm is not subjected to motion, and physical irritation is not, therefore, a valid objection to the use of metal sutures in these areas.

Silk (7-0 or 8-0) is the easiest suture for the surgeon to handle. The relatively high frictional resistance of silk can be reduced by passing it through subcutaneous fat several times before passing it through epineurium. Silk does not cut through flimsy tissue as readily as metal sutures and the knots are easier to form and do not come untied. The major disadvantage to silk is tissue irritation; there is no question that there is more deposition of fibrous tissue around natural fibers than around metals or synthetic fibers. There should not, therefore, be any argument about the advisability of using as few sutures as possible if a natural fiber is selected. If silk is preferred, as it is by many surgeons, the disadvantages should be reduced as much as possible by inserting the stitch in subcutaneous fat before passing it through epineurium, by using the smallest number of sutures possible, and by taking precautions to place the sutures accurately in the most superficial layers of epineurium only.

The greatest advantages of synthetic fibers are low coefficient of friction and nonreactivity, and their major disadvantages are difficulty in handling and "memory." Synthetic sutures are only slightly more difficult to handle than natural fibers, however, and should pose no problems for experienced surgeons. Memory, meaning that the knots tend to untie, is less important in repair of a peripheral nerve than in most other situations in which use of artificial fibers has been advocated. Since there must not be any tension on a peripheral nerve, untying of a knot once the skin is closed and the extremity is splinted is of less consequence than in replacing a heart valve, for example. The two ends of the nerve literally should lie together with no tension across the suture line. Nevertheless, the surgeon does not like to see a knot untie in front of his eyes within seconds after the suture has been placed; most surgeons, therefore, tie at least three knots in a synthetic fiber, and many find it irresistible to place four or five knots. The tendency to strangulate tissue and the small increase in foreign body reaction that multiple knots cause may not be valid objections to the use of synthetic sutures, which are becoming increasingly popular.

Catgut sutures are mentioned only to be condemned. High frictional resistance, large knots, and excessive tissue reaction make natural absorbable fibers undesirable.

Sutures should be placed with as little trauma as possible. Foreign body reaction is not, by any means, the only cause of excessive fibrous tissue proliferation. Every bite of the forceps produces a microwound which will heal by scar formation. Every scar appears to a stream of axoplasm as a keloid of impenetrable proportions. The nerve, therefore, should be handled as delicately and as infrequently as possible. Early during dissection, a traction suture should be placed in the relatively tough connective tissue surrounding the nerve at least 2 cm. proximal to the divided ends. This suture should not pass deep in epineurium but should be placed instead in surrounding loose connective tissue which, in this area, is not dissected off the nerve as it must be where the anastomosis will be performed. The nerve can be manipulated by this suture (or two sutures, if needed to prevent bobbling) so that forceps will be required infrequently. Some surgeons recently have advocated placing horizontal mattress traction sutures a centimeter or so proximal and distal to nerve ends and then tying the traction sutures to maintain nerve ends in approximation. In this technique, no sutures are used in epineurium and only a few sutures are used for funicular alignment. During dissection of nerve ends, longitudinally oriented blood vessels should be identified and protected. Blood vessels are undoubtedly of some value from the standpoint of nutrition and gas exchange, but even more important, they are useful in determining the proper rotation of nerve ends, particularly in a primary nerve repair but also in a secondary anastomosis. In the median nerve at the wrist, it is frequently possible to identify the motor funiculus on the deep surface of the nerve and the major longitudinal vein on the superficial surface to provide two reference points for controlling rotation. If it is advisable to control rotation with sutures, these two points can provide an accurate indication of correct alignment.

One advantage of a primary nerve suture is that the nerve does not have to be dissected out of a scarred soft tissue bed. During secondary repair, the natural plane between epineurium and loose connective tissue has been obliterated by new collagen synthesis during healing of the wound. The closer the surgeon comes to the distal neuroma in the proximal segment, the more indistinct the plane between surrounding soft tissue and epineurium becomes. Actually, perineurium also may contain more collagen and thus be thicker than normal over a distance too extensive to permit excision of all abnormal nerve. Surgeons have recognized that a thickened (scarred) epineurium makes repair technically easier, because it does not tear easily when grasped with forceps and sutures are less likely to pull out of it. Presence of a scarred epineurium means, however, that axons also will be passing through a scarred and somewhat constricted channel. It is possible to place a nerve under more tension when epineurium and perineurium are scarred but impediment to flow of axoplasm could be too high a price for a technical advantage. Neither ability to put the nerve under undue tension nor impediment to flow of axoplasm in a distal direction is advantageous from the standpoint of neurobiology.

Examination of the cut surface of the proximal end as soon as the neuroma has been excised provides a safeguard against suturing nerve endings that have more collagen in epineuruim or perineurium than is desirable. An immediate retraction of epineurium (or nerve sheath as it is often referred to by surgeons at this stage) should be obvious, and ideally, the appearance should be that of a cauliflower or mushroom bulge of the funiculi from the cut surface. If the cross-sectional appearance is one of a perfect horizontal plane with no retraction of the sheath or sprouting of funiculi, the inescapable conclusion has to be that section was made through an area of epineurium and perineurium that is rigid and fixed by new collagen deposition. The inference, of course, is that perineurium and endoneurium also are too dense to permit optimal funicular expansion. A secondary repair under such conditions may be technically easier than a primary one because fibrous tissue proliferation in and around the funiculi has bound them into an easily manageable, almost homogeneous mass. However, if the proximal surface appears homogeneous, like the cut end of a piece of spaghetti instead of a sprouting mushroom of individually identifiable funiculi, sections should be made more proximally until an area of normal collagen content in perineurium and epineurium is found. Expressed less accurately but more simply, if a secondary repair is technically easier than a primary one because funiculi are not sprouting out between sutures, the chances are good that an error in judging the level of section has been made.

Nerve ends should be sectioned with the sharpest possible blade, with the least amount of pressure, and while the nerve is free of any longitudinal tension. This is usually accomplished by breaking off a piece from a new, high-quality razor blade and inserting it in a hemostat to make a small bistoury. The nerve is placed on a piece of wood (broken tongue depressor) and held with a proximal traction suture if it does not lie without tension. A single bold cut is made without sawing motions. Repeated cuts, sawing motion, excessive pressure from a dull knife, and sectioning under tension produce undesirable fraying of

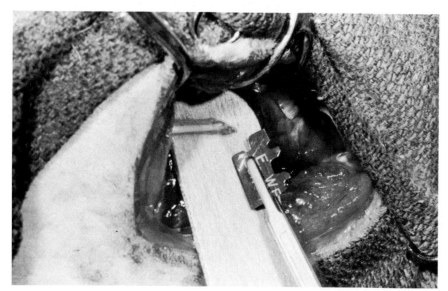

Figure 10–1. Proper position of lacerated digital nerve on tongue blade without tension. A clean section will be made with a segment of razor blade.

epineurium and distortion of the funicular pattern, making accurate coaptation of nerve ends difficult; moreover, ragged fragments of epineurium tend to turn in, so that they block axoplasm flow into distal tubes.

There really is no adequate test to determine when the distal end has been properly prepared in a secondary nerve repair. Fortunately the distal end may not be as badly distorted as the proximal one because a neuroma is not present. The distal nerve is between 30 and 40 per cent smaller in diameter than the proximal nerve and a funicular pattern may not be easily recognized, but usually some evidence of it can be detected; a completely homogeneous cross-sectional appearance should be avoided if possible. Homogeneous appearance in the distal end usually means that the section has been made through a longitudinally oriented area of connective tissue proliferation and not through the original nerve trunk. It may also mean that the knife has passed through an area so badly scarred by proliferation of perineurium and epineurium that there are no open channels to receive axoplasm. Because evaluation of the internal condition of the distal segment is so much less accurate than assessment of the condition of the proximal segment, most surgeons prepare the proximal end first and then merely excise as much of the distal segment as possible without placing the anastomosis under a significant amount of tension.

A number of reasons have been advanced recently for utilizing a low-power, wide-field dissecting microscope to observe the nerve during repair. One reason is that the condition of the nerve can be assessed more accurately under magnification than by gross inspection. We agree that this is true, but we are not convinced of its biological and clinical significance. Practically speaking, gross observation of nerve sheath retraction and axon sprouting provides adequate evaluation of the proximal section, and once this evaluation has been accomplished, the usual procedure is to sacrifice as much distal nerve as possible, regardless of the gross appearance. It is true that with microscopic inspection more extensive measures can be taken to mobilize distal or proximal nerve than would ordinarily be utilized if the appearance of the nerve under magnification was not satisfactory. But again, from a practical standpoint, we have not had enough experience in correlating the appearance of nerve ends under magnification with that in gross tests to state definitely that an extensive dissection of an extremity to gain a few more millimeters of nerve is justified on the basis of microscopic examination. Radical mobilizations have many disadvantages, and the decision for extensive mobilization of a nerve cannot be justified now on the basis of microscopic observations alone. It would seem, therefore, that use of the microscope for determining the level of nerve preparation is, at best, an investigational procedure and should remain so until more critical evaluation of the correlation of microscopic findings and surgical implications is possible.

Mobilization of nerve segments to overcome deficits in length is best accomplished by flexing or extending joints. It is important to remember that nerves are relatively nonstretchable structures and, although they have considerable resilience, they do not function well under significant longitudinal tension. Inexperienced surgeons often do not realize that the tissue surrounding nerves normally is not significantly restrictive; dissecting a nerve out of its aerolar tissue bed, therefore, does not provide as much additional length as theory might indicate. The most restricting element in stretch of a nerve is the arrangement of internal connective tissue, not the external loose connective tissue attachments. Peripheral tissues make a substantial contribution to the nourishment of a nerve, however, and when these tissues have been dissected away, neuronal regeneration and subsequent function are dependent entirely upon longitudinal blood supply. Moreover, dissection of a nerve out of its normal tissue bed means that wound healing will occur along the entire longitudinal surface of the exposed structure, not just at the anastomosis.

Neither interruption of segmental blood supply nor production of scar tissue along the course of an exposed nerve necessarily prevents a successful outcome following restoration of nerve continuity, but both are factors which militate against return of function and either or both can be ignored to the extent that they do prevent clinically significant return of function. Recent measurements indicate that when a nerve is dissected cleanly out of its soft tissue bed for a distance of over 14 cm., nutrition and oxygenation are compromised sufficiently to reduce return of function. This recommendation was based on clinical experience with relatively few cases. Our experience has been that considerably more than 14 cm. of a nerve can be dissected free — particularly if some perineural connective tissue is preserved. Although it is impossible to predict exactly how extensive longitudinal dissection must be before it interferes with function, there is a finite limit to the distance any nerve can be stripped out of its natural bed and still regenerate and function as well as if no longitudinal dissection had been performed. Because so little is gained by longitudinal dissection, therefore, it should be avoided when adequate length can be achieved by other means.

During secondary repair, scar tissue produced by previous exposure of the longitudinal surface of a nerve may be removed to gain length and release circumferential restriction. A nerve left free in an extensive soft tissue wound may become incarcerated in secondary scar while it is in a shortened or retracted position. When this has occurred, excision of surrounding scar will help to regain normal length even if no more than normal length can be achieved. Also, the original wound may have healed with a fibrous tissue cicatrix that cannot be converted into a site suitable for a definitive anastomosis; in such a case, longitudinal dissection permits transfer of the nerve to another location where subsequent scarring will be less severe.

An excellent opportunity to utilize the nerve transfer principle occasionally arises during emergency treatment of impending ischemic contracture of the forearm following a supracondylar fracture of the humerus (Volkmann's Ischemic contracture). This condition, which results in a peculiar conversion of forearm muscles to dense fibrous tissue, can also be produced by circumferential burns, crush injuries, and other injuries resulting in closed-space collections of blood, serum, or pus. The result is gradual compression of the median and ulnar nerves until no function remains. This complication can be prevented if the nerves are dissected out of the damaged muscle and transferred to a nonconfined space such as subcutaneous tissue superficial to forearm muscles and fascia.

Thus, even though longitudinal dissection of a nerve is to be avoided when possible, there are specific indications for it, such as emergency treatment of impending Volkmann's contracture or secondary treatment of a deep fibrous cicatrix. In most patients, however, the surgeon should keep in mind the cost of impaired nutrition and gas exchange as well as the inevitable formation of scar tissue, and he should look for every possible way to overcome a deficit in peripheral nerves without resorting to extensive longitudinal dissection.

Longitudinal dissection can produce a significant increase in length when it is done in conjunction with transplantation of a nerve. In fact, so little usually is achieved by longitudinal dissection alone that it probably should not be performed except as a preliminary step in transplanting a nerve out of an unsuitable environment or to the opposite side of a joint where subsequent flexion or extension can provide a relative increase in length. Examples include releasing the median nerve from the confines of the pronator teres and lacertus fibrosus or transplantation of the ulnar nerve from behind the epicondyle of the humerus to the anterior surface of the elbow.

From a technical standpoint, longitudinal dissection may carry one more hazard which, although subtle, may be pivotal in determining the outcome. It is very difficult for a surgeon to perform an extensive mobilization of a longitudinally oriented structure such as blood vessel, tendon, or nerve without putting the structure under some longitudinal tension. One of the oldest principles in surgery is, if a structure must be removed from the body, transect it as soon as possible, because once one end of a structure is under control it can be placed under longitudinal tension and dissected more easily. This, of course, is exactly what must be avoided in preparation of a nerve, particularly the proximal end. Unfortunately the nerve usually has already been transected and care must be taken to keep from putting it under tension by pulling, even gently, on the cut end.

After satisfactory length has been obtained and the nerve ends are prepared, they are coapted. Most surgeons prefer to use sutures for coaptation, but the theoretical advantage of a sleeve or sheath should not be forgotten. All studies now support the recommendation that multiple funicular grafts for large nerves and single free grafts for small nerves should be utilized if tension cannot be avoided by any other technique. The sural nerve appears to be the best graft.

In some conditions, for example, division of the facial nerve within the bony canal, a natural sheath such as the bony facial canal can be utilized. It is well known that the nerve should not be sutured within the canal; nerve ends should simply be aligned as well as possible. Placing sutures in the facial nerve in the area of the bony canal is extremely difficult. Moreover, the procedure usually is done under magnification, and exposure is so difficult that even though a suture can be placed adequately in the nerve sheath, tying it at the bottom of a narrow cavity puts vertical stress on the sheath, and the suture tears out of the sheath. To repeat the process seriously damages the sheath, and more fibrous tissue proliferation will occur inside and outside the nerve than if suturing had not been attempted. Regeneration of the facial nerve within the bony canal is to be expected, even if a segment is missing, unless damage has been produced by a long period of micromanipulation and abortive attempts to place sutures in the sheath.

Clinical observations such as those just outlined, when considered in the light of meager but rather conclusive evidence that the use and

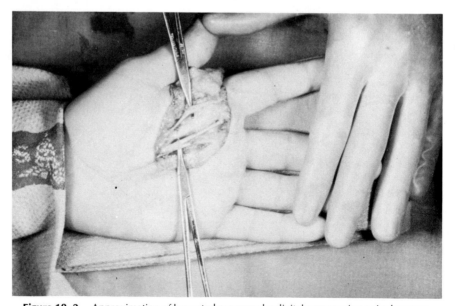

Figure 10–2.   Approximation of lacerated proper volar digital nerves using a single suture.

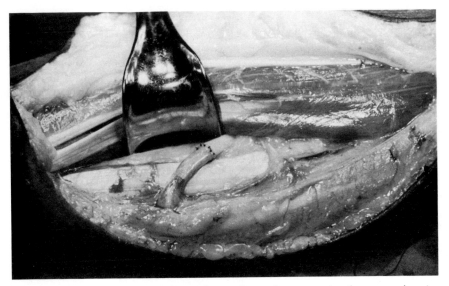

Figure 10–3. Typical mechanically perfect end-to-end anastomosis of nerve ends using multiple sutures.

placement of sutures increase measurably the amount of fibrous tissue reaction at the site of anastomosis, argue strongly for using no more sutures than absolutely necessary to coapt nerve ends. In the case of a digital nerve it is seldom necessary to use more than one suture, and it is possible that a single suture is all that should be used in repair of any nerve. One suture coapts nerve ends and thus produces the least amount of fibrous tissue proliferation, and it leaves unfixed the rotatory orientation of the nerve. If, indeed, biological forces are capable of correcting rotatory mismatch, two-point fixation with more than one suture will eliminate them. Another advantage to the use of only one or two sutures is that it provides automatic control over the surgeon's judgment about tension. If nerve ends lie perfectly coapted after placement of a single suture, one may be certain that adequate relief of tension was provided in the preliminary preparation and that regeneration will not be inhibited by the effect of longitudinal tension. Even when two sutures are used 180 degrees apart, one can be fairly certain that the nerve is not under undue tension if the shape of the anastomosis remains a cylinder. If two sutures are placed in nerve ends which have been stretched more than is desirable in order to make coaptation possible, the cylindrical shape of the trunks will be converted into an oval or flat shape from which funiculi will sprout uncontrollably while the neurolemma of both sides functions as a sphincter. Regeneration may occur to some extent under such conditions, even when a dozen or more sutures have been inserted to correct the shape of the nerve and force the wayward funiculi back into an endoneurial position. Such distortion is always a sign of undue tension, however, and if there are measures that still can be utilized to gain more length and release tension, it is better to resort to them than to insert more sutures to make the anastomosis physically stronger or correct the inaccuracy caused by physical distortion.

The most impressive argument against using only one or two sutures is that there are some nerve deficits which simply cannot be overcome unless a number of fine sutures are placed around the circumference of the anastomosis. Many times we have been confronted with a situation in which it was barely possible to get nerve ends together even though every available trick short of grafting had been tried. A deficit of around 13 cm. in the ulnar nerve is an example of such a defect. After extensive dissection of both ends, transplantation of the nerve anterior to the elbow, and flexion of every joint in the fingers, wrist, and elbow, sometimes nerve endings may be brought together only when strength is provided by a number of sutures. Two sutures simply will not hold the ends together and control the funicular spray. In these situations a number of carefully placed sutures will alleviate the problem from a mechanical standpoint even if the biological toll exacted by tension and excessive foreign material is high. Recent studies, basic and clinical, strongly suggest, however, that grafting is preferable to extensive mobilization and use of many sutures.

It seems advisable at this time to recommend that only one or, at the most, two sutures be used as a test for undue tension and to minimize intraneural scarring. If adequate coaptation of nerve endings cannot be accomplished with one or two sutures and no further measures are available to overcome tension, grafts should be utilized. It is possible that even with mild tension and with funiculi sprouting out at right angles to the anastomosis, multiple sutures cause more difficulty than benefit. Even though the anastomosis appears mechanically impossible, biological factors (as yet unidentified and unmeasurable) may be more influential than the mechanical manipulations of the surgeon if they are given an opportunity to act. The surgeon's belief that almost any mechanical manipulation or adjustment to fulfill the objective of creating an axoplasm-tight tube of epineurium is in order may be entirely wrong. Such a principle reflects an almost purely mechanical approach and strongly suggests that the surgeon believes that the flow of axoplasm is controlled primarily by physical confines or mechanical directives. Admittedly, the histological structure of nerve suggests that this may be true, but the fact that poor results occasionally follow mechanically perfect nerve repair and that good results sometimes follow mechanically horrible repairs raise some doubts that a purely mechanical concept is entirely adequate. In this regard, nerve stimulating factor, previously studied mostly in sympathetic nerve regeneration and the central nervous system, should be evaluated.

Closure of the soft tissue wound after nerve repair frequently is difficult if joints have been placed in an extreme position to make coaptation of nerve ends possible. Inversion of skin edges may be a problem when joint flexion has been necessary. An everting or vertical mattress suture may be required for accurate coaptation of skin edges. Skin healing should be uncomplicated; sections of inverted skin often form sinuses which delay healing and cause more deep scar than would have developed if skin had healed by primary intention. It is important that hemostasis be perfect; thus the tourniquet should be removed before the wound is closed. An acutely flexed extremity containing delicately approximated nerve ends, however, is not an ideal area for extensive clamping and ligation of small blood vessels, and if there is any possibility that vessels large enough to require ligation have been divided, the tourniquet should be removed just before coaptation of nerve ends so that hemostasis can be obtained. The profuse oozing from hyperemic tissue which occurs for approximately five minutes after release of a tourniquet will subside with nothing more than elevation and local pressure.

Following repair of a peripheral nerve, it is advisable to close the skin with a suture material other than silk. In very small children, 5-0 chromic gut (which produces considerably less skin reaction than plain gut) often is utilized so that suture removal can be avoided. Because the initial dressing should remain in place for three weeks, nonreactive sutures such as metal or synthetic monofilaments should be used. The extremity should be dressed (as described previously) and an external plaster splint should be applied to assure rigid immobilization. Unless signs of infection (drainage, lymphadenopathy, or fever) or signs of hematoma (inordinate or persistent pain and distal swelling) are found, the initial dressing should not be disturbed for three weeks. Three weeks is selected because this is the length of time needed for adequate collagen synthesis and deposition to splint the nerve internally, but it is not enough for collagen remodeling around the collateral ligaments and capsule of joints in extreme flexion or extension to produce permanent joint fixation.

By 21 days there has been adequate synthesis, deposition, and remodeling of collagen along the segment of the nerve which was exposed during surgery so that splinting of the anastomosis is adequate to prevent dehiscence. In addition, endoneurium, perineurium, and external sheath have healed by fibrous tissue proliferation and the nerve is virtually as strong as it was before injury. Strength of the anastomosis, of course, is not related to flow of axoplasm across the suture line. Flow of axoplasm into distal tubes does not occur immediately after coaptation of nerve ends, and the early synthesis of fibrous tissue which provides tensile strength may actually impede axon regeneration. The flow of axoplasm from a central source into the distal nerve undoubtedly is inhibited by edema, abnormal mechanical stresses produced by bringing nerve ends together, inflammation, and collagen synthesis. It has been estimated that no more than approximately 10 per cent of regenerating axons ever find their way into purposefully oriented neurolemmal tubes, and it is quite possible that even this does not occur until the primary effects of collagen synthesis and deposition have dispersed. In this regard, it is interesting that collagenolytic activity, measured by tissue culture techniques, has been found in human neuromas. Cell-mediated collagenolytic activity appears now to be associated with the presence of epithelial cells; it is interesting to speculate whether neurolemmal sheath or axoplasm may be endowed with substances such as acid hydrolases, cathepsins, and other enzymes capable of depolymerizing or digesting newly synthesized collagen. Such speculation brings to mind the marked sensitivity of anesthetic skin to degradation after seemingly insignificant mechanical trauma. Axoplasm or other cells of ectodermal origin in the sheath may have significant influence on control of collagen metabolism. It is startling how little is known about the effect of healing and regeneration of human peripheral nerves on other tissues—particularly now that some of the tools to investigate fundamental processes are available when the surgeon (who controls the experimental preparation) is curious enough to use them.

Although small joints become stiff after three weeks' immobilization—because of both collagenous tissue remodeling and pain of traumatic arthritis—the degree of inflexibility is not severe and, more important, not irreversible. Actually, pain and some inflexibility provide another seven days or so of partial immobility and keep the patient from making a sudden forced extension of a joint that was acutely flexed so that a divided nerve could be brought back together. If immobilization is continued for longer than three weeks or if some accident occurs that leads to an unusual amount of edema in the extremity, permanent joint stiffness in small joints may occur (interphalangeal joints are in most danger). Thus after three weeks of immobilization all restricting dressings and splints should be removed, sutures should be taken out, and gradual passive and active exercises should be begun. If a large joint such as the elbow or the wrist has been acutely flexed, it is a good idea to place the extremity in a sling for a week or ten days to avoid traumatic arthritis or excessive soft tissue reaction caused by gravity or forced manipulation.

The classic belief is that axons regenerate at a rate of approximately 1 mm. per day. It should be remembered, however, that in human beings such statements are based on no more refined or exacting measurements than changes in Tinel's sign. Moreover, such estimates are derived by averaging the results of many examinations at different times. Actually, the rate appears to change during the course of regeneration in a single nerve and is characterized by lag periods at the beginning and the end. As we have already described, axons apparently do not jump the gap of an anastomosis immediately; there is always a delay of five or six weeks before any evidence of regeneration can be detected. Thereafter, progress seems relatively rapid until return of function reaches the distal end of the nerve, where progress is measurably slower than in more proximal areas, particularly for return of sensation.

COMPLICATIONS OF NERVE INJURY OR REPAIR

It is often difficult to know when a secondary exploration of a repaired nerve is called for. Certainly as long as there is any objective evidence of continuing return of function the temptation to take a second look should be resisted. Development of a palpable and very sensitive neuroma suggests that a technical complication occurred or an inadequately prepared distal segment needs to be inspected and corrected, if possible. Some degree of hypersensitivity in the area of the anastomosis is normal; not all of the axons will be directed along distal longitudinal channels and some will form a sensitive neuroma. An excessively large, palpable neuroma with typical acute response to palpation is not normal, however, and should be ignored only if return of distal function is so good that there is no question that an adequate number of axons have reached distal end organs.

The most discouraging condition after repair of a peripheral nerve is the combination of inadequate distal function and absence of signs or symptoms of a neuroma. This syndrome strongly suggests that a more proximal injury existed and that a secondary exploration, although mandatory, may be unrewarding. If the nerve is found to be physically intact, the presence or absence of a neuroma provides the clue as to whether additional sacrifice of nerve should be performed proximal or distal to the previous anastomosis.

The most difficult problem of all is partial return of function that is less than was expected. The risk of losing what function has been gained must be weighed against the possibility of gaining more function. Secondary suture of a nerve may be a real gamble and probably should be avoided unless the surgeon knows positively that some mistake or complication occurred that he can prevent or control at a second operation. Neurolysis following repair of a peripheral nerve also is usually not successful unless a complication such as a hematoma or infection occurred and there is reason to believe that a similar fate can be avoided during a subsequent procedure. Scar that forms as a part of normal wound healing in an individual usually will re-form, possibly with greater severity, if neurolysis is performed within the time of the secondary healing phenomenon (probably about seven weeks). Unless a cause for excessive scar formation is identified and can be avoided during the second operation, excess scar formation should not be the reason for performing a secondary procedure, whether it be neurolysis or division and reanastomosis of the nerve.

Severe and persistent local pain or hypersensitivity distal to the site of injury or repair is more often associated with incomplete or partial injury than with complete division of the nerve. Persistent pain and disabling hyperesthesia should be investigated and treated vigorously. The longer these symptoms persist the more central a neurosurgical procedure to obliterate pain may have to be. Firm establishment of pain patterns should be avoided at all costs even if hospitalization and narcotics are required to interrupt for a short interval the unremitting pain. One of the more frequent sites for pain of this type is the radial side of the wrist and base of the thumb. Partial injury of the distal sensory radial nerve may follow Colles' fracture or careless retraction during removal of a ganglion or incision of the sheath of the long abductor and short extensor tendons. The development of Sudeck's atrophy adds to the severity of the condition. Many patients with Sudeck's atrophy and severe pain following Colles' fracture describe severe unremitting pain after application of the first cast. Experienced orthopedists recommend that as much of the cast as necessary be removed during the first few days after reduction if the pain cannot be relieved satisfactorily with drugs or change in position. The worst complication of such a fracture—loss of reduction—is insignificant compared to the prolonged and agonizing disability of a major pain syndrome after the bone has united.

When significant disability is the result of a partial nerve injury, one may have to decide whether the chance of recovering a substantial part of what has been lost outweighs the loss that sacrificing the entire nerve prior to an anastomosis will cause. Although diagrams and descriptions have appeared from time to time illustrating and extolling methods of partial nerve repair, repair of only half a nerve is more technically attractive than uniformly successful. In this regard, it should be noted that an extensive study of partial nerve injuries in human beings and primates by Kline, utilizing recordings of nerve action potentials, revealed more extensive damage to nerve conduction than the size of the partial laceration suggested. Thus, for all practical purposes, even though we can occasionally dissect a neuroma out of a partially damaged nerve and then suture the divided ends without damaging intact fasciculi, a partial nerve injury should not be explored unless the surgeon is prepared to divide the damaged nerve completely and perform a 360 degree anastomosis and the patient is willing to accept the consequences. Sometimes predominantly sensory or motor fibers remain in the partially damaged nerve. If motor function is intact in the ulnar nerve, the nerve should never be divided and resutured to obtain sensation because return of motor function is too unpredictable to risk a permanent intrinsic palsy, even if return of sensation could be guaranteed—and it cannot. Conversely, one usually would not be well advised to sacrifice median sensation with the idea of regaining thenar muscle power. Thumb opposition can be restored by tendon transfers, which are so simple to perform and so reliable in their outcome that jeopardizing the extremely important median nerve-mediated sensation is not justified. In the lower extremity, motor power is, of course, more important than sensation, although sensation is missed when it is lost.

NERVE REPLACEMENT

When a defect exists that mobilizing proximal and distal ends and flexing surrounding joints cannot overcome, the reconstructive surgeon must use his ingenuity to restore nerve continuity. Technical innovations reported in the surgical literature in recent years unfortunately have not been accompanied by sophisticated methods of evaluating the results; thus a review of methods for overcoming large defects is more encyclopedic than critical. One reason for this is that restoration of sensation usually is the goal in upper extremity reconstructions; available procedures for substituting normally innervated muscles to balance power deficits produce satisfactory results in most patients. If sensation cannot be recovered, however, further reconstructive surgery often is not warranted. This is particularly true when only one extremity is involved. Conditions such as leprosy which cause loss of sensation in all extremities, of course, are an exception. Reconstructive surgery to provide balanced power in the hands of patients with advanced leprosy has been of enormous value even though we do not yet have methods for restoring sensation. In the case of a unilateral traumatic loss of sensation, however, complex restorations of bone, tendon, joints, and so forth, simply are not warranted in most patients unless sensation can be restored. The damaged hand will only be used sporadically as a helper in the relatively few functions that the normal hand cannot perform satisfactorily.

In the lower extremity, when a simple anastomosis is not possible, a complex grafting procedure usually is not justified. Sensation, although valuable in preventing trophic changes in skin, is not as necessary for the function of weight bearing as it is for skilled use of fingers. Moreover, motor functions are relatively simple and can be substituted for by muscle transfers and stabilizing procedures.

Large defects in the facial nerve usually should be bridged with grafts since distal motor substitutions are not entirely satisfactory and regenerative capacity of the facial nerve is exceptional. Unfortunately, however, intentional removal of the facial nerve is usually done for tumor and often must be so peripheral in its extent that distal ends large enough to be identified and sutured to a central graft are not always available.

Therefore the upper extremity has been the most usual site for complex grafting procedures for major defects in peripheral nerves, and it is from these cases that most of our clinical information must be derived.

Before beginning a discussion on methods of free and pedicle nerve grafting, we should point out that remarkable progress was made during and just after the Korean conflict in methods of restoring sensation to important areas of the hand by island transfer of sensitive skin and by nerve transfer of intact digital sensory nerves. Before undertaking a long and often unrewarding series of peripheral neurological restorations, some of which may entail destructive complications at the donor site, a surgeon who is familiar with these latest procedures should keep distal transfer of sensation in mind when he evaluates an anesthetic hand. Some areas of the hand are relatively less important than others as far as the need for sensation is concerned, and if intact sensation exists in an unimportant area, it may be possible to transfer it to an area of greater importance by simpler and more reliable procedures than grafting a major nerve. Because grafting of large nerve defects in the upper extremity is always for sensory objectives (return of motor function should not be expected after grafting although it occasionally occurs), transfer of sensation by a single method can provide an ideal solution to a difficult problem.

An example of this principle can be found in either a pure ulnar nerve or a pure median nerve deficit. In the case of an ulnar nerve def-

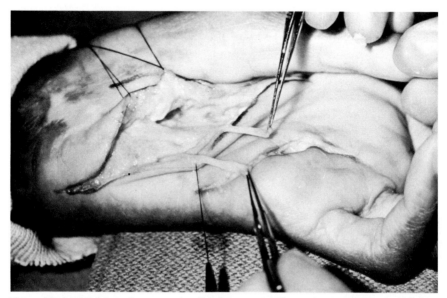

Figure 10–4. Division of proper volar digital nerves on ulnar side of small finger and radial side of long finger prior to transfer to radial side of index finger and ulnar side of thumb.

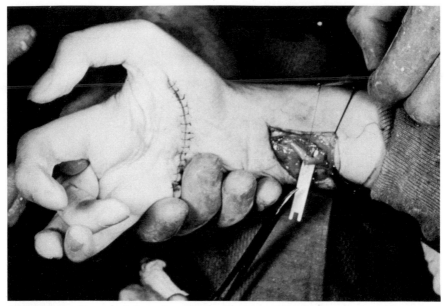

Figure 10–5. Transplantation of proximal ulnar nerve into distal median nerve to restore sensation to radial side of the hand. Motor branch of ulnar nerve was irreparably damaged in the palm.

icit, the most important loss of sensation is on the ulnar side of the small finger; this loss is far more disabling than the loss on the radial side of the small finger or the ulnar side of the ring finger because the ulnar side of the small finger amounts to the ulnar side of the hand. It is the fulcrum against which objects being grasped by all digits are centered. It is also the first surface to come in contact with objects when the hand is dropped in a natural position to a foreign surface. At the same time, there is little need for sensation within the interspace between the interior fingers. Transfer of sensation from the interspace between the ring finger and long finger or the long finger and index fingers to the ulnar side of the small finger moves sensation from an area of small importance to an area of greater functional significance. It is important to remember, however, that in ulnar nerve sensory deficit one should not transfer nerve or skin from the radial side of the ring finger, even though it is tempting to do so because it is the closest intact sensory skin or nerve. Taking skin or nerve from a digit that already has hemi-anesthesia is inadvisable because it makes the finger completely anesthetic. Removing sensation from one side of a finger that has normal sensation on the other side is less disabling than taking the last remaining sensation from a digit. The digit selected as a sensory donor, therefore, should be one in which removal of a nerve will produce only hemianesthesia.

The ulnar side of the thumb and the radial side of the index finger are of greater functional importance than the remainder of the hand. In restoring continuity in a median nerve sensory deficit, therefore, providing sensation to those areas is a large part of the objective. The interspace between the index finger and long finger or the long finger and ring finger often can be ignored if sensation can be restored to one-half of the thumb or one-half of the index finger or both. Nerve or skin transfer from the interspace between the ring finger and small finger can provide this in many patients.

Most surgeons prefer an island pedicle transfer to a nerve transfer in transferring sensation from one area of the hand to another, for several reasons. The most important is that sensation transferred by the island pedicle method is normal except for a slight loss of two-point discrimination (demonstrated only by careful and exacting measurements) and faulty localization. Although faulty localization is permanent, patients uniformly report that they have become accustomed to inaccuracy of this type and that it causes no significant disability. A second reason is that nerves are not divided in an island pedicle transfer, so that the possibility of failure of axon regeneration is avoided. A third reason is that some sensation will return to the skin-grafted donor site after removal of an island pedicle, whereas an area denervated by

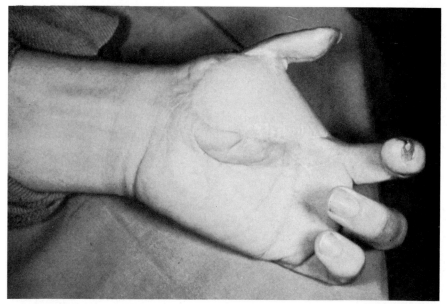

Figure 10–6. Severely damaged hand in which the ulnar neurovascular bundle was the only intact structure in the long finger. There was no sensation in the thumb as a result of avulsion of digital nerves from the pulp area. (Reproduced by permission from E. E. Peacock, Jr., Plast. Reconstr. Surg. 25:298, 1960. Copyright 1960, The Williams & Wilkins Co., Baltimore, Md. 21202, U.S.A.)

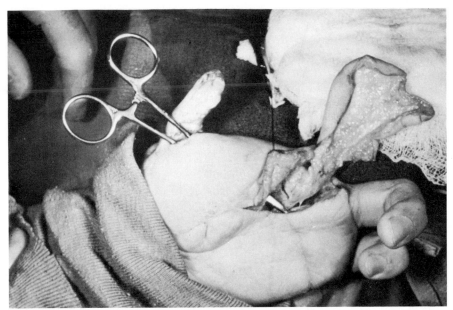

Figure 10–7. Conversion of irreparably damaged long finger into an island pedicle flap supplied by the ulnar neurovascular bundle. The anesthetic thumb has been denuded and a clamp is passed beneath the soft tissue to pull the island pedicle flap into the thumb area. (Reproduced by permission from E. E. Peacock, Jr., Plast. Reconstr. Surg. *25*:298, 1960. Copyright 1960, The Williams & Wilkins Co., Baltimore, Md. 21202, U.S.A.)

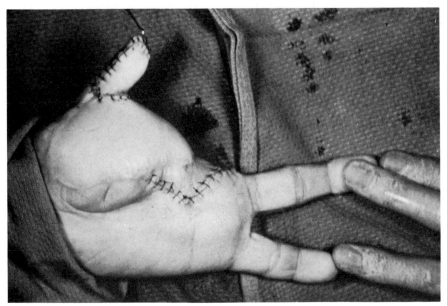

Figure 10–8. Thumb has been resurfaced with island pedicle flap shown in Figure 10–7 to bring sensation to thumb. Rotatory osteotomies at base of metacarpals of ring and small fingers will be needed to bring remaining digits into prehensile position. (Reproduced by permission from E. E. Peacock, Jr., Plast. Reconstr. Surg. *25*:298, 1960. Copyright 1960, The Williams & Wilkins Co., Baltimore, Md. 21202, U.S.A.)

dividing and transferring a digital nerve will remain permanently anesthetic.

With full- and split-thickness skin grafts, as well as composite pedicle grafts, usually some degree of sensory perception is regained, even though not a single intact nerve is preserved during their transfer. This fact, and the fact that skin rendered anesthetic by division of a peripheral nerve will never regain sensation, may be of some biological importance. The supposition has been that small peripheral nerve filaments in normally innervated skin surrounding the anesthetic area permeate a free graft and eventually provide some measure of sensitivity. This is especially striking in free split-thickness skin grafts although it can be demonstrated in composite flaps too. The unanswered question, however, is why, after proximal nerve injury, peripheral nerve filaments around an area of anesthetic skin fail to grow into a denervated area. Our answer has been that the one obvious difference between a denervated free skin graft and a denervated but otherwise normal area of skin is that one has been circumcised by a surgical incision whereas the other has not; the supposition is that division of terminal nerve filaments by surgical incision stimulates them to proliferate into the newly resurfaced area. When an incision has not been made, there is no such stimulation and therefore the anesthetic skin is not penetrated by proliferating nerve fibrils. Such a hypothesis

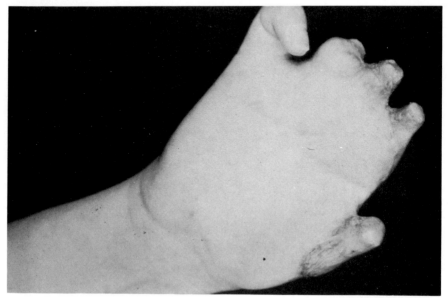

Figure 10–9. Severely damaged hand with first metacarpal covered only by a split-thickness skin graft. The only sensation in the thumb area was hypersensitivity secondary to inadequate coverage of metacarpal periosteum. (Reproduced by permission from E. E. Peacock, Jr., in *Hand Surgery,* edited by J. E. Flynn. Copyright 1966, The Williams & Wilkins Co., Baltimore, Md. 21202, U.S.A.)

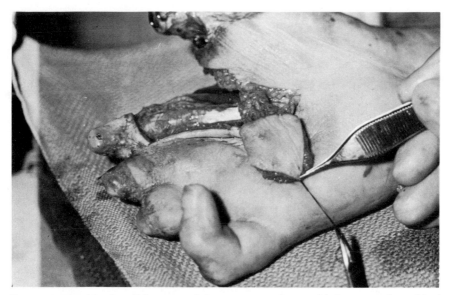

Figure 10–10. Island pedicle removed from metacarpal area of index ray and nourished by a single neurovascular bundle on radial side of index metacarpal. (Reproduced by permission from E. E. Peacock, Jr., in *Hand Surgery*, edited by J. E. Flynn. Copyright 1966, The Williams & Wilkins Co., Baltimore, Md. 21202, U.S.A.)

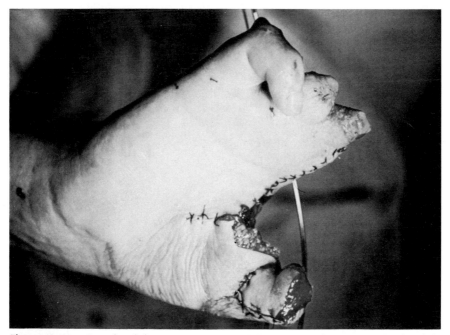

Figure 10–11. Same hand shown in Figure 10–9 following transplantation of island pedicle flap to volar surface of thumb metacarpal.

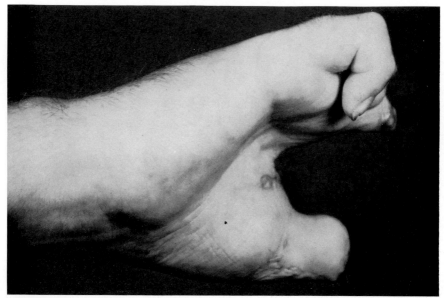

Figure 10–12. Final view of hand shown in Figures 10–9 to 10–11. The island pedicle flap provided sensation and a prehensile pad. (Reproduced by permission from E. E. Peacock, Jr., in *Hand Surgery,* edited by J. F. Flynn. Copyright 1966, The Williams & Wilkins Co., Baltimore, Md. 21202, U.S.A.)

might be tested by making an elective incision in the line of demarcation between skin innervated by the ulnar nerve and that innervated by the median nerve when one nerve is intact and the other is irreparably damaged. Controls for sensitivity measurements will be difficult but some useful data might be obtained.

The most important objections to the use of an island pedicle flap are disfigurement of the donor site and technical complexity of the operation. The most serious disadvantage to nerve transfer is that so much of the quality and quantity of sensory perception is lost during transfer. It has been hypothesized that only about 10 per cent of regenerating axons ever find their way along correctly oriented distal tubes to receptive end organs. To lose 100 per cent of sensitivity in a donor site and recover only 10 to 15 per cent in the recipient area is too high a price to pay in the judgment of many surgeons. Actually, the 10 per cent return of sensation, estimated on the basis of all types of nerve injuries, is not entirely correct in the case of an elective transfer, under optimal conditions, of a small, purely sensory nerve. The authors' patients have regained more nearly 50 per cent of normal sensation following this procedure although the risk of no return of function because of a technical complication exists, of course, in any nerve anastomosis. We should inject a word of caution regarding transfer of sensation regained by repair of a more proximal nerve injury. If, for example, median nerve sensation has been restored by means of a successful neurorrhapy in the midforearm but ulnar neurorrhaphy was impossible because of loss of nerve over too great a length, one might consider transferring a digital nerve from the interspace between the long and index fingers to the ulnar side of the small finger. To do so often will result in total anesthesia in the donor area and no significant return of sensation in the recipient area. Apparently after two anastomoses the number of successful axon regenerations is reduced below that which can transmit a centrally appreciated peripheral stimulus. This is one reason why subjective claims of patients following pedicle nerve grafting (two anastomoses are required) have been held suspect by many. Return of some sensation after nerve grafting of major nerves in the forearm by the pedicle method has produced some rather remarkable testimonials, however, and so it may be that a larger nerve provides so many opportunities for regenerating axons to find purposeful channels that two anastomoses do not defeat the overall objective.

When the defects in two major nerves are so extensive that the ends cannot be coapted, one should consider removing a segment of radius and ulna to shorten the forearm if approximation of nerve ends would then be possible. Approximately 2 inches of radius and ulna can be removed with virtually no functional disability. If an additional 2 inches of nerve will make a primary anastomosis possible, this is definitely preferable to nerve grafting by conventional free grafts of whole

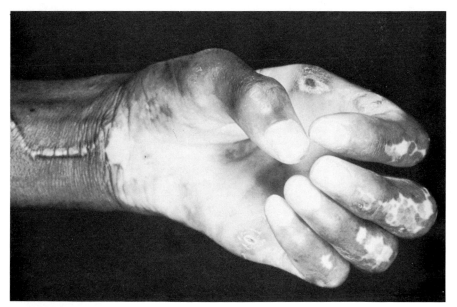

Figure 10–13. Typical trophic ulcers and skin changes in a totally anesthetic hand following unsuccessful repair of median and ulnar nerves in upper forearm.

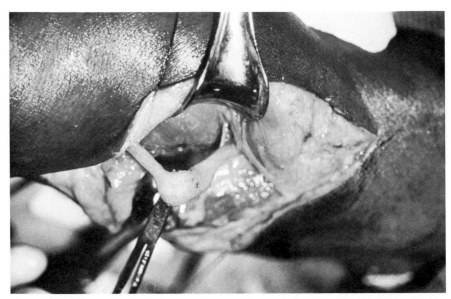

Figure 10–14. Appearance of neuroma in upper forearm of patient shown in Figure 10–13. Proximal enlargement suggests that distal nerve is fibrosed. Approximately 1 cm. distal to anastomosis, distal nerve is soft and pliable.

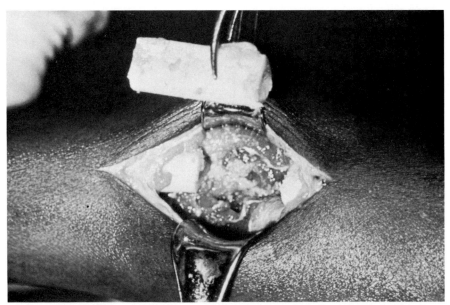

Figure 10–15. Because a large gap had been overcome during a previous operation, it was not possible to excise more nerve and still bring ends together without tension. Approximately 4 cm. of radius and 4 cm. of ulna were removed so that nerve could be anastomosed without tension.

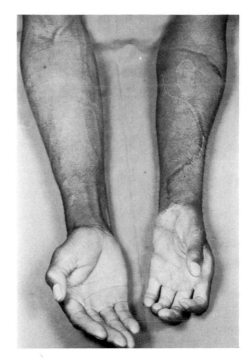

Figure 10–16. Shortened forearm following removal of segments of radius and ulna so that defects in median and ulnar nerves could be overcome. Note absence of trophic ulcers and normal appearance of skin in the hand following return of protective sensation.

nerve. Recent experience in funicular grafting suggests that this will become the nerve grafting technique of choice in the future. The greatest danger in shortening the forearm is nonunion of either or both bones. Exemplary technique, however, can result in a stable forearm. This procedure has not been advocated widely but, in our experience, it has been a worthwhile operation for selected patients. The procedure seems less justified now that excellent results are being reported on the use of multiple funicular sural nerve grafts. If a gain of 2 inches of nerve will not permit a perfect anastomosis without tension, shortening the forearm should not be done and a graft should be considered.

The two principal types of grafts are free grafts and pedicle grafts. Neither is as desirable as a single anastomosis without tension, if for no other reason than the fact that axons must cross two suture lines. Perhaps even more important, though, the amount of fibrous proliferation within a large free graft of any appreciable size is usually so excessive that axon regeneration is seriously inhibited. It appears that the amount of fibrous proliferation can be correlated with the diameter of the graft, and thus anoxia and malnutrition may be important contributing factors. A digital nerve or the sural nerve, being purely sensory and only a millimeter or two in diameter, can be utilized effectively as a free graft for another digital nerve or funiculus in a compound nerve. The opportunity to do so without producing an unacceptable anesthetic area in the donor site does not occur often,

however. When a digital nerve can be dissected out of a freshly amputated digit and utilized as a free graft for another finger, it should be
done. One should remember, however, that nerves being removed for
transfer or free grafts must never be retracted longitudinally. Every
tiny lateral filament must be carefully dissected so that the nerve can be
gently lifted out of its bed without longitudinal traction. In the case of
digital nerves, in spite of the fact that two suture lines are produced,
significant regeneration of axons apparently does occur in some cases.
In large nerves of the arm and forearm, however, the opposite is true.
Sural nerve grafts are, therefore, the best free grafts for most patients.

Use of a segment of median or ulnar nerve as a free graft to restore continuity of the other almost always results in central fibrosis of
the graft and absence of distal function. The explanation has been
given that deprivation of blood supply to a nerve of large diameter is
followed by central necrosis and replacement by fibrous tissue. Although such a hypothesis is tenable, data to support it are not available
at present.

Two alternatives to free grafting of large nerves have been advocated: utilization of multiple small grafts, and pedicle transfer of a
large graft. Multiple small nerve grafts from the sural nerve (1 or 2
mm. in diameter) can be removed with little loss of important sensibility in the leg. Several strands of sural nerve have been used to bridge a
gap in the radial or median nerves with the idea that gases and nutrients would diffuse into several nerves of small diameter more effectively than into a single large nerve. Occasional good functional results
reported in the past have now become relatively common. Notable suc-
cesses have frequently been reported after grafting the facial nerve
with combinations of central and peripheral divisions of the middle
cervical plexus and greater auricular nerve. This is a special condition,
however, as these grafts are of small diameter, the nerve to be grafted
is a pure motor nerve, and the facial nerve is known to have unusual
regenerative properties.

Recently, attempts have been made to reduce post-transplant
fibrosis and provide a more reliable source for nerve grafts than autogenous grafts can, by using irradiated nerve grafts from allogenic
sources. Radiation theoretically reduces the antigenicity of nerve grafts,
although it should be pointed out that the magnitude of antigenicity in
a peripheral nerve has not been studied intensively. It is possible that
superior results currently reported following the use of irradiated
allografts are due entirely to destruction of fibroblasts within the connective tissue framework of the nerve and not to any effect on tissue
rejection *per se*. In any event, radiation, immunosuppressive drugs,
lyophilization, and other procedures are currently being tested as ad-
juncts to the use of large peripheral nerve allografts in primates and
human beings. In the authors' judgment, the results are not convincing
that any real improvement in predictable axon regeneration is being

obtained. More data are needed, however, and undoubtedly will be forthcoming in the next few years.

The most interesting and most reliable nerve grafts yet proposed are those of the ulnar nerve in the cat prepared many years ago by Dr. Derek Denny-Brown. The axon was actually dissected out of the sheath of a segment of ulnar nerve, to produce an empty yet intact nerve sheath. As could be predicted, the sheath made a superb interposition graft. The ulnar nerve of a cat is ideally arranged internally for this type of preparation, however, and the principle has not yet been adapted to human beings.

Following the reasoning that reduction in internal scarring is related to oxygenation and nutrition and that a finite limit exists in the capacity of longitudinal blood vessels to provide adequate nutrition, attempts have been made to overcome long nerve gaps in parallel nerves (such as the median and ulnar nerve) by utilizing one as a pedicle graft with intact circulation to bridge a defect in the other. This procedure is most often applicable when a severe avulsion or electrical burn of the forearm has destroyed more than 15 cm. of both median and ulnar nerves. The proximal ends of both nerves are sutured end to end, and approximately 15 to 20 cm. proximal to the anastomosis of one nerve (usually the ulnar) a cut is made so that Wallerian degeneration will occur between the proximal cut and the more distal end-to-end anastomosis. This maneuver provides a nerve graft which, after Wallerian degeneration, can receive axons from the other nerve (through the anastomosis) and does not develop significant fibrous impediments because no period of anoxia occurs. Some 12 weeks later, after axons presumably have negotiated the anastomosis and most of the length of the graft, the arm is explored again and the graft is rotated distally into the defect. At this time all lateral vascular connections are severed, of course, but nutrition is not interrupted because longitudinal vessels are connected to the vessels of the proximal nerve and axoplasm has already appeared in the distal tubules. A distal anastomosis between the proximal end of the graft (now the distal end of the proximally grafted nerve) and the distal nerve in the wrist is performed. If both anastomoses are successful, and if the theoretical advantage of preserving lateral blood supply while longitudinal blood supply is being established is correct, sensation should be regained in a portion of the hand.

After World War II a number of patients were reported to have regained some sensation when this procedure was used (the authors also have had patients who have testified to some return of sensation), but several findings associated with reconstruction of nerves by this method have been bothersome. One problem is lack of positive identification of a typical neuroma at the distal end of the graft. Moreover, the size of the graft remains small throughout it length, regardless of how much time is allowed to elapse between primary anastomosis and reexploration. In addition, relatively enormous neuromas frequently are found at the site of the first anastomosis. These findings have led the authors to suspect that at least some of the return of sensation reported after major nerve restorations by the pedicle technique is due to mechanisms other than regeneration of axons in a retrograde fashion. Incomplete but interesting investigations in several patients have sustained this suspicion.

One interesting finding, reported in detail in 1963, was that axons were absent, on histological examination, in a pedicle nerve graft which apparently was successful in restoring sensation to the median side of the hand. Even more interesting was the fact that transection of the graft several months later failed to reduce sensation (which appeared after the second anastomosis). Because of these findings, we started to include in the procedure rotation of small segments of normal ulnar nerve proximal to the pedicle so that we would have a retrograde graft that could be removed for study when the pedicle graft was rotated into its final position. The finding of large neuromas without evidence of distal axon regeneration in these grafts raised the question of whether a graft that requires retrograde growth of axons is a biologically functional preparation. Subsequently we began to perform nerve transfers by rotating the median nerve to a more proximal position at the level of the proximal cut in the ulnar nerve and performing the first anastomosis at that level. This technical revision provides a pedicle graft with normal polarity. We have not had an opportunity to study axon regeneration histologically in these nerve grafts but we have noted that the proximal neuroma has appeared smaller than in retrograde grafts and that return of sensation has seemed more reliable. Similar observations have been made by others.

Evaluation of sensory perception can be very inaccurate as an assessment of the results of nerve repairs. This is unfortunate because so often the objective of peripheral nerve restorative surgery is restoration of sensation. Actual recovery of sensation or misinterpretation by the patient that sensation is returning can occur in a number of ways. Some are fairly well documented while others are only hypothetical at this time. There is no question, however, that a patient's affirmation that sensation is returning may be the result of many processes other than axon regeneration following a surgical restoration.

Studies in leprosy patients have provided some insight into how sensation may be appreciated without major nerve (median and ulnar) function. One of the authors (E.E.P.), with Dr. Paul Brand at the Christian Medical College Hospital in Vellore, South India, studied a patient who provided a vivid example of the complexities of evaluating sensory function. The patient had severe tuberculous leprosy involving all three (radial, ulnar, median) nerves; sections of all three nerves had been removed as surgical specimens. There was no question, therefore, that all of the major nerves in the upper extremity had been destroyed. His arm and hand had been operated on twice with no anesthesia. One night the patient complained of severe pain in the thumb, and examination revealed the presence of a typical felon. Drainage of approximately 0.5 cc. of pus produced immediate relief. In this case general visceral afferent fibers coursing along blood vessels must have provided a pathway for signals from stretch receptors to reach the central nervous system. In other patients with a similar triple nerve deficit, position sense occasionally is preserved even though the hand is completely anesthetic. In these patients, dramatic loss of position sense can be produced if the long flexor tendons to a digit are grasped with forceps and advanced to an abnormal position or fixed against a stable structure such as the radius. In spite of previous dictums, based on anatomical studies, about the location of kinesoreceptors in the hand, these findings cannot be explained unless kinesoreceptors are located in long motor units also.

Patients unconsciously use their eyes very effectively to make up for loss of sensation. Blindfolding the patient can reveal how significantly sight is contributing to his notion of return of peripheral sensation. Sensory organs in surrounding neurologically intact skin may become increasingly more sensitive to pressure transmitted mechanically from anesthetic skin. Finally, cerebral control over the intensity with which a peripheral stimulus is interpreted can be enormous. The patient's attitude toward doctor, operation, and injury can make a great difference in how he interprets sensation or lack of sensation in an injured extremity. All of these factors may enter into the patient's response when attempts are made to assess the results of a nerve restoration; it is no wonder, therefore, that testimonials can be found to substantiate almost every reconstructive procedure that has been devised. In no other area of restorative surgery is it more important to develop the science of measurement and a critical approach to the study of human patients.

SUGGESTED READING

Baker, P. F. The Nerve Axon. Sci. Amer. *214*:74, 1966.

Braun, R. M. Comparative Studies of Neurorrhaphy and Sutureless Peripheral Nerve Repair. Surg. Gynec. Obstet. *122*:15, 1966.

Cavanagh, J. B. Prior X-Irradiation and the Cellular Response to Nerve Crush: Duration of Effect. Exp. Neurol. *22*:253, 1968.

Denny-Brown, D. Importance of Neural Fibroblasts in the Regeneration of Nerve. Arch. Neurol. Psychiat. *55*:171, 1946.

Ducker, T. B., and Hayes, G. J. Experimental Improvement in the Use of Silastic Cuff for Peripheral Nerve Repair. J. Neurosurg. *28*:582, 1968.

Ducker, T. B., Kempe, L. G., and Hayes, G. J. The Metabolic Background for Peripheral Nerve Surgery. J. Neurosurg. *30*:270, 1969.

Grabb, W. C. Median and Ulnar Nerve Suture. An Experimental Study Comparing Primary and Secondary Repair in Monkeys. J. Bone Joint Surg. *50A*:964, 1968.

Guth, L. Regeneration in the Mammalian Peripheral Nervous System. Physiol. Rev. *36*:441, 1956.

Gutmann, E., and Sanders, F. K. Recovery of Fibre Numbers and Diameters in the Regeneration of Peripheral Nerves. J. Physiol. *101*:489, 1943.

Hirasawa, Y., and Marmor, L. The Protective Effect of Irradiation Combined with Sheathing Methods on Experimental Nerve Heterografts: Silastic, Autogenous Veins, and Heterogenous Arteries. J. Neurosurg. 27:401, 1967.

Kline, D. G., and Hackett, E. R. Reappraisal of Timing for Exploration of Civilian Peripheral Nerve Injuries. Surgery 78:54, 1975.

Kline, D. G., and Hayes, G. J. Experimental Evaluation of Effect of Plastic Adhesive Methyl Cyanoacrilate on Neural Tissue. J. Neurosurg. 20:647, 1963.

Lehman, R. A. W., and Hayes, G. J. Degeneration and Regeneration in Peripheral Nerve. Brain 90:285, 1967.

Marmor, L., and Hirasawa, Y. Further Studies of Irradiated Nerve Heterografts in Animals with Imuran Immunosuppression. J. Trauma 8:32, 1968.

Marx, J. L. Nerve Growth Factor: Regulatory Role Examined. Science 185:930, 1974.

McQuillan, W. M. Origin of Fibrosis after Peripheral Nerve Division. Lancet 2:1220, 1965.

Millesi, H., Meissl, G., and Berger, A. The Interfascicular Nerve Grafting of the Median and Ulnar Nerves. J. Bone Joint Surg. 54A:727, 1972.

Nathaniel, E. J. H., and Pease, D. C. Collagen and Basement Membrane Formation by Schwann Cells during Nerve Regeneration. J. Ultrastruct. Res. 9:550, 1963.

Peacock, E. E., Jr. Restoration of Sensation in Hands with Extensive Median Nerve Defects. Surgery 54:576, 1963.

Peacock, E. E., Jr. The Argument for Primary Repair of Injured Nerves. In: Controversy in Surgery. Edited by R. L. Varco and J. P. Delaney. Philadelphia, W. B. Saunders Co., 1976.

Peacock, E. E., Jr., Madden, J. W., and Trier, W. C. Transfer of Median and Ulnar Nerve during Early Treatment of Forearm Ischemia. Ann. Surg. 169:748, 1969.

Schenkein, I., Levy, M., Bueker, E. D., and Tokarsky, E. Nerve Growth Factor of Very High Yield and Specific Activity. Science 159:640, 1968.

Shanthaveerappa, T. R., and Bourne, G. H. Perineural Epithelium: A New Concept of Its Role in the Integrity of the Peripheral Nervous System. Science 154:1464, 1966.

Smith, J. W. Factors Influencing Nerve Repair. I. Blood Supply of Peripheral Nerves. Arch. Surg. 93:335, 1966.

Smith, J. W. Factors Influencing Nerve Repair. II. Collateral Circulation of Peripheral Nerves. Arch. Surg. 93:433, 1966.

Sunderland, S. The Connective Tissues of Peripheral Nerves. Brain 88:841, 1965.

Terzis, J., Faibisoff, B., and Williams, H. B. The Nerve Gap: Suture under Tension vs. Graft. Plast. Reconstr. Surg. In press.

Thomas, P. K., and Jones, D. G. The Cellular Response to Nerve Injury. 2. Regeneration of the Perineurium after Nerve Section. J. Anat. 101:45, 1967.

Van Beek, A., and Glover, J. L. Primary Versus Delayed-Primary Neurorrhaphy. J. Surg. Res. 18:335, 1975.

Wise, A. J., Topuzlu, C., Davis, P. and Kaye, I. S. A Comparative Analysis of Macro- and Microsurgical Neurorrhaphy Technics. Amer. J. Surg. 117:566, 1969.

Chapter 11

HEALING AND REPAIR OF BONE

Bone, like liver, is among the few organs that undergo regeneration rather than simple repair. The extent of regeneration of which bone is capable is limited, however. Removal of half of a long bone will not result in regeneration of the missing part. Thus, although the regenerative power of bone is considerably less than that of liver, its repair can be considered a regenerative phenomenon because the characteristic organizational structure is restored, including the marrow and its components.

Like many regenerative processes, the sequence of events in the repair of bone usually follows the pattern of embryonic development or the pattern that is followed in growth. In the case of bone this is a relatively complex process, and the mechanisms are still not well understood. In this chapter only the repair of the solid structure of bone will be considered. The regeneration of marrow components will not be discussed.

BONE STRUCTURE AND COMPOSITION

Bone is a complex structure. In long tubular weight-bearing bones, two types of structure are seen. At the ends is the so-called spongiosa, or cancellous bone. This name aptly describes its appearance, but not its properties. The structure is seen to be composed of columns of bony substance, called trabeculae, separated by large spaces. These columns follow lines of stress and are well adapted to load bearing. The shaft of bone is composed of a dense, compact mass of bony tissue, compact bone, which surrounds the marrow cavity. This compact bone is

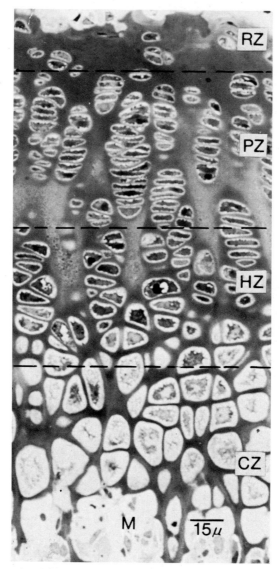

Figure 11–1. Levels of the epiphyseal plate (*top to bottom*): *RZ,* reserve cell zone; *PZ,* proliferative zone; *HZ,* hypertrophic zone; *CZ,* zone of overt calcification and chondrocyte disintegration. A portion of the metaphysis *(M)* is present at the bottom. × 600. (Reproduced by permission from H. C. Anderson, J. Cell Biol. *41*:59, 1969.)

traversed by numerous microscopic tubules, termed Haversian canals. Within these tubules are blood vessels, about the size of capillaries. These intercommunicate with each other and with larger tubules called nutritive canals. Around each Haversian canal, bone appears to be deposited in concentric layers and a well defined microscopic unit, the osteon, can be seen. Haversian canals are not found in cancellous bone.

Around bone is a fibrous sheet, periosteum. This is composed of two cell layers, the outer, or fibrous, layer and the inner, or cambium, layer, from which new bone cells arise. A similar fibrous sheet lines the marrow cavity and is termed endosteum. Joint surfaces of bones are covered by cartilage, over which the lining, or synovial membrane of the joint space, lies. In growing bone, at the ends, just under cartilage, is a more cellular and vascular area which joins the bone at a zone known as the epiphyseal plate. This is a zone of active bone growth. When growth is complete, this cellular zone disappears and the area is spoken of as a "closed epiphysis." In most bones, new bone formed during growth is formed at the epiphyseal plate by a process known as endochondral ossification. This type of bone formation, which will be discussed in more detail later, commences with cartilage formation, cartilage calcification, cartilage resorption, and bone formation.

In skull, the bones do not have epiphyses; nor does any part of these bones, except at the nose, at the junction of the spinal column, and at the maxillary-mandibular articulating surfaces, have adjacent cartilage. These bones are formed by direct ossification rather than by endochondral ossification. Direct ossification, also termed intramembranous ossification, is sometimes a feature in some cases of fracture repair in other bones of the body. As we shall see, the type of process used in repair depends upon certain critical environmental factors.

The composition of bone can be divided into the organic phase and the inorganic phase. The organic phase is termed matrix, and it gives form to bone and acts as the supporting structure on which inorganic salts are deposited and crystallized.

Composition of Matrix

The principal component of matrix is the fibrous protein, collagen. Bone collagen is type I; it consists of two $\alpha 1(I)$ chains and an $\alpha 2$ chain, and resembles skin and tendon collagen closely. Among various species there is a notable difference in the degree of hydroxylation of lysine residues. Rat bone collagen has a high proportion of lysine residues hydroxylated, but in human bone collagen the number of hydroxylysine residues is virtually the same as in human skin collagen. However, glycosylation of hydroxylysine residues in mature bone collagen is less than in other collagens. The relevance of this observation to mineralization of bone will be discussed later in this chapter.

It has been shown also that the distribution of polar and nonpolar residues in bone collagen is similar to that in skin collagen, although in certain locations along the peptide chain there are quantitative differences. The close similarity between bone and skin collagen makes it difficult to explain the observation that decalcified bone matrix can induce ossification, whereas other collagens do not. It is known, for instance, that only collagen in the native state (i.e., in triple helical conformation and assembled in the quarter-stagger arrangement) can be calcified. However, there is no indication that bone and skin collagen differ in any way in conformation or polymer assembly in formation of fibers.

In the cross-linking pattern of bone collagen, there are certain differences of a quantitative nature that may be important. It has long been suspected that cross-links in bone collagen may be different from those in other collagens because of the extreme insolubility of bone collagen as compared to other collagens. Less than 0.5 per cent of bone collagen can be solubilized in neutral salt solutions. Citrate buffers at pH 1.5 to 3.5 or 0.5M acetic acid will solubilize a further 6 to 10 per cent of collagen. Extraction with denaturing solvents, such as 5M guanidine, will solubilize an additional 17 per cent of bone collagen. Fractionation of this material indicates that some degradation of collagen peptide chains may occur, but the majority of solubilized material exists in β or γ forms. However, if animals are made lathyritic by administration of β-aminopropionitrile, as much as 40 per cent of bone collagen is soluble in neutral salt solution and consists primarily of α components. Since lathyrogens prevent covalent cross-linking as described in Chapters 4 and 5, the conclusion that insolubility of bone collagen is due to either a high degree of cross-linking or the fact that cross-links are of a different and more chemically resistant type than other collagens appears justified.

One group of investigators isolated from bone collagen a particular type of cross-link which they felt, on the basis of incomplete analytical results, to be an aldol formed by condensation of two hydroxylysine aldehydes. Subsequent studies by this same group, however, revealed that the cross-link was an aldimine involving one hydroxylysine and a hydroxylysine aldehyde, dehydrohydroxylysinohydroxynorleucine. Subsequent studies revealed that this cross-link was stabilized by spontaneous conversion, via an Amadori rearrangement, to the keto-al-

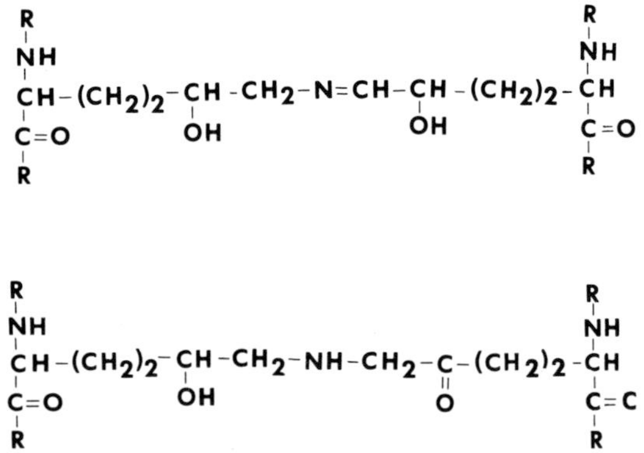

Figure 11–2. Major cross-links of bone collagen. The upper formula is dehydrodihydroxylysinonorleucine. It has been shown that this cross-link undergoes internal rearrangement to form the more stable keto-aldimine shown in the lower formula.

dimine, 5-keto-5-hydroxylysinonorleucine. This keto-amine has been shown to be stable to heat and acid, thus differing from other aldimine and aldol cross-links in collagen. One site of this cross-link has been identified as involving the NH_2-terminal region of one α chain with the COOH-terminal portion of an α chain of an adjacent molecule.

It also has been suggested, and evidence has been presented, that at least one and possibly two of the aldimine cross-links of bone collagen become reduced during maturation, thus becoming resistant to acid hydrolysis. It appears, therefore, that the great insolubility of bone collagen can be explained by the presence of keto-aldimine cross-links and other aldimine cross-links which become reduced during maturation. The presence of the keto-aldimine, 5-keto-5-hydroxylysinonorleucine, may be a feature which distinguishes bone collagens from soft tissue collagens of the type I configuration.

Matrix also has a small but important group of substances comprising ground substance. These account for less than 5 per cent of matrix and consist chiefly of a group of protein-polysaccharides and glycoproteins. In adult bone, the principal carbohydrate component of protein-polysaccharides is chondroitin sulfate A, although small amounts of keratosulfate may be present. Recent work suggests that the polysaccharide components of protein-polysaccharides may be more or less heterogeneous, and this can account for the difficulties experienced in experimental attempts to isolate and characterize components of ground substance. It seems probable that all chondroitin sulfate-protein complexes contain a few keratosulfate chains linked to the protein core.

A glycoprotein characterized by a high content of sialic, aspartic, and glutamic acids has also been reported in ground substance of bone. Similar glycoproteins have been found in dentin and in glomerular basement membrane, and it has been found that they are covalently linked to collagen via a hydroxylysine residue. Whether a similar situation exists in bone is not yet known. Some investigators believe that highly charged glycoproteins and protein-polysaccharides play a role in the calcification mechanism.

Cellular Components of Bone

Three principal cells are identified with bone formation and remodeling. These are the osteoblast, osteocyte, and osteoclast. Similar cells are also identified with cartilage formation and are called chondroblasts, chondrocytes, and chondroclasts. Osteoblasts are considered matrix-building cells. There is also evidence that they play an important role in calcification. Osteocytes can, apparently, act both as bone-forming cells and as bone-destroying cells. Their role is less clear, since during most of their existence they appear to be relatively quiescent, like fibrocytes. Osteoclasts are primarily responsible for bone resorption at exposed surfaces and play an important role in remodeling and shaping of bone.

The origin of bone cells and their relationship to other connective tissue cells are still matters of controversy. Most of the classification of cells and the resulting nomenclature is based on morphological considerations as determined by light microscopy. Cell morphology is a notoriously poor criterion for judging a cell's antecedents or its future activity. Morphology can be markedly influenced by physical and chemical environment in which a cell finds itself and by functional demands placed upon it.

Functionally, the osteoblast resembles the fibroblast. It synthesizes collagen, presumably by a process identical to that discussed in Chapter 4. It is thought that it also elaborates the glycoproteins and protein-polysaccharides. The principal functional difference between an osteoblast and a fibroblast is in the involvement of the osteoblast in the calcification process and in the fact that it appears to be under a dual hormonal control. These subjects will be elaborated upon later in this chapter.

As has been mentioned, the osteocyte is a relatively quiescent cell, and whether it is derived from a common precursor or whether it represents a resting stage of the osteoblast has not been definitely settled. It is usually associated with the Haversian system in compact bone, and the osteocyte can be seen to lie in a lacuna communicating with a Haversian canal through which it obtains its nourishment and oxygen supply. The fact that in new bone formation the osteoblast lays down the collagen matrix around it, and that it eventually lies in the lacuna of the Haversian system, strongly suggests that the osteocyte is merely a late functional form of the osteoblast.

The osteoclast is a multinuclear cell, usually found on the periphery of bone substance. It appears to be responsible for bone resorption. Presumably it elaborates a variety of enzymes, mostly proteases and hydrolases, including a collagenase. It also may be involved in decalcification, perhaps by lowering the pH locally.

In fracture repair, osteoblasts appear to be derived from cells of the cambium layer of periosteum and from endosteum. These cells have been termed osteoprogenitor cells, fibroblasts, and undifferentiated mesenchymal cells. The name is probably not important. The important thing to recognize is that periosteum and endosteum contain cells that give rise to osteoblasts. Surgical manipulation of bone, therefore, must always include careful protection of these valuable membranes or healing will be delayed or prevented.

The work of several investigators has shown that mesenchymal cells from so-called somatic connective tissue can be induced by appropriate stimuli to differentiate into osteoblasts. Thus, this type of differentiation is not unique to cells of periosteum.

Studies on differentiation of mesenchymal cells revealed that a culture of chick embryonic tibia cells subjected to various mechanical forces and oxygen tensions could be transformed into osteoblasts and would produce bone directly. If cells were subjected to compression at low oxygen tensions, they were transformed into chondroblasts and cartilage was formed. If cells were given adequate oxygen, but were put under tension rather than compression, they become fibroblasts and produced dense fibrous tissue which did not form either bone or cartilage.

These observations are very important in explaining what happens during the healing of a fracture and may account, *partly*, for failures of bony union in some patients. In healing of a fracture, as in other wounds, the proliferating cells — osteoblasts in the case of bone — migrate ahead of new capillaries. Thus the leading cells are in an area of low oxygen tension and tend to lay down cartilage. As the blood supply catches up to the cartilaginous area, oxygen tension increases and conversion of cartilage to osteoid and eventually to bone occurs.

Inorganic Constituents of Bone

Originally it was thought that the principal inorganic salt in bone was a form of calcium phosphate. When its crystalline nature was recognized, it became apparent that it was a form of apatite, hydroxyapatite, $Ca_{10}(PO_4)_6(OH)_2$. It has also been postulated that calcium carbonate may also be a mineral constituent. The possibility exists that carbonate ion can enter vacant positions in an incomplete crystal lattice in the hydroxyapatite crystal. It is known that fluoride, strontium, and certain other ions can do this, either by entering a vacant position or, more frequently, by exchange reactions.

Mineral crystals are minute tablets, 25 to 50 Å thick, about 400 Å long and nearly as wide. The shape and extremely small size of these crystals makes the specific surface area of bone mineral enormous, in the neighborhood of 100 square meters per gram. Because of crystal lattice imperfections and large surface area, the chemical behavior of bone mineral is dominated by surface phenomena, such as ion exchange.

Bone crystals form in a very definite relationship to collagen fibrils. The long axis of the crystal is oriented parallel to the longitudinal axis of the fiber. Crystals are seen to start their formation at a particular band in the collagen fibril. As the crystal grows, these relationships become obscured. Two explanations have been offered for this rather specific relationship between bone crystal and collagen fiber. One is that crystal formation is initiated in a region of specific charge on the collagen fiber and is held there by electrostatic forces. The other is that a direct physical bond exists between initial apatite crystallites and

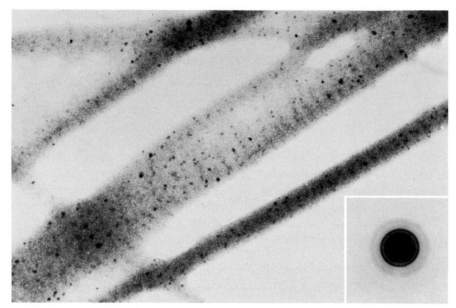

Figure 11–3. Electron micrograph of an unstained, unshadowed preparation of an early stage of *in vitro* calcification of collagen fibrils. Note regular and periodic distribution of crystals along the collagen-fibril axis corresponding to the intraperiod fine structure of fibrils and occurring primarily once per axial period. In the lower righthand corner is a selected-area electron-diffraction pattern of a preparation similar to the one shown in the electron micrograph, showing characteristic apatite reflections. There is no evidence of preferred crystal orientation, even though the diffraction pattern was obtained from an area where fibrils were well oriented. × 80,000. (Reproduced by permission from M. J. Glimcher, Rev. Mod. Physics *31*:359, 1959.)

collagen fibers. This last concept is supported by the results of electron paramagnetic resonance studies.

VASCULAR RESPONSE TO INJURY

When a bone is fractured, small blood vessels traversing the area of the fracture are severed. This has important consequences on the subsequent course of healing. As with any other form of trauma which interrupts the integrity of the vascular system, hemorrhage into surrounding tissue occurs and a blood clot is formed. Depending on the nature and extent of trauma that produced the fracture, adjacent soft tissues may be damaged and also contribute to hemorrhage and clot formation.

The blood supply to osteocytes in the Haversian system in cortical bone, as we mentioned previously, is derived from the small vessels traversing the Haversian canal. These anastomose with other similar vessels. If the fracture is proximal to this anastomosis, the cell will soon die since the dense tissue surrounding the cell does not permit nourishment by diffusion. Thus, there is a zone of necrotic bone at the fracture site.

It has been generally assumed that blood clot formed at the fracture site is organized and removed in a manner similar to clots in other tissues. It has been shown, however, that the clot is not invaded by granulation tissue or callus, but advancing callus pushes the clot ahead of it. If the clot cannot be pushed into marrow or surrounding soft tissue where fibrinolysis and phagocytosis can remove it, it appears to interfere with healing. Whether the clot always behaves this way has been questioned. Some believe that enzymatic and phagocytic activity removes the clot early in healing, but that in fractures in which absolute immobility is difficult to achieve, as in ribs, slight movement may reopen delicate vascular channels, leading to continued clot formation.

About two-thirds of the blood supply of cortical bone is derived from vessels in the nutrient cavity and about one-third from vessels traversing periosteum. Following a fracture, the existing arterial and arteriolar channels open up throughout injured bone. The new periosteal and endosteal bone that begins to appear three to four days after the fracture is highly vascularized. Most of the blood supply for revascularization of devitalized bone comes from the medullary circulation.

In long bones such as the femur, the periosteal vascular system is mostly efferent; that is, vessels in the outer cortex and periosteum are predominantly capillaries and venules. Thus it has been observed that after medullary reaming and tight nailing, only the outermost cortex remains viable around the anterior and lateral aspects of the femoral diaphysis. The posterior portion of the cortex is supplied with arterioles from posterior fascial attachments and thus will remain viable, unless trauma has severed these vascular connections.

In a fracture with concomitant soft tissue injury, the external callus that forms derives much of its blood supply initially from vascular ingrowth from surrounding soft tissue. This vascular system is not part of the normal osseous supply and can be considered only as a temporary vascular system. As healing and remodeling occur, this supply is lost and more and more of the vascular supply is derived from the afferent system of the medullary canal. This may be why one sometimes observes delay in revascularization of necrotic cortex at fracture ends following intramedullary nailing.

The major source of blood for uniting callus also appears to be the medullary cavity. This is anastomosed later with the lesser circulation coming from periosteum. In cases of delayed union, it appears that the periosteal circulation is the principal source of blood to the external callus. Initially, the external callus receives all of its blood supply from periosteal vessels but, in normal healing, medullary vessels penetrate uniting callus and contribute substantially to the circulation of external callus.

As stated earlier, the healing of fractures duplicates in most essentials the morphological and biochemical events that occur during normal endochondral ossification at epiphyses of long bones during growth. Fractures involving the diaphysis of long bones heal both by the process of endochondral ossification and by intramembranous bone formation. The relative contributions of each to final repair appear to depend to a great extent on the presence or absence of an adequate blood supply. Thus, a brief discussion of vascular events occurring during normal bone growth at the epiphyseal plate can shed light on the less well studied events occurring during fracture repair.

The vessels supplying the epiphyseal side of growing cartilage differ in origin, size, and distribution from those of the metaphyseal side. They cover the entire area under the bony plate separating the epiphysis from the growth cartilage. Interruption of this blood supply by vascular section or compression will inhibit further differentiation and dissolution of chondrocytes and halt calcification of cartilage. The same phenomenon is seen in rickets, and this suggests that inhibition of calcification is the causative factor in stopping chondrocyte differentiation and death, and that intact blood supply is essential to calcification.

Capillaries invading cartilage are possibly concerned with calcification and, subsequently, resorption of cartilage. It appears that the ends of many of the invading capillaries are open. As they invade chondrocyte capsules, blood elements are seen to be lying free in the capsule. These capillaries penetrate into each column of hypertrophied cartilage and simultaneously the matrix between cell columns begins to calcify. As soon as blood supply to this area is well established, a partial decalcification of matrix occurs, new matrix is laid down, and ossification proceeds. The important point to observe at this stage is the direct influence of the newly forming microcirculation on calcification of cartilage and its conversion to bony tissue.

Although no true epiphyseal plate is involved in fracture repair, the developing blood supply in the fracture callus is important in determining the kind of healing that takes place. Where a good blood supply already exists, as at the endosteal surface and at the periosteal collar adjacent to the fracture site, osteogenic cells differentiate immediately to osteoblasts and form bone directly. However, as the periosteal collar of callus expands and advances away from its blood supply, osteogenic cells differentiate into chondroblasts and form cartilage. As capillaries invade this tissue, cartilage first calcifies, and then is converted to bone. As mentioned previously, it is well established that low oxygen tension favors cartilage formation and higher oxygen tensions favor bone formation. Even after osteogenic cells have differentiated into osteoblasts, their functional activity is influenced by oxygen tension. In cultures of osteoblasts at low oxygen tension, collagen is synthesized faster than degradation occurs. However, at oxygen tensions of 50 per cent the rates of synthesis and degradation are equal. This, of course, has an important bearing on bone remodeling, both during growth and during fracture healing.

From a very practical point of view, it is evident that the extent of damage to the vascular system in and around a fractured bone has an important bearing on the rate and character of healing. Furthermore, disturbance of newly forming vascular supply at the fracture site as a result of inadequate immobilization will have a profoundly adverse effect on the rate of bony union.

MORPHOLOGY OF REPAIR

Inflammation and edema are the immediate results of injury to any tissue, including bone. Within a very short time after fracture, mobilization and proliferation of fibroblasts occurs in the outer layer of periosteum, and also perhaps in neighboring connective tissue. Simultaneously osteogenic cells in the cambium layer of periosteum commence to migrate and proliferate. Similar cell migration and proliferation occur on the bony surface in the marrow cavity. There is a

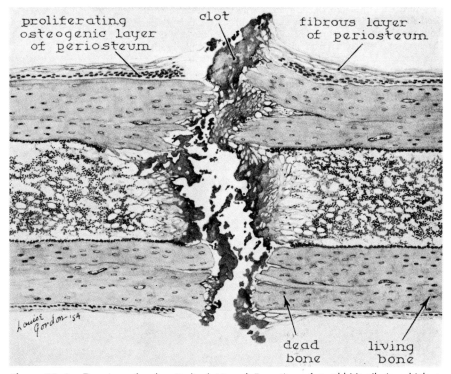

Figure 11–4. Drawing of a longitudinal H and E section of a rabbit's rib in which a fracture had been healing for 48 hours. (Reproduced by permission from A. W. Ham and W. R. Harris, in *Biochemistry and Physiology of Bone*, edited by G. Bourne, New York, Academic Press, 1956.)

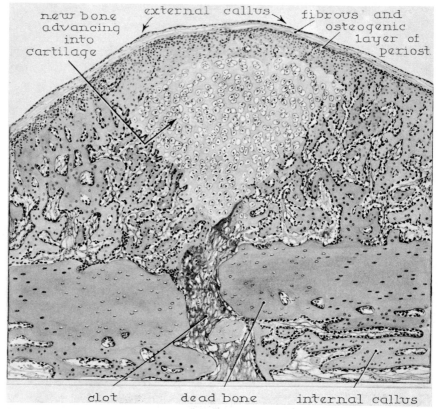

Figure 11–5. Drawing of part of a longitudinal H and E section of a rabbit's rib in which a fracture had been healing for two weeks. (Reproduced by permission from A. W. Ham and W. R. Harris, in *Biochemistry and Physiology of Bone,* edited by G. Bourne, New York, Academic Press, 1956.)

dispute as to whether osteogenic cells are derived from endosteum or represent migrating osteoblasts that line spaces in the spongy bone at ends of the shaft.

These proliferating cells, as they advance toward the area of injury, lay down a fibrous matrix of collagen. This newly formed tissue is termed callus. It originates not at the fracture line but at a short distance distal and proximal to it in relatively undamaged periosteum and endosteum. Within a few days, a collar of callus tissue is formed around each bone fragment and it lifts the overlying fibrous layer of periosteum. Usually, osteogenic cells closest to the bone surface modulate directly into osteoblasts and lay down a collagen matrix which quickly calcifies into bone. This initial layer is usually thin and evenly distributed, but as callus grows, ossification occurs in trabeculae with vascular spaces between them. This is so-called spongy bone.

As proliferating osteogenic cells move farther from an established blood supply, they modulate, not into osteoblasts, but into chondroblasts. These begin to form cartilage. Thus, periosteal callus is formed into three merging parts: the innermost is new trabecular bone, the intermediate zone is composed of cartilage, and the outermost consists of rapidly proliferating osteogenic cells covered by a fibrous layer

As fibrocartilaginous callus bridges the fracture site, the peripheral and distal edges of cartilage are gradually replaced by new spongy or trabecular bone.

At the same time external callus is being formed, a similar process is occurring in the marrow cavity. Here fibrous tissue, which quickly calcifies, fills the marrow cavity at the fracture site. This is formed from the endosteal layer proximal and distal to the fracture line. Because of good blood supply, cartilage formation seldom occurs and fibrous or spongy bone is formed directly.

As phagocytosis removes debris at the fracture site, dead bone at the fracture line is resorbed and new trabeculae develop in this region. Simultaneously, some of the trabeculae of internal and external callus are resorbed. Gradually, spaces in the trabeculae of bone bridging the fracture site are filled in by appositional growth, and cancellous or spongy bone is converted to compact bone indistinguishable from normal.

A prime example of healing of cancellous bone, as contrasted to that of compact bone, is afforded by events taking place in healing of a fracture of the neck of the femur. A large portion of the blood supply to the head of the femur is derived from medullary shaft via the major nutrient artery. Fracture at the neck may sever this blood supply and bone and marrow of the head may die rather quickly. Articular cartilage usually remains viable and it is believed that it derives its nourishment from synovial fluid.

If good apposition is obtained between fragments, osteogenic cells of endosteum and capillaries from marrow invade the necrotic head and replace dead bone. New trabeculae are formed. Under ideal circumstances, the head is replaced with new cancellous bone indistinguishable from old. Ideal healing, however, depends on accurate apposition with some compression and, above all, development of a good blood supply from the distal fragment. Such conditions are particularly difficult to obtain in the elderly, and this accounts for frequent failure to heal in fractures of the neck of the femur.

Parietal bones do not heal with formation of bulky callus as do other bones of the body. Even drill holes are frequently not closed by bony union, even though a small callus forms around the edges. Although parietal bone forms by intramembranous ossification, cartilage may form in the callus of repair. This is not commonly observed and may occur only when there is some interference with blood supply. One may speculate that different healing of parietal bone is due to the fact that compression at the defect cannot be obtained. Teleologically speaking, it is extremely fortunate that intramembranous bone in the facial skeleton does not heal by callus formation. Elective surgery such as rhinoplasty and mandibular recession would be unthinkable, and facial fractures would produce hideous deformities if facial bones healed in the same manner as long bones.

It is important to recognize that in some instances callus may be laid down at a fracture site, but because of a failure of bone induction or in the calcification mechanism, it does not calcify. This can happen, for instance, in animals deliberately placed on a low-calcium, low-phosphorus diet. On x-ray examination such fractures frequently give the appearance of nonunion. This is quite a different situation, however, from nonunion. The latter is a failure of matrix formation and is rare. Noncalcification is much more common and is usually due either to a metabolic abnormality or to some circulatory abnormality.

CALCIFICATION OF BONE

The mechanism by which bone matrix becomes mineralized has been the subject of much investigation and a large amount of theorizing. The precise mechanism is still not known, although some aspects seem to be established with reasonably certainty. The greatest obstacle that must be overcome in devising an acceptable mechanism of calcification is to explain why this process is confined to bone matrix and does not occur spontaneously in other connective tissues which, superficially at least, appear to be similar in composition to bone matrix.

Before it was recognized that the inorganic constituent of bone is composed of minute crystals of hydroxyapatite, it was supposed that the bone salt was formed by precipitation of $CaHPO_4$. A simple precipitation theory would not hold for formation of hydroxyapatite, however, since this would require simultaneous interaction of 18 ions, a highly improbable event.

The precipitation idea was replaced by the concept of crystal nucleation as the initial step, followed by crystal growth. The idea of crystal nucleation requires, however, some particular set of conditions or some particular site which brings calcium and phosphate ions into proper spatial arrangement so that an initial crystal lattice can be formed. The constituents of matrix and associated ground substance are logical choices in the search for initiators of nucleation. Observations on staining reactions, supposedly indicating the presence of mucopolysaccharides during bone formation, led some workers to postulate that protein-polysaccharide complexes might be involved in calcification. It was observed that just prior to calcification of cartilage, the concentration of protein-polysaccharides is high. As calcification proceeds, there is an apparent drop in their concentration, and more important perhaps, there appears to be a depolymerization of mucopolysaccharides. It was observed that calcium is strongly bound by highly charged protein-polysaccharides, but as they depolymerize the net charge drops. It was thought that this change in charge might release calcium ion, creating a high local concentration which would favor nucleation.

Many of the observations relative to changes in local concentrations of mucopolysaccharides are open to question. Relatively nonspecific staining reactions were used to make these observations, and the interpretation of variations in staining intensities or disappearance of metachromasia depends as much on the particular bias of the observer as upon demonstrable specific chemical changes. However, studies with ^{35}S tended to confirm at least the concentration changes of mucopolysaccharides that occur during calcification.

The fact that the solubility product, Ca $\times$ P, in serum has to be above a certain value for calcification to occur, and that calcification does not occur in soft tissues at a time when it is in active progress in bone and cartilage, suggests that some local factor is present in calcifiable matrix which is responsible for fixing the minimal solubility product, Ca $\times$ P, at which calcification would occur. Such a concept appears necessary, since serum Ca $\times$ P solubility product is the same in soft tissues as in bone. It was suggested that chondroitin sulfate might be important, particularly when complexed to protein. It had been observed that destruction or alteration of protein decreases the calcifiability of the matrix.

The observation that hydroxyapatite crystals appear to form on and within fibers of collagen matrix, that they appear to be oriented in a specific direction relative to the fiber axis, and that they appear to be associated, initially, with a particular portion of the collagen band pattern suggests strongly that collagen matrix is the nucleation site. It was suggested that this organic matrix binds either calcium or phosphate ions in the proper space relationships to form the hydroxyapatite crystal. It was further pointed out that serum is undersaturated with respect to $CaHPO_4 \cdot 2H_2O$, but is supersaturated with respect to hydroxyapatite; and, in the presence of a nucleation center, spontaneous crystal precipitation occurs. Thus, what is actually happening in bone formation is a phase change from a solution containing Ca^{++}, $HPO_4^{=}$, and a large number of other ions, to a solid crystalline state involving $Ca_{10}(PO_4)_6(OH)_2$ and possibly minor amounts of other closely related crystal forms. A phase diagram showing conditions for such a transition would be highly complex, indeed.

It was also suggested from physical-chemical studies that the presence of citrate, which is always found in bone, limits the size of crystals by chelation of excess calcium ions. Another limiting factor in crystal growth is the space available for the crystal and the dynamic state of the crystal surface, where ion exchange may be extremely active.

The development of the nucleation concept and observations on

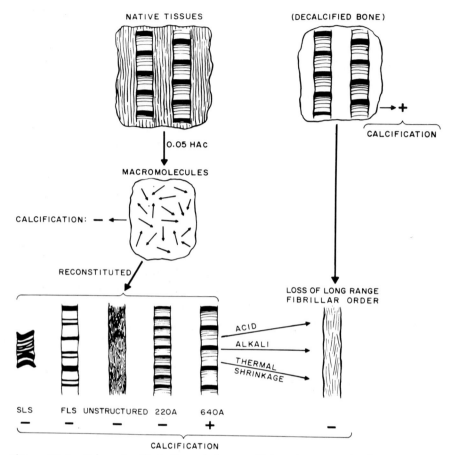

Figure 11–6. Schematic illustration of the specificity of macromolecular aggregation state of collagen in the *in vitro* nucleation of apatite crystals. Note that only collagen fibrils with the "native" 640 Å band pattern will calcify. (Reproduced by permission from M. J. Glimcher, in *Calcification in Biological Systems,* edited by R. F. Sognnaes. Copyright 1960 by the American Association for the Advancement of Science.)

the close and specific relationship of bone crystals to collagen fibers made it logical to assume that organic matrix of bone is intimately involved in calcification. Utilizing reconstituted collagen, it has been demonstrated that only fibers with the 640 Å periodicity are capable of being calcified. None of the other forms of collagen aggregation, the segment-long-spacing (SLS), fibrous-long-spacing (FLS), 220 Å, or amorphous forms, can be calcified. Thus, the spatial arrangement in the quarter-stagger, native form of collagen is essential for nucleation to occur. However, the native-type arrangement is not the sole determining factor since many fresh, undenatured collagen fibers with 640 Å periodicity fail to calcify until put into solution and reconstituted.

This suggests that failure to calcify may be due to the presence of some noncollagenous component that is removed in the process of being dissolved and reconstituted, or that calcifiable matrix has some subtle structural difference from noncalcifiable matrix.

One of the earliest theories regarding the mechanism of calcification involved the idea that a local increase in concentration of phosphate ions might be produced by hydrolysis of ester phosphates by a phosphatase. This theory foundered because of the low concentration of ester phosphates in body fluids. A brief revival of the theory was occasioned by the observation that hypertrophic cartilage cells at the epiphyseal zone contain great quantities of glycogen which appear to be utilized at about the time of calcification. This suggested that these cells supply both enzyme and substrate, hexosephosphate, needed for local liberation of phosphate ion. Unfortunately for this hypothesis, it was found that cartilage would calcify *in vitro* after all enzymes were destroyed.

The phosphatase theory was again revived when it was found that small amounts of pyrophosphate can be formed *in vitro* in rachitic cartilage if adenosine triphosphate is added. Such cartilage was shown to contain adenosine triphosphate pyrophosphatase.

More recently, it has been shown that in calcifying rat costal cartilage there is an increase in inorganic pyrophosphatase activity associated with uptake of ^{45}Ca by cartilage. Magnesium ion is essential for enzymatic activity and when enzymatic activity is greatest there is an accumulation of calcium, inorganic phosphate, and magnesium. Measurements of alkaline phosphatase activity did not show a direct relationship between this activity and onset of calcification.

Another calcification mechanism has been proposed on the basis of the finding that adenosine triphosphate (ATP) will bind calcium in stoichiometric proportions *in vitro*. The proposed mechanism involves formation of an ATP-calcium complex as the first step. In step 2, ATP-ase hydrolyzes the complex to form adenosine, sodium acid phosphate, and calcium acid pyrophosphate ($CaH_2P_2O_7$). This calcium salt undergoes further hydrolysis to hydroxyapatite and orthophosphoric acid. Orthophosphoric acid then reacts with adenosine to regenerate ATP. The evidence to support this mechanism is still largely circumstantial, but it does fit in with a number of concepts to be discussed in this chapter.

The fact that reconstituted collagen fibers appear to calcify readily seemed to argue against the existence of local factors, such as phosphatases, in calcifying cartilage or bone. However, the Ca × P product necessary for such *in vitro* calcification is very much higher than that at which calcification occurs *in vivo*. This, therefore, argued in favor of some booster mechanism. Such a mechanism would require energy and the most obvious choice of an energy-donating substance would be ATP.

Simultaneously with the search for local factors or booster mechanisms in calcification, other investigators were attempting to identify specific sites in matrix that could be shown to be involved in crystal nucleation. Identification of such a site and demonstration of the mode of binding of calcium or phosphate might suggest the nature of local factors controlling calcification.

A significant observation that opened up a fruitful line of inquiry into the site of nucleation was made in studies of decalcification of dentin (which resembles bone in many respects). It was observed that as decalcification proceeds, the number of free ϵ-amino groups, as determined by dinitrofluorobenzene, increases. The same kind of increase was observed in demineralization of ox bone. This immediately suggested that ϵ-amino groups of lysine and hydroxylysine in collagen matrix are in some way essential to the calcification mechanism. This observation was followed by a demonstration that either blocking ϵ-amino groups with dinitrofluorobenzene or esterification of carboxyl groups in dentin collagen prevents calcification of dentin. It was suggested, without proof, that in soft tissue collagens, these reactive sites are in some way blocked, and thus calcification is prevented. In bone, presumably, there is a local mechanism which either prevents such blocking or removes the blocking agents. This will be discussed in more detail after consideration of other experiments on the calcification mechanism.

The observation that blocking or inactivation of phosphatase in serum ultrafiltrates inhibits calcification in calcifiable collagen when the ultrafiltrate is added to the system again pointed to some involvement of phosphate esters in the nucleation mechanism. Extremely low concentrations of phosphate ester seemed to be inhibitory and this suggested that the ester might block nucleation centers. This would agree with the findings of older workers that pyrophosphates and ATP block calcification. It was postulated that *in vivo* the inhibitor, a polyphosphate present in plasma, prevents calcium phosphate nucleation, except in bone and ossifiable cartilage which contain enzymes that destroy polyphosphates.

These observations led several investigators to the idea that phosphate, rather than calcium, is the key ion in the nucleation mechanism. Although it might seem that these data indicated that phosphate might be transferred to a free amino group in collagen from ATP by a specific phosphatase, it has been pointed out that this might be an oversimplification of the true mechanism. However, these suggestions did serve to point out that bone cells, osteoblasts and osteocytes, and corresponding cartilage cells probably play an active role in calcification. These cells were shown to have an active aerobic glycolysis with release of ATP.

Purified collagens will bind 150 to 170 moles of phosphate per mole of collagen. Part of the bound phosphate seems to be incorporated as organic phosphate which appears to be bound not to an amino acid but to a sugar. Separation of α chains of phosphate-treated collagen reveals the $\alpha2$ chain to contain relatively more phosphate than the $\alpha1$ chains, and the phosphate-containing fraction may be a glycopeptide.

Calcification, however, can proceed normally in collagens which have been deaminated, but the presence of carboxyl groups is essential. It is argued, therefore, that calcium is the controlling ion in nucleation and not phosphate. Calcium binding by matrix is alleged by some investigators to be an important phase of the process. These workers argue that phosphate is bound to calcium and not to matrix, and that a conglomeration of such calcium phosphate-protein complexes are nucleation centers.

Most workers, but not all, have come to the conclusion that ϵ-amino groups are not involved in calcification, but that blocking them with bulky groups like dinitrofluorobenzene or carbobenzoxy chloride inhibits calcification because of steric hindrance of actual nucleation site. It becomes possible, in the light of what is now known about collagen structure, to suggest that the nucleation center resides in the monosaccharide or disaccharide attached to a hydroxylysine residue of collagen. Formation of a sugar phosphate at this point could readily be hindered by attaching a bulky group to the ϵ-amino group of hydroxylysine.

In opposition to the hypothesis that the nucleation center resides in the mono- or disaccharide side chains of collagen is the observation that type II collagen with a high content of mono- and disaccharides does not calcify. Furthermore, bone collagen, which has a higher number of hydroxylysine residues than most other soft tissue collagens, actually has a lower number of glycosylated hydroxylysine residues. It has recently been suggested that rather than acting as a nucleating site for mineralization, glycosylation of hydroxylysine residues inhibits mineralization by steric hindrance in "hole" regions of polymerized collagen. It is suggested that these "hole" regions are nucleation sites and that the presence of unglycosylated hydroxylysine may be the key factor in nucleation.

The fact that important intramolecular cross-links in bone collagen appear to be those involving hydroxylysine residues raises the question of whether such cross-links can serve as nucleation sites. This must await further study. It should be noted, however, that there is no indication that lathyritic bone collagen, in which cross-linking is inhibited, will not calcify normally. All of this suggests that perhaps the key factor in nucleation is the presence of the hydroxyl group of hydroxylysine in the "hole" region of bone collagen. Much more experimental work is needed before the precise nucleation site can be identified.

Very recently, an entirely new site for nucleation and subsequent calcification of bone and cartilage has been proposed. Discovery of the nature of "osmiophilic bodies" or "cytoplasmic fragments," seen in the extracellular space in calcifying bone and cartilage, as being membrane-bound extracellular particles, and recognition that the first signs of calcification occurred in or on these "matrix vesicles" opened an entirely new era in the study of calcification.

The origin of matrix vesicles is still a matter of dispute. These tiny (approximately 1000 Å) particles consist of a double-layered membrane with the electron microscopic appearance of a cell membrane surrounding a granular cytoplasmic material. Four possible origins of matrix vesicles have been investigated and the weight of the evidence favors formation by budding or detachment of elongated cellular processes derived from hypertrophic chondrocytes or, possibly, osteocytes. Other theories regarding their origin suggest that they may be extruded from cells as fully formed intracellular structures, that they may be assembled from fragments of disintegrating chondroblasts or, finally, that they may be formed by secretion of subunits from cells, which aggregate extracellularly.

Matrix vesicles have a high lipid content and contain a number of enzymes, notably ATPase, alkaline phosphatase, and pyrophosphatase. The principal lipid components that appear to be involved in some way with calcification are the phospholipids, particularly serine and inositol phospholipids.

It has been shown that the presence of matrix vesicles enhances precipitation of calcium phosphate. In the absence of matrix vesicles, a $Ca \times P_i$ product of 70 mg. per 100 ml. or higher is needed for precipitation. Addition of matrix vesicles to the calcifying medium reduces this product to 30 mg. per 100 ml.

Phosphatidylserine has a strong affinity for calcium in the presence of phosphate. Calcium thus accumulates either in the vesicle or on its membrane. A local increase in phosphate concentration within or on the vesicle is thought to be brought about by the actions of phosphatases. Although the substrate has not been defined, it is suggested that pyrophosphate may be broken down by pyrophosphatase, and this would provide substrate and remove the inhibiting influence of pyrophosphate. As the $Ca \times P$ product rises within the vesicle, calcium phosphate precipitation occurs, forming crystals which serve as a site for formation of hydroxyapatite. Exposure of hydroxyapatite crystals to surrounding matrix fluid then leads to crystal growth and further calcification.

Matrix vesicles are found predominantly in the longitudinal septa of growth cartilage at about the time calcification commences. They also are found in all calcifying tissue, including the aorta. They may be intimately associated with collagen matrix, and this is probably why it was long thought that collagen in some way acted as the nucleation site for hydroxyapatite formation. Collagen still may play a role, and much remains to be learned about the mechanism of bone formation. The discovery of matrix vesicles and the current work on their role in the process of bone formation have opened an exciting new horizon.

At this time it is difficult to estimate the significance of phosphate groups in relation to nucleating properties of collagen. The organic phosphate content of bone collagen has been reported to be from 0.5 to 1 mg. per mole of tropocollagen. However, the hexose content of most collagens, other than that of cornea or basement membrane, is also quite low. Thus, if phosphate is bound to hexose, the amount bound per tropocollagen molecule also would be quite low.

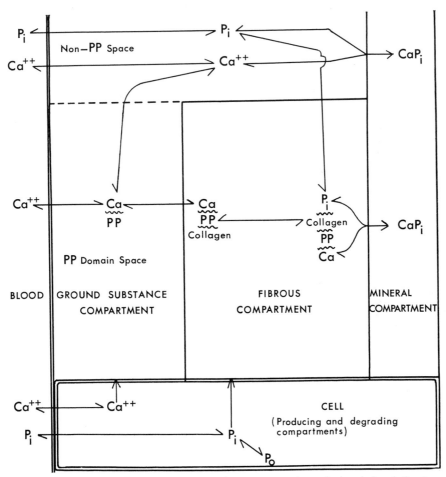

Figure 11–7. Suggested compartments and components in endochondral calcification. PP, protein polysaccharide; P_i, inorganic phosphate; P_0, organic phosphate; the wavy line represents an interaction of unspecified type. This scheme represents one theory, among many, of the manner in which bone matrix, ground substance, cells, and inorganic constituents may interact in osseous tissue to produce calcified bone. Note particularly the suggested interaction of protein polysaccharide with calcium and the further interaction of this complex with calcium, followed by binding of inorganic phosphate with collagen. This type of interaction may provide the "nucleation" center for formation of hydroxyapatite crystals. It is to be emphasized that this is purely hypothetical at this time. (Reproduced by permission from J. M. Bowness, Clin. Orthop. 59:233, 1968.)

The question of the role of protein polysaccharides in the calcification mechanism has also been a matter of considerable debate. One group has suggested that chondroitin sulfate inhibits calcification by limiting ion diffusion and by calcium binding. At the time of calcification, depolymerization of chondroitin sulfate occurs, lowering the binding capacity and increasing the diffusibility of ions. More recent evidence suggests that mucopolysaccharide in the ossifying zone closest to bone is of a higher molecular weight than that in the resting or transforming zone. Another group has proposed that chondroitin sulfate, together with collagen, is necessary for initiating calcification through formation of nucleation centers, where crystal growth could begin. Finally, another group has recently suggested that, in fact, chondroitin sulfate-protein complexes supply a critical grouping necessary for calcification, but that these exist in separate compartments and interact with calcium and phosphate in different ways. This is shown in Figure 11-7.

Thus, various theories for calcification, at the moment, suggest that phosphate ion is transferred from a phosphate ester, possibly ATP, by a phosphokinase to a hexose in a strategic location in collagen. Alternatively, the hydroxyapatite crystal may be formed by a two-step hydrolytic reaction involving ATP-calcium complexes. However, this latter theory leaves unexplained the close and specific association of hydroxyapatite and collagen fibrils. Phosphate ester, and probably the enzyme, may be produced locally by osteoblasts and chondroblasts. Calcification is hindered or promoted by mucopolysaccharides, and, in fact, these may interact with inorganic constituents in different ways according to the particular compartment being observed. Polyphosphates in tissue fluids may also inhibit calcification, and bone cells produce phosphatases to neutralize the inhibitor.

It is likely that calcium binding to protein also must occur for nucleation to ensue. However, it is more likely that a particular steric configuration must exist between bound calcium and bound phosphate for the crystal lattice to form. Subsequent crystal growth occurs in the same manner as crystal growth elsewhere.

It can be seen that much more work must be done before we can obtain a complete understanding of the complex process of calcification.

REMODELING OF FRACTURE CALLUS

Internal and external callus that forms during repair of a fracture is qualitatively and quantitatively different from bone originally present. Qualitatively, it is a highly vascular, trabeculated, spongy bone, whereas if the fracture was in a long bone shaft, the original bone was dense, relatively avascular, compact bone. Quantitatively, there is a great overproduction of calcified tissue, particularly around the external surfaces of the fracture site, but within the marrow cavity the internal callus may also fill the marrow lumen.

When callus is well formed, a process of remodeling occurs which eventually results in its replacement by dense compact bone and the removal of excessive external and internal overgrowth. If the alignment of bone fragments is done accurately, and the position maintained by adequate splinting, the remodeling process will eventually contour the bone at the fracture site so that it may be difficult to recognize where the fracture occurred. If there is displacement or misalignment of fragments, remodeling will produce a smooth contour, albeit a crooked one, best adapted to unite misaligned fragments.

The process of remodeling involves both synthesis and degradation of bony tissue. Since the mechanism of synthesis has already been discussed, our emphasis here will be on bone resorption.

It has been recognized for more than a century that the process of bone resorption, whether it is that which results from various diseases or that with which we are concerned in fracture healing, is closely associated with certain large, destructive, multinucleated cells termed osteoclasts. These are typically motile cells and exhibit ruffled membranes which are associated with cell movement. Like most motile cells, their shape is quite variable and tends to conform to environmental factors. Their most characteristic feature is the several nuclei they contain, the number varying from three to as many as 100, the average being about 30. The extensive cytoplasm shows a striated border, particularly where the cell membrane is in close apposition to bone.

The osteoclasts can be seen frequently wrapped around a bone spicule, or it may be flattened out against a bone surface or occupy an erosion pit. These pits, or lacunae, termed Howship erosion pits after the man who first described them, are characteristic findings on the surface of absorbing bone. When new bone is laid down on a surface which has undergone partial absorption, a scalloped line, or seam, persists, marking the boundary between old and new bone. That the process of absorption and new bone formation is a continuing one throughout growth is evidenced by the many scalloped seams seen in normal adult bone.

The osteoclasts appear to phagocytize bone mineral. Matrix is removed by enzymatic action. A specific collagenase has been demonstrated in resorbing bone by several investigators. Remodeling of fracture callus involves simultaneous dissolution of collagenous matrix by enzymatic attack with a specific collagenase elaborated by osteoclasts, and possibly also by osteocytes, and phagocytosis of bone crystals by osteoclasts. New bone formation occurs in the trabeculated area between bone fragments, leading to a change from cancellous to compact bone and to a contouring at the fracture site which restores, as nearly as alignment permits, the original contour of the bone.

HUMORAL CONTROL OF BONE METABOLISM

It was mentioned at the beginning of this chapter that bone, in contradistinction to other connective tissues, except that of uterus, is directly under the influences of certain hormones. This is not to say that other connective tissues do not respond to changes in the level of various hormones; they do, and bone also responds similarly to these hormones. However, hormones directly involved in bone metabolism exert the primary and main effect on bone tissue and have little or no action on other connective tissues.

Parathyroid Hormone

That the parathyroid glands are primarily concerned with bone resorption and that excessive secretion of the parathyroid glands produces hypercalcemia, the excess calcium being derived from bones, has been known for many years. The mechanism by which this effect is brought about was not thoroughly explored until relatively recently. It has been shown that parathyroid hormone has an immediate and direct effect on those osteoclasts already present in bone. An injection of parathyroid hormone causes a stimulus of RNA synthesis in osteoclasts within one and a half hours, followed by a rise in cytoplasmic RNA production at about 7 to 12 hours after the injection. Increase in RNA production is accompanied by increased protein and mucoprotein synthesis. These events parallel the rise in serum calcium concentrations. About 24 hours after injection of parathyroid hormone the number of osteoblasts increases, but this can be considered as secondary to the initial cellular stimulation caused by parathyroid hormone.

The observations just mentioned indicate that the site of parathyroid action is within the cell. However, it is not at all established that only the osteoclast is the target. In fact, much evidence is available that all bone cells are affected to a greater or lesser extent by major variations in parathyroid gland activity. When excess parathyroid hormone is given, collagen synthesis is depressed temporarily, and collagen degradation is decreased. The depression of collagen synthesis may not, however, be due to a direct action of parathyroid hormone on osteoblastic cells, since neutral salt extracts of bone from parathyroid-treated animals stimulate hexosamine synthesis and depress collagen synthesis in bone fragments from normal rats. In other words, the effect on osteoblasts may be mediated through a negative feedback mechanism.

The effect of parathyroid hormone in depressing collagen synthesis by the osteoblast is only temporary. Even while collagen matrix destruction is proceeding at an increased rate under the influence of parathyroid hormone, collagen synthesis also begins to increase. These effects can be well demonstrated by pulse labeling with radioactive proline.

Hydroxyproline-containing peptides are normally found in urine. It was thought that, since bone is the most metabolically active connective tissue, this excretion of hydroxyproline peptides represented a measure of collagen synthesis. Radioactive tracer studies have shown, however, that urinary hydroxyproline is derived from insoluble collagen of bone and thus represents collagen catabolism. It has also been shown that hydroxyproline excretion increases following parathyroid administration, and that the level of excretion is dose-dependent.

Although the main action of parathyroid hormone is on bone, it also decreases renal tubular resorption of phosphorus and increases the resorption of calcium and magnesium. This accounts for differences in effects on serum calcium and serum phosphorus seen after parathyroid hormone administration.

Considerable evidence has been obtained showing that parathyroid hormone has an action on osteocytes as well as on osteoclasts. Under the stimulus of parathyroid hormone, these cells produce a perilacunar absorption. This is significant because osteocytes are typically located within the Haversian system, and this is where older bone would be broken down. As was mentioned, the increased amount of hydroxyproline excreted in urine has been shown to come from the older bone and not from recently synthesized matrix.

In summary, it would seem fair to say that parathyroid hormone has a direct effect on osteoclasts and osteocytes. It increases the number of osteoclasts and stimulates their remodeling actions. Similarly, the hormone also stimulates osteolysis by osteocytes deep in compact bone. It was formerly thought that only osteoclasts were involved in bone resorption, but good evidence now exists that such absorption occurs within lacunae of the Haversian system where only osteocytes exist. It can also be shown that these cells respond morphologically to parathyroid hormone. An indirect effect on osteoblasts is produced by parathyroid hormone; new synthesis of bone is depressed by high local concentrations of the products of bone destruction. This effect is only temporary and collagen synthesis eventually resumes in response to a demand for bone formation. However, with high levels of circulating parathyroid hormone, synthesis cannot keep up with destruction and a net loss of bone results.

Calcitonin

Since the discovery of a polypeptide in the secretion of the thyroid gland that reduces serum calcium levels, originally called thyrocalcitonin but now referred to simply as calcitonin, its effects on bone metabolism have been under intensive study. Most of the studies on this hormone have been designed to show its antagonistic action to the effects of parathyroid hormone. For instance, adequate dosage with calcitonin will inhibit bone resorption induced by parathyroid hormone. However, calcitonin will decrease serum calcium levels in parathyroidectomized rats and this, of course, suggests that calcitonin is not just a simple competitor of parathyroid hormone, but probably acts directly on the cellular mechanism of resorption.

Calcitonin will also decrease urinary excretion of hydroxyproline. Since it has been shown that the major portion of urinary hydroxyproline is derived from lysis of mature bone matrix, this is further evidence of an action on cells involved in bone destruction. It has also been shown that calcitonin increases production of both cancellous and compact bone and that there is a direct dose-response ratio between total dose of calcitonin and amount of new bone formation. Tracer studies have shown that the effect of calcitonin on resorption is greatest for old bone. Thus, the evidence points to a common site for parathyroid and calcitonin action; however, it does not necessarily mean that there is a direct antagonism.

Our knowledge of the precise mechanism of calcitonin action is far from complete. However, the finding of two hormones acting specifically on the same target organ in an opposite fashion argues strongly that subtle balances between them could provide an ideal regulatory mechanism. It also suggests that manipulation of this balance might be a useful means of increasing the rate and extent of bone repair, particularly in those instances in which bony union is delayed.

NUTRITIONAL CONTROL OF FRACTURE REPAIR

The deficiency disease rickets, due to an inadequate intake of vitamin D, has its principal effects on bone. Other nutritional disorders, too, are frequently associated with bone changes; this fact testifies to the high metabolic activity of this tissue, which is particularly striking when one considers the relative inertness of other connective tissue structures.

Vitamin A

Although the action of vitamin A is generally associated with epithelial tissues, it does have effects on bone. Severe vitamin A deficiency produces an apparent overgrowth, or thickening, of bone which is particularly noticeable in the calvaria. Conversely, severe hypervitaminosis A results in thinning of cortical bone to the point at which it cannot withstand normal mechanical stresses.

It has been reported, however, that low doses of vitamin A shorten the period of fracture healing by promoting cellular proliferation and matrix formation. The mechanism of action of vitamin A on bone is not understood, but it may induce mesenchymal cell differentiation, with a more marked effect on osteoclast differentiation in excessive doses.

Vitamin C

The role of vitamin C in hydroxylation of proline and lysine has been discussed in Chapter 4. It will be recalled that evidence suggests that the role of vitamin C is more important where the demand for new connective tissue is great and that other electron donors may be involved in normal growth. This is probably true in bone. Thus, the greatest requirement for vitamin C is during the process of bone repair; without it, matrix synthesis may not occur.

In any event, there is good evidence that bone repair will not occur in vitamin C deficiency and that it resumes promptly when this substance is supplied in adequate amounts.

Vitamin D

Vitamin D is absorbed from the intestine and transported to the liver where it undergoes hydroxylation in the 25-position, becoming 25-hydroxycholecalciferol (25-HCC). 25-HCC then circulates to the kidney where tubular cells hydroxylate the 1-position, forming 1,25-dihydroxycholecalciferol (1,25-DHCC), which is the active form of vitamin D. 1,25-DHCC enters brush-bordered intestinal epithelial cells and triggers nuclear DNA to initiate the synthesis of a calcium-binding protein. Calcium absorbed by these cells from the intestine is bound to this specific protein and the calcium is released into the portal circulation as ionic calcium. Thus, one of the major functions of vitamin D is to facilitate intestinal absorption of calcium.

That the effect of vitamin D on serum calcium levels may not be due solely to an action on intestinal absorption and renal excretion is suggested by the observation that bone from animals pretreated with vitamin D, when incubated in modified Krebs-Ringer media, maintained a significantly higher Ca^{++} and PO_4 concentration in surrounding fluid than did normal bone. It would appear that vitamin D affects bone cell metabolism by increasing the passive solubility of bone minerals through increased lactate production.

That an effect on bone cells is one of the mechanisms of vitamin D action is supported by the observation that actinomycin D will suppress the hypercalcemic effects of vitamin D as well as those of parathyroid hormone. However, the effect of actinomycin D is probably confined to suppression of synthesis of calcium-binding protein in intestinal epithelial cells. Excessive doses of vitamin D produce hypertrophy of osteoblasts with increases in Golgi apparatus and endoplasmic reticulum. It must be noted that these visible effects on bone cells are seen only with toxic doses of vitamin D, and thus there is some doubt as to whether these changes occur at all under physiological conditions.

Earlier in this chapter it was shown that bone cells produce citrate, this ion forming a nonionized complex with calcium. Excessive citrate production, therefore, lowers ionized calcium content of serum. This in turn creates a demand for ionic calcium, which is furnished by transfer of calcium from bone to tissue fluids, so that internal homeostasis is maintained.

Citrate has been shown to be derived as a by-product of the Krebs cycle. Vitamin D appears to stimulate conversion of pyruvate to oxaloacetate, which, in turn, is converted to citrate. Parathyroid hormone, on the other hand, interrupts the Krebs cycle by inhibiting conversion of isocitrate to oxalosuccinate, thus permitting citrate to accumulate. Thus, vitamin D, stimulating one portion of the Krebs cycle, and parathyroid hormone, inhibiting another part of the cycle, both produce the same end result, namely, an increase in citrate in extracellular fluid.

Even in severe calcium and vitamin D deficiency, administration of vitamin D alone will increase mobilization of calcium from bone to serum. Concomitantly there is a rapid rise in bone citrate and a much slower rise in serum citrate. This is additional evidence that vitamin D directly affects citrate metabolism in bone cells.

It would seem, therefore, that vitamin D has a threefold effect on calcium levels in serum. First, it increases active transport of calcium and phosphorus from intestine to blood. Second, it regulates movement of these ions across renal tubular epithelium. Finally, it increases citrate production in bone cells by stimulating conversion of pyruvate to oxaloacetate and its subsequent conversion to citrate in the Krebs cycle. Citrate chelates calcium and removes ionized calcium, promoting mobilization of this ion from bone. This last action of vitamin D can play a role in the remodeling phase of bone repair.

COMPLICATIONS IN BONE REPAIR

Earlier in this chapter, the effect of oxygen tension on the differentiation of bone cells was discussed. It was shown that low oxygen tensions favor ossification by the endochondral route, whereas high oxygen tensions favor direct ossification. It can be appreciated, therefore, that maintenance of an adequate blood supply in handling fractures is of great importance in determining the rate and outcome of the healing process, and that infection could be very influential in its effect on pH, oxygen delivery, and oxygen utilization.

Denervation

In severe injuries to the extremities, not only may fractures be present, but major nerves may be damaged or severed. The question arises: Is healing of a fracture influenced by its nerve supply? Bone atrophy has been observed in severe poliomyelitis and in lesions resulting in loss of innervation to a limb. How much of the bone atrophy is due to direct loss of nerve connections to bone and how much is secondary to muscle atrophy and disuse of the limb are difficult to assess.

Delayed union of tibial fractures in rats following partial sciatic resection has been reported. Osteoporosis was noted in denervated bone, but whether delayed healing was due to a direct effect on bone, or to an effect on its blood supply, or to loss of muscle tone around the fracture site was not determined. Other workers, using combined motor and sensory denervation produced by spinal root section, have concluded that denervation has little effect on normal bone growth. Sensory denervation alone appeared to have an adverse effect, but this was probably due to trauma of an anesthetic limb with intact motor innervation.

The apparent contradiction between effects of denervation by sciatic section and by spinal root section can probably be explained by the fact that spinal root section does not sever nerve pathways to blood vessels, whereas peripheral nerve section also denervates local blood vessels. It has been shown that peripheral nerve section affects appositional growth of bone rather than epiphyseal growth. This, of course, would be consonant with a decreased blood supply, since cortical bone is less richly endowed with vessels than the epiphyseal growth zone.

It can be concluded that slow and poor healing of fractures in some paralyzed limbs is due to alterations in vascular dynamics plus loss of muscle tone with its splinting and compressing force at the fracture line. It should be noted that healing of long bone fractures in patients with paraplegia and tetraplegia sometimes is remarkably efficient in spite of poor immobilization and obvious severe osteoporosis. There is no reliable or predictable correlation between nerve supply to an extremity and the rate of fracture healing in a long bone. Loss of sensation in a fractured limb, without loss of motor innervation, will usually not delay healing, but may lead to other complications secondary to the loss of sensation.

Compression

Although it has long been recognized that good apposition of bone fragments is necessary for optimal healing and that, if immobilization can be maintained, early weight bearing may also be beneficial, the exact role of compression in bone healing has not been fully explored.

Compressive forces of 12 to 18 pounds applied across the fracture line in the ulna of the dog have been reported to give optimal healing. Pressures of 30 pounds or more produced necrosis of the cortex. It will be recalled that tension on bone cell cultures resulted in production of fibrous tissue only. Whether this is the sole explanation for the occasional instance of fibrous union of fractures has not been proved. Probably other factors enter into the picture also. It has been suggested, however, that poor healing noted in bone defects in the skull may be due to a lack of compressive force.

The effect of compression, *per se*, on fracture healing is still unsettled. It is entirely possible that the only significant effect of compression is to provide firm interaction of bony spicules and thus increase immobilization of the fracture. There are also data which strongly suggest that, particularly during later stages of healing of a fracture, compression forces are extremely important in development and remodeling of regenerating bone. Piezoelectric effects, in particular, have been measured in bone, and these studies strongly suggest that the crystalline nature of bone is responsible for a sort of stress-transducer effect when bone is subjected to mechanical stress. Polarity is maintained and the amplitude of potential generated, as measured by current output, is roughly proportional to the degree of deflection under load. Many studies have shown that unidirectional currents of less strength can exert a significant biological effect. Polarization and alignment of collagen fibrils, for instance, are examples of such an effect. The possibility that the two basic components of bone (apatite and collagen) form multiple PN junctions which are exceedingly sensitive to minute amounts of stress is intriguing; the physical properties of bone appear ideally suited for such an effect. Bone definitely is a semiconductor and the stress sensitivity of multiple PN junctions is such that measurable electrical currents with potentials proportional to the magnitude of stress and polarity determined by the direction of stress are produced. Tropocollagen molecules in solution are oriented into linear parallel structures by application of electrical fields equivalent to those produced by bone under stress. It is not difficult to speculate, therefore, that regenerative growth during fracture healing of a long bone might be influenced, beneficially or harmfully, by stress-induced currents, perhaps controlled by a negative feedback system. A direct constant-current cathode will cause bone to form at a site remote from traumatized tibia in a rabbitt. The osteogenic response is dependent upon the amount of current delivered. Approximately 20 microamperes of current produces optimal osteogenesis. Excessive current or voltage produces osteonecrosis.

There is also no doubt that compression forces can exert a serious inhibitor effect on healing of bone. Even under the most ideal circumstances there is always some necrosis of important cells at the interface between fractured bone and hematoma. This may be nothing more than confirmation of the importance of periosteal and endosteal vessels including the potential osteogenic induction powers of blood vessel walls as postulated previously by Trueta. There is also resorption of apatite and measurable collagenolytic activity in this area. A gap will inevitably develop, therefore, between two fracture fragments, and gaps reduce significantly the effectiveness of any immobilization scheme. Too much compression of a fracture during the early period when collagen degradation processes are particularly prominent increases the ultimate size of a gap and thus reduces the effectiveness of immobilization and increases the amount of regeneration needed for solid union.

Realization that some compression definitely is beneficial — although how much and by what mechanism are still not clear — and that too much compression definitely is detrimental has been responsible for development and utilization of the basic engineering principle of stress loading in the form of slotted plates and intramedullary nails. The Eggers slotted plate, in particular, has been designed to maintain some compression or physical stress on an area of regenerating bone, but it also insures that the magnitude of stress is within physiological limits by allowing readjustment in response to changes such as hematoma, edema, bone necrosis, and callus development. Application of a walking cast at certain stages during the relatively slow healing of a tibial fracture is a clinical application of the principle of stress loading which often appears to produce a marked increase in the rate of healing. The use of screws, plates, and crossing Kirschner wires can have exactly the opposite effect. These appliances maintain the distance between grossly approximated bone fragments with unerring accuracy. Even though two bone ends may have been placed in what appeared to be perfect approximation at the time a mechanical fixative was inserted, subsequent reabsorption of bone and necrosis of cells at the interface may produce a gap that is rigidly maintained by the fixation device. This is particularly true in an arthrodesis when multiple-plane fixation is utilized. A single Kirschner wire, comparable to an Eggers plate or a Kuntscher nail, or two Kirschner wires running parallel are definitely superior to multiple Kirschner wires in several planes or screws or plates which prevent any compression effect from soft tissue wound contraction or other physiological changes during healing.

Infections

Although the development of antibiotics has modified treatment of osteomyelitis considerably during the past 20 years, the old adage — once osteomyelitis, always osteomyelitis — still has a great deal of practical significance for those who treat this condition in human beings. The problem, from a biological standpoint, is somewhat analogous to radiation necrosis in that the blood supply to the affected tissue is often not adequate to assure that normal defense mechanisms or processes of repair and regeneration can proceed to an orderly conclusion. Although many processes involved in chronic infection in bone have been studied and described extensively in the past and will not be repeated in this chapter, the contribution of soft tissue has not always been appreciated and does not appear prominently in descriptions of therapeutic principles or the analysis of failure of bone healing. This aspect of the pathophysiology of osteomyelitis is a product of modern biological investigation and is responsible for new approaches to the problem of bone infection — from both a preventive and a therapeutic standpoint.

Bone covered with normal periosteum has reasonable defense mechanisms against invading organisms. Bone only partially covered with periosteum because of surgical or traumatic damage is extremely susceptible to invading organisms. Part of the prevention of osteomyelitis is, therefore, the prevention of damage to periosteum. It is important to emphasize that this statement does not refer to the direct contribution of periosteum to bone healing. This is another subject which will be treated separately. In certain compound fractures such as those of the middle or lower third of tibia, however, there is a relatively high incidence of osteomyelitis and nonunion, and orthopedic practice in the past has been directed primarily toward preventing soft tissue infection by forcing the soft tissue wound to heal secondarily. This is usually accomplished by placing a pack of some description in the wound after it has been debrided. Gradually removing the pack allows the wound to heal secondarily from the bottom up. Immobilization is usually obtained by traction or a cast with a window, not by insertion of foreign materials through the fracture site. Such practice, although it entails a prolonged course of surgical management, is successful unless some complication involving periosteum occurs. If packing is too forceful or prolonged, so that adequate wound drainage does not occur, or if the pack or surgical manipulation physically damages periosteum, or if an extremely virulent organism is present, or if immobilization is not completely satisfactory, conservative management fails and chronic osteomyelitis and nonunion may develop. When this happens, and it still does happen in spite of the use of antibiotic therapy and skillful soft tissue management, one can only surmise that the treatment contributed to the complication and that periosteal complications were at least partially responsible. Such reasoning leads one to the conclusion that secondary healing of overlying soft tissue, particularly if the wound is in an area with diminished blood supply (naturally or because of trauma to blood vessels), is not the best approach to a problem in which preserving segmental blood supply and natural defense mechanisms is of critical importance. From a theoretical standpoint, successful wound closure by immediate surface restoration, so that healing will occur by primary intention, would offer the best possible insurance that a secondary complication in the periosteum would not occur. Although all the details of the preparation and exacting technique necessary to convert a badly contaminated or secondary healing wound into a surgically clean or primary healing wound will not be repeated here, there is probably no place in the practice of surgery where these principles are more essential than in managing a compound fracture of a long bone.

One reason why soft tissue wounds complicating fractures of the tibia have not been treated in the same way as soft tissue wounds elsewhere is that there is always a relative, and sometimes an actual, shortage of soft tissue. As was pointed out in Chapter 6 in the discussion of treatment of soft tissue wounds around the malleoli, the lower leg is an area where there is not 1 mm. of extra skin or subcutaneous tissue. When even a small amount of skin has been lost and edema of the leg is becoming extensive, it may be extremely difficult for a surgeon of average experience and training to perform an adequate debridement. To treat such a wound as a neoplasm and excise it completely, as was advocated for soft tissue wounds in areas such as the buttocks or thigh, is extremely difficult unless one has great confidence in his ability to shift local tissue or bring distant tissue into the defect which will be created. When faced at 3:30 A.M. with a patient who has other injuries requiring emergency treatment, the surgeon is much more apt to depend upon secondary healing following limited debridement and packing of the wound than to perform a radical debridement which will then require a complex shift of soft tissue to close the defect. Thus, if one depends upon normal physiological defense mechanisms in a secondary healing wound, deep infection in the soft tissue may be avoided unless a pack is inserted too vigorously. Wound closure will occur by contraction and epithelization which is, for the surgeon, a much easier method of obtaining a healed wound than a complicated shift of tissue which would be required if an extensive debridement had been conducted.

Such thinking does not always lead to uncomplicated fracture healing, for several reasons. One reason is that soft tissue techniques (even though generally regarded as conservative) which lead to healing by contracture and epithelization simply do not provide adequate coverage for a healing fracture. Another reason is that wounds healing by secondary intention and requiring continual attention may be very difficult to immobilize. Less than adequate immobilization is a contributory factor to inhibition of natural host defense mechanisms and possible development of osteomyelitis.

Surgical therapy of compound fractures based on modern wound-healing biology and directed primarily at protecting natural defense and regenerative potential of periosteum leads the surgeon to another approach in some patients. That such an approach is practical for the average surgeon practicing alone in hospital with average equipment is far from conclusive at this time, however. The reasoning behind the approach is biologically sound, and experimental results in animals strongly suggest that the hypothetical basis is sound. A few courageous surgeons who have utilized the experimental data in clinical practice are reporting results superior to those obtained by classic therapy in many patients. The plan encompasses all of the principles outlined in treatment of soft tissue wounds and is based upon two fundamental premises: that the biology of periosteal tissue is essential in prevention of osteomyelitis and that uncomplicated primary soft tissue healing and perfect reduction and immobilization of hard tissue are fundamental to preserving the normal structure and function of periosteum. Such reasoning leads one to the inescapable conclusion that open reduction, internal fixation, wide debridement, and primary closure of the soft tissue wound, regardless of what is required to accomplish this, provide ideal circumstances for uncomplicated healing and regeneration of soft and hard tissues.

The major weakness of this approach is that it may be very difficult to execute perfectly in a patient with multiple injuries or by a surgeon with average training and equipment. This, of course, argues strongly for continuing what may theoretically be second-best treatment because complications of inadequate primary closure and internal fixation may be horrendous compared to complications of more conservative therapy. Experimental and clinical evidence to date, however, does not indicate that there is a great risk of osteomyelitis when a well trained surgeon with modern equipment treats a lower leg wound by wide debridement, replacement of excised tissue with a local or distant flap, and perfect, internal reduction and fixation of the fracture. It does indicate that the incidence of osteomyelitis and nonunion of such bones as the tibia can be substantially reduced and that the procedure will provide an extraordinary saving of time and expense for the patient. Enough data to take a firm position on this approach are not available in human beings yet; such an approach certainly is not recommended for all patients with compound tibial fractures or for all surgeons or hospitals where they are treated. Application of the principles of the approach is fraught with hazards; the techniques for excising a large lower leg wound adequately and replacing soft tissue immediately are very demanding. Failure to execute these techniques properly will invariably result in enlargement of difficult wounds or increased susceptibility to infection because of inadequate soft tissue management. The ideas are biologically sound and may result in decided improvement in uncomplicated healing of complex, compound fractures, but it should be emphasized strongly that these ideas (like all ideas emanating from modern human biology) must be applied under carefully controlled and ideal conditions where the results can be assessed accurately. In spite of the limitations of the approach at the present time, there is reason to predict that the principles embodied in it may change surgical practice significantly as the age of surgical biology continues.

Biological principles of treatment of chronic osteomyelitis also entail preservation of natural defense mechanisms rather than use of external weapons to combat bacterial invasion. Of course, proper selection and introduction of adequate amounts of antibiotics are extremely important, and provision of adequate preliminary soft tissue drainage is fundamental in the treatment of these infections. Osteomyelitis is seldom cured by adequate soft tissue drainage and antibiotic therapy, however. Antibiotics cannot reach all of the organisms because of lack of perfusion, and soft tissue drainage exposes noninfected bone to the effects of drying and bacterial contamination. The result is usually a continued progression of osteomyelitis. Instability, if an ununited fracture also is present, adds to the progression of osteomyelitis, just as osteomyelitis exerts an inhibitory effect on healing of the fracture. In a stable bone, where failure of a fracture to heal is not a problem, biologically oriented surgeons have recently approached the problem of osteomyelitis by radically removing involved bone and immediately replacing soft tissue to protect the cut surface of freshly exposed bone. In an area of persistent osteomyelitis of the tibia, this might be accomplished by first saucerizing the wound in a conventional manner to establish adequate soft tissue drainage and remove sequestra. At the same time a delay procedure on a large cross-leg flap on the opposite extremity might be begun. After drainage has become minimal, new cultures are taken, sensitivity studies are performed, and the best antibiotic is administered in maximal dose and course. Shortly before completion of adequate antibiotic therapy, the patient is operated upon again in an attempt to excise radically all of the clinically infected bone without cutting through areas of natural defense activity. In effect, the zone of osteomyelitis and surrounding reaction is treated like a malignant tumor and is extirpated by a bloc dissection; as much tissue as necessary should be removed, but not enough to produce instability, if possible. Immediately the defect in soft tissue and bone is resurfaced with a local or distant flap so that all exposed bone is covered by full-thickness skin and subcutaneous fat set in to provide soft tissue coverage and wound healing by primary intention. Actually, a split-thickness skin graft may take on exposed bone under these conditions but take is uncertain and the type of coverage provided by a split-thickness skin graft is not as reliable as that with a full-thickness pedicle that includes a cushion of fat.

When osteomyelitis complicates an ununited fracture of the tibia, similar principles are called for, plus the addition of stability and bone induction. Both stability and bone induction can be obtained by utilizing a posterior approach (if the principal drainage in the soft tissue wound is anterior) and adding an autogenous cancellous bone graft from the ilium. Anterior drainage is not a contraindication to this procedure, although if soft tissue is deficient anteriorly, this should be corrected, even though the sinus is not closed completely, before bone grafting by a posterior approach is attempted. The results of treating osteomyelitis in human beings by radical excision, soft tissue replacement, and bone grafting, where necessary, are not known completely at this time. From a biological standpoint, however, the principles are sound and the first results reported are very encouraging, particularly those of treatment of persistent osteomyelitis in old patients. Results have shown that it is possible to eradicate the disease and obtain union by such an approach. The rate of success or failure and the long-term results are not available at this time, however. Undoubtedly, experienced surgeons, working under favorable conditions where as many factors as possible can be controlled and considered during analysis of results, will continue to evaluate these principles as they apply to treatment of fractures in human beings.

In developing the biological thesis for modern treatment for osteomyelitis, the tibia was used as an example of a well known site of persistent osteomyelitis and nonunion of fractures. The tibial area is also an area where soft tissue management and replacement often are beyond the capabilities of the surgeon. It is a perfect example, therefore, of a problem in which modern biological knowledge and interdisciplinary technical skill can improve clinical results over those obtained by classic techniques which have dominated thinking and management for so many years. The same principles are adaptable, usually more simply, to other areas. A word of caution should be introduced, however; the radical approach to osteomyelitis cannot be applied in all bones, and it is strongly contraindicated in the hand and face. Osteomyelitis in membranous bone of the facial skeleton or in the small cancellous bones of the hand is a different problem from osteomyelitis in compact bone of the tibia or femur. Persistent osteomyelitis in bones of the hand is rare (and was rare even in preantibiotic days), and adequate soft tissue drainage to permit natural sequestrectomy, or simply lifting out a piece of naturally sequestered bone, is all that is usually required in the rare cases of osteomyelitis of carpal or phalangeal bones. As described in detail in the discussion of management of osteomyelitis of the mandible, it is often preferable to permit gradual fibrous replacement of an infected mandible rather than to excise radically a significant portion of that bone. Midfacial bones usually will sequestrate rapidly when infected. Only exposed bone needs to be mechanically debrided, except under unusual circumstances.

Chronic osteomyelitis and chondritis of the sternum, costal cartilages, and anterior ribs is an extremely serious condition which occurs most frequently after external fixation of a flail chest wall and may defy treatment by soft tissue drainage and debridement of bone and cartilage. In this area the principles of protecting exposed bone and periosteum by causing primary soft tissue healing to occur as an adjuvant to radical excision of affected bone can be utilized in the following way. Preliminary incisions over the ribs several inches lateral to the infected bone and cartilage (including the most lateral extent of soft tissue recesses and sinuses) are made for the purpose of excising approximately 2 inches of normal rib. After segments of the ribs have been excised, the soft tissue wounds are sutured and allowed to heal by primary intention. Only after these wounds have healed, and the infected bone and cartilage are isolated from remaining rib by the healed soft tissue, are infected cartilage and bone in the center of the thorax excised. The wound of excision thus does not expose the cut end of noninfected ribs and, if all of the infected bone and cartilage can be removed without exposure of uninvolved bone, soft tissue healing will occur by secondary intention.

Successful treatment of trophic ulcers that have infected bone in the depth of the wound also is dependent upon radical excision of bone and involved soft tissue followed by immediate coverage of exposed uninfected bone with a large rotation flap of full-thickness skin and fat. The reason these principles, long recognized as being necessary for successful closure of large defects complicated by persistent osteomyelitis in the axial skeleton, have not been applied to the lower extremity is that blood supply is less profuse, technical execution is more demanding, and the problem of transplanting soft tissue is so complex that it has been avoided even though basic biological considerations strongly suggest that such factors cannot be ignored.

Nonunion

The principal causes of nonunion are inadequate reduction, especially when there is interposition of soft tissue; distraction of fragments because of too powerful traction, or inaccuracy of internal fixation; loss of bone; impairment of blood supply; infection; metabolic disturbances; local neoplasm; and improper immobilization.

Interposition of soft tissue usually can be corrected only by internal reduction. Application of too much traction usually can be corrected easily if the diagnosis is made promptly. Occasionally distraction of fragments goes unsuspected, as when a hand or arm is suspended from an overhead support immediately after open reduction of a fracture or an elective osteotomy. Hanging an upper extremity to an intravenous fluid pole or Bradford frame is not good practice for several reasons. In addition to the danger of distracting bone fragments, skin grafts can be displaced and edema increased by the constricting effect exerted by a dressing that is tight enough to support the arm without letting it slip out. This is particularly true for small children, in whom the dressing must bear, in addition to the normal weight of the arm,

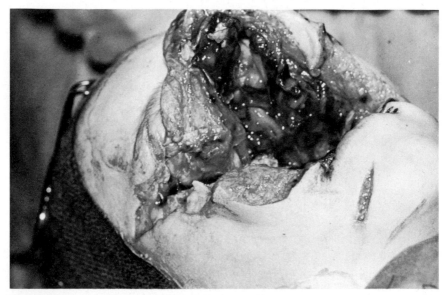

Figure 11–8. Severe injury of midface with multiple comminuted fractures of all facial bones. (Reproduced by permission from E. E. Peacock, Jr.: Amer. Surg. *24*:639, 1958.)

the child's muscular action against the restraining dressing and overhead support. Small children consciously and subconsciously attempt to pull away from an immovable restraint and very often succeed in pulling an extremity out of even the most accurately applied full-arm

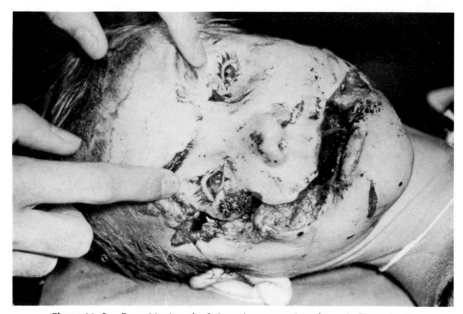

Figure 11–9.   Repositioning of soft tissue in same patient shown in Figure 11–8.

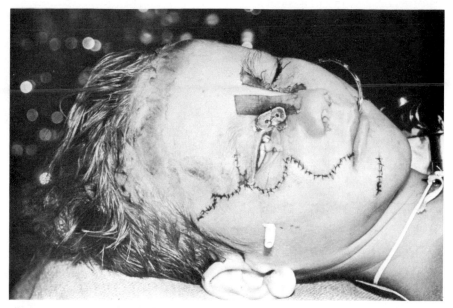

Figure 11–10. Use of multiple internal and external Kirschner wires to stabilize midfacial skeleton so that soft tissue can be draped over it and repaired accurately.

dressing or cast. Consequently, we never suspend an arm or hand from an overhead support. In adults, the extremity is elevated by placing the semiflexed elbow on pillows and stabilizing the arm or hand laterally against a padded solution pole or bed rail. Thus the elevated extremity

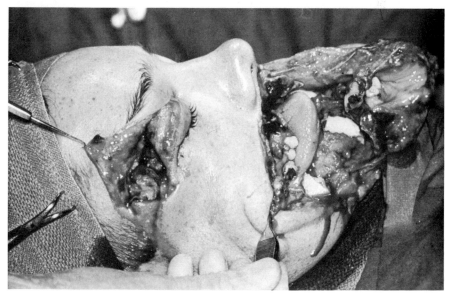

Figure 11–11. Severe injury of mandible with loss of 4 cm. of bone.

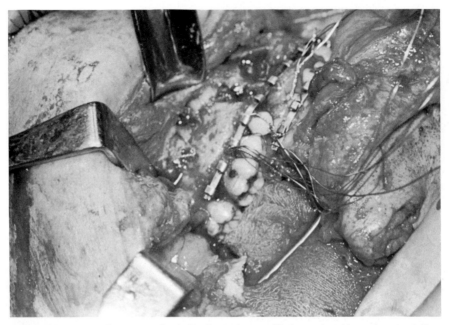

Figure 11–12. Replacement of missing bone in mandibular arch with an intramedullary Steinmann pin. Fixation of upper alveolar arch has been accomplished with an Erich arch bar. Occlusion of remaining teeth is being carried out by interdental wiring.

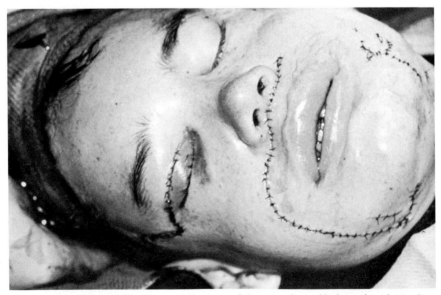

Figure 11–13. Closure of soft tissue following stabilization of mandibular arch with Kirschner wire.

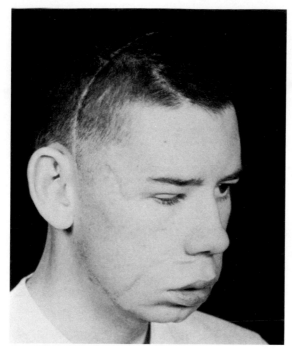

Figure 11–14. Appearance of patient following removal of Steinmann pin and insertion of cancellous bone graft in mandibular defect.

rests on its support—it does not hang from it. Children are kept in bed and the dressing or cast is not attached to any external object.

If single or parallel Kirschner wires and Steinmann pins are used instead of crossing wires, and if the stress-binding principle is applied by means of slotted plates and intramedullary nails, internal fixative devices will not hold fracture fragments distracted after inaccurate reduction or postreduction absorption of bone at the fracture site. Use of Kirschner wires has been particularly valuable in the hand and face. Numerous descriptions outlining important technical details involved in the use of these devices are available and should be studied carefully by restorative surgeons. Although Kirschner wires and Steinmann pins can be left protruding through skin in patients who are responsible enough to take care of them so that infection does not occur in the pin tracts, it is usually possible to cut off the Kirschner wires just beneath skin so that none of the wire is exposed. The ends of the wires can be located by flexing or extending a joint so that skin is tented up, and then the wire can be forced through skin far enough so that it can be grasped with pliers. In the hand, the use of Kirschner wires is aimed primarily at immobilizing just the fracture site and not adjacent joints. Modern fracture treatment, especially in the hand where malunion or nonunion is not nearly so serious as development of small joint

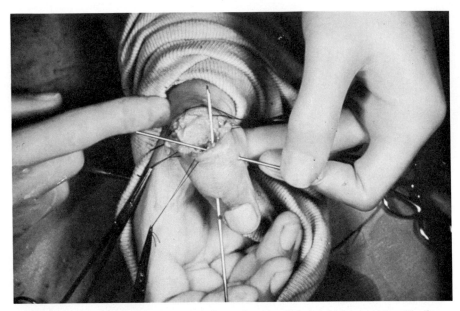

Figure 11–15. Fusion of metacarpophalangeal joint of thumb using crossing Kirschner wires to stabilize arthrodesis. Note that wires do not cross exactly at the bone interface. Off-center position of wires prevents rotation of fragments. When crossing Kirschner wires are used, bone segments must be in close apposition and cancellous bone chips should be used to pack the arthrodesis. When two wires are used, nonunion is more frequent than if a single wire stabilizes the bony union.

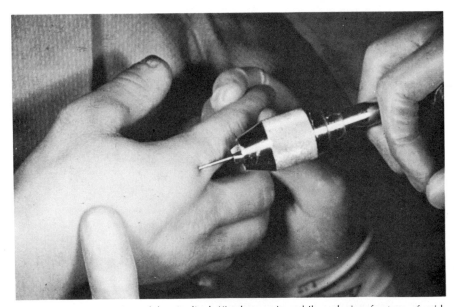

Figure 11–16. Insertion of longitudinal Kirschner wire while reducing fracture of mid-shaft of index metacarpal. (From E. E. Peacock, Jr., Surg. Clin. N. Amer. *33*:1297, 1953.)

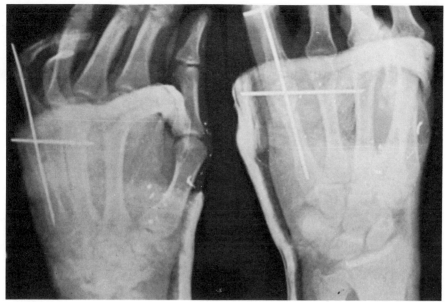

Figure 11–17. Longitudinal and transverse Kirschner wires used to stabilize a fracture of the small metacarpal. Rotatory deformities are less common in central rays than in marginal ones.

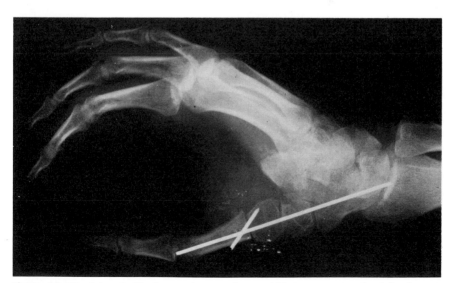

Figure 11–18. Internal Kirschner wires used to stabilize osteotomy site following re-construction of the thumb with a transplanted index finger. (Reproduced by permission from E. E. Peacock, Jr., in *Hand Surgery,* edited by J. E. Flynn. Copyright 1966, The Williams & Wilkins Co., Baltimore, Md. 21202, U.S.A.)

stiffness, has as its objective stabilizing the fracture while still maintaining active and passive motion in adjacent small joints. Because there is little in the way of effective treatment for patients with severe stiffness of proximal interphalangeal joints (the most important joints in the hand), preservation of motion is the key to a successful result.

Joint Stiffness

In many respects development of joint stiffness following immobilization is a biological problem closely related to wound healing. Recent studies on the fundamental pathological processes involved in this problem have shown that such basic wound healing mechanisms as collagen synthesis, collagen degradation, and rapid remodeling of mature collagenous tissue in joint capsules and collateral ligaments are the fundamental steps in development of a stiff joint. In the case of proximal interphalangeal joints in the hand, new collagen synthesis on the lateral side of the head of the phalanx prevents tangential movement of the collateral ligament over the head of the articular surface. It should be emphasized that proximal interphalangeal joints are simple diarthrodial joints and that collateral ligaments arise and insert from the axis of rotation of both phalanges participating in joint motion. This arrangement is quite different from that in metacarpophalangeal

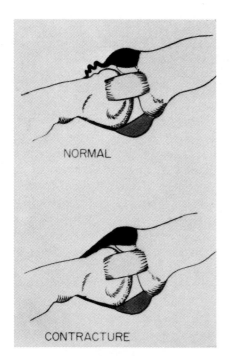

NORMAL

CONTRACTURE

Figure 11–19. Diagram of changes in dorsal capsule of an interphalangeal joint following development of an extension contracture. (Reproduced by permission from E. E. Peacock, Jr., Ann. Surg. *164*:1, 1966.)

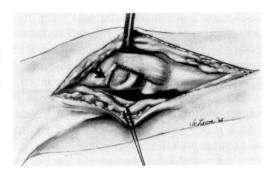

Figure 11–20. Arrow points to site where new collagen synthesis fixes collateral ligaments so that tangential movement across the lateral surface of the proximal phalanx is impossible. (Reproduced by permission from E. E. Peacock, Jr., Ann. Surg. 164:1, 1966.)

joints where collateral ligaments arise from a point dorsal to the axis of rotation on the metacarpal heads and insert inferior to the axis of rotation on the proximal phalanx. Such an arrangement in metacarpophalangeal joints provides lateral instability during extension of the joint and lateral stability during flexion.

Proximal interphalangeal joints have equal lateral stability regardless of the position of the joint. This is possible only if collateral ligaments arise and insert from the axis of rotation of both bones. It also means that flexion and extension are dependent upon some tangential movement of the collateral ligament across the lateral surface of the phalanges. It is at this critical point that collagen synthesis can bind the collateral ligament to the phalanx and restrict flexion and extension of the joint. Although most experienced hand surgeons strongly recommend that excision of collateral ligaments not be performed on proximal interphalangeal joints in human beings because of the danger of producing severe lateral instability, it is possible to excise them if the remaining retinacular structures such as Landsmere's ligament and the lateral bands of the extensor mechanism are carefully preserved.

Understanding the fundamental biology of production of joint stiffness makes it unnecessary to excise collateral ligaments of simple diarthrodial joints; only newly synthesized collagen adjacent to the insertion of the collateral ligament and the phalanx need be excised if adequate volar or dorsal capsulotomy also is performed.

The major restricting influence in a joint which has become stiff following immobilization relates to remodeling of the dorsal or volar capsule. A relatively wide excursion of one bone over the surface of the other is required for normal range of motion in the proximal interphalangeal joint. Such an excursion requires redundant volar and dorsal capsules to accommodate the relatively wide amplitude of motion of joint surfaces. When the joint is in extension, the dorsal capsule is pleated in loose folds; the same is true of the volar capsule when the joint is in flexion. If the joint remains in either extreme flexion or extension for longer than seven to ten days, collagenolytic activity results in absorption of excess connective tissue in the pleated capsule, and

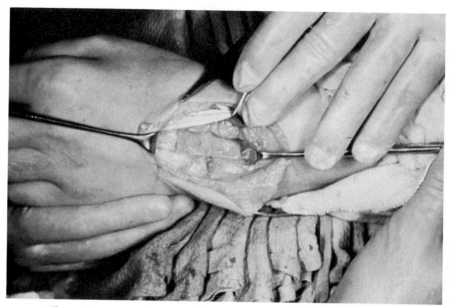

Figure 11–23.   Bone graft shown in Figure 11–15 crossing radiocarpal joint.

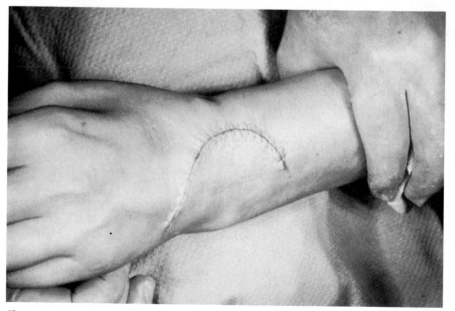

Figure 11–24.   Closure of wrist fusion wound with a continuous wire which can remain for several months.

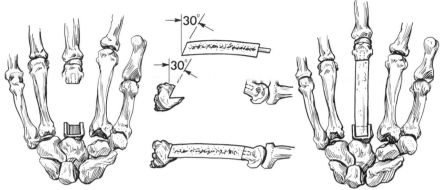

Figure 11–25. Architectural design of metacarpal bone graft according to method of J. W. Littler.

sufficient to polarize cells and collagen and also is adequate to induce cells to differentiate along specialized lines.

Although cancellous bone seems to have the most certain inductive properties and is, therefore, the graft of choice in treating nonunion in human beings, compact bone also is useful, as it can be cut more accurately to form splints, dowels, interlocking surfaces, and so forth, and may be preferable for conditions in which bone is missing and in which mechanical stability is of prime importance. An example is restoration of central defects of metacarpals. The inexperienced surgeon often is tempted to insert a small interposition cancellous bone graft into a small defect in the center of the shaft of a metacarpal. Nonunion

Text continued on page 602

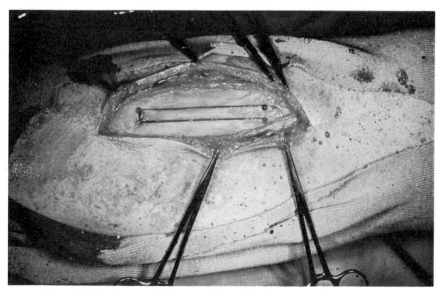

Figure 11–26. Removal of bone graft from tibia for metacarpal reconstruction.

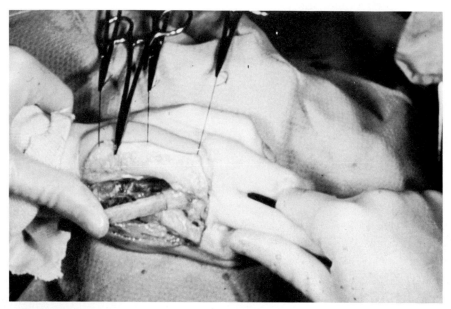

Figure 11–27. Bone graft dowel has been inserted into head of metacarpal. Proximal end of graft is being snapped into base of metacarpal while traction is placed on long finger and wrist is brought into extension.

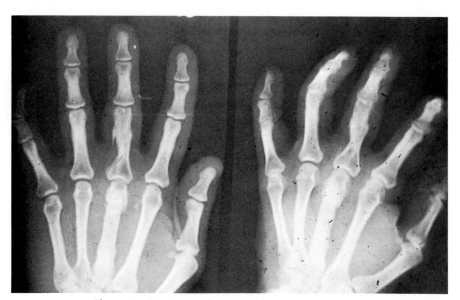

Figure 11–28. Union of bone graft shown in Figure 11–20.

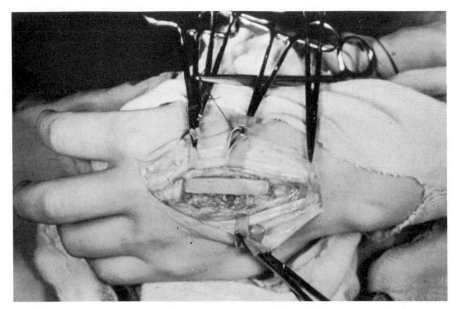

Figure 11–29. Tibial bone graft spanning defect in long metacarpal.

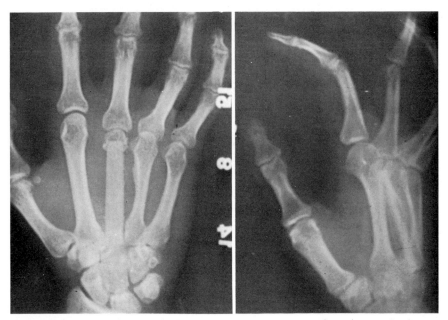

Figure 11–30. Tibial bone graft shown in Figure 11–22. Note that when neck of meta-carpal is missing, a dowel is not carved on end of graft. Entire graft is inserted into head of metacarpal so that penetration of metacarpal head will be unlikely. (From E. E. Peacock, Jr., in *Surgery: Principles and Practice,* 4th edition, edited by C. A. Moyer, J. E. Rhoads, H. N. Harkins, and J. G. Allen, Philadelphia, J. B. Lippincott Co., 1970.)

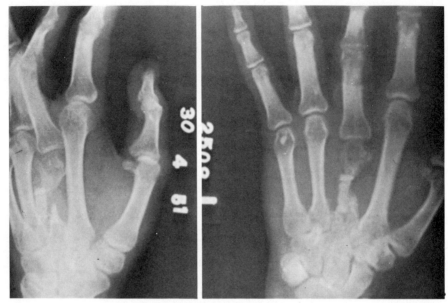

Figure 11–31. Incorrect use of small medullary or cortical bone graft in metacarpal defect. Graft is too small and too unstable to result in union.

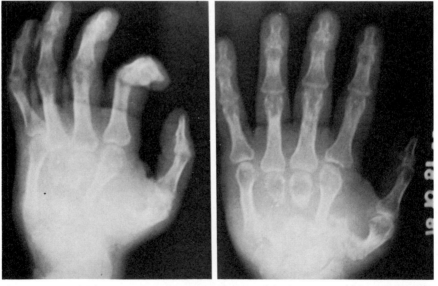

Figure 11–32. Dislocation of small metacarpal, major defects in ring and long metacarpals, and fracture of index metacarpal in gunshot wound of hand.

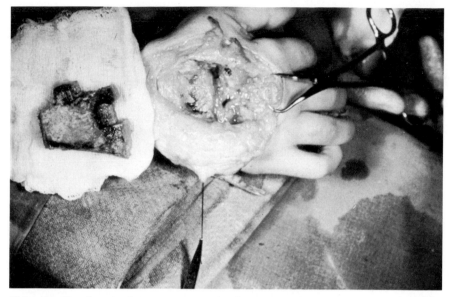

Figure 11–33. Complex bone carpentry utilized to reconstruct all of the metacarpals with a single graft. Note insets and platforms on graft to accommodate metacarpal fragments of various lengths. Proximal end of graft will rest in notch in radius.

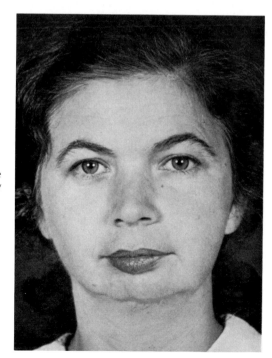

Figure 11–34. Deficiency of bone in symphysis of mandible secondary to osteomyelitis.

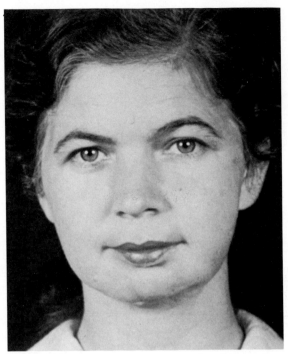

Figure 11–35.　Restoration of mandible with onlay cancellous bone graft removed from ilium.

because of continued instability is a frequent complication of this procedure. The keystone of an arch must be much more secure than that produced by an interposition graft of cancellous bone in the center of the fixed longitudinal arch of the hand. Proper immobilization is very difficult to obtain following insertion of such a graft. It is much wiser to remove most of the metacarpal shaft and replace the entire arch with a long bone graft so as to get rid of the keystone effect and make it possible to immobilize the site of bone junction with Kirschner wires or the action of intrinsic muscles. Cancellous bone from the ilium can be used in this type of graft provided one cortical surface is maintained for mechanical stability. More often, however, a compact graft from the anteromedial surface (never the anterior spine) of the tibia is selected because the dense bone from this area can be shaped into interlocking surfaces, dowels, and so forth, so accurately that once the graft is locked into place, the effect of intrinsic muscle action will maintain excellent immobilization and union without internal or external support other than a volar wrist cock-up splint. Accurate interlocking surfaces cannot be cut and maintained in cancellous bone, and Kirschner wire or casts or both are needed if a cancellous graft is used in a metacarpal defect.

Bone grafts heal primarily by a process known as "creeping substitution." Fundamentally this means that most of the transplanted cells do not survive the short period of ischemia required for transplantation. Cells are replaced by mesenchymal cells from the host bed which apparently differentiate into mature osteocytes and osteoclasts. Such bone grafts are an excellent example of a homostatic (compared to a homovital) graft. They perform function (architectural stability) while they are being replaced even though there are no living cells within them. After new cells find their way into the various interstices of matrix, they begin the slow but measurable task of remodeling matrix to resist stress indigenous to the recipient area. They also appear to promote healing by new bone formation between the graft and the fragments they are connecting. The process is a complex one, often requiring six to nine months in large defects. Superb immobilization is mandatory for a successful outcome. Although heterologous bone can be used and other biological and nonbiological materials have occasionally been reported to provide a homostatic scaffold for new bone to develop in and around defects while architectural stability is provided, autogenous cancellous bone is by far the material of choice to restore

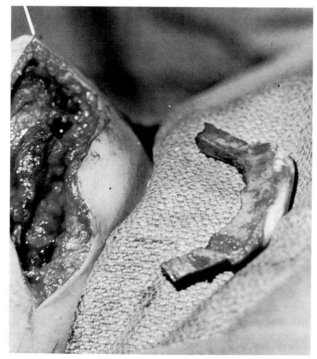

Figure 11–36. Massive cortical bone graft from ilium prior to insertion into symphysis defect of mandible. Center third of mandible was removed during treatment of malignant tumor.

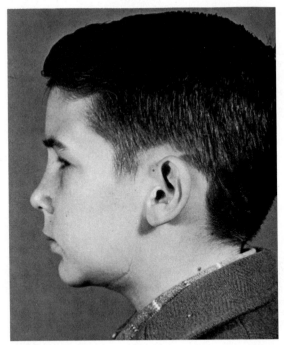

Figure 11–37.   Lateral profile of patient shown in Figure 11–36 one year after reconstruction of center third of mandible with free ilial bone graft.

bony defects. Heterologous bone and various bone substitutes are not nearly as dependable as autologous bone and should be used only as a last resort.

Metabolic Disturbances

General metabolic disturbances usually are not responsible for delayed fracture healing. The effects of vitamin deficiency have been outlined previously. It is interesting to the surgical biologist that vitamin C deficiency is by far the most important vitamin deficiency as far as delayed fracture healing is concerned. Fractures will heal in patients with rickets but they do not heal well in patients with scurvy. Moreover, bone healing cannot be accelerated by increasing serum levels of calcium, phosphorus, or vitamin D. Fractures should always be considered as a specialized type of healing wound and it will be recalled that the healing wound, in many respects, is comparable to a fetus. It seems to have first call on body substances which serve as raw materials for regeneration or healing. Because the amounts of these materials required to synthesize a scar or callus are relatively small compared to the size of the body pool (even during a relative deficiency state), it is extremely unusual for wound healing ever to be inhibited by deficiency of raw materials. When wound healing is delayed, it is usually because a critical catalyst for a basic biological or chemical reaction is missing. Optimal levels of important catalysts can be extremely critical. As such they are far more important in the course of delayed healing of wounds, including fractures, than are deficiencies in raw material.

The effect of cortisone on healing fractures is the same as in healing of soft tissue wounds. Cortisone decreases the inflammatory response, inhibits fibrillogenesis for a realtively short time, and thus delays fracture healing by about the same amount of time that fibrogenesis is active during the bone healing process. The delay in fracture healing caused by cortisone experimentally is in the range of two to four weeks and is the same for all fractures. Permanent inhibition of fracture healing in laboratory animals or human beings has not been reported.

Local pathological conditions affect bone healing and are an important clinical factor which must be taken into consideration in every fracture. Common local pathological causes of delayed healing and nonunion are tumors (metastatic and primary), Paget's disease, osteogenesis imperfecta, and osteoporosis. Metastatic tumor, in particular, if it is radiosensitive often can be treated successfully in bone by radiation; healing of a pathological fracture often will ensue. It is a tragedy to miss the diagnosis of a pathological fracture and thus lose the opportunity to provide this important palliative therapy.

Secondary Wounding

Secondary wounding in bone is usually the result of delayed manipulation of an improperly reduced fracture. It is similar to making a secondary wound in soft tissues and does not delay fracture healing during the cellular proliferative stage. Secondary manipulation of a fracture after the primary cellular stage (seven to ten days) significantly delays and may even prevent normal healing. Biologically speaking, secondary manipulation, either intentional or unintentional because of poor immobilization, produces a mechanical stimulation for formation of a joint surface. Fractures which normally heal without cartilage formation can be induced to form large amounts of cartilage and actually proceed to pseudarthrosis if the fracture is manipulated after the primary cellular proliferation stage of healing. The wry saying that some surgeons seem to obtain their best fusions when they are trying to perform arthroplasties and that their best arthroplasties occur when they are trying to achieve fusion may be based on nothing more complex than errors in the control of mechanical stimulation of a healing wound of bone at a critical time. Other factors (oxygen concentration, for instance) in experimental preparations such as tissue culture can cause the same effect, but in most patients development of pseudarthrosis or firm union probably relates more to accuracy of reduction and fixation than to local or general metabolic derangements.

CONCLUSION

The repair of bone is a complex process. It involves removal of necrotic tissue, exudate, and other products of the trauma that produced the effect. There occur concomitantly a proliferation and differentiation of osteoprogenitor cells which proceed to form matrix that is subsequently ossified, either directly or by the more complex process of endochondral ossification. Formation of a trabeculated callus is followed by a process of remodeling which involves osteolysis and new bone formation. In fractures of the shafts of long bones, trabeculated bone is converted, during the process of remodeling, to compact bone.

Experimentally, bone repair is extremely sensitive to inadequacies in blood supply, to oxygen tension, to mechanical forces, to the balance between parathyroid hormone and calcitonin, and to nutritional requirements, particularly vitamins C and D. Although optimal healing will occur only when all of these controlling factors are maintained at optimal levels, the biology of fracture healing is amazingly well protected in the human body. Unless a separate disease process such as metastatic or primary bone neoplasia is overlooked, fracture healing can best be assured by meticulous attention to accurate anatomical reduction and rigid immobilization. Overemphasis of mechanical factors can inhibit biological systems and thus defeat the objective of bone regeneration, but if mechanical principles are not fulfilled, all of the biological processes we presently know about and can control will not result in a mechanically stable reconstitution of the skeletal system.

SUGGESTED READING

Alcock, N. W., and Shils, M. E. A New Mechanism for the Calcification of Skeletal Tissues. Association of Inorganic Pyrophosphatase Activity with Normal Calcification of Rat Costal Cartilage in Vivo. Biochem. J. 112:505, 1969.

Ali, S. Y. Analysis of Matrix Vesicles and Their role in the Calcification of Epiphyseal Cartilage. Fed. Proc. 35:135, 1976.

Bassett, C. A. Environmental and Cellular Factors Regulating Osteogenesis. In Bone Biodynamics. Edited by H. M. Frost. Boston, Little, Brown & Co., 1964.

Bassett, C. A. L., and Herrmann, I. Influence of Oxygen Concentration and Mechanical Factors on Differentiation of Connective Tissue in Vitro. Nature 190:400, 1961.

Bassett, C. A. L., and Ruedi, T. P. Transformation of Fibrous Tissue to Bone in Vivo. Nature 209:988, 1966.

Bonfiglio, M. Repair of Bone-Transplant Fractures. J. Bone Joint Surg. 40A:446, 1958.

Bowness, J. M. Present Concepts of the Role of Ground Substance in Calcification. Clin. Orthop. 59:233, 1968.

Buring, K., and Urist, M. R. Effects of Ionizing Radiation on the Bone Induction Principle in the Matrix of Bone Implants. Clin. Orthop. *55*:225, 1967.

Chase, S. W., and Herndon, C. H. The Fate of Autogenous and Homogenous Bone Grafts. A Historical Review. J. Bone Joint Surg. *37A*:809, 1955.

Cohen, J. Biomaterials in Orthopedic Surgery. Amer. J. Surg. *114*:31, 1967.

Dubuc, F. L., and Urist, M. R. The Accessibility of the Bone Induction Principle in Surface-Decalcified Bone Implants. Clin. Orthop. *55*:217, 1967.

Felix, R., and Fleisch, H. Role of Matrix Vesicles in Calcification. Fed. Proc. *35*:169, 1976.

Flanagan, B., and Nichols, G., Jr. Metabolic Studies of Bone in Vitro. IV. Collagen Biosynthesis by Surviving Bone Fragments in Vitro. J. Biol. Chem. *237*:3686, 1962.

Fleish, H., and Neuman, W. F. Mechanisms of Calcification, Role of Collagen, Polyphosphates and Phosphatase. Amer. J. Physiol. *200*:1296, 1961.

Foster, G. V., Doyle, F. J., Bordier, P., and Matrajt, H. Effect of Thyrocalcitonin on Bone. Lancet *2*:1428, 1966.

Friedenberg, Z. B., Zemsky, L. M., Pollis, R. P., and Brighton, C. T. The Response of Non-Traumatized Bone to Direct Current. J. Bone Joint Surg. *56A*:1023, 1971.

Furlow, L. T., Jr., and Peacock, E. E., Jr. Effect of Beta-Aminopropionitrile on Joint Stiffness in Rats. Ann. Surg. *165*:442, 1967.

Glimcher, M., Francois, C., and Krane, S. M. Studies on the Mechanism of Calcification, II. Possible Role of Phosphate in the Calcification of Collagen and Enamel Proteins. In *Structure and Function of Connective and Skeletal Tissues.* Edited by S. F. Jackson, S. M. Partridge, R. D. Harkness, and G. R. Tristram. London, Butterworth & Co., 1965, p. 344.

Harris, E. D. J., and Sjoerdsma, A. Effect of Parathyroid Extract on Collagen Metabolism. J. Clin. Endocr. *26*:358, 1966.

Hartles, R. L. A Reappraisal of the Evidence Linking Vitamin D, Parathormone, and Citrate with Bone Resorption and Remodeling. In *Calcified Tissues.* Edited by L. J. Richelle and M. J. Dallemagne. Université de Liège, 1965, p. 93.

Heiple, K. G., Chase, S. W., and Herndon, C. H. A Comparative Study of the Healing Process Following Different Types of Bone Transplantation. J. Bone Joint Surg. *45A*:1593, 1963.

Herring, G. M. Chemistry of Bone Matrix. Clin. Orth. *36*:169, 1964.

Hoaglung F. T., and States, J. D. Factors Influencing the Rate of Healing in Tibial Shaft Fractures. Surg. Gynec. Obstet. *124*:71, 1967.

Hurley, L. A., Zeier, F. G., and Stinchfield, F. E. Anorganic Bone Grafting. Amer. J. Surg. *100*:12, 1960.

Irving, J. T. Interrelations of Matrix Lipids, Vesicles, and Calcification. Fed. Proc. *35*:109, 1976.

Jibril, A. O. Proteolytic Degradation of Ossifying Cartilage Matrix and Removal of Acid Mucopolysaccharides Prior to Bone Formation. Biochem. Biophys. Acta *136*:162, 1967.

Kaufman, E. J., Glimcher, M. J., Mechanic, G. L., and Goldhaber, P. Collagenolytic Activity during Active Bone Resorption in Tissue Culture. Proc. Soc. Exp. Biol. Med. *120*:632, 1965.

Ketenjian, A. Y., and Shelton, M. L. Primary Internal Fixation of Open Fractures: A Retrospective Study of the Use of Metallic Internal Fixation in Fresh Open Fractures. J. Trauma *12*: 756, 1972.

Laitinen, O. The Metabolism of Collagen and Its Hormonal Control in the Rat. With Special Emphasis on the Interactions of Collagen and Calcium in the Bones. Acta Endocr., Suppl. 120, 1967.

Leonard, F., and Scullin, R. I. U.S. Army Biomechanical Research Laboratory, Walter Reed Army Medical Center, Technical Report 6906, April 1969.

MacLennan, D. Some Aspects of the Problem of Radionecrosis of the Jaw. Proc. Royal Soc. Med. *48*:1017, 1955.

Marmor, L. How to Treat the Infected Ununited Fracture of the Tibia. Amer. J. Surg. *113*:475, 1967.

McLean, F. Bone. Sci. Amer. *192*:84, 1955.

Miller, E. J., and Martin, G. R. The Collagen of Bone. Clin. Orthop. *59*:195, 1968.

Nogami, H., and Urist, M. R. Explants, Transplants, and Implants of a Cartilage and Bone Morphogenetic Matrix. Clin. Orthop. *103*:235, 1974.

Pappas, A. M., and Radin, E. The Effect of Delayed Manipulation Upon the Rate of Fracture Healing. Surg. Gynec. Obstet. *126*:1287, 1968.

Peacock, E. E., Jr. Some Biochemical and Biophysical Aspects of Joint Stiffness: Role of Collagen Synthesis as Opposed to Altered Molecular Bonding. Ann. Surg. *164*:1, 1966.

Piez, K. A. The Amino Acid Chemistry of Some Calcified Tissues. Ann. N. Y. Acad. Sci. *109*: 256, 1963.

Rabinovitch, A. L., and Anderson, H. C. Biogenesis of Matrix Vesicles in Cartilage Growth Plates. Fed. Proc. *35*:112, 1976.

Ray, R. D. Vascularization of Bone Grafts and Implants. Clin. Orthop. *87*:45, 1972.

Shamos, M. H., and Lavine, L. S. Piezoelectricity as a Fundamental Property of Biological Tissues. Nature *213*:267, 1967.

Sheldon, H., and Robinson, R. A. Electron Microscope Studies of Crystal-Collagen Relationships in Bone. IV. The Occurrence of Crystals within Collagen Fibrils. J. Biophys. Biochem. Cytol. *3*:1011, 1957.

Sobel, A. E. Local Factors in the Mechanism of Calcification. Ann. N.Y. Acad. Sci. *60*:713, 1955.

Sobel, A. E., Burger, M., and Nobel, S. Mechanisms of Nuclei Formation in Mineralizing Tissues. Clin. Orthop. *17*:703, 1960.

Trueta, J. An Experimental Study of the Vascular Contribution to the Callus of Fracture. Surg. Gynec. Obstet. *120*:731, 1965.

Urist, M. R. Recent advances in Physiology of Calcification. J. Bone Joint Surg. *46A*:889, 1964.

Urist, M. R., and Adams, J. M., Effects of Various Blocking Reagents upon Local Mechanisms of Calcification. Arch. Path. *81*:325, 1966.

Urist, M. R., Dowell, T. A., Hay, P. H., and Strates, B. S. Inductive Substrates for Bone Formation. Clin. Orthop. *59*:59, 1968.

Urist, M. R., Silverman, B. F., Buring, K., Dubuc, F. L., and Rosenberg, J. M. The Bone Induction Principle. Clin. Orthop. *53*:243, 1967.

Chapter 12

HEALING AND REPAIR OF VISCERA

PERITONEUM

The two most important clinical considerations in healing of peritoneum are failure to heal normally, which may be significant in the development of hernia or dehiscence or both, and overhealing, which may be involved in the production of intra-abdominal adhesions. Hernia formation and dehiscence as biological variations of normal wound healing involving peritoneum have been considered in previous chapters. This section will deal with the other end of the hypothetical healing scale—complications caused by production of scar tissue during healing of a peritoneal wound. Although abdominal adhesions are not classically thought of as scars, present meager knowledge suggests that the term "traumatic scars of peritoneum" might be useful in a biological analysis of the cause and effect of these serious complications of an abdominal exploration. Considered as such, the concept developed repeatedly in this book, that all healing is not necessarily good and that healing by scar tissue, in particular, may be bad, takes on additional meaning in terms of gastrointestinal physiology.

Peritoneal Adhesions

The first point to be made in such a treatise is that the problem that concerns practicing surgeons taking care of human beings is decidedly different from the problem that has been reproduced and studied in laboratory animals by experimentalists. Expressed in the simplest terms, the laboratory preparation is one of formation of

609

fibrous adhesions between viscera and viscera and between viscera and peritoneum; the problem in human beings is *intestinal obstruction.* Before any consideration is given to available laboratory data which might be useful in surgical practice, it must be made clear that intestinal obstruction secondary to formation of peritoneal adhesions is a disease limited to human beings. As such it stands in support of the thesis that wound healing is a perfect example of a real and independent discipline known as human biology. Just as surface wounds in fur-bearing animals do not heal in the same manner as wounds in human beings, peritoneal wounds in common laboratory animals apparently do not heal in the same way, or at least with the same complications, as in man. Moreover, there is a known difference among animal species in the reactivity of peritoneum to mechanical, chemical, and pharmacological influences. This is particularly true among the laboratory animals commonly used to study peritoneal healing—rats, rabbits, and dogs. In addition, there is a marked individual difference within species, and we do not have to go beyond clinical observations in people to illustrate this point. Study of patients undergoing a second abdominal operation strongly suggests that nearly every individual whose peritoneum has been wounded has abdominal adhesions to some extent. Mercifully, only a few have intestinal obstruction. Intestinal obstruction is most often caused by peritoneal adhesions, however. Thus, we are probably concerned with a problem of individual variations in the synthesis and remodeling of scar tissue that may be similar to the kinetic differences hypothesized for production of a keloid or hypertrophic scar. In any event, we must caution that present data measuring the effect of an agent or procedure on development of adhesions in the peritoneal cavity of animals may bear no relation to the fundamental mechanism in human beings leading to intestinal obstruction following healing of a peritoneal wound.

It is possible that development of peritoneal adhesions is predictable, in fact, a normal consequence of suturing peritoneum, whereas development of intestinal obstruction is related either to chance location of adhesions or to the physical properties of collagen and what happens to collagen during secondary remodeling or maturation. Should this hypothesis be correct (and there is some evidence that it may be), prevention of abdominal adhesions might not be nearly as rewarding an approach to control of intestinal obstruction as manipulation of the secondary metabolism of collagen. At the moment, however, the best available biological data which can be utilized by the practicing surgeon are related to prevention of adhesions and, thus, clinical repair of peritoneum at present must be governed by these data.

The known causes of peritoneal adhesions can be separated into three major groups: infection, foreign bodies, and vascular insufficiency. It should be noted that trauma, *per se,* is not listed as a cause of adhesions. In both experimental animals and human beings there is a great deal of evidence that trauma alone, even to the point of removal of large areas of visceral or parietal peritoneum, does not necessarily produce adhesions unless an additional factor such as one or more of those listed above is introduced. Expressed differently, trauma is more correctly defined as an initiating influence, while foreign material, infection, and ischemia are promoting factors. It is not only possible, but apparently usual, for a large defect in the peritoneal surface of the abdominal or pelvic wall or abdominal viscera to heal rapidly with no evidence of adhesions of the type which causes intestinal obstruction, unless an additional factor such as sepsis or foreign body is introduced.

There are essentially two types of peritoneal healing. One occurs after an injury to or removal of peritoneum, and its end result is a reconstituted surface without fibrous adhesions. The other type of healing is caused by an injury or defect plus addition of a foreign body, vascular abnormality, or severe inflammation. Healing following this combination usually results in formation of dense fibrous adhesions. The next step, secondary remodeling of fibrous adhesions to form a tendinous band capable of obstructing bowel, may or may not be related to any currently recognizable factors.

Adhesions produced by injury plus a promoting agent or factor may be of three types: fibrinous, which apparently undergo lysis and disappear; fibrous, which may subsequently be remodeled to form dense organized connective tissue or be degraded and disappear; and omental, which, teleologically speaking, seem to develop primarily for the purpose of increasing the vascular supply to viscera and then either disappear or persist without causing any great difficulty. Although data from human beings are sparse and inconclusive, deductive reasoning based on data from animal experiments strongly suggests that there are methods now available to the clinician which will influence markedly the healing process following parietal or visceral peritoneal injury. Perhaps even more important, we also have data on some measures which theoretically might have helped but are known now to have no practical value, and even may be detrimental. Such measures are more numerous than 35 years ago when Hertzler wrote, "Fibrous adhesions are the bogey of most surgeons and a central factor in diseases of all abdominal viscera; the idea of preventing adhesions led to the introduction of everything under the sun that could be bent, poured, or powdered, with the usual result of making things worse." Fortunately, the biologically oriented surgeon is in a much more favorable position today to evaluate these claims and may even be on the verge of controlling the evolution of adhesive peritonitis.

CONTROL OF ADHESIONS. As in the search to control the healing process elsewhere in the body, clinical approaches to controlled peritoneal healing can be classified as inhibition of collagen synthesis, manipulations of the physical properties of collagen, and stimulation of collagen-degradative processes. As in the case of skin and tendon healing, the most promising approach from a clinical standpoint at this time appears to be control of the physical properties of postoperative scar tissue.

Attempts to control synthesis of collagen in healing wounds of peritoneum in laboratory animals have been disappointing for the same reason that they have been unsuccessful in skin or fascial wounds—lack of specificity. Although such powerful agents as alkylating drugs, externally administered radiant energy, and other general inhibitors of protein synthesis such as actinomycin and puromycin will inhibit significantly the synthesis of fibrous protein in a peritoneal adhesion, the effect is not limited to collagen synthesis alone, and doses large enough to be clinically significant in peritoneum dangerously inhibit synthesis of protein throughout the body. Agents which theoretically might have a specific effect on protocollagen hydroxylase and thus specifically inhibit collagen synthesis include trace element chelators and monoamine oxidase inhibitors. These agents have not been evaluated specifically for their effect on development of abdominal adhesions, with the possible exception of one agent which will be discussed in another section. Although cortisone, administered at the time a foreign body is introduced, does have a measurable although quantitatively small effect, it is questionable if this is of clinical significance in preventing the development of fibrous adhesions. The timing and degree of the effect appear to be correlatable much more accurately with the initial inflammatory response and subsequent disappearance and absorption of foreign bodies than with collagen synthesis and intermediate metabolism. At best, cortisone and its derivatives exert only a delaying influence on collagen synthesis during wound healing. Microscopic and ultrastructural changes in peritoneum during adhesion formation are essentially those described elsewhere in the body during fibrosis and healing. An interesting observation from peritoneal studies has been that when eosinophils are numerous, little proliferation of fibroblasts and reduction of fibroplasia are seen. Conversely, in sites where fibroblast proliferation and accelerated fibroplasia are seen, virtually no eosinophils can be identified. It may be that the presence of eosinophils and their associated antihistamine activity hold in check the proliferation of fibroblasts while new mesothelium is formed. Such a process might retard fibrous adhesion formation. Thus, at this time, protein-synthesis inhibitors do not seem to be particularly useful in prevention of fibrous adhesions.

Several other groups of agents theoretically might affect development of adhesions or the physical properties of collagen within adhesions. Most have not proved to be useful clinically. Drugs include anticoagulants such as heparin, Dicumarol, Ancrod, and fibrinolysin, and streptococcal products such as streptokinase (but not hyaluronidase, which does have a significant effect in rats). Mechanical agents such as saline, amniotic fluid, siloxane, and polyethylene, agents which increase peristalsis such as prostigmine and early feeding, and biological replacements such as grafts of peritoneum, amnion, or mesothelium-lined tissue either show no effect at all, or have an effect on only one species and then only on initial fibrous tissue formation and not on adhesions producing secondary obstruction. An increase in the number and character of adhesions or production of dangerous side effects such as hemorrhage or toxicity has resulted from the use of all of these agents. Two approaches, however, have been effective. These are the elimination of foreign material and the simultaneous introduction of a powerful antihistamine (Phenergan) plus a cortisone derivative. A third influence, avoidance of ischemia, has an effect primarily on development of omental adhesions; venous obstruction appears to increase fibrous adhesions. Decreased pO_2, increased pCO_2, and increased rate of oxygen consumption within the peritoneal cavity have been measured consistently during production of experimental adhesions in animals. Finally, causing adhesions to form in a place where they will not produce obstruction of the intestine has prevented this major complication of adhesions in human beings.

Foreign bodies, which every surgeon recognizes now as producing fibrous adhesions of the type that causes intestinal obstruction, include talcum powder, lycopodium, sulfonamide powder (particularly when introduced in lumps), and petrolatum. Other materials which are not always recognized as foreign bodies but which may produce fibrous adhesions in some patients under some conditions are cotton lint from gauze sponges and abdominal packs, cornstarch when used improperly, and most important, suture material of any kind.

Peritoneal Healing

The most important fundamental principle in the healing of peritoneum, which distinguishes it from many other tissues, is the rapid reconstitution of the surface following injury or removal. Regardless of the size of the defect, a mesothelial surface with physical characteristics essentially indistinguishable from normal peritoneum will be reconstituted within three to five days. The fact that a mesothelial surface is restored rapidly in large or small defects, and that covering the defect with a polyethylene shield retards restoration, strongly suggests that desquamated or shed mesothelial cells from remaining visceral or parietal peritoneum rain down upon the denuded surface. Because there is some basal activity in surrounding mesothelium and because a polyethylene cover does not prevent completely reconstitution of the peritoneal surface, it may also be assumed that centripetal movement of uninjured cells is involved, but to a lesser extent. Stem cells in the base of the wound or defect also contribute to the remesothelization process. The fact that ascorbic acid depletion significantly retards the process suggests that the fibroblast may be actively involved; other studies have suggested that macrophages also are important in the healing of peritoneal defects. Recent work clearly shows, however, that blood cells do not become fibroblasts in wounds as was previously thought.

The important principles for practicing surgeons are that wound contraction is not an outstanding feature of peritoneal healing and that reconstitution of even the largest defect is certain within a relatively rapid time provided mechanical interference with normal restorative processes is not introduced. The second fact, one with enormous clinical implication, is that one of the most certain ways to interfere with normal healing of peritoneum is to insert foreign bodies such as sutures. Under controlled conditions, in every species which has been studied, the fibrous band produced between the peritoneal scar and some other structure takes origin from and apparently is oriented by a peritoneal suture. Other foreign bodies such as lumps of drugs, retained cotton lint from sponges and packs, drains, and so forth, are not as clearly related to development and orientation of adhesions but the evidence strongly suggests that they have the same effect as sutures. Obviously we do not have controlled observations in human beings, but a large number of uncontrolled observations also suggest that sutures are the primary stimulus for development of a fibrous band in an otherwise uncomplicated (no infection, necrosis, drains, and so forth) peritoneal repair. An example is a patient recently operated upon by one of the authors (E.E.P.). She had been operated upon eight times previously for intestinal obstruction and each time was found to have tendinous bands of fibrous tissue between abdominal viscera and various incisions in her abdominal wall (see Fig. 12-2). Small bowel obstruction was relieved in this patient by dividing the bands; closure of the abdominal wall was performed without placing a single suture through peritoneum (see Fig. 12-3). Previous closures had been performed by placing sutures through the entire thickness of the abdominal wall, including peritoneum. For three years the patient has not had any symptoms or signs of intestinal obstruction; she had been chronically ill with recurrent small bowel obstruction for six years before the last operation. Such observations are uncontrolled and offer little more than anecdotal information. Accumulation of such information, however, does make it important to continue studies based upon the concept that suture material in peritoneum may be one of the leading causes of secondary remodeling of fibrous tissue of a type which causes intestinal obstruction.

The therapeutic implications of these recent biological observations are more than most surgeons are willing to accept at this time. Some of the reluctance may be justified by the notion that complications, such as dehiscence, would be more certain and more horrendous than adhesions if no sutures were used in peritoneum during closure

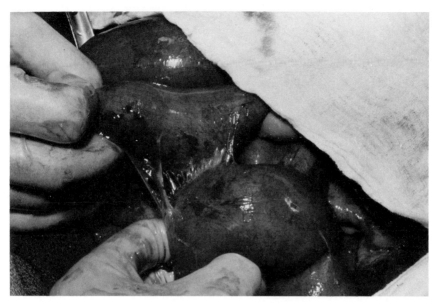

Figure 12–1. Adhesions between viscera. These collections of loose areolar connective tissue are part of normal wound healing in abdominal cavity and seldom cause intestinal obstruction.

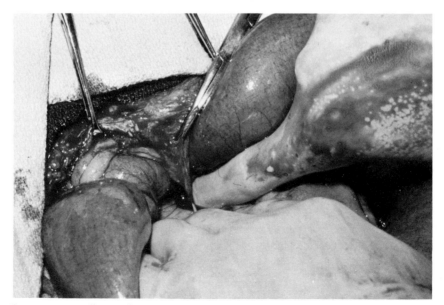

Figure 12–2. Adhesion between viscera and incisional scar on abdominal wall at point where a large suture passed through peritoneum. This is the result of secondary remodeling of loose connective tissue to form dense connective tissue bands that frequently cause intestinal obstruction. Note distended bowel.

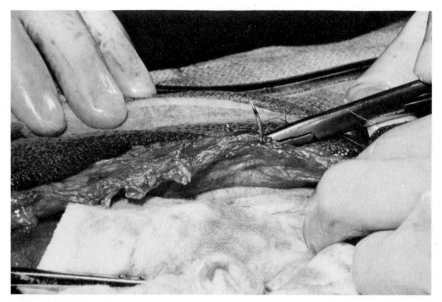

Figure 12–3. Placement of abdominal wall sutures so that peritoneum is not pierced. This maneuver is thought to reduce potential reaction and secondary remodeling of adhesions to form tendinous bands between abdominal viscera and anterior abdominal wall.

of an abdominal wound. The authors know of no data or evidence that this is true. Indeed, some surgeons virtually never place sutures through peritoneum when closing the abdominal wall. It is generally supposed that dehiscence begins as a small protrusion of omentum or viscera through an opening in peritoneum. Regardless of the weakness which present lack of controlled data imposes on the thesis that sutures should not penetrate peritoneum during closure of an abdominal wound, the data on reconstitution of peritoneum by natural means cannot be ignored in making the decision to close the pelvic or abdominal floor after major extirpative surgery. In studies performed on laboratory animals from three species and in studies of human beings being operated upon a second time (uncontrolled observations), there is a great deal of evidence to support the suggestion that no attempt should be made to reconstruct a defect in the abdominal or pelvic peritoneum, as will be discussed in more detail later. Reluctance to accept this principle, although understandable, is not defensible on the basis of modern knowledge of wound healing biology, in our judgment.

PERITONEAL REPAIR. Only a few surgeons have had the courage to depart from the time-honored principle that any denuded area on the posterior abdominal wall or pelvic floor should be reconstructed immediately by suturing peritoneum. The results which they have published give an exciting preview of how surgical practice can be improved in this decade by merely utilizing biological knowledge which is now available. Insofar as can be determined now, the incidence of postoperative herniation of bowel through a partially dehisced wound of posterior peritoneum, and intestinal obstruction from postoperative adhesions can, for all practical purposes, be eliminated in patients undergoing abdominoperineal resection or excision of the colon. The advantage of saving time by not performing a complete, and often difficult, closure of posterior peritoneum cannot be measured but is of some benefit also. In the opinion of the authors, prevention of a postoperative hernia requiring emergency surgical correction, and prevention of chronic or acute mechanical intestinal obstruction secondary to fibrous adhesions are excellent examples of the benefits awaiting patients and surgeons when surgical technique is based upon modern biological principles. Again, it is important to emphasize that such a statement in no way diminishes the importance of the many valuable technical improvements which master surgeons have developed and taught through the years. It does imply strongly, however, that the age of reason by biologically oriented surgeons is here and that, just as major advances in physical sciences have improved diagnostic accuracy to a level undreamed of by those who developed the fine art of physical diagnosis by clinical observation, so some of the technical skills such as the ability to close pelvic peritoneum rapidly even though it is under considerable tension may not be necessary if we are willing to utilize our knowledge in the field of human biology.

The question of whether surgeons should avoid placing sutures in anterior parietal peritoneum has not been studied in human beings except by uncontrolled observations. From the data collected in animal experiments there is no doubt that potentially dangerous fibrous adhesions can be eliminated almost completely if no sutures are placed through peritoneum. There is also no question, however, that, in dogs, the most certain way to insure postoperative evisceration is not to close the incision in anterior peritoneum as accurately as possible. Many surgeons have had similar notions about closing anterior peritoneum in human beings. It seems likely, however, that if the hypothesis is true that a suture passing through anterior parietal peritoneum serves as an inductor or nidus for rigid fibrous bands producing intestinal obstruction, some means of closing peritoneum from the anterior side without disturbing the visceral surface should be utilized. Undoubtedly those who have advanced and proved the hypothesis in animals will carry their work to human wound closure in the future.

Treatment of Peritoneal Adhesions

Assuming that it is possible to eliminate postoperative hernias of small bowel through a rent in a posterior suture line, and also eliminate small bowel obstruction from adhesions originating in a wound in the anterior abdominal wall, what can be done about the patient who was operated upon before the era of biological enlightenment and now has an abdomen or pelvis containing numerous hypertrophic scars coursing between every conceivable surface? Such patients are candidates for partial or complete mechanical obstruction which may be chronic or acute and require emergency surgery as many as ten times in a single year. There are two approaches to this problem—mechanical and biological. The mechanical approach is, for the moment, the more certain as measured by past experience in human beings; the biological approach is the more exciting as far as our imagination can take us now.

None of the mechanical approaches to *prevention* of secondary adhesions after an operation for intestinal obstruction has been helpful except that of avoiding penetration of peritoneum by sutures. In fact, many have been not only not helpful but actually detrimental. These include installation of all sorts of liquids to hold intestinal loops apart, introduction of natural and artificial substances to prevent denuded surfaces from adhering, and attempting to decrease formation of adhesions by increasing mobility of the bowel. There is a physical manipulation which has been effective (according to most reports) in reducing the incidence of postoperative obstruction from adhesions, however. It is based upon exactly the same principle as that discussed under the section on development of composite tissue allografts for restoring the flexor mechanism following adhesive tendinitis. Because adhesion formation cannot at present be selectively prevented, the surgeon's efforts should be directed toward making the scar form in a place where it will not restrict function. In the case of tendons, adhesions can be made to form in an area where they will not restrict motion; in the case of intraperitoneal healing, adhesions can be made to form so that they do not produce intestinal obstruction. This analysis emphasizes again that, unlike most animal experimental end points, the problem in human beings is not formation of adhesions but development of intestinal obstruction caused by adhesions. As long as a loop of small bowel does not become incarcerated within an aperture created by dense unyielding fibrous tissue, the average patient cares not at all whether an adhesion is present or not. In an operation commonly known as the Noble plication, the small bowel and its mesentery can be permanently arranged in an orderly, nonobstructing pattern by the use of a few strategically placed sutures. Wound healing with subsequent intraperitoneal fibrosis permanently cements the loops together in an orderly pattern. Similar objectives recently have been obtained by the use of an internal splint in the form of a semiflexible gastrointestinal tube which can be removed after adhesions have formed.

Everyone has not had as uniformly successful results with small bowel plication as Noble and his associates, but the principle is a simple one, and probably will provide reliable relief of repeated small bowel obstruction if technical performance is accurate. The greatest disadvantage to the procedure is that the operation is technically horrendous in patients who need it most. All of the scarred and distorted bowel must be released before plication is started (see earlier chapters for discussions on the importance of re-creating surface wounds and undoing all that the healing process has accomplished before beginning a restoration). Hours of tedious and technically demanding surgery may be required and in some patients it may be impossible to achieve complete release of all of the adhesions. Rents in the bowel must be recognized and closed and some loops may even have to be resected; this, of course, affects morbidity and mortality.

A report that a combination of Phenergan and cortisone effectively prevents fibrous adhesions in rats and dogs is of special interest, as it introduces the possibility of a new approach which is neither preventive nor mechanical in concept. Although both agents were advocated because of their anti-inflammatory effect, it is possible that the result they produce is at least in part the result of another mechanism. Phenergan, in addition to being a powerful antihistamine and thus properly classified as an anti-inflammatory agent, is also similar in structure to some very powerful lathyrogenic agents and has been shown to have mild lathyrogenic qualities. Although no study of the potential lathyrogenic effect of Phenergan has been done as far as its ability to alter the physical properties of newly synthesized scar tissue is concerned, further investigation of this possibility may be worthwhile for two reasons. First, the effect in preventing fibrous adhesions in several species of laboratory animals was pronounced; the drug is relatively nontoxic in human beings, and should be evaluated in them for a similar effect. More interestingly, however, the concept that physical properties of adhesions are more important than whether they actually are present or not also can be studied by determining whether the incidence of internal obstruction is diminished after alteration of the physical properties of intraperitoneal scar tissue. Thus an attack on the primary problem of intestinal obstruction in human beings could be directed specifically at influencing intermolecular and intramolecular cross-linking of newly synthesized collagen, instead of trying to prevent collagen from being synthesized, or mechanically preventing it from obstructing the gut.

Another approach to the problem of intestinal obstruction from peritoneal adhesions could be based on the recent discovery that the type and amount of intraperitoneal scar tissue is influenced by oxygen tension in surrounding tissues. This is particularly true following venous obstruction which experimentally can produce dense fibrous tissue adhesions in otherwise normal visceral peritoneum. With increasing ability to measure and control tissue and blood gases, the biological approach to control of intraperitoneal scar tissue should include further investigation of these phenomena.

The most recent approach has utilized the phenomenon of fibrinolysis to prevent fibrous adhesions. Experiments in dogs have suggested that, if fibrinous adhesions are prevented, fibrous adhesions also may not form. These data must not be falsely construed to mean that fibrin ever becomes transformed into collagenous fibers. As far as is known now, proteins are individually synthesized upon specific RNA templates and one protein does not turn into another protein after extrusion from cells. The data cited above, however, do suggest that fibrous or collagenous adhesions may require a fibrinous scaffold or template and, if the scaffold is removed, secondary formation of fibrous adhesions may be diminished.

GASTROINTESTINAL TRACT

Lips

Technical details on the repair of wounds of the lips are to be found in abundance in plastic surgery texts. The most difficult wound of the lips to repair is an electrical burn of the commissure; the next most difficult wound to repair is a congenital wound: cleft lip. In the opinion of the authors, one of the real advancements made in the last few decades in this area has been in devising a technique for the repair of congenital clefts based almost entirely on the concept of the cleft as a healed intrauterine wound. The most successful surgical procedures have been designed on the basis that the cleft is not only a wound but a wound which has undergone healing with all of its complications. The concept that the original defect must be re-created (or the results of wound healing removed or corrected) before surgical reconstruction has been the most important contribution of the rotation-advancement technique described so eloquently by Millard. In addition to the fact that the rotation-advancement concept has made it possible to reduce the deformity to the congenital cleft more than any other previously devised procedure, it is enthusiastically recommended by us to all students of surgical biology as an example of the benefit to patients which accrues from combining technical excellence with sound biological principles. It should also be pointed out that there are other congenital deformities such as hypospadias and congenital contraction bands which also can be considered intrauterine wounds that have healed by contraction and fibrous protein synthesis. In spite of the relatively enormous regenerative capacity of developing tissue, simple wound healing by all of the processes presented in the first few chapters does occur *in utero*. Scar formation and tissue distortion from contraction, rather than tissue regeneration, are essential parts of these deformities and must be dealt with just as in a traumatic wound during later life if best results are to be obtained. It is not uncommon to find patients with every sign of a previously repaired cleft lip or palate who have never seen a physician before. In these individuals the congenital wound of the lip healed before the child was born and, as a result, the lip may contain scar tissue, an uneven vermilion, a small fistula, or any of the usual signs of wound healing that we are accustomed to see after an adequate or inadequate surgical repair. Thus, the complications of healing, as well as the concept that a wound existed during the formative months, can provide an important biological foundation for tissue adjustments during correction of congenital deformities. In correcting the defect produced by congenital wounds and wound healing, one of the most fundamental principles in reconstructive surgery should be recalled — to re-create the defect before beginning the constructive stage of the procedure. Contractures must be released and the products of healing such as epithelium and scar tissue must be removed before tissue planes are adjusted and new tissue brought into the defect.

Oral Mucous Membranes

Wounds of the oral mucosal and submucosal tissue are generally thought to heal unusually well without suturing. Rapid healing has been presumed to be the result of the mild antibacterial properties of human saliva and the beneficial effect of having a continually wet surface. Evidence to support these assumptions is far from overwhelming, even though uncomplicated healing of surface defects within the oral cavity is to be expected under most circumstances. It should be remembered that the usual uncomplicated healing may not be all that is required when the dental surfaces of the lips and buccal mucous membranes are involved. It is not generally appreciated how accurately the lip and buccal mucous membranes fit against the teeth and jaw and how important a small ridge of scar tissue in these areas can be. Specifically, if a permanent ridge of scar tissue develops, or an uneven approximation of tissue persists on the medial side of the lips or cheek, several undesirable complications may be produced, including restriction of normal movement and distortion of normal position of the lips which is visible on the external surface. In addition, the scar or uneven surface can be a source of irritation during occlusion so that the patient either distorts his normal occlusion, causing temporomandibular joint arthritis, or continually bites the scar so that an area of chronic inflammation and persistent wound healing is produced. Both, of course, have potentially serious long-term implications. It is probably desirable, therefore, to repair, as accurately as possible, lacerations of the buccal and labial mucous membrane in dentulous patients in spite of the fact that it is also technically difficult (particularly in small children) and usually unnecessary as far as simply obtaining a healed wound is concerned. Repair of deep lacerations, especially those crossing lines with

changing dimensions, should include a local revision, such as placement of darts, or a Z-plasty. Relatively simple adjustments of this type
will usually prevent an external visible distortion or an internal functional disability.

When mucous membrane is missing in the oral cavity one must assume that healing will occur by contraction and epithelization. Which
process will predominate, however, depends upon the position of the
wound and may differ considerably from that in an external wound. It
is commonly taught that oral mucous membrane has unusual regenerative possibilities and that almost any defect will close spontaneously by
growth of new mucous membrane. As far as can be determined by actual measurement, however, there is no evidence that this is so, and the
concept (in violation of some of the most fundamental principles of the
biology of wound healing) has been responsible for a great deal of
preventable intraoral deformity. Such erroneous concepts of intraoral
healing are due, in large measure, to the mobility of mucous membrane and submucous tissue.

Redundant mucous membrane is found in several places in the
oral cavity and most of it is only loosely attached to submucous tissue.
This arrangement—ideally suited for a wide range of jaw and tongue
movement and for the change in dimensions of the oral cavity required
for normal phonation and eating—means that wound contraction is
possible over a relatively large area. An examiner can easily get the
false impression that regeneration of mucous membrane has occurred
when, in fact, wound contraction has been responsible almost entirely
for restoring surface integrity, and a significant diminution of oral cavity function may have occurred. Often, loss of function is inconsequen-
tial, and healing by contraction is permissible. Occasionally, however,
such abnormalities as malocclusion, subtle changes in expression, and
temporomandibular joint abnormalities are the result of deficiencies of
oral mucous membranes secondary to a local shift of tissue caused by
wound contraction.

Although extensive shift of tissue is possible in most tissues of the
oral cavity, there are some areas where tissue is attached firmly to
periosteum and wound contraction cannot occur. In these areas healing of the mucous membrane is almost entirely by epithelial regeneration. The notion that one usually does not need to graft a mucosal
defect over the hard palate or alveolar ridge is correct and grafts
should be avoided, when possible, in these areas. The reason why grafting need not be done, however, is that soft tissues are superbly splinted
so that contraction cannot occur and epithelization provides an adequate means of restoring surface continuity. Skin grafts will take nicely
in oral cavity wounds but they should be avoided whenever possible for
two reasons. Junctions between epithelial and subepithelial tissue of
different types are not biologically quiescent. Although skin and oral
cavity are both lined with stratified squamous epithelium, there are dif-

ferences between the two tissues and grafting frequently results in a low-grade inflammatory reaction or excessive scar production beneath or surrounding the graft. Experimental confirmation of this observation has been presented in Chapter 2. Secondly, a skin graft within the oral cavity usually forms a relatively rigid plaque which may not be pliable enough for normal function. It is best, therefore, to use mucous membrane grafts from the posterior buccal fornix or tongue to graft mucosal defects in the mouth.

Palate

Healing in the soft palate and mucoperiosteum of the hard palate is based on the same three biological principles as healing of bowel: avoidance of tension, preservation of blood supply, and accurate approximation of healing surfaces. In the case of palatal mucosa, however, only one surface, the submucosal surface, had adequate potential for uncomplicated healing; inversion of the oral mucosal surface invariably produces a fistula. Tension is avoided in palate wounds by development of freely movable flaps, usually based on the posterior palatine artery, and by fracturing (greenstick) the hamular process of the palatine bone so that the circuitous route of the tensor palatine tendon will be shortened and the effect of the muscle on the new suture line will be lessened. Blood supply is assured by identifying and preserving the posterior palatine artery. To move flaps adequately, it is sometimes necessary to dissect the artery out of its bony foramen by removing the posterior wall of the palatine foramen. An island pedicle flap of the whole posterior palate and anterior mucous membrane can be created by partially dissecting the posterior palatine artery off the deep surface of the flap. If the palatine artery is inadvertently cut it is usually best to stop the dissection and return the flap to its original position. The procedure up to that point should be considered as a delay (see Chapter 7). Three or four weeks later, the flap can be elevated again with a safer blood supply than at the time the artery was damaged. Advanced techniques have taken into consideration the need to line the nasal surface of palatal flaps so that wound contraction on the nasal surface will not occur. This is frequently accomplished with a small local island pedicle of mucoperiosteum rotated 180 degrees and placed on the nasal surface of a posteriorly positioned mucoperiosteal flap.

Fistula formation following palate repair is usually the result of inaccurate approximation of mucosal edges. The natural tendency for palatal edges to invert into the nasal cavity, bringing oral surface mucosa into contact with nasal surface mucosa, must be prevented. This is usually accomplished with everting vertical mattress sutures inserted as close together as necessary to assure that there is not a single millimeter of mucosal surface inverted. Postoperative care includes liquid diet, strict use of arm restraints, and other measures to prevent introduction of foreign bodies into the mouth. Restraint on the part of physicians in inspecting or culturing the suture line and nasopharynx is mandatory. Opening the mouth excessively or inserting tongue depressors or culture swabs increases tension across the suture line and may produce retching or vomiting followed by dehiscence of the wound.

Tongue

Sutures should be used to approximate edges of a deep tongue wound even though healing of the tongue is generally thought to be extremely rapid without them. Deep lacerations of the tongue may produce serious hemorrhage; excessive scar tissue may produce deformity when wounds heal by secondary rather than primary intention. Special features about the tongue which must be remembered during placement of sutures are uncontrollable continuous muscle action and profuse blood and lymph supply. Sutures should be placed wide and deep, and should be tied very loosely. A large stout needle (adequate to pass through a large mass of muscle without danger of breaking) and a fairly heavy suture (silk or chromic catgut) should be inserted and tied loosely. It is helpful to place an instrument such as a closed hemostat or the handle of a knife between the suture and the tongue while the knot is being tied. Edema is so severe during the first 48 hours that sutures will either cut through tissue too quickly or produce deep necrosis and excess scar tissue if they are tied in the usual way. Monofilament synthetic sutures should not be used in a muscular structure such as the tongue; they become untied too rapidly. Postoperative care includes copious use of mouthwash to keep the suture line free of food particles and blood. Swelling may be so severe as to require tracheotomy but this is not usual for wounds in the anterior two-thirds of the tongue.

Oral Cavity

Wounds of the oral cavity which extend to the external surface, such as those intentionally produced by a combined radical neck dissection and removal of an intraoral tumor, have a notorious tendency to develop orocutaneous fistulas during the period of initial healing. There are three reasons why this annoying complication develops. Two of the causes are mechanical in nature: they are splinting of tissues by insertion of artificial materials and inaccurate coaptation of soft tissue. The third cause is biological in nature and is the result of interference with blood supply by the surgical procedure or preoperative radiation.

Orocutaneous fistulas are most common after the so-called "pull-through" procedure involving a neck dissection and excision of an intraoral tumor with preservation of the mandible. There are many reasons (technical as well as biological) why this procedure should not be performed as far as curing the tumor is concerned. In addition, when a pull-through procedure is performed or when the equivalent is produced by reconstructing the mandibular arch immediately with a metallic or other artificial prosthesis before soft tissue is healed, the effect of the preserved mandible is to hold minimally sufficient external soft tissue away from internal tissue which has a tendency to retract medially. Internal muscular action pulls the tongue and other soft tissue in a medial direction while an inadequate amount of skin on the external surface has a tendency to stretch across the wound so that a dead space between deep tissue and skin is produced. The space between "tented" skin and internally retracting tissue held open by the mandible or a prosthesis fills with fluid and ultimately leads to dehiscence and an orocutaneous fistula. This complication can be prevented by not performing the pull-through procedure and by being certain that a Steinmann pin, or other mandibular replacement, does not act as a splint holding skin away from deep tissues. A mandibular replacement at the time of jaw-neck dissection should be utilized to stabilize the remaining mandible, minimize malocclusion, and reduce respiratory complications. It should not be inserted to restore cosmetic appearance. Even if no skin is removed during the neck dissection there will always be a relative shortage of skin after the contents of the anterior triangle have been removed. It takes a great deal more skin to line a cavity than to stretch across it. Removing the contents of the anterior triangle of the neck produces a cavity; therefore more skin will be required to cover the surface than was needed before lymph nodes and muscles were removed. The external skin flaps must be permitted to drape loosely over the deep tissues and should not be held away from them by a horizontal bar in the shape of the mandible. Cosmetic deformity is the price one must pay for such biological considerations but the advantages of having a rapidly healed wound without a fistula are worth it. Cosmetic defect, of course, can be repaired by secondary restorations which do not involve the simultaneous production of mucosal and skin defects. Mercifully, such mutilating procedures as excision of the symphysis of the mandible are not being performed very often now. It is hoped that continued improvement of high voltage externally administered radiation will reduce the necessity for this type of surgery to zero.

A second cause of orocutaneous fistulas following jaw-neck dissection is the use of a continuous suture in the mucous membrane. Such a suture frequently produces inversion of the mucous membrane and compromises blood supply. The surgeon is tired and is thinking in terms of extirpative surgery at the end of a jaw-neck dissection; it is natural to choose the most rapid method possible for closing the defect. A continous mucosal suture accomplishes this but also produces a wound with a high propensity for developing an orocutaneous fistula.

The incidence of such fistulas can be lessened by first suturing the sub-mucous tissues accurately with interrupted absorbable sutures. Absorb-able sutures are preferable to nonabsorbable sutures because retained foreign bodies are undesirable if a fistula should develop. Proper inser-tion of eight or ten such sutures actually causes the submucosal tissues to be gathered together in such a way that the mucous membrane becomes everted into the oral cavity. After this has been accomplished, a continuous mucosal stitch will not have nearly so much tendency to invert the mucosal edges and thus increase the possibility of an orocu-taneous fistula.

Radiation-induced ischemia is better avoided than treated. The subject will not be discussed again in this chapter other than to make a plea for surgeons and radiologists to consider, from the standpoint of fundamental wound healing and oncological biology, all aspects of what they are attempting to accomplish before starting a patient on some combination of preoperative radiation therapy and surgery. The concept that a little radiation should be combined with a little surgery or that the therapeutic effects of both are additive often results in less than adequate radiation and less than adequate surgery. Such thinking often is the result of the understandable desire to try something new when dealing with a condition as discouraging as advanced intraoral cancer. There really is nothing very new about combined therapy, how-ever, and the lesson which has to be relearned with almost every gener-ation is that the very best surgery or the very best radiation usually is the best that can be done for these unfortunate patients. Combining the two may result in less than the best of either without any additive effect compensating for failure of either. At this time there are no good (controlled) data to support the notion that combined radiation and surgical therapy of head and neck neoplasms is superior to expert treatment by either alone.

Development of a postoperative fistula is not a serious complica-tion unless complete dehiscence of the external flaps also occurs. With proper care, fistulas will close predictably unless there is a foreign body or cancer in the tract. A fistula which has a circuitous course will close more rapidly than one whose internal aperture is directly over the ex-ternal one. If cancer or foreign body is not responsible, therapy is directed toward keeping the patient clean and encouraged, and pre-venting malnutrition. Fistulas will heal by wound contraction, which seldom is interfered with by local or systemic abnormalities. While wound contraction is occurring the patient should be encouraged to eat just as if the fistula did not exist. While he eats a pad should be held against the opening to prevent loss of food and soiling of bed clothes and linen. A small, easily changed pad should be applied between meals, and care of the surrounding skin should be meticulous. Recog-nition that the fundamental biological process in healing of this partic-ular wound is contraction, and that wound contraction is not easily interfered with, prevents an overzealous surgeon from starving the patient or making him more miserable by attempting to reduce salivary excretion pharmacologically. The most important contribution a surgeon can make is continual reassurance that wound contraction will occur and concentration on measures which help the patient lead as normal a life as possible until the fistula is closed. Complete dehiscence with exposure of the internal carotid artery requires more complex therapy. Details of the biological principles involved and the technical considerations which have evolved are found in Chapter 7.

Mandible

Radiation effect within the oral cavity is most serious when radiation necrosis of the mandible has occurred. It should be emphasized at the beginning that symptomatic radiation necrosis can be one of the most painful and debilitating conditions a human being is required to endure and that every precaution must be taken to prevent it. Many patients have testified that cure of their cancer was not an achievement of note because the price they had to pay in terms of constant pain of radionecrosis of the mandible and mucous membrane kept the life which was saved from being productive or enjoyable. The surgeon and the radiologist have responsibility for preventing radionecrosis; the surgeon may have to assume all of the responsibility for treating it. Biological principles which can be utilized include realization that with present equipment and techniques it is not possible to cure cancer in bone without also destroying the reparative and regenerative mechanisms. Carcinoma cells in bone usually are not more sensitive to radiation than stem cells or even mature osseous cells. It takes only a few thousand roentgens of soft radiation to render bone incapable of regeneration or repair. Thus, the dose of radiation required to produce radionecrosis of bone is less than that necessary to kill neoplastic cells.

The surgeon should keep in mind that radionecrosis of the mandible itself is not painful. There is an intermediate stage in the progression of events which can be arbitrarily classified as asymptomatic. The key to helping patients with this condition is realization that a radiation-damaged mandible can be asymptomatic until an injury is superimposed. It is not the death of cells alone that makes patients miserable, it is an injury—even a slight one—superimposed on radiation damage that leads to severe pain and ulceration. Extraction of a tooth and abrasion of the alveolar ridge with a hard object, such as a denture or some external object, are typical examples of relatively insignificant injuries which will not heal in a radiation-damaged area and thus start the symptomatic stage of the disease with all its consequences. A fundamental principle in radiation and wound healing biology is that stem cells necessary for healing are not replaced when destroyed. In addition, reduction of blood supply, so important in the healing process, adds further to the problem. Finally, bacterial invasion and osteomyelitis may have to be contended with.

Hemimandibulectomy may be necessary for control of pain and closure of the wound. Most surgeons begin with local excision of exposed bone only, if removal of a small amount of bone will permit overlying soft tissue to fall together without tension. Excision of exposed mandible, where surrounding soft tissues have been irradiated, seldom results in anything more than extension of the wound including development of a large area of exposed mandible and eventually osteomyelitis. Melted butter or Petrogalar can be used to soothe pain of exposed mandible; narcotics should not be started early. Drug addiction is common in patients with radiation effect in the oral cavity; thus the surgeon should be aggressive in recommending excision of larger portions of bone and bringing permanent blood-carrying pedicles (as described in Chapter 7) into the area if minor procedures are not successful. Realization of what the patient is enduring is the most important factor in the surgeon's decision to be aggressive in treating this miserable complication of cancer therapy.

Osteomyelitis of the mandible without radiation is an entirely different problem from osteomyelitis in a radiation-damaged mandible and should be approached from a different biological basis. The wound healing process is not abnormal in patients with simple osteomyelitis, and usually the blood supply to the area is adequate. The fundamental biological problem is one of host versus organism, and when the tissue involved is the mandible, the cosmetic and functional costs of extirpative surgery are so great that most surgeons approach the problem conservatively, particularly when treating youngsters. We agree with this reasoning. The key to treatment of chronic osteomyelitis of the mandible is adequate and prolonged soft tissue drainage. If this can be provided by placing semipermanent soft tissue drains in the submandibular area where they and the scar they produce will not be conspicuous, the pathological process in the bone eventually will be corrected by natural processes without loss of function or alteration of appearance. Normally, the blood supply to the mandible is excellent, and if good soft tissue drainage is provided over a long period, sequestration of infected bone followed by regeneration or fibrous tissue replacement will occur so that appearance and function are not seriously altered. The only debridement of bone which is permitted, when such a course is followed, is removal of sequestra which are completely detached and can be lifted out of the wound without cutting across viable bone. The fundamental biological principles are that infected areas of mandibular bone eventually will separate and that healing of membranous bone is primarily by fibrous replacement and not by production of callus. Localization and sequestration of infected mandible are far better performed by natural mechanisms than by cutting across involved bone.

The surgeon only extends the process when he excises large fragments of mandible for osteomyelitis; the cosmetic and functional costs are too great even if immediate cure of osteomyelitis could be promised. The authors have seen patients in whom most of the mandible was replaced by a combination of fibrous tissue production and bone regeneration over a two year period when adequate soft tissue drainage was provided. Removal of a significant portion of the mandible produces a cosmetic or functional defect which is not necessary in most patients.

Pharynx

The only important and different biological principle which is of therapeutic importance in wounds of the pharynx is that pharyngeal mucous membrane can be stretched to extraordinary dimensions and may even have regenerative potential which is stimulated by physical stress. The authors have removed so much of the pharyngeal mucous membrane while excising extensive cancers that only enough mucosa remained to encircle a large feeding tube. Aphagia has not been a permanent problem in these patients and within six weeks the pharyngeal aperture is large enough to permit swallowing and talking. Whether enlargement of the reconstructive pharyngeal aperture represented actual regeneration or only an unusual ability for tissue to stretch with repeated physical stimulation is not certain. Practically it implies, however, that the surgeon should not become involved in a complicated shift of local or distant tissues if enough mucous membrane remains to close the pharynx around a feeding tube. It also means that some cause, other than lack of mucous membrane, must be found for persistent dysphagia in patients who have had extirpative surgery in the pharyngeal area. Frequent causes of dysphagia are removal of the glossopharyngeal nerve, suturing the base of the tongue too far forward while reconstructing the oral cavity, and restricting the motion of the base of the tongue in other ways so that closure of the epiglottis is not possible during swallowing. Therapy usually should be directed toward these and other causes of persistent dysphagia, not toward enlarging the pharyngeal aperture.

Esophagus

Healing in the esophagus is of special interest to the surgical biologist because of two clinical objectives. They are: leak-proof healing of a primary anastomosis, and dilatation of a restricted aperture caused by chronic inflammation and synthesis of a fibrous scar. In the case of the primary wound or anastomosis, there is a great deal of information concerning the various factors responsible for failure to heal adequately, but vexatiously little that can be done about them. In the chronic wound there is a shortage of biological knowledge to explain clinical observations, yet there are some rather effective therapeutic manipulations which, incredibly, seem to improve the ability of people to swallow.

ESOPHAGEAL ANASTOMOSIS. The major problems in a primary wound or anastomosis of the esophagus are leaking and dehiscence. Leaking is by far the most common complication. As late as 1950, mortality rates as high as 23 per cent were reported following replacement of a segment of the esophagus; half of the deaths were due to leakage at the site of the anastomosis. Biological considerations responsible for this serious complication involve anatomical position of the esophagus, lack of a tough fibrous protein layer (the esophagus has no serosa), barely adequate segmental blood supply, constant motion of external organs and surfaces, movement of food or saliva through the anastomosis, and absence of a movable surrounding structure such as omentum which can be used to patch or seal an opening externally. There is not much that can be done about the anatomical location of the esophagus except that selection of a substitute procedure occasionally is influenced by the knowledge that a suture line in the neck is safer than one in the mediastinum. Thus a right or left colon replacement based on a midcolic vascular pedicle is frequently selected over other procedures for defects of the middle or upper third of the esophagus so that the superior anastomosis can be placed in an area where leakage can be drained more directly than it can within the thoracic cavity. Special care and protection are afforded submucous tissues as they contain the most fibrous protein and are therefore the tissues through which a suture is most effective in maintaining physical integrity until cellular migration and globular protein aggregation occur. Blood supply must be kept in mind continually while selecting the level of reconstruction, dividing the esophagus, and reconstructing the defect. Blood supply is so critical and so easily made inadequate during anastomosis of the esophagus that selection of interrupted sutures instead of a continuous suture is advisable even though a continuous suture would be more likely to produce a watertight anastomosis. Although cervical and dorsal sympathectomy have occasionally been recommended to increase the blood supply of the esophagus, there is no sound biological basis for such an approach. The circulatory problem is one of segmental distribution of a small number of small-caliber vessels; it is not a problem of smooth muscle spasm in otherwise adequate arteries. Section of the phrenic nerve on the side where the anastomosis lies may be of considerable value in reducing mechanical factors caused by movement of the diaphragm. Finally, rotation of the omentum so that a local pedicle flap of abdominal fat can be placed around the suture line occasionally may be possible if the anastomosis is in the lower thorax. Usually, however, the omentum should be removed as part of the extirpative procedure.

Nutrition probably has been overemphasized in the past as a factor responsible for poor healing of the esophagus. Although patients with esophageal obstruction characteristically are dehydrated and undernourished at the time they are admitted to a hospital, present knowledge about fibrous protein synthesis, mucopolysaccharide interaction, and epithelial migration (the principal biological mechanisms responsible for successful healing in the esophagus) indicates that these basic processes are not affected by protein depletion except that of an extremely severe order. The wound, like a fetus, seems to have first call or receive preferential treatment in the distribution of protein building blocks even though they are measurably depleted by usual clinical standards. Moreover, it is inexcusable now, in an age when nutrition of the surgical patient by artificial openings in the gastrointestinal tract or parenteral alimentation is so well developed, to start a major extirpative or reconstructive procedure of the esophagus in a malnourished patient.

Finally, the question of an indwelling tube has to be considered. The surgeon, from time immemorial, has had an uncontrollable urge to put a tube through every aperture or circular structure he operates upon — particularly when an anastomosis has been performed. From a general standpoint, the authors would like to state that the biological foundations of wound repair strongly suggest that a great number of such tubes exert deleterious influences on healing and that considerable damage has been produced in tubular organs because of such practices. Whether this is the case in esophageal anastomosis is not entirely clear, as will be discussed in succeeding paragraphs. Scar tissue in the esophagus does not react to mechanical stretching in a manner predicted by behavior of scar tissue elsewhere in the body. It is possible that placement of a tube in a clinically scarred esophagus may produce specific benefits for patients which simply do not apply to other structures. The effect of a tube in a primary healing wound, or during the healing of an esophageal anastomosis, is another matter, however; there is no question that such a tube is deleterious to the basic mechanisms of wound healing. Whether the practical and theoretical advantages of a tube in the esophagus outweigh its effects on wound healing is a question which the authors will not try to answer definitively. From the standpoint of fundamental principles of basic healing mechanisms, however, it would seem that, if defunctionalizing the esophagus is a major reason for inserting a tube, the objective might better be accomplished by inserting an esophageal tube to within a few centimeters of the anastomosis (but not through it) while decompressing the stomach or intestine from below with a gastrostomy or retrograde jejunostomy. The experimental evidence justifying such a recommendation reveals that, although placing a tube through an esophageal anastomosis in an animal does not interfere significantly with the rate of gain of tensile strength in the organ as a whole, it does cause spot areas of significant weakness so that "blow-out" or leak pressures are below clinical safety standards. Even though the entire circumference of the anastomosis, considered as a single wound, gains tensile strength at the same rate whether a tube is inserted or not, isolated spots within the circumference may be seriously weakened and leaks will occur more frequently when a tube is passed through the area than when it is not.

Antibiotics definitely are indicated for prevention of infection around sutures in the submucosa. Suture-line necrosis is inevitable in the mucosa and submucosa, and prevention of infection, even if it is a matter of no more than small stitch abscesses, may be extremely important in preventing a potentially fatal leak. The need for adequate external drainage after an esophageal resection of any kind is obvious.

ACUTE WOUNDS OF THE ESOPHAGUS.   Acute wounds of the esophagus leading to chronic stricture formation include those caused by chemical poisons or corrosives of which lye is the most common. The effect of alkali burns is destruction of epithelium and submucosal structures in small injuries which are treated rapidly, and deep necrosis of muscle in more severe injuries which are not treated rapidly. Destruction of epithelium is not followed by stricture in most patients. Epithelium is a tissue with excellent regenerative capacity and the healing of a superficial lye burn involving epithelium only is comparable to the healing of a split-thickness skin graft donor site. Epithelium which regenerates in a superficially damaged esophagus is not exactly the same as that which was lost but the major functions of esophageal epithelium are replaced and the factors which alter wound healing mechanisms such as wound contraction and fibrous protein synthesis are not introduced. An alkali burn which destroys the full thickness of epithelium and extends into the submucosa or muscle, however, is equivalent to a loss of full-thickness skin on the surface, and the damage produced results in a wound of a compound organ which, like most compound organs, does not have significant regenerative capacity. In the esophagus, wound contraction and fibrous protein synthesis predominate in the healing mechanism and the result may be extremely serious from the standpoint of esophageal function. The major function of the esophagus, swallowing, is dependent upon rather specific physical qualities and physiological functions such as distensibility and coordinated smooth muscle contraction and relaxation. An area of dense connective tissue, physically woven and intermolecularly and intramolecularly cross-linked to resist deforming forces, such as the scar which we depend upon when repairing a hernia or tendon, interferes seriously with both mechanical and physiological function of the esophagus. In addition, other epithelium-lined organs such as skin have a much better anatomical arrangement for resisting injury than does the esophagus. The tough dermis of skin, interposed between epithelium and subcutaneous tissue, provides an important physical and biological barrier and surface wounds of this type heal by epithelial regeneration and are not complicated by fibrous protein synthesis and wound contraction.

Skin-lined esophageal replacements are grossly inadequate, however, for many reasons, one of which is that predominantly fibrous protein dermis is not mechanically or biologically suitable as a conduit for a large bolus which must be transported by smoothly coordinated wave-like muscular action. Thus, the concept that healing without fibrous protein synthesis could introduce an entirely new vista of reconstructive surgery in some areas of the body is stimulated by the problem of healing following chemical burns of the esophagus. Limited but definite regenerative capacity of muscle and marked regenerative capacity of stratified squamous epithelium are present in the esophagus. If the elements of wound contraction and fibrous protein synthesis could be selectively eliminated, healing might not take such a terrible toll in loss of function.

Modern therapy of acute chemical burns of the esophagus takes two forms—mechanical and biological. To the modern student of human biology, both approaches may seem crude and illogical, so much so that it is always a source of wonderment when a beneficial effect is obtained. Actually, however, it is possible that no beneficial effect is obtained by modern treatment of alkali burns with mechanical dilation, cortisone, and anti-inflammatory drugs, but the notion that these agents are effective in reducing or preventing stricture is so firmly implanted in the minds and practice of surgeons that a treatise on the subject would not be complete without discussing them—even if the only conclusion is that very few good data are available. After all, many thousands of uncontrolled observations are of no more value than, and probably not as much value as, a small number of carefully controlled observations under experimental conditions. One of the reasons why the study of human biology is so extremely difficult is that we are unable to set up controlled experiments. The only knowledge we have on the effect of many therapeutic regimes is a compilation of so many random reports and observations that scientifically valid conclusions often cannot be made. The study of the treatment of esophageal burns is no exception. Nevertheless, clinicians who treat alkali burns of the esophagus, particularly in children, have strong impressions that corticosteroid therapy prevents subsequent stenosis and that it should be used, particularly if esophagoscopy reveals more than epithelial damage. If this is true, the explanation may be that transient inhibition of fibrous protein synthesis permits cellular healing to proceed to an extent that stimulation of fibrous protein synthesis does not occur. This is the most plausible explanation at the moment for the apparent beneficial effect of steroids. In other organs where fibrous tissue healing is prominent, treatment by steroids only delays fibrous tissue synthesis and never actually prevents it from occurring. Scar formation is the same in these organs whether cortisone is used or not. The esophagus is different, however, by virtue of having stratified squamous epithelium, without an organized dermis, lying directly on submucosal loose connective tissue. Healing may be more simple and rapid than in a complex organ such as skin and early retardation of fibrous protein synthesis could make a significant difference in the quality and quantity of the final scar.

The apparently effective method of treating strictures of the esophagus by dilatation or stretching is even more difficult to explain on the basis of present biological data. Mature connective tissue does not stretch significantly under physical tension unless it actually breaks, and this of course produces a new wound that usually will heal with more rigid and voluminous scar tissue. The temporary, and sometimes permanent, improvement of acquired achalasia, produced by mechanical dilatation of a stricture with a bougie or hydrostatic instrument, may be due to the relation of the scar to a movable base such as submucosa or muscle. Scar tissue in the esophagus, of course, is not attached to immovable structures as it often is in the abdomen or extremities. Thus response to stretching may be related to stretching or movement of the tissue to which the collagen is attached more than to any actual changes in the scar tissue itself. The mechanism by which mechanical stretching and corticosteroids exert their effect is open to research, however, and the possibility exists that recent discoveries of mechanisms by which the physical properties of recently synthesized collagen can be controlled selectively could introduce exciting possibilities for controlling scar tissue and preserving natural physical properties of esophageal tissues. Work on this problem presently has passed into Phase II (animal testing) and has been concerned primarily with induction of controlled lathyrism by the use of purified β-aminopropionitrile (BAPN). When BAPN is administered for three to six weeks to dogs following an acute alkali burn of the esophagus, prevention of a contracting scar is at least as effective as traditional therapy with cortisone and mechanical dilatation. An important difference in the long-term course of animals treated with BAPN, however, is that BAPN therapy can be discontinued in six weeks without development of a stricture thereafter. Apparently, once epithelium regenerates without development of scar tissue and occurrence of wound contraction, the danger of a chronic stricture is passed. In animals treated conventionally with steroids and dilatation, some form of mechanical dilatation is necessary for very long periods of time, if not permanently. The old clinical expression "once a bougienage patient, always a bougienage patient" is not without some truth in animals as well as human beings. Phase III (human testing) extension of this encouraging work may be delayed because of the frequent occurrence of esophageal stenosis in young children. Evaluation of new experimental drugs in youngsters is almost impossible at this time.

CHRONIC WOUNDS OF THE ESOPHAGUS.   Chronic inflammation, ulceration, and wound healing in the lower esophagus are usually the result of acid corrosion of the lower esophagus secondary to achalasia, hiatus hernia, or functional disturbances at the esophagogastric junction. Healing in this area is chronic and features fibrous protein synthesis and wound contraction which worsen the state of affairs as more obstruction develops. Treatment by mechanical dilatation may produce more small wounds which heal with scar, leading to more obstruction which causes more chemically induced inflammation. The cycle can be interrupted only by correcting the functional and mechanical aspects of the condition. The Heller procedure (designed to alleviate spasm and enlarge the esophagogastric junction), correcting interabdominal pathological conditions in the gastrointestinal or biliary tract, and relieving emotional problems which may have functional reflections in the mechanism of swallowing and regurgitation all can be effective if properly timed and performed.

The most serious complication of chronic healing in the esophagogastric area is development of a neoplasm. Just as any chronically healing wound is subject to neoplastic change, and just as any area where one type of epithelium changes to another is a likely site for neoplasms to develop, the chronically inflamed and intermittently healing lower end of the esophagus is a prime site for development of epidermoid carcinoma. Failing in medical management, the physician must include the danger of malignant change as a reason for recommending rather serious extirpative surgery unless scar formation is not so severe that another type of therapy will suffice.

An operation which has been advocated in the past and which is decidedly safer than extirpative surgery in animals is enlargement of the esophageal contracture by incision of the constricted area and insertion of a skin-lined pedicle flap of gastric or small bowel tissue. This is achieved by placing a skin graft on the serosal surface of nearby stomach or even distant small bowel, opening the constricted area of the esophagus, and applying the grafted surface (skin graft internally) as a permanent pedicle flap to enlarge the diameter of the opening. Serosa seems as good as skin to some individuals; the use of a skin graft, therefore, can be questioned. Either new tissue must be added or the old permanently scarred area excised if wound healing has progressed to the point where mature dense connective tissue has rigidly constricted the opening of the esophagus. Resection and reanastomosis, or replacement of the area, is a dangerous operation with a relatively high morbidity and mortality. It should be possible to develop less dangerous and simple methods but, until this has been accomplished, the danger of cancer in the esophagus is sufficiently high to justify excision and reconstruction of the affected area in many patients.

Stomach

On first examination it might seem incredible that healing of any type could occur in wounds of the gut. A continually wet surface, bathed with enzymes, acid, and bacteria of varying pathogenicity, is hardly conducive to healing of a type considered in the first few chapters of this book. Factors indigenous to gastrointestinal tissues such as extraordinarily profuse blood supply, rapidly regenerating epithelium, and external defense mechanisms against infection provided by peritoneum and omentum, however, make healing predictable and satisfactory unless something is done or occurs to interfere with natural processes. The study of healing and surgical repair in the gastrointestinal tract is, therefore, the study of these processes. They are, in order of importance, control of blood supply, control of infection, and control of hydrodynamic forces by mechanical and biological methods. These factors may be influenced by the design of the extirpative and reconstructive procedures, attention to detail and technique of holding bowel and mesentery together, and preparation (mechanical and bacteriological) of the bowel. Before analyzing these factors in the light of modern wound healing biology and gastrointestinal physiology, it is important to emphasize the shortcomings of a common method for evaluating healing in the wall of a hollow viscus. The usual measurement of tensile strength, or bursting strength, actually is of little practical importance in the study of the effect of most of the factors the surgeon controls at this time. As pointed out by Halsted, the submucosal layer is the only layer where fibrous protein is found in sufficient quantity and physical array to support sutures. Any technique which includes passing a suture through the submucosa, regardless of the eventual arrangement of the tissue, will provide sufficient longitudinal breaking strength so that dehiscence is not a serious problem. The crucial measurement in evaluating clinical reliability of anastomotic techniques, however, is resistance to rupture or leak from increase in intraluminal pressure. An accurate analysis of the effect of various techniques and biological factors on this clinical parameter requires rather formidable biomathematical and physical principles, beyond those which have been commonly utilized by clinical surgeons. Distention of a viscus by either compressible or noncompressible media is a useful measurement of anastomotic competence only if the shape and diameter of the viscus are continually controlled as required by Laplace's law. Even more important, the rate of distention of a viscus also must be controlled since slow distention is tolerated without leakage at a much higher pressure than is rapid distention. When these variables are not controlled, in addition to others such as the presence or absence of external adhesions, condition of sutures, and accuracy of placement of sutures, it may appear that circumferentially healed gut is actually stronger than uninjured gut. Although such a finding may be true it is also possible that the circumferential scar, being less elastic than normal uninjured gut, does not increase in diameter during inflation as much as normal gut, and thus the internal force is not as great and leakage or rupture occurs in distensible uninjured gut before it occurs at the site of a repair. Very few studies on the comparison of different types of anastomotic techniques and preoperative and post-operative drug regimes have been carried out with sophisticated biomathematical and biophysical techniques. Thus we have to turn for most of our information on the biological basis of gastrointestinal healing to crude analysis of uncontrolled mortality and morbidity data and to the descriptive sciences.

The stomach has the thickest wall of any gastrointestinal organ, owing largely to the variable thickness of the mucous membrane. One of the most difficult problems in operating on the stomach is control of hemorrhage. When an incision is made, retraction of the seromuscular coat makes the mucous membrane protrude or evert, and hemorrhage always is profuse. A great deal of the time involved in making a gastrotomy incision or anastomosing the stomach is spent in identifying and ligating the numerous bleeding vessels which are always present. Post-operative hemorrhage also is a problem, which attests to the technical difficulty in identifying and ligating all of the numerous blood vessels in the stomach wall. This, of course, is one reason why large crushing clamps and stapling devices have been popular with busy surgeons; the profuse blood supply in the stomach, however, is probably one reason why one can use such brutal instruments and still obtain excellent healing. Excellent healing is to be expected whether mucous membrane is inverted or everted; the diameter of the stomach is such that the advantages and disadvantages of inverting or everting a cuff of tissue are not as important as in the small or large bowel. The relatively rigid wall and the weight of the stomach cause it to control the shape of an aperture when it is joined to another viscus such as the esophagus or jejunum. This is why additional tacking or supporting sutures or a gastrotomy should be utilized to support the stomach when it is being anastomosed or hung from a more flimsy organ such as the esophagus.

Erosions of the mucous membrane of the stomach heal rapidly by epithelial regeneration. Even removal of the entire mucous membrane of the stomach from a cat or a rat does not result in permanent anacidity. Apparently the regenerative capacity of cells deep within the crypts of mucus- and acid-secreting glands is exceptional, and both functional and morphological integrity is established rapidly by epithelial proliferation, provided the submucosa or tunica muscularis is not injured also. When injury involves more than a simple tissue such as epithelium, healing proceeds as in a wound made in any other compound organ, except that fibrous protein synthesis predominates over wound contraction. The result often is a deeply scarred ulcer which may be so rigid that wound contraction is impossible and mucous membrane coverage is delayed or prevented. No work has been done to investigate the effect of acid, pepsin, or mucus on the healing process; an interesting experience with important clinical applications awaits investigations of this type. A great deal of work, of course, has been done on the physiological forces responsible for production and continued existence of typical ulcers.

As every serious student in the field knows, gastric ulceration is a different disease from duodenal ulceration. Although the hypothesis (based on sound physiological data and brilliant deductive reasoning) that gastric ulceration is the result of stimulation of the antrum by food retained because of pyloric spasm secondary to a duodenal ulcer can be shown to be true for some gastric ulcers, it is not a satisfactory explanation for all gastric ulcers. Hyperacidity simply is not present in all patients with gastric ulcer, and other causes must be found to explain these chronic wounds in some patients. The effect of local ischemia due to acquired or congenital abnormalities of microcirculation has appeared attractive to some investigators. Other important work has been done on the effect of drug-induced changes in the mucus (particularly the sialic acid moiety) which protects the stomach from autodigestion.

Most of the principles of management of surface wounds can be applied to some extent to management of gastric ulcers. In addition, physiological alterations, such as removal of the antrum, division of the vagus nerves, or treatment of a duodenal ulcer, can be added if hyperacidity is present. The principle of resection of the defect (removal of the results and products of wound healing) and closure of the wound and submucosal tissues, so that excessive fibrous protein synthesis will not occur again, are reliable general principles. Although a gastric ulcer should be excised for pathological examination as well as to assure uncomplicated wound healing, occasionally the condition of the patient, location of the ulcer, and involvement of contiguous structures may be such that it is inadvisable to resect a portion of the stomach during an emergency operation for gastric hemorrhage. In these patients, the combination of reducing acidity and putting the stomach to rest by dividing the vagus nerves, providing adequate drainage by pyloroplasty or gastrojejunostomy, and decreasing arterial pressure by ligating major blood vessels is safer than a gastric resection. Ligation of major arteries such as the left gastric artery can be done with any type of ligature, but local suturing of the base of an ulcer, which is frequently necessary, should not be performed with an absorbable suture. Peptic digestion occurs rapidly in the stomach and secondary hemorrhage is common if an absorbable suture is used to control hemorrhage in a bleeding surface of the gastrointestinal tract.

The most common type of postoperative ulcer following gastric or duodenal surgery is a stomal jejunal ulcer. Recurrent gastric ulceration also occurs; the rarest postoperative ulcer is a suture-line ulcer. Suture-line ulcers almost always are due to use of a continuous nonabsorbable suture during the anastomosis. Some portion of the suture inevitably will become exposed in the wound but the entire suture cannot be extruded into the lumen, whereas a single or interrupted nonabsorbable suture can. Suture-line ulcers can be prevented by not using a continuous nonabsorbable suture in the gastrointestinal tract. The surgeon should always keep in mind that the mucous membrane of the gastrointestinal tract is almost gelatinous in consistency. Sutures cut through it easily and there is no resistance to the passage of a needle from the external surface of the bowel when only a submucosal suture was intended. Thus exposure of sutures in the lumen of the gastrointestinal tract is to be expected, and if nonabsorbable sutures are used they should be single interrupted sutures which ultimately can be extruded into the lumen.

Duodenum

One of the most difficult problems in applied wound healing biology is to provide closure and leakproof healing of the duodenal stump following gastrectomy. Mortality from general biliary peritonitis is high; thus the stakes are high for obtaining uncomplicated healing in this organ. Adequate drainage is about the only insurance or safeguard the surgeon has to protect his patient from a potentially fatal complication if healing in the duodenal area is not 100 per cent leakproof. Healing of the duodenum is subject to many complications, and elaborate drainage of the right upper quadrant is a must in surgery of this area. Inadequate tissue (because of both the effects of long-term healing in the area and extirpative surgery) and synthesis of considerable fibrous protein which cannot be removed to re-create the defect or eliminate the effects of healing, as is done in other organs, are the fundamentals of the problem. Some surgeons follow the old premise "If you can't lick them, join them" and avoid the problems of a difficult duodenal closure by intentionally converting the wound into a controlled external fistula. This is usually accomplished by placing a tube into the duodenum and converting the wound into a freely draining duodenum-abdominal wall fistula. Enthusiasm for this technically simple although physiologically complex solution to wound healing problems in the duodenum has diminished. Death from intraperitoneal leakage around the tube, in addition to the well known problems of maintaining electrolyte and fluid balance in a human being with an open duodenal fistula, has contributed to waning enthusiasm. As a result, the search has been reactivated for methods to insure healing of the badly scarred, tissue-deficient duodenal stump. The old biological analysis of "State the problem accurately and the solution may be easier than it appeared" has been of some help to the authors. The basic problem in many duodenal wounds is lack of tissue. It is certainly not the only problem, and in many patients fibrous protein synthesis may be more of a problem than inadequate tissue. If vital organs such as pancreas, common bile duct, and liver are involved in the healing process, however, there simply may not be anything that can be

using inverting mattress sutures. The mucosa trapped between the sutures or staples undergoes necrosis with the result that mucosal continuity is actually reconstituted more quickly than when submucosa, tunica muscularis, and mucosa are inverted by other techniques. A fibrin seal cements the mucosal layers almost immediately after eversion techniques, and early regeneration and fibrin aggregation provide a watertight mucous membrane anastomosis within three days. Carbon particles and other markers have been shown to traverse the mucosal and submucosal suture line through vascular or lymphatic channels more rapidly after everting anastomosis than after inverting anastomosis. Rate of gain of longitudinal tensile strength or burst strength is approximately the same following inverting and everting anastomoses but the internal hydraulic pressures required to produce a leak of gas or liquid are less in everting than in inverting anastomoses. The significance of this finding does not seem to be great from a clinical standpoint, however, as all anastomoses apparently leak to some extent, and surgical technique is completely dependent upon the natural resistance provided by peritoneal and omental function for bacteriological success. Any anastomosis isolated from the general peritoneal cavity by a plastic or other synthetic wrapping will become infected and necrotic and ultimately will dehisce. This is true for inverted, end-to-end, and everted anastomoses. Thus the slightly lower hydraulic leak pressure of everted anastomoses is apparently not of clinical significance because of the important and reliable defense mechanisms peritoneum provides.

Histologically the healing process appears to be delayed following an everted anastomosis. The inflammatory reaction persists longer, presumably because of degenerating trapped mucosa. Again, however, this is probably of more biological than clinical importance because the length of time inflammation persists in the cuff does not affect intestinal motility. Sustained or excessive inflammation outside the lumen does produce one undesirable factor, however, and that is overhealing of peritoneum. As might be predicted, visceral peritoneal adhesions are much more pronounced after an everted anastomosis than after conventional inversion techniques.

At present, the conventional inverted technique, habitually repeated daily by 99 per cent of the world's surgeons, is referred to as the Halsted closure. The everting technique is called the Navy technique because of the excellent work done by a group in the San Diego Naval Hospital; a compromise between the two, which is really an end-to-end anastomosis, is called the Gambee technique. Variations of the Gambee technique have been described which include invagination of the entire thickness and circumference of the bowel, or only of a seromuscular coat. The important clinical advantages of the everting or end-to-end technique are that postoperative obstruction is reduced, less time is required to perform an anastomosis, and a difficult anastomosis can be performed with relative ease. At the moment, the only measurable disadvantage is a greater increase of abdominal adhesions around the suture line when mucous membrane has been everted. Adhesions are rat or dog type of adhesions, however, and whether they have any significance in human biology as far as producing intestinal obstruction is concerned has not been determined. In all probability the adhesions reported following everted anastomosis of the bowel are similar to the adhesions found in animal experimental techniques, such as dropping liver fragments into the peritoneal cavity, or scrubbing the small bowel with a wire brush. It appears that such adhesions are a part of normal wound healing and that collagen produced normally is subject to remodeling, with the end result that permanent adhesions leading to intestinal obstruction are not produced. It is possible that the adhesions produced in laboratory animals by an everting anastomosis are quite different from those produced by a permanent foreign body in the peritoneal cavity of human beings in that they undergo extensive remodeling and do not produce postoperative intestinal obstruction. A few surgeons who have performed everting anastomoses in human beings report excellent results. There has not been an increased incidence of intestinal obstruction to date. Like so many themes taken from textbooks of authoritative teaching in the past, however, preservation of the concept that bowel must be inverted to heal properly continues to be another way surgeons can pay honor to the technical masters of yesteryear. Every biological fact we have at the moment strongly suggests that the hypothesis of the inverting anastomosis is not correct, and that both patients and surgeons can be greatly benefited if present-day techniques for anastomosis of the bowel are based on modern biological information rather than the comfortable security of past clinical dogma. In other words, there is a perfectly sound biological basis for continued development of mechanical stapling devices, cements, and even surgical techniques which are not based upon serosa-to-serosa approximation. Obviously, however, additional data in human beings are needed before any hypothesis can be proved or disproved. Certainly the data which animal experimentation has provided so far can serve only to open up new vistas of human biological research; they cannot be used to substantiate dogmatic statements about what may or may not turn out to be good surgical practice.

Colon

All of the technical principles and problems discussed in the preceding sections are applicable to anastomosis or repair of the large bowel. In addition, however, the problem of sepsis must be taken into account when wound healing in the large bowel is considered; the biological basis for wound repair in the colon actually is concerned most with control of this important process. Lest any beginning student's interest in sepsis following colonic surgery be dulled by the notion that introduction of sulfonamides and flavines relieved surgeons of concern about peritoneal sepsis, it should be pointed out that intraperitoneal sepsis occurs in at least one of five colonic anastomoses today. In addition, wide use of intestinal antibiotics has increased the incidence of such serious postoperative complications as staphylococcal enterocolitis and, even more important, undoubtedly has been responsible for laxity in technique on the part of some busy surgeons.

The most important point to be made in this section is that the usual cause of postoperative wound or intraperitoneal infection following anastomosis of the colon is contamination with bowel contents. Although sepsis often is not evident externally for a week or more after surgery, particularly if postoperative antibiotics were used, study of the temperature chart and leukocyte response indicates that the process started within 48 hours of the time the bowel was opened and is clearly related, from a chronological standpoint, to the surgical procedure. The organisms involved almost always are those found in the large bowel — coliforms, clostridia, bacteroides, and, less commonly, *Staphylococcus aureus.*

The second most important point is that introduction of sulfonamides has not eliminated septic complications. Intestinal antibiotics, along with more attention to and better methods for mechanically cleansing the bowel, have made a significant contribution to large bowel surgery. They do *not,* however, sterilize the bowel and thus reduce the need for superb technical performance, and they *do* introduce other complications such as staphylococcal enterocolitis if used indiscriminately or improperly. Advanced age, debility, obesity, diabetes, obstruction, open versus closed techniques, operative time, and many other judgment and technical details are just as important in the postantibiotic period as they were in the preantibiotic era. Actually, some argument still remains as to whether intestinal antibiotics should be used at all. This argument is based on evidence that antibiotics are no more effective in reducing bacterial flora of the intestine than is good mechanical cleansing. Antibiotics do change the bacterial flora, however, and the result may be dangerous proliferation of organisms such as staphylococci. Some experienced surgeons have stopped using preoperative intestinal antibiotics for this reason. The case against postoperative intestinal antibiotics is even more convincing. Examination of data from a large number of cases of both elective and emergency treatment of colon wounds indicates that the incidence of overgrowth of bacterial flora not affected by common antibiotics is significantly greater when postoperative antibiotics are used. At present, most successful large bowel surgery does include judicious use of preoperative antibiotics, but not postoperative intestinal antibiotics, in conjunction with every effective means of mechanically cleansing the bowel. In addition, every effort is expended to avoid soiling of the peritoneal cavity.

Colostomy is performed if there is any question about the suitability of the bowel for direct anastomosis. From a biological standpoint, the contribution of the peritoneum to the success of colonic wound repair remains one of the most important, most interesting, and least well understood factors in successful large bowel surgery. Excellent experimental work on this subject has shown that, although distant trauma such as a femur fracture apparently does not affect colon healing, local trauma such as extensive peritoneal healing in the retroperitoneal area has a significant effect upon primary healing in a colon anastomosis. From a practical standpoint, extraperitoneal wound repair of the large bowel must be considered more dangerous than intraperitoneal repair; thus external drainage is more important in extraperitoneal wounds than in intraperitoneal ones.

Side-to-side anastomosis, although possibly unavoidable in special conditions such as anastomosis of the colon following reconstruction of congenital defects in young infants, is mentioned with the recommendation that it be avoided whenever possible. Side-to-side anastomosis may be appealing to the inexperienced surgeon because it assures an adequate aperture between two segments. It also produces a blind pouch which subsequently causes complications of great biological importance. There is a rather wide variation in the length of time required for symptoms or signs to develop, but the sequelae from stasis of intestinal contents in a blind pouch are progressive and predictable. They include cramping abdominal pain, nausea and vomiting, abdominal distention, palpable mass, recurring partial or total obstruction, melena, fever, diarrhea, anorexia, failure to gain weight, and failure of the young to develop normally. As far as we know now these findings are all related to stasis and infection in the blind pouch. Treatment, therefore, should be directed toward elimination of the pouch by resection and end-to-end anastomosis. The anemia which develops in patients with a blind pouch is especially interesting in that it is not accounted for either in type or in severity by the melena which occasionally occurs. It has been suggested that the organisms which proliferate in the pouch, like organisms which proliferate in multiple diverticuli, compete for intestinal metabolites and thus produce deficiency syndromes leading to primary anemia. A cause-and-effect relationship of this type has not been proved but the hypothesis fits many of the clinical observations in the gastrointestinal tract and the reticuloendothelial system.

Continued improvement in parenteral alimentation techniques raises the question of whether more predictable healing can be obtained in the colon by improving nutrition. The answer now is that improvement can be attained in some measurable modalities such as burst strength and collagen content of healing wounds. That such improvements are in a range to make any significant difference in complications in human patients undergoing intestinal surgery has not been shown as long as all patients are reasonably nourished prior to surgery. Of course, surgical procedures should not be performed upon badly malnourished patients and, if they are, wound healing as well as other aspects of general health and recovery will be complicated. Modern nutritional techniques, however, make this problem less important than in previous years. It is still fair to state, therefore, that major complications of wound healing in the large bowel are, for the most part, related to sepsis and that internal sepsis is the chief offender in most patients. Reduction in complications of large bowel surgery most likely will follow more sophisticated understanding and control of internal sepsis.

Rectum

All of the biological principles involved in wound healing of the intestine and colon apply to the rectum. The problem of infection is, of course, even more dangerous because of more solid intraluminal contents, higher bacterial count, and extraperitoneal location. An acute small wound of the colon, such as a laceration from a sigmoidoscope or small stab wound, treated quickly, can be closed without extensive drainage or a proximal colostomy. A similar wound, or for that matter any wound, of the rectum, requires extensive soft tissue drainage after repair. Chronic wounds of the rectum must be suspected of having specific and sometimes unusual parasites or organisms; diagnostic studies should include an exhaustive search for unusual parasites, viruses, and bacteria.

A wound in the rectum which requires special attention is radiation proctitis with or without rectovaginal or rectovesicular fistula. Special attention is deserved not only because of the incidence (decreasing fortunately) but also because the location of the wound frequently is responsible for surgeons' ignoring the basic biological mechanisms of radiation damage which must be corrected in the rectum, as elsewhere, if wound healing is to occur. The basic principles of defunctionalizing both organs, excising the products or results of healing, and repairing tissues in such a way that primary healing is assured are, of course, fundamental in the rectal area as in the treatment of any fistula. If radiation damage also has occurred, additional biological considerations must be included. Above all, the basic concepts that wounds produced by radiant energy produce severe vasculitis with resulting ischemia, and that important stem cells, indigenous to tissues which have the capacity to heal, are very susceptible to radiation and usually have been destroyed, must be considered in the treatment plan. As in skin, bone, and any other tissue, the cells responsible for fibrous protein synthesis and wound contraction are stem cells, which are not replaced by blood elements when destroyed by radiation. Deficient blood supply from radiation-induced vasculitis does not improve with time or local care of the wound. The inescapable conclusion from such biological reasoning is that repair of radiation-induced rectovesicular or rectovaginal fistulas must follow the same basic principles as repair of radiation-affected tissue elsewhere. The most important principle is that a new permanent blood supply must be brought into the area and that stem cells with propensity to divide and participate in the wound healing process must be transplanted if healing is to be successful. Technical details of how this is accomplished have been published in detail, but the general principle which fulfills the biological objectives outlined above is the same principle advocated before — development of a permanent blood-carrying pedicle (grafting of new blood vessels). This is usually achieved by excising completely the radiated section of rectum or colon and bringing down a proximal segment of bowel with intact mesentery to pass through the radiated pelvis and be anastomosed to undamaged distal rectum or anus. Of course, other principles such as defunctionalization of the fistula and proper preparation of both organs are mandatory.

Prolapse of the rectum is more complex than is often appreciated and the large number of technical approaches which have been advocated attests to the lack of understanding and the problem of diagnosis of the fundamental disorder in every patient. The symptoms and signs of a protrusion of mucosa from the anus can be due to polyps or other tumors, mucosal redundancy, change in course and direction of the distal colon or rectum, a sliding hernia of the pouch of Douglas, and numerous other conditions. Correct diagnosis of what is actually protruding and the route through which it protrudes is usually followed by selection of the proper procedure to correct the defect and a successful outcome for the patient. The solution to the problem, dictated by the fundamental defect which allowed protrusion, may be no more complicated than excision of mucous membrane, or it may be as complex as reconstructing the pelvic diaphragm and changing the direction of the rectum. Symptomatic therapy and procedures utilized because of respect for the man whose name they bear have been unsuccessful so many times that repair of rectal prolapse has become a sort of *bête noire*, which need not be the case if diagnostic accuracy is achieved.

The soft tissue wound following combined abdominoperineal excision of the rectum is an extensive one. The external or perineal wound will heal as any other soft tissue wound, by contraction and fibrous protein synthesis, if mechanical impediments such as large packs, improper use of sutures, huge drains, and unskilled use of wet applications and damaging drugs are not introduced. The external wound, of course, must be drained adequately to insure that collections of blood and serum do not become infected and converted into a large abscess. This can be accomplished with relatively small tubes or rubber drains if the wound is properly sutured and the drains are accurately placed and cared for. Healing should be almost entirely by primary intention with only a small drain tract requiring secondary care and healing.

Anus

Wounds of the anus are often converted from primary healing wounds which could and should heal like any incision of soft tissue to chronic secondary healing wounds with a deeply scarred base. An important cause for this transition is uncontrolled spasm of the external sphincter. A fundamental consideration, therefore, in aiding healing of an anal wound is relief or prevention of external sphincter spasm. The common notion that a chronic fissure-in-ano must be excised for healing to take place, or that dilatation of the sphincter to produce temporary paralysis is necessary for healing, is not true for all patients. Simple relief of pain can relieve spasm in the external sphincter just as relief of spasm can relieve or prevent pain. Experienced surgeons avoid placing sutures in skin of an anal wound following a hemorrhoidectomy for just this purpose. The reason such practice is effective is that it reduces the pain of the incision and therefore lessens the spasm of the external sphincter. Avoidance of packs and drains in the sphincter area following hemorrhoidectomy also is effective in relieving pain and assuring uncomplicated wound healing; these agents all contribute to spasm of the external sphincter. Relief of pain and spasm by local use of anesthetic cream can be enough to produce healing in a chronic fissure. Of course, if the ulcer has been present for a long time and deeply scarred base or internal openings have developed, the same principle of successful wound management must be followed in this area as elsewhere. These include excision of the products of wound healing and protection of the wound during the primary healing process.

Wounds of the sphincter also can be helped to heal successfully by utilizing the fundamental biological principles outlined in the first four chapters. An acute wound can be made to heal by primary intention if the tissues are put at rest until tensile strength has been regained. If healing does not occur by primary intention, particularly if there is more than one wound in the circumference of the anal sphincter, incontinence may be produced. Correction of incontinence is, of course, most satisfactory if the external sphincter wound can be excised, the products of attempted healing removed, and normal tissues approximated so that healing can occur by primary intention. Replacement of a paralyzed or mutilated sphincter with local muscle transfers has not been satisfactory because transplanted skeletal muscle does not retain adequate blood and nerve supply to maintain reliable voluntary control. Continence does not always depend on a normal external sphincter under voluntary control, however. If the direction of the rectum is posterior rather than vertical so that a column of feces is not directly above the sphincter, if the consistency of the feces is regulated by diet, and if a competent internal sphincter exists, continence may be perfectly satisfactory without a normal external sphincter. Unless some other way to substitute for a paralyzed sphincter is developed, the biologically oriented surgeon is more likely to think in terms of assuring posterior direction of the rectosigmoid and controlling bowel habits than to transplant or revise scars of skeletal muscle when it is impossible to repair and obtain primary healing of the external sphincter.

Liver

REPAIR IN ACUTE LIVER INJURY. The liver is a complex organ. It has two afferent blood supplies: the low-pressure portal system draining the gastrointestinal tract, and the hepatic artery bringing high-pressure arterial blood to the organ. The efferent drainage is through the hepatic vein, but the biliary ductal system and extensive lymphatics are also efferent systems.

The cell types present in the liver are varied. Parenchymal cells, or hepatocytes, constitute about 60 per cent of the cell population. The remaining 40 per cent of cells comprise vascular endothelium, ductal endothelium, Kupffer cells, which belong to the reticuloendothelial system, and mesenchymal cells associated with liver septa, capsule, and other supporting structures. Hepatocytes can be considered the "functional" cells of the liver, but other elements are certainly needed to make the functional activity available to the body.

The unit structure of the liver is the lobule, and although this is not necessarily easily seen microscopically, it assumes considerable importance and is more visible in chronic hepatic injury. In the center of a lobule is a venule which drains into the hepatic vein and thence to the vena cava. Hepatic cells are arranged more or less radially around this central venule in "plates" one cell thick. Between these plates are sinusoids connecting the portal circulation, on the periphery of the lobule, with the central vein. Between cells are bile canaliculi which drain into bile ductules. Kupffer cells are found in sinusoids; mesenchymal cells are more frequently seen at the periphery of the lobule near portal venules and hepatic arterioles, which run close to each other.

The biology of repair and regeneration of liver is different from that of most other organs. Technical measures to insure healing without complication are different from those used in other organs, therefore, when placed on a biological foundation. Three such differences in the morphology and biology of liver compared to other organs are especially important in the present approach to repair of a liver injury: relative absence of connective tissue stroma, marked susceptibility to relatively small changes in blood flow and cellular oxidation, and regenerative capacity exceeding that of any other compound organ in the body. These conditions are so profound in their influence on healing of the liver and therefore upon survival of the patient that such basic surgical principles as sharp dissection, packing to obtain hemostasis, accurate localization and ligature of small blood vessels, and careful suturing with sharp needles and small sutures simply cannot be utilized effectively. Most of these techniques are mechanical adjustments which are simply unusable in the liver because of sparsity of fibrous protein (almost nonexistent except in Glisson's capsule). As a result, sharp dissection in the substance of the liver results in retraction of blood vessels and bile ducts within a friable cellular substrate; this creates a situation that is not unlike trying to tie bleeders in cottage cheese, as far as physical consistency is concerned. Ligation of structures after they have been cut is extremely difficult, and placing a pack sufficiently firmly against the cut surface to stop external hemorrhage or bile leak results in ischemia and mechanical compression of unprotected cells. Immediate hemorrhage or biliary leak can be stopped by applying a pack, but within five days the cells which were compressed will be necrotic and another severe hemorrhage will begin. Also, the liver of some species normally harbors varying concentrations of pathogenic anaerobes which proliferate and produce internal and external sepsis when blood supply to the liver is decreased. During healing of a liver wound, Glisson's capsule is reconstituted very slowly; collagen is not synthesized until after the seventh day and liver (particularly cirrhotic or healing liver) shows the most consistently elevated collagenolytic activity of any mammalian tissue except uterus. Collagenolytic activity in the liver has been shown to be of lysosomal origin and can be separated from catheptic activity by temperature variations. The collagenolytic activity in liver tissue appears to be typical of tissue collagenase in epithelium.

The mechanical and biological hazards to successful surgical repair and healing of the liver are partially balanced by the fact that the liver has unusual regenerative or compensatory qualities which make surgical care more challenging than in other organs where a healed wound means only homeostasis, not replacement of what has been lost or return to normal function. If a liver wound will heal and the complications of an acute injury such as hemorrhage, biliary peritonitis, or abscess can be prevented, the enormous regenerative capacity of the organ usually assures that the patient will not be disabled from inadequate liver function—even if 80 per cent of the organ was removed or destroyed. The biological mechanisms responsible for regeneration of this order are not clear, but it should be pointed out that they are neither as simple nor as effective as pure regeneration or embryonic development. There are some alterations in the microscopic architecture of the regenerated liver. Many of the plates of hepatocytes become two cells wide rather than one cell wide. This is a condition seen in the fetal liver and it is not known whether the adult architecture is ever regained in the regenerated liver. However, in the fetal liver, the hepatocytes are normally diploid cells, but in the adult liver, polyploidy of liver cells is the rule. A large number of hepatocytes are tetraploid and perhaps 5 per cent are octaploid. On regeneration, polyploidy is retained and the ratio of diploid to tetraploid to octaploid cells in the regenerated liver is the same as in the normal adult liver. Thus, in this respect the regenerated liver is adult in form.

Hepartrophy, as it is occasionally more accurately referred to, is a combination of mitotic activity and a great deal of hypertrophy of remaining cells with the end result that the gross mass of the liver is very nearly or completely restored and liver function is adequate. Careful examination of the microscopic and ultrastructure architecture, however, reveals that complete morphological reestablishment of an organized triad with normal duct and lymphatic drainage and normal cell arrangement has not occurred. Nevertheless, liver function is restored and reconstitution of the gross mass of the liver exceeds that seen in any other organ, and is, therefore, a phenomenon worthy of more study. Some cross-circulation experiments have yielded data strongly suggesting that a circulating substance during hepatic regeneration could affect liver growth and cell mitosis in an uninjured liver. There have been other experiments which suggested that this might not be true. Our experiments to see if wound healing in fascia and skin could be affected during liver regeneration revealed that there was no effect in distant tissue from liver regeneration. The most exciting possibility, of course, to those who have been fascinated by the concept that healing without fibrous tissue synthesis and cross-linking might open a new vista of surgical practice, is that one of the rewards of controlling the fibrous protein synthesis portion of healing might be the ability to take advantage of or utilize regenerative potential which is never expressed in the presence of excessive scar formation. This hypothesis is supported by study of healing in the liver because the normally small connective tissue component, the insignificant contribution of fibrous protein synthesis to healing, and the relatively high collagenolytic activity of normal and healing liver may be responsible for the enormous regenerative activity. That any of these factors have anything to do with the regenerative capacity of liver is highly theoretical at this time, however, and present studies suggest that a great deal of the regenerative activity in healing liver may be correlatable only with blood flow. The possibility that portal blood flow is the only important factor, however, has been disproved. Although total blood flow has seemed to correlate with regenerative capacity in some animals, the origin of blood (mesenteric circulation as opposed to blood reaching the liver from other sources) does not seem to make any great difference in regeneration.

Liver injury has a relatively high mortality, primarily because of hemorrhage and secondarily because of infection. Lacerations have the best prognosis, and fractures or blunt injuries have the worst. Gunshot wounds are intermediate between these two types of injuries. Mortality is strongly influenced by the conditions of surrounding organs and, of course, liver injury associated with other injuries carries a worse prognosis than an uncomplicated injury of the liver. Although thoracic injuries occurring simultaneously with liver injury were almost overwhelmingly fatal until thoracoabdominal surgery and hypothermia became technically and biologically feasible, associated abdominal injuries carry a worse prognosis now than thoracohepatic injuries. Injuries to the colon complicating a liver injury have the worst prognosis of all.

The object of surgical repair of the liver is to stop hemorrhage and biliary leak and align cellular surfaces into reasonable approximation without producing a dead space or compromising cell oxygenation while protein aggregation is occurring internally and regeneration and reconstitution of Glisson's capsule are occurring externally. Repair of Glisson's capsule is critical as this fibrous protein sac surrounds an organ which is composed almost entirely of cells. The biological and physical limitations which such objectives place on present surgical techniques are extensive. A great deal has been written on the subject; only general concepts which have a sound biological basis will be summarized in this chapter.

Lacerations of the liver should be closed when it is technically feasible to do so. They should be closed without creating an internal pocket of bile or blood, and without producing ischemia or inordinate pressure on cells. This is best achieved, in our experience, by using sharp, slender needles, rather than large, round, blunt needles as usually recommended. A large suture with high frictional resistance such as 0 chromic catgut should be used. The suture is usually placed as a wide horizontal mattress suture which is tied on both sides over a bolster of surgical gauze, Gelfoam, reconstituted collagen sponge, omentum, or some other resilient substance, so that some cushioning effect is provided and swelling does not produce ischemia. Although a few surgeons have recommended drainage of a liver incision, it would seem that the fundamental biological aspects of healing in this organ would be more likely impaired than helped by insertion of a drain. Consequently, if suturing does not produce a wound without a dead space or without excessive internal or external drainage, resection in the past has been considered advisable rather than insertion of an intrahepatic drain. Recently it has been shown that ligation of the hepatic artery can be performed safely as an emergency measure to control hemorrhage from extensive liver lacerations and that this is probably the procedure of choice rather than excision of large areas of the liver.

Of course, necrotic or devitalized liver must be excised, but resection of entire hepatic lobes to stop severe hemorrhage usually is not necessary if ligation of the hepatic artery is performed first.

Large fractures of the liver with radiating extensions and large areas of necrosis and contusions simply cannot be sutured in most instances. The emergency treatment of these injuries often has been packing. Packing occasionally has been successful in stopping a severe hemorrhage but such an accomplishment is only temporary. Often, unless the surgeon is very careful, the fracture is actually extended during insertion of the pack. If the pack is inserted firmly enough to stop a serious hemorrhage, the cells adjacent to the pack undergo ischemia and necrosis. When the pack is removed, or autolysis occurs (depending upon which happens first), another serious hemorrhage is inevitable. Attempts to prevent secondary hemorrhage by leaving the pack in for a long period, or continuing to insert more pack to keep up with persistent oozing, ultimately will result in severe infection, more autolysis, general sepsis, and death. Thus, packing a complex liver injury does not meet any of the criteria for successful healing, and should not be considered as part of the surgeon's approach to injury of the liver.

Complex fractures and severe contusions in either the right or left lobe of the liver should be treated by hepatic lobectomy if ligation of the hepatic artery does not result in hemostasis. It is important to emphasize, however, that the term lobectomy, as used during these discussions, applies to surgical anatomy (planned according to the blood supply of the liver) and not to external gross anatomy. In general, the central portal and biliary distribution area must be avoided; resection is possible on either side but not in the central area, medial to the gallbladder, and surrounding the portal vessels. Although surgical anatomy, as it pertains to resection of the liver, has been covered adequately in the past, three points are worthy of reemphasis. These are: The dividing line between the right and left lobes is an oblique one, which extends from the gallbladder fossa to the inferior vena cava; the middle hepatic vein lies in the lobar fissure, and in resection of the right lobe care must be taken not to injure this sole source of venous drainage to the medial segment of the left lobe; several small hepatic veins pass directly from the liver to the vena cava and, if they are inadvertently avulsed, they may provide a source of major blood loss and require placement of a suture in the vena cava.

The hepatic artery must be identified carefully before ligation is performed. There is great variation in this vessel, and in as many as 25 per cent of patients, the branch to the medial segment of the left lobe takes origin from the right hepatic artery. Catheters placed in the biliary ducts can be helpful in identifying their arborization in the liver mass. Emergency control of hemorrhage may require cross-clamping of the portal triad. This usually can be done without producing serious hypotension, particularly if the patient is under hypothermia. Extension of an abdominal incision into the thoracic cavity may be necessary, particularly if there is associated diaphragmatic injury, or if the liver injury extends in a posterior direction. Dissection of liver parenchyma should be performed in a blunt fashion using the handle of a knife or the tip of the small finger. When resistance is encountered the structure producing it should be clamped in continuity, divided by sharp dissection, and ligated. It is important to plan resection on the basis of biliary and vascular anatomy and to adhere to the plan as the dissection proceeds. It is important not to select or determine a plane of resection on the basis of the appearance of the external hepatic veins. After the lobe or segment has been excised, a wound is produced which is best characterized as having a deficiency of Glisson's capsule. Omentum, diaphragm, and peritoneum have all been used as a patch graft to replace missing fibrous tissue. Drainage of the biliary tract apparently is of measurable value in the treatment of controlled experimental wounds of the liver in dogs. Experienced surgeons are divided in their opinion about the necessity for draining the common bile duct after repair of a liver injury in human beings. Review of others' experience suggests that drainage of the common duct does not make a significant contribution to healing in the liver.

Drainage of the abdominal cavity is a problem worthy of special consideration. It has been said that drainage may not be needed if the liver has been repaired accurately and, if drainage is needed because accurate repair was not possible, the usual methods of inserting Penrose drains in an abdominal wound are not adequate. Special attention must be directed toward providing direct free drainage of the right upper quadrant; posterior subcostal drains are one method of accomplishing this. Extraordinary accuracy in placing and taking care of large drains and soft tubes is mandatory. Coughing and vomiting should be inhibited when possible. Selection and administration of antibiotics and external care of the wound must be exemplary. It must be remembered, particularly in the upper quadrants of the abdomen, that drains are two-way streets. They provide a route for bacteria to infect hematomas and create subhepatic and subdiaphragmatic abscesses as well as assist in removal of blood and bile.

A biological approach with several theoretical advantages which we developed several years ago may be practical in the future. It has been evaluated primarily in controlled liver injuries in animals and traumatic injuries which extend into surgical "no man's land" (central or portal area) in human beings. Wounds characterized by exposure of large areas of liver parenchyma deficient in Glisson's capsule have been the object of most of our studies. The technique is based on the same reasoning described for other organ wounds where a specific tissue deficiency exists. In the case of extensive liver wounds, the deficiency is primarily in fibrous protein; thus an obvious solution to the problem is a graft of fibrous protein with properties similar to Glisson's capsule. Although many experiments with various fibrous protein membranes have been performed, a graft of reconstituted collagen sponge was found by us to be most satisfactory. Collagen sponge, unlike foam products, has open interstices which can be permeated by connective tissue and cellular elements which need a fibrous stroma in which to proliferate. The material can be used in rolls or pads so that resiliency can be produced to accommodate swelling or hemorrhage during the immediate postoperative period. Collagen sponge can be applied as an external (never internal) pack by attaching it to the liver with a large suture. Reconstituted collagen tapes were very effective in our experiments and proved more useful than the usual suture materials. Nonfatal wounds in a large number of dogs, and potentially fatal central wounds in human liver injuries, were successfully treated by this technique. Unfortunately, collagen sponge with the physical and biological properties needed to resurface broad expanses of exposed hepatic parenchyma is not available commercially at this time. The laboratory preparations used in our experiments were formulated specifically to introduce the concept that an artificially prepared biological dressing could be utilized to meet the specific deficiency of inadequate Glisson's capsule.

In the postoperative period, the surgeon must be familiar with, and on the lookout for, all of the metabolic effects of massive loss of liver substance. These fall into three major categories: carbohydrate, protein, and lipid metabolism. Blood glucose levels must be maintained by constant infusion of glucose; serum albumin levels must be maintained by administration of plasma or human albumin, and other protein metabolic derrangements such as those which affect blood clotting may be so extensive that treatment with fresh whole blood, fibrinogen, or fresh frozen plasma may be required. If fibrinolysis is prominent, treatment with ε-aminocaproic acid may be indicated. Serum nonesterified fatty acids usually are elevated for a few days and then return to normal without treatment.

REPAIR IN CHRONIC LIVER INJURY. Chronic liver injury is a surgical problem only when it becomes necessary to perform emergency or palliative procedures to correct immediate life-threatening events which are the consequence of the disease process. Examples of such procedures are ligation or other treatment of bleeding esophageal varices and portacaval shunt operations to control portal hypertension. It is not proposed to discuss the etiology or treatment of chronic liver injury or its complications. This type of injury is described briefly to illustrate the evil consequences of repair of a cellular organ by fibrous proliferation rather than by true regeneration. The sequence of events in chronic liver injury is seen in all parts of the body where a repeating sequence of injury and repair occurs over a long period of time.

Chronic injury of the liver is characterized by simultaneous cell necrosis and cell regeneration. Cell necrosis frequently begins around the portal venules and progresses toward the central venule. The space left by dead cells around the portal venule and hepatic arteriole is occupied by collapsed ductal and septal tissue. If necrosis involves all of the cells between a portal venule and a central venule, the subsequent collapse brings the portal and hepatic vein systems into contact and shunting occurs. One might surmise that this would prevent any rise in portal pressure, but since progression of the disease causes collapse and compression of the hepatic vein system proximal (relative to the heart) to the shunt, the ultimate effect is to cause portal hypertension.

Regeneration of hepatocytes occurs around the areas of necrosis. Condensations of fibrous septa and ductal tissue force regenerating cells to establish themselves in nodules, surrounded by areas of fibrous repair. Although well supplied by sinusoids and bile ducts, these nodules no longer resemble the normal liver lobule in architecture.

As the disease progresses, the ratio of hydroxyproline to DNA begins to rise, indicating the progressive victory of collagen fiber synthesis over new cell formation. Formation of these fibrous areas around portal and central venules as a result of lobular collapse leads to increasing portal pressure. This, in turn, results in congestion and increased periportal necrosis, further collapse, and further fibrosis, and a chain of events commences that, since it involves the whole liver, becomes irreversible.

As the amount of viable liver tissue decreases, and as the portal pressure increases, all the sequelae of chronic liver disease appear. Because of the enormous reserve capacity of the liver and because, in the early stages, significant regeneration occurs, the serious ill effects of chronic liver disease do not become manifest until it is too late to reverse the course. Only palliative measures will ease the patient as relentless fibrous scarring of the liver progresses.

The contrast between the regeneration seen in acute liver injury and the repair seen in chronic liver injury is only a dramatic instance of the type of competition that goes on in many injured tissues and organs. If an organ's regenerative capacity is great, and the injury is acute and not prolonged, true regeneration may occur. However, if the regenerative capacity is low, or the injury becomes chronic, then fibrous repair may gain ascendancy over regeneration. In some tissues this may be of little consequence, but in a compound organ such as the liver it can be fatal.

Biliary Tract

About the only statement which can be made with certainty about the biology of healing of the extrahepatic biliary tree is that healing will occur unless obstruction is present. Because treatment of wounds of the gallbladder usually is cholecystectomy, the study of wound healing in the biliary system is primarily the study of regeneration or repair of extrahepatic ducts. Healing of extrahepatic ducts is primarily a process of rapid and efficient reepithelization which is characterized by more mitotic activity than has been recognized in other epithelium-lined structures. Fibrous protein synthesis also is prominent during later stages of healing of the biliary tree. Rather extraordinary mitotic activity in the biliary tract is of some interest to surgical biologists because of the remarkably high mortality from cancer of the gallbladder and bile ducts. All cancers of the gallbladder are fatal when diagnosed preoperatively and most are fatal when found incidentally following cholecystectomy, even though no metastases are visible during the operation. Epithelial growth potential, both controlled and uncontrolled, is of a different order from that encountered in most epithelium-lined surfaces. Additional study of this phenomenon undoubtedly will produce potentially useful data concerning the mechanisms of control of epithelial regeneration.

In some patients and under some conditions, of which infection is the most notable, wound contraction becomes an important feature of the healing process in the biliary tree. Wound contraction is not, however, the only cause of postoperative obstruction, as many surgeons have thought it to be. Careful observers have pointed out repeatedly that what may appear by clinical examination to be complete or near complete obstruction of the common bile duct following repair of a wound is not the result of a contracting cicatrix or hypertrophic scar. A surprisingly adequate lumen may be found, after repair of the entire circumference of the common duct, even though the patient appeared clinically to have obstruction. Thus the hypothesis has been advanced that a physiological obstruction, due perhaps to lack of relaxation, or spasm of the sphincter of Oddi, may be the result of interruption of neurologically mediated reflexes following repair of an injury of the common duct. This hypothesis has been supported by studies in dogs measuring the effect of transection and healing of the duct on tone and control of the sphincter of Oddi. Such measurements cannot be considered definitive, at this time, however, and the hypothesis, even though strongly suggested by data obtained in dogs, is not necessarily transferable to human biology.

An interesting facet to the study of healing in the biliary tree is the effect of drainage. Most surgeons, although not all, have been taught and have almost religiously adhered to the concept that repair of an elective acute wound or reconstruction of an old stenosis or transection of the common bile duct must be splinted postoperatively with a tube of some description. On theoretical grounds, use of an internal splint might seem to be a certain way of increasing fibrous protein synthesis during primary healing and secondary wound contraction during secondary remodeling of the scar. In addition to mechanical stimulation and foreign body reaction, entrance of bacteria from the outside wound seems to increase probability of late failure directly attributable to use of a tube. About the only comment that can be made now is that use of a tube following repair of a surgical incision in the common bile duct is not necessary in human beings. Although approximately 99 per cent of the world's surgeons believe that internal drainage of the biliary tract is needed, the other 1 per cent or so do not, and the number of successful cases operated upon without insertion of a drainage tube into the biliary tract has been sufficient to state with confidence that drainage of the duct with a T tube or other device following elective exploration and repair of the wound is not necessary. Stenosis and obstruction are not caused by failure to drain the duct. (It is, of course, mandatory to drain Morrison's pouch for a few days following biliary tract surgery.) On the other hand, the fact that so many hundreds of thousands of internal drains have been inserted in biliary tracts over the years without a high incidence of stricture or other complications directly attributable to the tube emphasizes how very little we actually know about healing in the biliary tract, and the factors which influence it. Overuse or poor use of a drainage tube in the extrahepatic duct is a detriment to function. Tubes can obstruct ducts and failure to keep tubes clean and properly flushed invariably causes cholangitis and chronic duct obstruction.

In some patients, however, the effect of uncontrolled healing or overhealing in the biliary tract can be so disastrous that we are stimulated to find out why cicatrization and anatomical obstruction do occur in these unfortunate individuals. Biological control of fibrous protein synthesis and scar contraction could be extremely useful in biliary tract surgery, as it shows promise of being in other tissues. With the exception of infection, we simply cannot show a cause-and-effect relation at this time between factors such as foreign bodies, circumferential healing, and selection of sutures and the type of healing which is characterized by circumferential wound contraction or stenosis. Factors other than those which theoretically might cause a stenosing contracture must be involved; such factors have not yet been identified, and so the possibility of controlling the healing process is still open to those who are curious enough to investigate and attempt to control it. Clinical experience reveals that tension must be avoided at all costs if secondary contractures and stenosis are to be avoided. Ducts sutured under tension invariably become stenosis complications. Thus mobilization of the duct or gastrointestinal tract must be accomplished before reconstruction is started.

An extremely interesting and clinically provocative study on regeneration of the common bile duct in dogs has suggested that, if just a small strip of common bile duct wall remains intact, the duct will regenerate with amazing functional and anatomical reproduction of a normal structure. A similar phenomenon in human beings also has been suggested on the basis of a few uncontrolled observations. This important biological phenomenon has been explored clinically by using a vein graft to bring new tissue into a constricted area. If a tiny bridge of posterior duct wall remains, even though it is only a few millimeters in width, replacement of the vein graft will occur by epithelization, fibrous protein synthesis, and minimal contraction and stretching of the remaining bridge.

Most of our surgical efforts to date have been mechanical struggles to obtain adequate exposure so that two ends of a severed duct can be approximated without tension. Why an anastomosis without tension is so important in prevention of a secondary stricture is not entirely clear at this time. The phenomenon could relate to leakage of bile and external scarring or to some complex phenomenon such as the effect of longitudinal tension upon horizontal or circumferential remodeling of newly synthesized connective tissue. Whatever the mechanism, however, longitudinal tension on the suture line of a repaired biliary duct can be correlated with severe stenosis during the postoperative period. The method recommended at present by most experienced surgeons is to anastomose the proximal biliary tract to the duodenum or to the jejunum when possible. When insufficient proximal duct makes these procedures impossible, hepaticojejunostomy can be attempted. Such procedures are practically always followed by long periods (many months or years in some clinics) of internal splinting and external drainage. Although it seems miraculous to the student of wound healing, they appear to provide a semipermanent or permanent conduit for bile in some patients. Reconstruction with a long-term internal splint does not suffice for the majority of patients, however, and the occasional patient who develops disastrous circumferential stenosis following seemingly simple trauma or uncomplicated repair attests to the fact that further investigation of biliary tract healing and the factors which influence it could be extremely rewarding. Biological control of healing with inhibition or control of fibrous protein synthesis and wound contraction could have one of its greatest applications in surgery of the external biliary tract.

Finally, replacement of the duct continues to interest a few surgeons. The problem of internal clogging by precipitation of bile salts has been relieved considerably by introduction of silicone and other biologically nonreactive, conductive hydrophilic polymers such as Hydron. The problems of attachment of viable tissue at either end, functional considerations of distal sphincter control and reaction, and absence of self-regenerating capacity through the many years that such artificial conduits have to serve when they are placed in young individuals keep this approach from being quite as exciting as the possibility of a more biological approach based on utilization of normal regenerative powers which could be possible with the biological control of fibrous protein synthesis and wound contraction. Until major discoveries or breakthroughs of this type occur, however, the external biliary tree will remain an area where technical competence is extremely important and where manual dexterity, operative experience, and surgical judgment of the surgeon often are the most important factors we have to offer patients, the difference being that between survival and death from biliary obstruction.

Pancreas

Wound healing and management of wounds of the pancreas are more concerned with the direction and flow of pancreatic secretions than with cellular or fibrous protein aspects of repair. Wounds of the pancreas and pancreatic ducts heal by either primary or secondary intention, and (unlike the case with liver and spleen) there is enough fibrous protein stroma to hold tissues adequately until natural tensile strength has been restored. Wound contraction is not a prominent characteristic of healing in the pancreas; pancreatic duct obstruction is usually the result of parenchymal edema or pathological conditions of the sphincter of Oddi. Thus the pancreas may be repaired with sutures and will heal superbly by fibrous protein synthesis, epithelization, and aggregation and polymerization of fibrin.

The primary concern of the surgeon is not wound healing biology but the physiology and biochemistry of pancreatic secretion. Such a statement should not be interpreted as implying that pancreatic wounds are not extremely dangerous injuries. The pancreas lies deeper than many other organs in the abdominal cavity and is relatively firmly attached to immovable structures. A penetrating or blunt abdominal wound must be severe to injure the pancreas, and when such an injury occurs there is a 15 to 20 per cent chance of a fatal outcome. Mortality of such injuries cannot be correlated, however, with degree of injury of the pancreas, or with complications associated with wound healing; it is almost always due to associated injury such as damage to a major blood vessel (and hemorrhage) or to surrounding organs. Of course, development of such complications as pseudocysts and sinuses increases the morbidity of a pancreatic injury.

The morbidity of pancreatic wounds is related primarily to the effect of injury and healing on the flow and disposal of pancreatic secretion. Depending on where and how pancreatic secretion is directed, the result may be acute or chronic pancreatitis, pancreatic pseudocyst, pancreatic fistula, or a large abscess. Fistulas are more often the result of penetrating injuries, whereas pseudocyst, pancreatitis, and abscess are more often complications of blunt nonpenetrating abdominal injuries. Most complications can be prevented by performing subtotal pancreatectomy, and this is probably the treatment of choice following complete transection (relatively rare) or severe contusing or fragmenting injuries. Previous concern that health would be impaired by reduction of endocrine and exocrine secretion is known now to be unfounded if no more than 80 per cent of the pancreas is removed. Removal of the body or tail of the pancreas has another advantage in that it affords excellent exposure to areas of potentially serious hemorrhage in the splenic pedicle. Distal excision of a serious wound of the pancreas should not be undertaken if the general condition of the patient is not appropriate for a procedure of this magnitude, or if other more serious or life-threatening injuries require attention during the operative time permissible. Recent reports of performing total pancreatectomy and duodenectomy for extensive wounds of the body and head of the pancreas should not be interpreted as recommendations that this form of treatment is preferable to more conservative measures for most patients and for most surgeons under most conditions. Under most circumstances, adequate drainage of the lesser peritoneal sac and retroperitoneal area, combined with simple suture of the pancreatic parenchyma to stop hemorrhage, may be all that is advisable. Such treatment often is followed by development of a fistula or pseudocyst, either of which may resolve spontaneously, particularly if the pancreas is put to rest by use of large doses of atropine and gastric drainage. Operative diversion of pancreatic secretion into the gastrointestinal tract is a relatively simple and satisfactory method of managing persistent pseudocyst or fistulas. Because development of cysts and fistulas was believed in the past to be due partially to spasm or healing in the sphincter area, some surgeons have recommended sphincterotomy at the time of repair of the pancreatic wound. Duodenostomy and sphincterotomy add considerable operating time and trauma, however, and so the procedure has not seemed to be a wise one in the judgment of most surgeons. The same reasoning holds for the Roux-en-Y and other intestinal drainage procedures performed at the time of primary wound management. An alternate procedure which accomplishes the same objectives with considerably less operative time and trauma is simple cannulation of the proximal end of the transected duct with a small polyethylene catheter. If the distal pancreas is removed and a small polyethylene catheter is inserted into the distal end of the proximal duct, the remaining pancreas, including the important proximal segment which contains the common bile duct, will be decompressed or drained effectively in a retrograde manner. The polyethylene catheter will direct the pancreatic secretion through other tissues, such as skin, without damage and make collection simple so that the high-bicarbonate, low-protein secretion can be returned to the patient with ease. Withdrawal of the catheter after healing has occurred and edema in the pancreas has subsided usually will be followed by a transient fistula which will close spontaneously. In some respects, retrograde external drainage of the pancreatic duct system is equivalent to producing an intentional duodenal fistula at the time of gastrectomy. The physiological and biological significance of an external fistula of the pancreas, however, is vastly different from that of a duodenal fistula. Decompression of the biliary tree at the time of repair of pancreatic injuries also has been recommended. This does not seem necessary in our judgment, particularly if adequate drainage of the pancreatic duct system is provided. Primary reconstruction of the pancreatic ducts, although technically feasible, is often followed by unsatisfactory healing and probably should not be attempted in most patients.

Ingenious methods for producing pancreatic pseudocysts and chronic fistulas in dogs have been developed. The fact that so little experimental work has been done on the subject of wound healing and wound management of pancreatic injuries, however, suggests that general surgical judgment, particularly regarding institution of adequate retroperitoneal, lesser sac, and internal duct drainage, is all that is usually needed to insure excellent healing without serious complications. Associated injuries to other organs and blood vessels remain the most dangerous aspect of pancreatic injuries.

TRACHEA

Two serious problems complicate wound healing in the trachea. One is formation of granulation tissue in the subglottic area following tracheostomy. This distressing complication occurs most often in small infants after an emergency tracheostomy. Chronic presence of granulation tissue in these desperately ill infants can make closure of the tracheostomy virtually impossible or extremely dangerous for many months or even years. Control of granulation tissue is not possible or reliable by any known pharmacological, surgical, or biological method. Cortisone reduces somewhat and delays slightly formation of granulation tissue, but it does not eliminate the problem. The best therapy is preventive. It is seldom necessary to perform a tracheostomy in tiny infants; the procedure should be avoided unless absolutely necessary for survival. Forced bag insufflation, insertion of large needles below the larynx, and skilled intubation of the trachea all are superior alternatives to an emergency tracheostomy in a young infant.

A second and equally serious complication of wound healing in the trachea is chronic stenosis. A combination of formation of new fibrous tissue and wound contraction seems to be involved in producing this extremely serious complication of healing. As in treatment of common bile duct injuries, anastomosis of the trachea without tension is paramount in the surgical cure of tracheal stenosis. It was previously thought that no more than 2 cm. of trachea (four rings) could be removed and followed by a primary anastomosis which would not become stenotic. The brilliant work of Grillo in devising techniques by which as much as half of the trachea can be excised and a successful anastomosis performed without tension has expanded the possibilities of reconstruction of the trachea during the last few years. Foreign bodies and prosthetic tubes are mentioned only to be condemned. No prosthetic trachea has permanently solved the problem of stenosis. End-to-end anastomosis without tension must be achieved if the complication of stenosis is to be avoided. Thus the surgery of wound healing complications in the trachea is really an exercise in applied mediastinal and cervical anatomy. For details of operative management, the reader is referred to the monumental treatises by Grillo summarizing his experience in this area.

URINARY TRACT

Kidney

The kidney, like the liver, is primarily a cellular organ. Unlike the liver, however, it has a well developed fibrous capsule and is more generously endowed with fibrous stroma. The result is that repair of wounds of the kidney is not quite so difficult as repair in liver or spleen and healing usually is less complicated. On the other hand, injuries of the kidney are seldom clean lacerations leaving capsule or parenchyma which can be approximated neatly. Blunt contusions and ragged fractures often are not repairable by conventional suturing techniques. Mild contusions or fractures usually can be managed conservatively; healing occurs primarily by fibrous protein synthesis. A scar is produced which may replace some functioning nephrons, but wound contraction secondarily involving other units is not a predominant part of the healing process.

The decision to operate upon a wound of the kidney usually is based on injury to the major collecting system or great vessels. Such injuries are defined by pyelography and arteriography. Treatment consists of either amputation of a portion of the kidney (when a major portion with adequate vascularization and drainage can be preserved) or nephrectomy. Occasionally a clean laceration is found which can be repaired by approximating the capsule; sometimes a radiating fracture is not so extensive that closure is impossible. Complications of wound closure are continued hemorrhage, subcapsular hematoma, perirenal abscess, and severe fibrosis from organization of a hematoma or extravasation of urine. The likelihood of these complications is diminished if adequate suction drainage of the retroperitoneal area is provided. Methods of providing such drainage are described more completely in the section on management of injuries of the ureter.

Injuries of the renal medulla and major collecting system can be repaired in many patients. In the collecting system, particularly the ureteropelvic juncture, wound contraction is a more prominent feature of healing than it is in the cortex of the kidney. Stenosis is a common complication of healing in the ureteropelvic junction and secondary revision of stenotic areas often is needed to change the direction of scar tissue and contraction forces. The basic principles in revision of strictures at the ureteropelvic junction are the same as those outlined in the section on revision of cutaneous scar. Scars which cross lines of changing dimension interfere with peristalsis and drainage. Bringing more tissue into the area when the diagnosis is lack of tissue, or changing the direction of scar tissue when contraction is the cause of deformity, or doing both if the diagnosis reveals multiple causes for poor drainage, is successful in many patients. As in skin, failure to make a correct diagnosis and performing a secondary reconstructive procedure selected out of respect for the man's name attached to it or "what seemed to work last time" frequently are responsible for failure of reconstructive procedures at the ureteropelvic junction.

Subtotal excision of the kidney is the preferable method for managing fractures or contusions which are not so extensive as to require nephrectomy yet are too severe to be repaired primarily. Excision of a portion of the kidney can be performed through any plane which does not encroach upon the blood supply and drainage of the remaining portion. The immediate problem for the surgeon after subtotal nephrectomy is hemorrhage and closure of the wound. Hemorrhage can be managed by compression provided some material containing fibrous protein is available to repair the defect in the capsule. Renal capsule, if available, is the ideal material. Often, however, capsule is deficient when the injury is severe enough to require subtotal amputation, and free grafts of fascia or peritoneum and application of artificial substances such as hemostatic agents or reconstituted collagen have been utilized successfully to close the wound. We have found reconstituted collagen sponge ideal for grafting the cut surface of the kidney; others have had a similar experience with collagen film. Hemostatic foam preparations have been used; free or pedicle grafts of fat, fascia, and peritoneum have been reported as being successful also.

The use of monomeric tissue adhesives has appeared more practical for treating renal wounds than in almost any other organ. Although problems of quality control, distribution, and skill in applying adhesives have prevented these substances from being widely accepted for repair of renal injuries, their effectiveness in animal experimentation and a few human cases has been superior to that reported for tissue adhesives in other organs. This is probably because it is possible to control blood supply to the kidney for a long enough period to properly prepare the surface. Success is also due to the fact that the surgeon can deliver the kidney into the operative wound and isolate it from other tissues long enough to use the adhesives properly. Temporary complete hemostasis and isolation of wounds of other organs often is not possible. Experimental data are encouraging and further clinical experience is being obtained. Theoretically, the ideal substance to apply to the cut surface of a kidney would be monomeric collagen if it could be made to aggregate, polymerize, and form a tough replication of the renal capsule. All previous attempts to apply neutral cold collagen or acid-soluble collagen to wound surfaces have been disappointing as far as increasing the collagen content of the scar is concerned. Reconstituted collagen sponges or sheets of natural collagen such as fascia lata or peritoneum applied as free grafts are superior to reconstituted collagen from collagen solutions. The physical weave of small fibrils in naturally formed collagen is probably the single most important factor in providing the physical strength needed for immediate closure of a large wound, and most artificial collagen products lack the wet strength of naturally aggregated collagen. Among other factors, the stabilizing effect of various combinations of mucopolysaccharides, which contribute significantly to the physical properties of membranes, is absent.

Ureter

The ureters are of special interest because the incidence of injury is high and complications of repair are serious. As in the common bile duct, there is a high incidence of surgical accidents responsible for ureteral wounds; perhaps this is why the surgeon has a tendency to overtreat them. Also like the biliary tract, there is remarkable regenerative potential in the ureter and some of the physical manipulations which the surgeon may use in an attempt to guarantee patency of the conduit may actually diminish or prevent regeneration. As in so many organs, fibrous protein synthesis—out of control—may overwhelm regeneration and physically interfere with whatever function remains after continuity has been reestablished. Application of rather scant knowledge available at present in the field of ureteral wound healing is concerned mostly with the effect of urine flow on fibrous protein synthesis and wound contraction.

The problem is not obtaining a healed wound. Urothelium has enormous proliferative potential and epithelium, submucosal tissue, or a combination of the two unquestionably has inordinate inductive action on mesenchymal stem cells. The result is that soft tissues surrounding a wound of the ureter and bladder are frequently induced to form rather massive amounts of fibrous tissue. Sometimes, in both dogs and human beings, induction of fibrous tissue proceeds along lines of osteogenesis. In other cases, it follows lines of lymphoid and muscle tissue formation. Mature bone is often found in the retroperitoneal or abdominal tissues following management of a wound of the ureter or bladder. The clinically based assumption that a combination of urothelium and urine is required for bone formation has not been confirmed experimentally; considerable work has been done on the osteogenesis-inductive properties of urothelium and it can be stated that these properties are not dependent entirely upon the presence of urine. It is also quite definite, however, that urinary flow within a healing ureter in which urothelium has been exposed and repaired results in production of considerably more fibrous tissue than is found in similar wounds in which urine has been diverted. There may be a higher incidence of bone formation in wounds which are not drained properly; this has not been shown conclusively, however.

The healing process is a rather straightforward progression of biological events similar to those studied in other tubular organs. It consists first of rapid and effective proliferation of urothelium by mitosis and migration of dedifferentiated cells. The highly specialized epithelium (remarkably unaffected by changes in hydrostatic pressure, hydrogen ion concentration, or metabolic poisons released by invading organisms) effectively seals the leak within 48 hours provided nothing is done to prevent it. An early watertight anastomosis, seldom obtained because of the effect of sutures, does not guarantee unobstructed flow of urine into the bladder, however. This is why many urologists have been so concerned with diversion procedures when repairing ureteral wounds. Physical restoration of a draining conduit must be accompanied by return of peristalsis if drainage of the kidney is to be adequate. Peristalsis is absent in the distal segment of a completely transected ureter for at least 10 to 14 days after repair. Although return of distal peristalsis in a repaired ureter usually does occur, it seems to be independent of peristalsis in the proximal segment for some time. In some patients normal peristalsis seems never to return, as far as coordinated unidirectional propulsive action is concerned. This is one of several reasons why urologists prefer to sacrifice the distal segment of a ureter rather than repair it circumferentially when reimplantation into the bladder is possible.

Fibrous protein synthesis interestingly does not appear to be a prominent part of ureteral healing when complete diversion of urinary flow has been accomplished during the healing period. In animals, a ureteral repair followed by immediate nephrectomy does not result in significant scar; fibrous protein synthesis seems limited to reestablishing adequate longitudinal tensile strength and overhealing is not observed. Also, wound contraction is not so prominent when nephrectomy has been performed. In other laboratory preparations and occasionally in human beings, however, if all urinary flow is not diverted by proximal ureterostomy of some type, healing, primarily in surrounding tissues, and wound contraction result in a severely, if not completely, obstructed ureter. The problem has been so formidable that numerous opinions have been published, even in relatively modern urological literature, suggesting that repair of a complete 360 degree transection of the ureter will almost always be followed by hydronephrosis. Such experience, plus the natural tendency of the surgeon to put a tube in every hollow organ he manipulates or repairs, has been responsible for the widespread belief that healing of the ureter must occur over an internal splint to be successful and that the larger the splint and the longer it is kept in place, the better the effect on wound healing will be. At almost the same time that the first doubts were raised about a similar approach to biliary tract surgery, from the point of view of fundamental wound healing biology, emphasis shifted from internal drainage in repair of the ureter to external wound drainage and proximal diversion of urinary flow. Recent reports strongly suggest that improvement in functional results has been spectacular. Where biological principles of wound healing have directed the thinking of urologists, there has been a remarkable improvement in the results of ureteral reconstruction, both in laboratory preparations and in clinical practice. Progress has been so striking that a number of experienced urologists now recommend that ureteral splinting by an internal catheter not be done. Instead, they emphasize meticulous coaptation of the divided ureter, preservation of segmental blood supply, avoidance of fixation of the ureter to immovable structures, and diversion of the urinary stream. Diversion of urinary flow by a proximal ureterostomy certainly is not always necessary. Under favorable circumstances, simple anastomosis without proximal diversion has produced excellent results. Theoretically and practically, small plain gut sutures seem to be the most satisfactory suture material when repairing a ureter; Polyglactin-910 appears to be equally satisfactory, but experience with this new synthetic absorbable suture is limited. It was previously thought that chromic gut or nonabsorbable sutures should not be used because they serve as a nidus for deposition of urinary salts and development of a ureteral stone. Recent reports of successful repair of ureteral transections with fine silk sutures raise some doubt about the absolute interdiction of permanent sutures. Whether the anastomosis is end-to-end, everted, or inverted in type has not seemed to make an important difference. Stapling and gluing ureteral surfaces also have been accomplished successfully in laboratory animals. Again, the problem seems related more to what happens to surrounding mesenchymal tissues and what they will be induced to do than to what will happen in the actual suture line of the ureter or how it can be controlled by adjustment of the edges. An oval anastomosis provided by cutting the ureter obliquely or making a small longitudinal slit to increase the circumference of the cut edge, thus producing an oblique suture line, seems to be somewhat better than a circular suture line, however.

An important point, as far as function is concerned, is the observation that ureters normally lie on a cushion of retroperitoneal fat. Apparently, satisfactory unidirectional propulsion of urine is dependent, to some extent, upon freedom of movement of the ureter on such a cushion. Surgical maneuvers or complications of healing which fix the ureter to an immovable structure such as the spine or lumbodorsal fascia seriously inhibit return of effective peristalsis and unobstructed flow of urine. The retroperitoneal fat pad should be carefully protected and all possible measures taken to be sure that the ureter is not left adjacent to an immovable structure. Urinary diversion is probably best performed by making a longitudinal ureterotomy at least 5 cm. proximal to the anastomosis. Some urologists recommend removing an oval segment of ureter to insure that the path of least resistance for urine is via the proximal ureterostomy and not the anastomosis. If the procedure has been performed through a transperitoneal approach, the retroperitoneal space must be freely drained posteriorly; the peritoneum should be closed tightly anteriorly. If a retroperitoneal approach was used, drainage of the ureterostomy should be provided by the use of large rubber drains or suction catheters placed in a dependent position. Periureteral and peripelvic fascia should be widely split to permit adequate egress of urine without internal dissection along tissue planes. Suction drainage is preferred and catheters should be placed alongside but not against the reconstructed ureter. The position of catheters is so important that a few small absorbable sutures should be used to insure that they are in the proper plane and position. Drainage should be continued for at least nine days to insure an adequate soft tissue drainage tract while watertight healing of the ureter is occurring. Closure of the ureterostomy usually will occur in a few days after drains are removed. Ureteroneocystostomy should always be performed if a ureteroureterostomy repair cannot be performed under ideal circumstances.

Repair of a ureteral injury utilizing the general principles outlined above eliminates problems involved with internal splints. These problems include introduction of bacterial infection, the need for frequent acid irrigation, overhydration, and use of acid-ash diets. A serious complication of internal ureteral splints—stenosis in previously undamaged ureter at the end of the splint—also is eliminated.

Replacement of a ureter has been the subject of considerable study; the results have been interesting but not particularly useful for human reconstructive surgery. The most satisfactory ureteral substitute has been a bladder flap tubed to form a conduit and rotated superiorly to replace the lower one-third of the ureter. Actually, a divided ureter, with a 2 cm. gap, left free in the retroperitoneal space will be reconstituted with time. Epithelium will bridge the gap but in the process sacculations, double lumen, or other inadequate conduits are produced. A point of considerable interest has been whether the smooth muscle at either end of the ureter has regenerative potential and can be counted upon in unidirectional propulsion of urine. The few good studies which have been completed suggest that regeneration of smooth muscle in a transected ureter is very small. There is some hyperplasia of smooth muscle but regeneration is usually more the effect of wound contraction pulling the muscular coat from each end of the ureter into the repaired area. There is little evidence that mitosis and proliferation of smooth muscle cells occur. More data about this interesting subject will be given in the discussion of regeneration of the bladder; here we shall simply say that audioradiography and cell labeling studies on regenerating ureter strongly suggest that proliferation of smooth muscle, although present to a small extent, is not an important or dependable part of the healing process.

The fibrous proliferation stage of ureteral regeneration produces a remarkably well polarized and morphologically appealing adventitia. Almost invariably, however, a stricture occurs during secondary remodeling of the fibrous tissue scar; stenosis will be severe in every case if an internal splint is used to direct regenerative processes. Unidirectional, unobstructed propulsion of urine is not possible following regeneration of the ureter in human beings. Studies of regeneration in animals have been of interest more from a regenerative biological standpoint than from the possibility of clinical application. A fundamental biological study with considerable clinical emphasis, however, has been concerned with regeneration after subtotal loss of the circumference of a ureter. The sum and substance of this study is that if at least 50 per cent of the circumference of the ureter remains, a relatively long defect will be closed by natural processes of epithelization, fibrous protein synthesis, and longitudinal (not circumferential) wound contraction. Thus a relatively large patch of ureter may be removed in performing a proximal diverting urethrostomy to assure complete diversion of the urinary stream without fear of stenosis after wound healing is complete. As in the case of repair of transections, diversion of urinary flow and avoidance of internal splinting increase the likelihood of a successful functional result.

Bladder

Incised and sutured wounds of the bladder heal with almost the same sequence of biochemical and morphological steps as other compound tissues. Collagen content is diminished temporarily in the area of wound repair but collagen synthesis is measurable by the fifth day and continues until adequate tensile strength is regained. Although actual rupture strength of the scar tissue and bladder have not been determined under controlled conditions, clinical observations suggest that the strength of a scar not only does not reach that of uninjured bladder but that the difference can be responsible for rupture through an area of previous healing. As in bowel, a scar is the point of least resistance to rising intraluminal pressure and, if rupture of a repaired bladder occurs, it invariably will be at the point where healing took place. This is particularly true for large scars in small bladders such as those produced during repair of exstrophy or closure of remnants of the bladder following subtotal cystectomy. When signs of abdominal or pelvic inflammation appear in patients who have had bladder surgery, a small dehiscence of the scar should be suspected. Closure of bladder incisions should be by means of rather large through-and-through absorbable sutures. The tendency of sutures to become the nidus for deposition of urinary salts or formation of bone is adequate reason to use only plain catgut sutures. Closure of bladder wounds is sometimes accompanied by suprapubic drainage to assure maximal rest of bladder tissue and adequate soft tissue drainage overlying the bladder wound.

Mucosal defects in the bladder heal by extraordinarily effective epithelization. In fact, the process is so effective that if the entire bladder is denuded of urothelium, regeneration from ureteral sources (possibly urethral sources also) occurs within 30 days. The process involves more mitotic division of cells than is usually seen in restoration of other epithelium-lined surfaces. PAS-positive mucopolysaccharides are produced in large quantity; the presence of urine seems to accelerate this process. After the bladder is reepithelized following total removal of epithelial lining, the dome is often covered with a thinner layer of cells than the trigone; this indicates that migratory activity exceeds mitosis. The normal mixture of clear cells and compact cells is changed with compact cells predominating after reepithelization. Physiological and biological effects of denuding a portion or all of the bladder are surprisingly few. Absorption of urinary products does not exert a pronounced effect on general health; voiding and bladder capacity are not significantly altered. An interesting complication of reepithelization is a high incidence of some degree of ureteral reflux; this strongly suggests that regeneration does not leave a bladder with perfectly normal function even though morphologically it may appear completely restored. In many patients ureteral reflux is not clinically significant, but if it is followed by hydronephrosis of any degree, it can be severe and should be a positive indication for frequent examinations of the urinary tract.

A study of reepithelization of the totally denuded bladder is of more scientific than clinical interest at this time because there is seldom any need to strip the bladder of its epithelial covering. Interest in removing urothelium from the bladder, therefore, stems primarily from attempts to treat multiple papillomas. Although stripping all of the mucous membrane from the bladder solves the immediate problem of multiple papillomas, epithelium that regenerates appears to be affected by the same factors that were responsible for papillomatosis originally. Reepithelized bladder develops multiple papillomas as if an inductor substance in urine or adjacent tissue was responsible. A possible solution to this problem is resurfacing the denuded bladder with another type of epithelium such as squamous or columnar epithelium provided by a free graft of skin or intestinal mucosa. Although such replacements have been shown to be technically possible and to provide a surface which is morphologically and physiologically compatible with storing urine under changing hydrodynamic pressures, we do not have biological data on the fate of transplanted epithelium in human beings. The danger of neoplastic changes, in particular, has not been measured.

Most surgeons have thought that the bladder is an exception to the general principle that only tissues (usually not compound organs) regenerate. The idea that the bladder is a compound organ with amazing regenerative capacity is probably due more to the fact that patients and animals can be made to store urine after cystectomy than to any sophisticated studies on the regenerative biology of bladder wall. If a mold or stent is placed in the proper position and intermittent storage and expulsion of urine are continued, the enormous regenerative capacity of uroepithelium and the propensity for urine to stimulate fibrous tissue reaction in mesenchymal tissues can be combined to produce a fairly satisfactory storage sac for urine. That anything more than a urothelium-lined hollow scar is produced after total cystectomy, however, has not been proved by modern techniques for studying regenerative activity. There is no question that a substantial portion of the bladder (more than 75 per cent) can be excised and, particularly if the trigone remains, closure of the remnant around a stent no larger than a 5 cc. Foley bag will be followed in a few weeks by development of a 30 cc. capacity. Within three months the capacity of the pseudocyst may be as much as 300 cc. and voiding may be amazingly effective. Whether or not ureteral reflux, the *bête noire* of all bladder surgery, will be present, however, seems to be dependent more on the state or condition of the ureters at the time the bladder was reconstructed than on how much bladder was removed or what type of reconstructive procedure was selected. Ureters that were dilated or scarred at the time of cystectomy usually will be found to reflux postoperatively; in normal ureters there is only insignificant reflux without hydronephrosis or no reflux at all following subtotal bladder reconstruction. Apparent regeneration of the bladder following subtotal cystectomy is a combination, therefore, of epithelial regeneration, synthesis and remodeling of scar tissue, hypertrophy and proliferation of smooth muscle, and stretching of the bladder remnant. Function can be superb following these processes, particularly if the trigone was preserved and the ureters were round.

Regeneration of the bladder following total cystectomy is another story. If urinary diversion is carried out, no evidence of regeneration is seen in experimental animals. If a stent is inserted and urinary flow is preserved with the aid of ureteral and urethral catheters, a pocket lined with urothelium and surrounded by typical fibrous tissue induced by foreign body or extravasated urine will be formed. The functional results range from dismal failure to a reasonably effective reservoir which will hold from 50 to 300 cc. of urine with some degree of continence and only a small degree of hydroureter or hydronephrosis. Continence, of course, is due entirely to voluntary skeletal muscle contraction in the pelvic diaphragm. It tends to be more satisfactory at the beginning of the day than in the afternoon or during sleep. Patients who have undergone this operation have understandably been extremely interesting to urological surgeons, and the bladder has been assigned regenerative capacities which on critical analysis do not seem completely warranted.

Urothelial regeneration and fibrous tissue synthesis are components of wound healing similar to those described in other tissues; appearance or lack of smooth muscle in a bladder which is thought to have regenerated, however, is pivotal in determining whether regeneration actually occurred. Smooth muscle regeneration, of course, does occur in other organs such as the uterus. It also is found surrounding blood vessels which are actively proliferating. About all that can be said at this time about smooth muscle regeneration in bladder, however, is that careful examination of bladder wall which is thought to have regenerated following total or subtotal cystectomy reveals only that some smooth muscle fibers can be identified. As in fibrous tissue components, there is no consistent or purposeful weave to the smooth muscle in regenerated bladder. There is very little evidence that the isolated muscle cells that are occasionally found in scar tissue surrounding an implant are arranged or innervated to produce coordinated contraction. The cells appear to be the result of random induction or differentiation of totipotent cells rather than an organized attempt to reduplicate the structure of the detrusor muscle.

The enormous capacity for regeneration which urothelium shows has already been observed and utilized clinically in such situations as resurfacing of a large prostatic urethra after prostatectomy. The combination of urothelial proliferation and synthesis of organized connective tissue is only beginning to be explored as far as clinical applications are concerned. The biological control of the amount and type of scar tissue induced could be useful in further studies of means to utilize these natural phenomena in reconstructing the urinary tract. Fortunately, the physiological and mechanical requirements for excretory function are relatively simple. Combined utilization of the natural regenerative processes of urothelium, the biological control of the amount and physical properties of scar tissue, and improvement of technical methods for revising and altering the tissue produced offer exciting possibilities during the years ahead for those interested in reconstruction of the urinary tract.

Urethra

Posterior Urethra.   The posterior urethra heals readily by epithelization, fibrous protein synthesis, and scar contraction. Primary treatment of a complete transection is directed toward realigning as accurately as possible the two cut ends of the urethra. This is usually accomplished without difficulty through a combination retroperitoneal and intravesicular approach. Short-term use of a catheter serves to direct the course or channel or reepithelization. Fibrous protein synthesis in the submucosal tissue is not excessive and usually does not result in any serious narrowing of the lumen. Fibrous protein synthesis in surrounding tissue, particularly the corpus spongiosum, can be excessive, however, and even more important, it undergoes secondary remodeling of a type which may lead to progressive and unrelenting stricture. Such strictures may be deceiving by the usual methods of investigation. Only the most carefully performed urethrograms accurately portray the true longitudinal extent of a posterior urethral stricture and thus provide accurate information for the surgeon contemplating a reconstructive procedure. Because tissue other than mucous membrane is involved in production of a posterior urethral stricture, it is probably important to combine accurate apposition of mucosal edges with superb hemostasis and external drainage to minimize scarring of surrounding soft tissue and thus lessen the severity of a secondary stricture.

Treatment of stricture of the posterior urethra, like treatment of stricture of other conduits in the body, has been dominated for over 2500 years by a mechanistic approach with the objective of immediate enlargement of the channel. Fundamental biological considerations of the mechanisms of fibrous protein synthesis, cross-linking, and remodeling of collagen and the possibilities of controlling these processes have not been prominent in the clinician's approach. The same can be said for the other important contribution to stricture formation — wound contraction. The two oldest approaches to correction of a posterior urethral stricture, forcible dilatation and incision of the stenosed area, are excellent examples of a nonbiological approach to a problem which has a simple biological basis and an even sounder biological means of exploration for long-term failure of mechanical treatment. Only recently have the most basic fundamentals of reconstructive surgery — accurate diagnosis of what is missing, re-creation of the defect by excision of the products of healing, and transplantation of missing tissue with similar physical properties — been introduced into urological thinking. In so many ways, the story is similar to that of the history of surgery of stenosis of the esophagus or common bile duct.

Mechanical dilatation of a fibrous stricture of the posterior urethra results in several biological events. The most immediate (and perhaps most damaging) is rupture of collagen fibers and fibrils to enlarge the internal diameter of the urethra. If dilatation is done gradually and over a long enough period of time, the best that one can hope for is longitudinal slippage of individual fibrils so that permanent lengthening of collagen bundles occurs. Collagenolytic activity is stimulated by mechanical forces in some areas and under some conditions, and it is possible that softening of scar in the corpus spongiosum (reported following gross observation by some observers) occurs by this mechanism and is responsible for further enlargement of the internal diameter. Permanent enlargement, which is occasionally reported, must be the result of remodeling of the external scar in response to stretching so that a permanent increase in the diameter of the urethra occurs. More often, however, after a few weeks of measurable enlargement, constriction of the lumen begins again and may progress to an even more severe stenosis than was present before dilatation was performed. This is also the course of events if an incision is made with an intraurethral instrument. In these cases one can only surmise that collagen synthesis (also known to be stimulated by mechanical forces) exceeds collagen degradation and that remodeled scar tissue becomes more restrictive from the standpoint of accommodating urinary flow. There can be no doubt that the secondary wounding phenomenon also is drawn into play by the frequent use of a sound. This is undoubtedly why most urologists have found that if relief is not obtained for at least 60 days following dilatation, repeated use of a sound should not be resorted to.

Just as it is possible to obtain permanent lengthening of a flexor tendon adhesion by waiting for or perhaps stimulating remodeling of deep scar tissue, it also may be possible to force changes in the dimensions of a posterior urethral scar by mechanical means. The secondary healing effect and the fine balance between collagen synthesis and collagen degradation apparently are much more delicate in the posterior urethra than in tissue of the hand during healing of a flexor tendon graft. Hundreds of years of experience attest to the unsatisfactory overall results of the mechanical approach to urethral scarring, even though an occasional good result is undeniable. Urologists have become more interested, therefore, in applying techniques which have successfully controlled scar tissue elsewhere in the body to the problem of stricture of the urethra. The results so far have been encouraging. It is hoped that this treatise and other discourses on the possibility of greater success by the biological control of physical properties and amount of scar tissue during healing may open an even greater vista of urological service.

Application of modern principles of reconstructive surgery to the problem of posterior urethral strictures has been based on the following general considerations. The defect (caused by trauma, necrosis, infection, or congenital abnormalities) is found less in mucosa than in elastic properties of submucosa and corpus spongiosum. The undesirable effects of wound healing are measured not so much in wound contraction as in loss of elasticity caused by excessive new collagen production. Treatment aimed specifically at this aspect of the problem includes complete excision of newly synthesized collagen and introduction of tissue which is more elastic than organized scar tissue. Dangers of this type of surgery are that impotence may be produced and that too long a segment will be involved to make primary reconstruction by anastomosis possible. Transplantation of elastic tissue is fraught with so many technical and biological difficulties that a compromise consisting of enlarging the channel and extending the extraluminal tissues beyond the place where elasticity is needed has been substituted. Skin, amnion, peritoneum, and nonbiological substances have been used. None appear as satisfactory now as non-hair-bearing skin. Skin can be introduced in the form of a free full-thickness graft or a local pedicle flap; it is important not to use hair-bearing skin. Because qualities of elasticity are being sought primarily, split-thickness skin should not be used in lieu of a full-thickness graft. What little elasticity exists in skin grafts is due to the presence of elastic fibers and the physical weave of collagen in layers of dermis. A split-thickness graft leaves most of this desirable stratum behind. Of course, all that can possibly be done to prevent the factors responsible for overhealing should be taken into consideration. Prevention of infection, minimal use of foreign material in the wound, and free drainage of serum, blood, and urine are obviously very important.

Utilization of reconstructive principles to meet specific biological deficiencies or replace undesirable biological phenomena in the healing process has been rewarding in the genitourinary tract. Utilization of biological methods to control collagen synthesis and cross-linking could be even more useful. Lack of a satisfactory experimental model has hampered fundamental research in this area but potentially dangerous research in human beings is becoming less dangerous as increasing experience with induced lathyrism from administration of β-aminopropionitrile and penicillamine is gained. In addition, more experience with trace metal chelators in human beings rapidly is bringing us to the point where inhibition of fibrous protein synthesis may be practical in patients with urethral strictures. Once enough is known about the basic pharmacology and toxicity of these agents and the physiological and biochemical changes they evoke in human beings, clinical investigations will be possible by those who are interested in an entirely new approach to one of the oldest problems in urology.

ANTERIOR URETHRA.   Wounds of the anterior urethra are either traumatic or congenital. Traumatic wounds are usually lacerations or missile wounds characterized primarily by interruption of tissue integrity. Congenital wounds are caused by developmental abnormalities and are characterized by deficiency of tissue. Healing of traumatic wounds usually is not complicated and is primarily the result of epithelial proliferation and minimal fibrous protein synthesis. Healing of congenital wounds is primarily by fibrous protein synthesis and severe wound contraction. Repair of traumatic wounds is only occasionally complicated by stenosis; repair of congenital wounds is often complicated by fistula formation. The major portion of this section, therefore, will be devoted to biological considerations in healing and repair of congenital wounds.

The concept of a typical hypospadias deformity as a healed and contracted congenital wound of the urethra is fundamental to the surgical restoration of the penis and urethra. In many respects the considerations are similar to those outlined in the section on congenital clefts of the lip. All of the steps in a reconstructive plan can be logically based on the concept that hypospadias is the end result of an intrauterine wound characterized by deficiency of urethral tissue and healed by fibrous protein synthesis and wound contraction. Thus, as in any reconstructive procedure, the basic principles which must be followed are accurate analysis of what is missing, re-creation of the defect, excision of the products of wound repair, and transplantation of missing tissue. Hypospadias with typical ventral chordee is the result of a deficiency of urethral mucosa and ventral skin. Fibrous protein synthesis produces a band of collagenous scar tissue and wound contraction leads to axial deviation or chordee. Successful restoration includes excision of abnormal collagenous tissue, dorsal extension of the ventrally angulated penis, and resurfacing of the denuded urethral area with full-thickness skin. Reconstruction of the urethra involves more complex transplantation of additional soft tissue and this is usually delayed until a second procedure.

Most reconstructive surgeons recommend that chordee be released as soon as is practical, usually between one and two years of age. The authors have not seen any compelling reason to release chordee at any particular age, however, and have, therefore, usually waited until the penis is large enough to permit meticulous surgery to be performed easily. In order to complete the reconstruction before the child begins school, we generally release chordee when he is four or five years of age, and complete the urethral reconstruction during the ensuing year. Release of chordee requires a meticulous dissection and excision of all ventral fibrous bands without entering the corpus spongiosum. One of the major complications of a first stage (chordee-correction) urethroplasty is hematoma formation with subsequent fibrosis or loss of a skin flap. Such a complication is always followed by wound contraction and reappearance of the chordee. This can be prevented by meticulous attention to detail with special emphasis on not entering the corpus spongiosum. Individual ligation of even the smallest bleeding point is mandatory. Techniques for excising all of the fibrous tissue scar or ventral bands so that complete release of the angulation is achieved have been described repeatedly and will not be reviewed in this chapter.

In addition to excising all restraining fibrous tissue during release of the chordee, another objective — opening the space between the two corpora, particularly in the glans section — can be achieved without causing excessive hemorrhage. The reason for recommending that this be done is that as large a denuded area as possible should be created on the ventral surface so that the largest possible flap of skin can be inserted. To reconstruct the urethra easily during the second stage, as much skin as possible is needed on the ventral surface. Even though the glans is temporarily distorted or flattened when the space between the corpora is opened on the ventral surface, the corpora will roll together smoothly over the reconstructed urethra during the last stage of urethral construction. Preparation of skin flaps, preferably from un-folded foreskin or from scrotal skin, should be carried out so that the ventral defect can be resurfaced without tension. A staggered line of approximation of the skin flaps is simple to arrange so that a longi-tudinal scar on the ventral surface is not produced. Most urologists do not recommend reconstruction of hypospadias defects which do not ex-tend more distal than the coronal sulcus. They also do not carry urethral reconstruction more distal than the sulcus (in complete de-fects). It is not difficult to carry the reconstructed urethra to the distal tip of the glans, however, provided the glans is opened out and enough skin is brought into the ventral surface at the first operation. Skin flaps are maintained firmly against the corpora by a stent fixation which also serves as a longitudinal splint to hold the penile shaft in a straight posi-tion. Urinary flow is diverted with a urethral catheter in the proximal urethra until distal wound healing is complete.

Reconstruction of the urethra can be accomplished by surgically "tubing" a longitudinal flap of skin (Byars), allowing normal wound contraction to "tube" a buried flap of skin (Denis Browne), or utilizing a free skin graft turned inside out over an indwelling urethral catheter. The greatest advantage of surgically "tubing" a flap is that the distal end or spigot can be accurately formed at the tip of the penis under direct vision. The most outstanding advantage of allowing wound con-traction to "tube" a buried flap is technical simplicity. Assurance of hav-ing an adequate amount of skin for the urethra is the greatest advan-tage of using a free graft. Few procedures in reconstructive surgery are as dependent upon exacting technique for successful healing as recon-struction of the urethra. Fistulas almost always are due to small tech-nical errors in selection, placement, and adjustment of sutures. There is no way to describe all of the subtleties of urethral reconstruction; one must be shown how and supervised by a master surgeon to appreciate all of the fine points in preventing a postoperative fistula.

As in other tubular reconstructions, consideration of the basic bio-logical phenomena involved in healing leads one to the inescapable conclusion that an indwelling catheter should be avoided during an-terior urethral reconstruction. Much more important is urinary diver-sion which can be accomplished successfully with a proximal perineal urethrostomy. Small fistulas which are detected immediately after the urethrostomy tube is removed can be prevented from enlarging and often be made to heal spontaneously if urinary flow through the fistula is controlled. This is accomplished by teaching the patient immediately to hold the fistula edges while urinating so that no urine passes through the abnormal opening. A small early fistula which is allowed to conduct a large volume of urine will almost always become a larger fistula which will be permanent or require operative revision. A small fistula which is held closed during urination so that all of the urinary stream must pass through the distal meatus often will heal without further operative manipulation.

Operative correction of a urethral fistula which does not close spontaneously must await subsidence of all inflammation and maturation of surrounding scar tissue. An additional few months of having to sit to urinate is not disastrous (slightly less than half of the world's population do so normally). Meticulous technique required to correct urethral fistulas cannot be carried out on inflamed, edematous, or dense scar tissue. Repair is based on the same general principles as with other fistulas. These are defunctionalization, excision of the products of wound repair, and avoidance of contiguous suture lines. Diversion of the urinary stream is accomplished by a proximal urethrostomy (not an indwelling catheter); scar tissue is excised and the urethra and overlying skin are repaired separately using fine absorbable sutures for one and nonabsorbable sutures for the other. A maneuver which is occasionally effective in keeping the urethral and skin suture lines from being in contact with each other is to leave some of the urethral sutures long and pass them beneath skin so they can be brought out at a distance from the skin suture line. These sutures can be tied snugly, but without excess tension, over a bolster; the effect is to deviate and rotate the ureter so that the suture line in skin and the suture line in the ureter are not adjacent to each other. Even if a second fistula develops following such a maneuver, it will have a much more devious course than before and will, therefore, be more likely to heal spontaneously.

SUGGESTED READING

Peritoneum

Belzer, F. O. The Role of Venous Obstruction in the Formation of Intra-abdominal Adhesions: An Experimental Study. Brit. J. Surg. *54*:189, 1967.
Bridges, J. B., Johnson, F. R., and Whitting, H. W. Peritoneal Adhesion Formation. Acta Anat. *61*:203, 1965.
Buckman, R. F., Bordos, D., Bell, W. R., and Cameron, J. L. Prevention of Experimental Postoperative Adhesions by Ancrod Defibrinogenation. J. Surg. Res. *18*:377, 1975.
Ellis, H. The Cause and Prevention of Postoperative Intraperitoneal Adhesions—Collective Review. Surg. Gynec. Obstet. *133*:497, 1971.
Ellis, H., Harrison, W., and Hugh, T. B. The Healing of Peritoneum under Normal and Pathological Conditions. Brit. J. Surg. *52*:471, 1965.
Frey, C. F., Thorpe, C., and Brody, G. Silicone Fluid in the Prevention of Intestinal Adhesions. Arch. Surg. *95*:253, 1967.
Glucksman, D. L., and Warren, W. D. The Effect of Topically Applied Corticosteroids in the Prevention of Peritoneal Adhesion. An Experimental Approach with a Review of the Literature. Surgery *60*:352, 1966.
Hubbard, T. B., Jr., Kahn, M. Z., Carag, V. R., Jr., Albites, V. E., and Hricko, G. M. The Pathology of Peritoneal Repair: Its Relation to the Formation of Adhesions. Ann. Surg. *165*:908, 1967.

Johnson, F. R., and Whitting, H. W. Repair of Parietal Peritoneum. Brit. J. Surg. *49*:653, 1962.

Milligan, D. W., and Raftery, A. T. Observations on the Pathogenesis of Peritoneal Adhesions: A Light and Electron Microscopical Study. Brit. J. Surg. *61*:274, 1974.

Mott, T. J., Ashby, E. C., and Ellis, H. Studies in Peritoneal Healing—A Review. Abdominal. Surg. *11*:110, 1969.

Myllarniemi, H., and Karppinen, V. Vascular Patterns of Peritoneal Adhesions. Brit. J. Surg. *55*:605, 1968.

Renvall, S., and Niinikoski, J.: Intraperitoneal Oxygen and Carbon Dioxide Tensions in Experimental Adhesion Disease and Peritonitis. Amer. J. Surg. *130*:286, 1975.

Ryan, G. B., Grobéty, J., and Majno, G. Postoperative Peritoneal Adhesions. A Study of the Mechanisms. Amer. J. Path. *65*:117, 1971.

Schade, D. S., and Williamson, J. R. The Pathogenesis of Peritoneal Adhesions: An Ultrastructural Study. Ann. Surg. *167*:500, 1968.

Villavicencio, J. L., and Gross, R. E. Critical Thrombolytic Dosages of Human Fibrinolysin in the Treatment of Peritoneal Adhesions. Surg. Forum *13*:348, 1962.

Gastrointestinal Tract

Akiyama, H. Esophageal Anastomosis. Arch. Surg. *107*:512, 1973.

Azar, H., and Drapanas, T. Relationship of Antibiotics to Wound Infection and Enterocolitis in Colon Surgery. Amer. J. Surg. 115:209, 1968.

Borgstrom, S., and Lundh, B. Healing of Esophageal Anastomosis: Animal Experiments. Ann. Surg. 150:142, 1959.

Canalis, F., and Ravitch, M. M. Study of Healing of Inverting and Everting Intestinal Anastomoses. Surg. Gynec. Obstet. *126*:109, 1968.

Cohn, I., Jr., and Nance, F. C. Small Bowel Resection. Surg. Clin. N. Amer. 46:1179, 1966.

Cronin, K., Jackson, D. S., and Dunphy, J. E. Changing Bursting Strength and Collagen Content of the Healing Colon. Surg. Gynec. Obstet. *126*:747, 1968.

Crowley, L. G., Anders, C. J., Nelsen, T., and Bagshaw, M. Effect of Radiation on Canine Intestinal Anastomoses. Arch. Surg. 96:423, 1968.

Goldsmith, H. S., Kiely, A. A., and Randall, H. T. Protection of Intrathoracic Esophageal Anastomoses by Omentum. Surgery *63*:464, 1968.

Goligher, J. C., Morris, C., McAdam, W. A. F., de Dombal, F. T., and Johnston, D. A Controlled Trial of Inverting Versus Everting Intestinal Suture in Clinical Large Bowel Surgery. Brit. J. Surg. *57*:817, 1975.

Hamilton, J. E. Reappraisal of Open Intestinal Anastomoses. Ann. Surg. *165*:917, 1967.

Hastings, C., Van Winkle, W., Barker, E., Hinds, J., and Nichols, W. Effect of Suture Material on Healing Wounds of Stomach and Colon. Surg. Gynec. Obstet. *140*:701, 1975.

Healey, J. E., Jr., McBride, C. M., and Gallagher, H. S. Bowel Anastomosis by Inverting and Everting Techniques. An Experimental Study. J. Surg. Res. *7*:299, 1967.

Irvin, T. T., Goligher, J. C., and Johnston, D. A. Randomized Prospective Clinical Trial of Single-Layer and Two-Layer Inverting Intestinal Anastomoses. Brit. J. Surg. *60*:457, 1973.

Irving, T. T., and Hunt, T. K. Effect of Malnutrition on Colonic Healing. Ann. Surg. *180*:765, 1974.

Irving, T. T., and Hunt, T. K. The Effect of Trauma on Colonic Healing. Brit. J. Surg. *61*:430, 1974.

Kilam, S. K., Jackson, F. L., and Williams, H. T. G. Bacterial Peritonitis and the Bursting Strength of Intestinal Anastomoses. Canad. J. Surg. *18*:372, 1975.

Loeb, M. J. Comparative Strength of Inverted, Everted, and End-On Intestinal Anastomoses. Surg. Gynec. Obstet. *125*:301, 1967.

Nakanishi, H. Experimental Gut Anastomoses and Their Revascularization. Aust. N. Zeal. J. Surg. *45*:309, 1975.

Nelsen, T. S., and Anders, C. J. Dynamic Aspects of Small Intestinal Rupture with Special Consideration of Anastomotic Strength. Arch. Surg. *93*:309, 1966.

Nora, P. F., Vanecko, R. M., and Bransfield, J. J. Prophylactic Abdominal Drains. Arch. Surg. *105*:173, 1975.

O'Connor, R. J. Mucosal Repair in the Rectum. Brit. J. Surg. *44*:93, 1956.

Poth, E. J., and Gold, D. Technics of Gastrointestinal Suture. Curr. Probl. Surg. October 1965, p. 1.

Ravitch, M. M. Observations on the Healing of Wounds of the Intestines. Surgery *77*:665, 1975.

Ravitch, M. M., Canalis, F., Weinshelbaum, A., and McCormick, J. Studies in Intestinal Healing: III. Observations on Everting Intestinal Anastomoses. Ann. Surg. *166*:670, 1967.

Sanders, R. J. The Management of Colon Injuries. Surg. Clin. N. Amer. 43:457, 1963.

Schrock, T. R., Deveney, C. W., and Dunphy, J. E. Factors Contributing to Leakage of Colonic Anastomoses. Ann. Surg. *177*:513, 1975.

Small, W. P., Smith, A. N., Falconer, C. W. A., Sircus, W., and Bruce, J. Suture Line Ulcer after Gastric Surgery. Amer. J. Surg. *115*:477, 1968.

Temple, W. J., Voitk, A. J., Snelling, C. S., and Crispin, J. S. Effect of Nutrition, Diet and Suture Material on Long Term Wound Healing. Ann. Surg. *182*:93, 1975.

Tsukamoto, M., and Thal, A. P. Correction of Experimental Esophageal Stricture with the Use of the Skin-lined Fundic Patch. J. Thorac. Cardiov. Surg. *52*:682, 1966.

Whitaker, W. G., and Shepard, D. Late Complications of Side-to-Side Intestinal Anastomosis: Case Reports. Ann. Surg. *161*:824, 1965.

Wise, L., McAlister, W., Stein, T., and Schuck, P. Studies on the Healing of Anastomoses of the Small and Large Intestines. Surg. Gynec. Obstet. *141*:190, 1975.

Liver, Biliary Tract, and Pancreas

Aust, J. B., Root, H. D., Urdaneta, L., and Varco, R. L. Biliary Stricture. Surgery 62:601, 1967.

Becker, F. F. Restoration of Liver Mass Following Partial Hepatectomy: "Surgical Hepartrophy," Amer. J. Path. 43:497, 1963.

Belzer, F. O., Watts, J. M., Ross, H. B., and Dunphy, J. E. Auto-reconstruction of the Common Bile Duct After Venous Patch Graft. Ann. Surg. *162*:346, 1965.

Bradley, B. E., Vineyard, G. C., Defalco, A., Lawson, D., and Hayes, J. R. An Evaluation of Silicone Rubber Tubing as a Replacement of the Common Bile Duct. Amer. J. Surg. *113*:501, 1967.

Cameron, G. R., Hassan, S. M., and De, S. N. Repair of Glisson's Capsule after Tangential Wounds of the Liver. J. Path. Bact. 73:1, 1957.

Carroll, C. P., Cass, K. A., and Whelan, T. J. Wounds of the Liver in Viet Nam. A Critical Analysis of 254 Cases. Ann. Surg. *177*:385, 1973.

Condon, R. E., Callen, P., Bettz, W. R., Van Meter, S. W., Pissiotis, C. A., and Nichols, R. L. Serosal Onlay Repair of Common Duct Stricture. Amer. J. Surg. *127*:13, 1974.

Frankland, D. M., and Wynn, C. H. The Degradation of Acid-Soluble Collagen by Rat-Liver Preparations. Biochem. J. *85*:276, 1962.

Lane, C. E., Sawyers, J., Riddell, D., and Scott, H. W. Long Term Results of Roux-En-Y Hepatocholangiojejunostomy. Ann. Surg. *177*:714, 1973.

Lane, T. C., Johnson, H. C., and Walker, H. S. J., Jr. Extrahepatic Biliary Decompression in Traumatized Canine Livers. Surgery 62:1039, 1967.

Levowitz, B. S., LaGuerre, J., and Calem, W. S. A New Hydrophilic Polymer as a Common Duct Replacement. Arch. Surg. 98:251, 1969.

Lucas, C. E., and Walt, A. J. Analysis of Randomized Biliary Drainage for Liver Trauma in 189 Patients. J. Trauma *12*:925, 1972.

Mackie, D. B., Haynes, J., and May, R. E. Unabsorbable Suture Material—A Rare Cause of Recurrent Stones in the Common Bile Duct. Brit. J. Surg. 60:23, 1973.

Mays, E. T. Management of Severe Liver Trauma. Surg. Gynec. Obstet. *123*:551, 1966.

Mays, E. T. The Hepatic Artery. Surg. Gynec. Obstet. *139*:595, 1974.

McMinn, R. M. H., and Johnson, F. R. Wound Healing in the Gall-Bladder of the Cat. Brit. J. Surg. 46:76, 1957.

Northrup, W. F., and Simmons, R. L. Pancreatic Trauma: A Review. Surgery *71*:27, 1972.

Owens, M. P., and Wolfman, E. F. Pancreatic Trauma: Management and Presentation of A New Technique. Surgery 73:881, 1973.

Peacock, E. E., Jr., Seigler, H. F., and Biggers, P. W. Use of Tanned Collagen Sponges in the Treatment of Liver Injuries. Ann. Surg. *161*:238, 1965.

Sparkman, R. S., and Fogelman, M. J. Wounds of the Liver. Review of 100 Cases. Ann. Surg. *139*:690, 1954.

Sturim, H. S. The Surgical Management of Pancreatic Injuries. Surg. Gynec. Obstet. *122*:133, 1966.

Thorbjarnarson, B., Bostrom, P. D., Smith, G. L., Tucker, D. N., and Cortese, A. F. Experimental Common Bile Duct Conduits. Arch. Surg. 92:818, 1966.

Way, L. W., and Dunphy, J. E. Biliary Stricture. Amer. J. Surg. *124*:287, 1972.

Wyatt, A. P., Belzer, F. O., and Dunphy, J. E. Malfunction without Constriction of the Common Bile Duct. Amer. J. Surg. *113*:592, 1967.

Trachea

Grillo, H. Reconstruction of Trachea. Thorax 28:667, 1973.
Grillo, H., Dignan, E. F., and Miura, T. Extensive Resection and Reconstruction of Mediastinal Trachea without Prosthesis or Graft. An Anatomical Study in Man. J. Thorac. Cardiovasc. Surg. 48:741, 1964.
Grillo, H. C. Tracheal Anatomy and Surgical Approaches. In General Thoracic Surgery. Edited by T. W. Shields. Philadelphia, Lea and Febiger, 1972.

Urinary Tract

Baker, R., Maxted, W. C., and Dipasquale, N. Regeneration of Transitional Epithelium of the Human Bladder after Total Surgical Excision for Recurrent Multiple Bladder Cancer: Apparent Tumor Inhibition. J. Urol. 93:593, 1965.
Bartone, F. F., and Shires, T. K. The Reaction of Kidney and Bladder Tissue to Catgut and Reconstituted Collagen Sutures. Surg. Gynec. Obstet. 128:1221, 1969.
Catino, D., Torack, R. M., and Hagstrom, J. W. C. Idiopathic Retroperitoneal Fibrosis: Histochemical Evidence for Lateral Spread of the Process from the Midline. J. Urol. 98:191, 1967.
Hastings, C., Van Winkle, W., Hinds, J., Barker, E., and Nichols, W. Effect of Suture Material on Healing of Wounds of the Bladder. Surg. Gynec. Obstet. 140:933, 1975.
Hinman, F., Jr., and Oppenheimer, R. Smooth Muscle Regeneration in Repair of Experimental Ureteral Defects: The Significance of the Double Lumen. J. Urol. 75:428, 1956.
Hoch, W. H., Kursh, E. D., and Persky, L. Early Aggressive Management of Intraoperative Ureteral Injuries. J. Urol. 114:530, 1975.
Liang, D. S. Late Results in Bladder Regeneration. J. Urol. 95:215, 1966.
Matsumoto, T., Pani, K. C., Hardaway, R. M., III, Leonard, F., Jennings, P. B., and Heisterkamp, C. A., III. Higher Homologous Cyanoacrylate Tissue Adhesives in Injured Kidney. Arch. Surg. 94:392, 1967.
Rasmussen, F. Biochemical Analysis of Wound Healing in the Urinary Bladder. Surg. Gynec. Obstet. 124:553, 1967.
Ross, A., Jr., Thompson, I. M., Bynum, W. R., and Thompson, E. P. The Role of Smooth Muscle Regeneration in Urinary Tract Repair. J. Urol. 95:541, 1966.
Zinman, L., and Libertino, J. A. Surgical Management of Urethral Strictures. Surg. Clin. N. Amer. 53:465, 1973.

INDEX

683